Emergency Care and Transportation
of the Sick and Injured

Emergency Care and Transportation of the Sick and Injured

Second Edition, Revised

BY

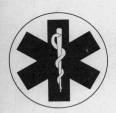

THE COMMITTEE ON ALLIED HEALTH
American Academy of Orthopaedic Surgeons

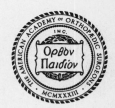

This textbook is intended solely as a guide to the appropriate procedures to be employed when rendering emergency care to or transporting the sick or injured. It is not intended as a statement of the standards of care required in any particular situation, since circumstances and patients' physical condition can vary widely from one emergency to another. Nor is it intended that this textbook shall in any way advise emergency personnel concerning legal authority to perform the activities or procedures discussed. Such local determinations should be made only with the aid of legal counsel.

Library of Congress Catalog Card No. 76-3157

© 1977 by American Academy of Orthopaedic Surgeons. All rights reserved

430 North Michigan Avenue, Chicago, Illinois 60611

First edition published 1971. Second edition 1977

Printed and bound by George Banta Co., Inc., Menasha, Wisconsin

Contents

v

BOARD OF EDITORS

CONSULTANTS

CONTRIBUTORS

GEORGE N. ALDREDGE, JR., M.D., Dallas, Texas
HENRY ALSOBROOK, New Orleans, Louisiana
GEORGE T. ANAST, M.D., Chicago, Illinois
HAP ARNOLD, Washington, D. C.
PHILIP J. BAILEY, Ottawa, Illinois
RICHARD K. BENJAMIN, Olympia, Washington
Lieutenant D. BEST, Washington, D. C. Fire Department
RALPH O. BLACKWOOD, Akron, Ohio
JUDY B. BONTRAGER, R.N., Phoenix, Arizona
NOEL C. BUFE, Lansing, Michigan
WILLIAM E. BURNETTE, Chicago, Illinois
D. W. CALDWELL, M.D., Linden, New Jersey
C. ROBERT CLARK, M.D., Chattanooga, Tennessee
DOUGLAS R. COOKSEY, South Charleston, West Virginia
MRS. JOAN DAVIDSON, St. Petersburg, Florida
PAUL DE MARTINI, Livonia, New York
DONALD A. DUKELOW, M.D., Chicago, Illinois
JAMES J. DUNNE, M.D., Richmond, Virginia
DAN C. EDWARDS, Commerce City, Colorado
GLEN H. EGSTROM, Ph.D., Los Angeles, California
TOM ELO, M.D., San Diego, California
JOSEPH T. FUCIGNA, Darien, Connecticut
Sergeant WILLIAM C. GARTEIZ, Carson City, Nevada
ROBERT W. GILLESPIE, M.D., Lincoln, Nebraska
GEORGE A. GATES, M.D., San Antonio, Texas
ARCHER S. GORDON, M.D., Dallas, Texas
JOHN E. GOULD, Dallas, Texas
JAMES R. GRISHAM, Chicago, Illinois
JOEL R. GUILLORY, JR., M.D., Chicago, Illinois
PAUL R. HAITH, Lincoln, Nebraska
MARSHALL E. HALL, M.D., Miami, Florida
OSCAR P. HAMPTON, JR., M.D., St. Louis, Missouri
JOHN T. HANNA, Richmond, Virginia
Captain WILLIAM D. HARVEY, Washington, D. C.
SAMUEL M. HAWKEN, M.D., Washington, D. C.
HENRY J. HEIMLICH, M.D., Cincinnati, Ohio
S. S. HELLMAN, Richmond, Virginia
THOMAS K. HOOD, M. D., Elko, Nevada
BERTRAM E. HOWARD, M.D., New Bedford, Connecticut
D. HOWE, M.D., Washington, D. C.
A. E. HUNTER, Des Moines, Iowa
Lieutenant DAN IRVINE, Glen Echo, Maryland, Fire Department
RONALD W. JENSEN, Honolulu, Hawaii
RONALD C. JONES, M.D., Dallas, Texas
JAMES W. JUSTICE, M.D., Tucson, Arizona
RICHARD P. KING, Carson City, Nevada
MAX KLINGHOFFER, M.D., Elmhurst, Illinois
SARAH H. KNUTTY, M.D., Bethesda, Maryland
LOUIS C. KOSSUTH, M.D., Phoenix, Arizona
RALPH H. KUNSTADTER, M.D., St. Croix, Virgin Islands
DUSTIN F. LEER, Mid Valley, California

CHARLES R. LEONE, JR., M.D., San Antonio, Texas
JAMES LICH, Washington, D. C.
G. G. LINDQUIST, Chicago Heights, Illinois
ERNEST LITTLEJOHN, Columbia, South Carolina
D. H. H. MACKENZIE, M.D., Toronto, Canada
Lieutenant KEITH B. MALLEK, Millersville, Maryland, Fire Department
Sergeant J. MARTIN, Washington, D. C. Fire Department
WILLIAM C. MAXTED, M.D., Washington, D. C.
WAYNE MCKENNA, R. S., Lansing, Michigan
J. JUDSON MCNAMARA, M.D., Honolulu, Hawaii
ROBERT L. MECKELNBURG, M.D., Hockessin, Delaware
J. W. MIKOS, Baltimore, Maryland
ROBERT K. MILLS, Indianapolis, Indiana
EUGENE D. MINDEL, M.D., Chicago, Illinois
JOHN A. MONCRIEF, M.D., San Antonio, Texas
RICHARD D. MULROY, M.D., Brighton, Massachusetts
KEN MUTTER, Richmond, Virginia
EUGENE L. NAGEL, M.D., Miami, Florida
W. R. OLSEN, Manassas, Virginia
WILLIAM L. ORRIS, M.D., La Jolla, California
STEFAN A. PASTERNAK, M.D., Washington, D. C.
V. F. PEKAREK, M.D., New York, N. Y.
WILLIAM H. PETERSON, R.Ph., Bethesda, Md.
JOHN PIERCE, M.D., St. Louis, Missouri
G. A. PODA, M.D., Aiken, South Carolina
JOHN RADCLIFFE, Madison, Wisconsin
JAMES RANSOM, Ph.D., Los Altos, California
ROBERT M. REISS, M.D., Huntington, New York
JOHN E. ROWLAND, Harrisburg, Pennsylvania
ANDREW C. RUOFF, III, M.D., Salt Lake City, Utah
KENNETH H. RUSCH, M.D., Madison, Wisconsin
PETER SAFAR, M.D., Pittsburgh, Pennsylvania
PHILIP R. SALYERS, Chicago Heights, Illinois
JUSTUS J. SCHIFFERES, Ph.D., Livingston, New Jersey
RICHARD C. SCHNEIDER, M.D., Ann Arbor, Michigan
LEO R. SCHWARTZ, Washington, D. C.
DON A. SLEEPER, Washington, D. C.
Captain S. J. STEPHANY, Washington, D. C.
ROBERT E. STREICHER, M.D., Hyattsville, Maryland
HUGH B. TILSON, D.D.S., San Antonio, Texas
JOHN B. TITUS, Batesville, Arkansas
LAWRENCE A. TRISSEL, R.Ph., Bethesda, Maryland
ARTHUR ULLRICH, Grand Terrace, California
HENRY L. VERHULST, Washington, D. C.
ROBERT G. WAGGENER, Ph.D., San Antonio, Texas
GEORGE E. WEBB, M.D., San Antonio, Texas
BERNARD W. WEBBER, Minneapolis, Minnesota
GEORGE W. WEINSTEIN, M.D., San Antonio, Texas
WILLIAM A. WHITELEY, Sacramento, California
G. R. WHITNEY, Baltimore, Maryland
PHILIP C. WHITNEY, Sterling, Massachusetts
JOHN A. WOODCOCK, M.D., Bangor, Maine
JAMES J. WOODRUFF, M.D., Los Angeles, California
CARL B. YOUNG, JR., Corpus Christi, Texas

Foreword to Second Edition

The American Academy of Orthopaedic Surgeons is pleased to provide the second edition of this textbook. It has been extensively revised to include updated and new information and has also been reorganized to provide a more effective method of teaching.

Since 1971, publication date of the first edition of this textbook, *Emergency Care and Transportation of the Sick and Injured*, there has been a significant improvement in the quality of emergency care in the United States. Formal educational programs have been established in all the states, and graduating students are granted certification upon successful completion of a comprehensive examination. They are required to maintain their competence thereafter by continuing education and periodic recertification. The men and women who serve these educational programs, both administrators and teachers, deserve a great deal of praise.

The major credit for this revised edition belongs to Charles A. Rockwood, Jr., M.D. of San Antonio, Texas. As chairman of the Academy Sub-Committee on Emergency Medical Care Text, he and his committee, consisting of Marshall B. Conrad, M.D., J. D. Farrington, M.D., George W. Hyatt, M.D., and Raoul P. Rodriguez, M.D., spent countless days of their busy professional careers to complete this enormous task. The caliber of the textbook and its accompanying workbook attests their dedication and devoted service.

A number of individuals and professional organizations representing all the concerned medical disciplines were contributors. Without their professional expertise and assistance the manuscript would never have been completed. The American Academy of Orthopaedic Surgeons extends its gratitude for their unselfish participation.

The Academy is confident that this textbook will be used by many students of emergency medical care throughout the country and that it will serve well the educational purpose for which it was designed.

WALTER A. HOYT, JR., M.D.
Akron, Ohio
December, 1976

Foreword to First Edition

The emergency medical technician performs a unique service which cannot be rendered by any other individual or group. Through effective application of his skills at the scene of an accident or illness, he is in the enviable position of being able to save lives and prevent or alleviate suffering. Although there are many competent emergency medical technicians, their numbers are by far too few to fill the national need for their services. It is most important not only to increase their numbers but also to provide a standardized educational approach for them that will help establish a uniform standard of competency in this vital allied medical profession. With this goal in mind, the American Academy of Orthopaedic Surgeons decided to develop a standard textbook for use by both student and teacher.

In 1964, Samuel Banks, M.D., then chairman of the Committee on Injuries of the Academy, initiated a series of concentrated three-day courses for training emergency medical personnel, which the Committee on Injuries has conducted each year since then and which it plans to continue. By 1967 certain lessons had been learned and an obvious, but formidable, undertaking presented itself as being essential to overcome difficulties encountered in conducting the courses. The undertaking which was proposed to the Academy was that the Committee members compile and write a text to provide a standard educational reference for those engaged in this work, particularly for those just entering it. Requirements for such a text were agreed to be: (1) that it be comprehensive enough to meet the full requirements of the training course; (2) that it be clear enough to be understood by those with limited previous training; and (3) that it be sufficiently illustrated to provide not only basic factual information but in some degree to teach the skills involved.

The broad spectrum of medical subjects to be presented demanded that knowledgeable specialists be involved to insure the major objectives of accuracy and completeness. It was recognized that no one organization could furnish all the necessary personnel. The names of the contributors, consultants, and task forces participating attest to the thoroughness with which the objectives were pursued. Medicine and its allied services joined together unselfishly to provide this textbook, the need for which they recognized to be vitally important.

It was the consensus of those involved that a text alone would be of limited value. All agreed that it must be implemented within the structure of an educational system. In my own opinion, the educational system needed should parallel the arrangements of those already in existence for various allied medical services. It must embody the necessary subject material and must be taught by those with recognized teaching ability. The instructors must be professionally familiar with the information to be presented and be aware of the educational level and methodology needed to alter significantly the behavior patterns of the individual to be taught.

A formal educational program of sufficient depth and duration is necessary to achieve vocational status for the emergency medical technician. The ultimate goal, of course, is a core curriculum for a community college whose graduates' competency would be greater than that required by minimal standards. It is hoped that this text, along with lesson plans which have been developed in concert with it, will be utilized on a national basis for this purpose.

It has been medicine's responsibility to develop the methods of education, to create the certifying process, and to recognize the vocational status of persons trained as emergency medical technicians. It is, however, the responsibility of those at state and local levels of government to provide facilities for both initial and continuing education in order to meet minimum standards of certification.

Many individuals have served this cause beyond any demands made of them. First, and most important, is Charles A. Rockwood, Jr.,

M.D., present secretary of the Committee on Injuries, who assumed sole responsibility for putting the manuscript in final form. Were it not for him this would never have been accomplished. I am deeply grateful to him for seeing through to completion the enormous project passed on to him.

I am personally indebted to Mr. Carl Udall, photographer; Mr. Tom Campbell, medical illustrator; and my secretary, Mrs. Lois Pennington.

I extend my special gratitude to my wife, whose understanding has transcended the disruption of an orderly life.

WALTER A. HOYT, JR., M.D.
Akron, Ohio
1971

Preface to Second Edition

Five years have passed since publication of the first edition of this book. Although the basic principles of emergency medical care remained unchanged, the American Academy of Orthopaedic Surgeons agreed that a new and revised second edition was required to keep pace with the concepts, techniques, and ideas which have been developed in emergency medical care in those five years. This textbook is designed for basic emergency care, as opposed to one including expanded training required for the EMT-Advanced Paramedic. The text is designed to be used in conjunction with the Basic Training Program for the Emergency Medical Technician (EMT) developed for the National Highway Traffic Safety Administration of the Department of Transportation by Dunlap and Associates, Inc.

This edition offers a completely revised and expanded text. The chapters have been reorganized and assembled into twelve separate, identifiable sections. Each section combines chapters on interrelated subjects and brings to the student a correlated review of the major topics in them. In addition, new chapters have been added: Basic Life Support, Alcohol and Drug Abuse, Oxygen Therapy and Equipment, and a new section on the triage of injured patients.

A valuable innovation has been the development of goals and objectives for each chapter and the creation of a student workbook. The goals and objectives, listed at the beginning of each chapter, outline the most important concepts that the student should learn and remember. The workbook, through a series of questions to be answered and illustrations to be labeled, evaluates the student's ability to understand concepts. The material in the workbook is taken directly from the text and the two books can be used together in scheduled classes or in a self-teaching process.

Since the first edition was published in 1971, the AAOS has maintained a file of the letters and comments received concerning the book. Each of these communications has been carefully considered and corrections and suggestions have been incorporated into this edition. Your help and interest in all the detail concerning the teaching of emergency medical care is deeply appreciated. The item requested most frequently was a glossary. Therefore, at the end of the present text, we have compiled a list of definitions of the medical terms and other specialized words used in this edition.

On behalf of the Academy, the Board of Editors offers its sincere appreciation to:

The medical organizations of the United States and their representatives who have been of major assistance in preparing this text.

The consultants, contributors, and members of the Manuscript Review Committee.

The American Heart Association and Arnold Sladen, M.D., of the University of Pittsburg, for their valuable cooperation on the new chapter entitled Basic Life Support. This chapter contains the current concepts and standards being taught by the American Heart Association.

Arthur S. McFee, M.D., professor of Surgery of The University of Texas Medical School at San Antonio, who served as special consultant to the Board of Editors and was a major contributor in the development of the textbook, the workbook, and the answer booklet.

Margarette Sharpe, of The University of Texas at Austin, who served as before as a dedicated, highly appreciated special assistant to the Board of Editors.

Betty Montgomery, former coordinator of Graphic Arts at The University of Texas Health Science Center at San Antonio, who provided excellent, clear, and precise illustrations.

Walter A. Hoyt, Jr., M.D., whose unfailing interest and guidance were heartening to all who worked with him. He was always on call and always ready to lend assistance.

The Board of Directors of the Academy, for generous backing and encouragement. Their vision and identification with emergency care has made this text a reality which we feel will in no small way help to improve emergency medical service in our country.

I should personally like to express my special appreciation to Colleen Mann, my indispensable administrative assistant; to the Board of Editors for the splendid cooperation they have given; and finally to the members of the Academy who made this text possible.

CHARLES A. ROCKWOOD, JR., M.D.
San Antonio, Texas
December, 1976

Preface to First Edition

This text on emergency care owes its existence to the dedicated efforts of Walter A. Hoyt, Jr., M.D., who undertook the task of editorial supervision in 1967, when he was chairman of the Committee on Injuries of the American Academy of Orthopaedic Surgeons. By April of 1969 Dr. Hoyt had assembled a preliminary manuscript consisting of sixty chapters which were the work of many contributors and consultants. This manuscript was submitted to the Executive Committee of AAOS, whose decision was that it should be reviewed by representatives of other interested medical organizations.

A special Task Force for this purpose, appointed by S. Benjamin Fowler, M.D., then president of the Academy, consisted of the following men:

GEORGE T. AITKEN, M.D., AAOS

J. D. FARRINGTON, M.D., American College of Surgeons

S. BENJAMIN FOWLER, M.D., AAOS

JOSEPH T. FUCIGNA, Dunlap and Associates

OSCAR P. HAMPTON, JR., M.D., American College of Surgeons

IRVIN E. HENDRYSON, M.D., American Medical Association

CHARLES H. HERNDON, M.D., AAOS

JOHN J. HINCHEY, M.D., AAOS

WALTER A. HOYT, JR., M.D., AAOS

FLOYD H. JERGESEN, M.D., AAOS

ROBERT M. OSWALD, American National Red Cross

JOSEPH K. OWEN, PH.D., U. S. Public Health Service

CHARLES A. ROCKWOOD, JR., M.D., AAOS

SAM F. SEELEY, M.D., National Research Council–National Academy of Sciences

GEORGE E. SPENCER, JR., M.D., AAOS

In addition, a special ad hoc text review subcommittee of the Committee on Injuries was appointed which consisted of George E. Spencer, Jr., M.D., chairman of the Committee on Injuries; Charles S. Neer II, M.D.; Norman D. Logan, M.D.; William S. Stryker, M.D.; and me. This subcommittee was assigned the task of critically reviewing and correcting the text and having each chapter reviewed by a consultant. The revised manuscript was submitted to the Task Force, which collectively met on three occasions and reviewed the text line for line, made minor and major chapter modifications, and utilized the expertise of more consultants. In September of 1969, a rough draft was delivered to Mrs. Margarette Sharpe, Austin, Texas, for literary editing and preparation of copy for the printer. Mrs. Sharpe undertook the task of editing a manuscript that had been written by many different contributors, matching numerous illustrations to text, and satisfying the sometimes contradictory requests and demands of a final Editorial Advisory Board. Everyone involved in this project is indebted to Mrs. Sharpe for her work throughout all phases of her involvement with this major editorial assignment.

I should like to thank the Department of Medical Communications of The University of Texas Medical School at San Antonio for their support in photography and art work. I especially thank Arthur S. McFee, M.D., Associate Professor of Surgery at UTMS at San Antonio, for his assistance in collating the final corrections and suggestions made by the Editorial Board. Dr. McFee rewrote many of the preliminary chapters for the Task Force, proofread the entire book, and responded both energetically and brilliantly to endless demands on his time and talents.

The medical organizations listed below have authorized the following statement:

"The materials in this text are endorsed as reflecting current established principles of emergency care."

AMERICAN COLLEGE OF SURGEONS
AMERICAN MEDICAL ASSOCIATION
AMERICAN NATIONAL RED CROSS
NATIONAL RESEARCH COUNCIL–NATIONAL ACADEMY OF SCIENCES

The men and women of the American medical community deserve and are extended the thanks of the AAOS for their interest and unfailing support in this undertaking.

CHARLES A. ROCKWOOD, JR., M.D.
San Antonio, Texas
1971

Emergency Care and Transportation of the Sick and Injured

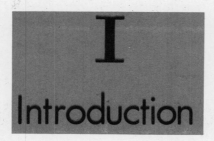

Introduction

CHAPTER 1

Orientation of the Emergency Medical Technician

GOAL I. Understand the elements of total emergency medical care.

OBJECTIVES

A. Identify the members of the emergency medical care team.
B. Describe a proper disaster plan for a community.

GOAL II. Understand the importance and effect of proper training for the EMT.

OBJECTIVES

A. Describe the characteristics of a properly trained EMT.
B. List the responsibilities of an EMT.
C. Classify the capabilities necessary for an EMT to assume responsibility for the sick and injured.
D. Describe the qualities of character necessary for the EMT to cope with the emotional problems of the sick and injured.
E. Describe the proper management of relatives, bystanders, and passersby at the scene of the sick and injured.
F. Describe the correct handling of handicapped patients who are sick or injured.
G. Describe the difference between first aid and emergency medical care.
H. Identify the national organization responsible for the certification of Emergency Medical Technicians.

Introduction

Emergency medical technicians serving on ambulances have the greatest opportunity of any segment of society to alleviate human suffering at the scene of accidental injury or sudden illness and during transportation to a hospital. With proper training and experience, ready availability of equipment and supplies, radio communication with the hospital and medical staff, and a vehicle designed to meet the needs of the sick or injured, the Emergency Medical Technician (EMT) is equipped to serve as the most valuable lay member of the emergency medical care team outside the hospital.

Emergency medical care is a team effort, provided by a team consisting of those among the general public who are trained in first aid, the

EMT, personnel of the hospital Emergency Department, allied health personnel, and administrative authorities of the hospital, the emergency service, and the municipality.

Whether injury or sudden illness occurs at home, at work, on the highway, or at a recreational area, there is rarely a physician, a nurse, or a trained EMT at hand to provide initial care. Even though parents, friends, or bystanders may have had instruction in first aid, they—and even policemen, firemen, workers in public utility agencies, and others who may have undergone more extensive training—are limited in their ability to maintain patients with life-threatening conditions until professional assistance becomes available. The limitation is due in large part to the fact that they do not have the equipment, supplies, or means of transportation that may be necessary to save a life and safely deliver an individual to a hospital. It is thus essential that the well-qualified EMT be able to assess the quality and effectiveness of first aid already rendered by those with less training and to assume primary responsibility immediately and tactfully, enlisting the assistance of others to the extent that it may be required.

The major portion of this textbook is devoted to instruction in the actual care of patients with specific injuries or illnesses, from initial pickup through transportation to a medical facility. To learn to administer proper care efficiently, the student must constantly be mindful of the ways in which instructions contained in a number of chapters not directly concerned with specific injuries or illnesses are important to the goal of saving lives; he must learn to avoid or reduce the complications that might prolong recovery or result in additional disability. Thus, in the emergency medical care of any patient, to be able to judge the care that is needed and to render that care with the equipment and supplies at hand is not enough. The EMT must also be thoroughly familiar with the usefulness and limitations of the transportation vehicle, the communication equipment, and every item of supplies and equipment available to him. He must combine tact and firmness with his medical skills and practices in every case that comes to his attention.

Disaster Plan

To lessen the inevitable confusion and often chaos that exist when mass casualties occur, as for example, in a catastrophic accident or a natural disaster, a comprehensive, written disaster plan should be developed in advance for every area in the community with a potential hazard, and every Emergency Medical Service region must have an overall plan. These plans must involve all agencies, organizations, and resources concerned with Emergency Medical Services. Prior designation of overall authority is essential. Ambulance services are a vital element in any disaster plan and thus EMTs must be deeply and vocally involved in the development of these plans, which should be an expansion of adequate day-to-day operations.

Attributes of the Emergency Medical Technician

The attitude and conduct of an Emergency Medical Technician must at all times reflect a sincere dedication to serving fellow human beings. His moral and ethical standards should be high. He must seek always to increase his knowledge and skills, to perform to the best of his ability with full recognition of his own limitations, and to accept and benefit from constructive criticism and advice.

The EMT must earn the respect and recognition of others as a responsible member of the emergency care team. He must take pride in his personal appearance, his technical knowledge, and his ability to render care. He must perform under pressure with composure and self-confidence. He must discipline himself to control his emotions, to be sympathetic to the abnormal or exaggerated actions of those under stress, and to exert reasonable and firm leadership in carrying out measures that insure the survival, safety, comfort, and confidence of the patient from the time of arrival on the scene until the patient is delivered to medical members of the team.

Assumption of Responsibility

Regardless of the circumstances encountered when he responds to an emergency call, the

EMT must recognize that from the moment he first attends a patient he assumes a responsibility to provide emergency care to the fullest extent of his ability until a physician or other qualified person at the scene or at a hospital assumes responsibility for the continuation of care.

Among the EMT's responsibilities are:

Careful evaluation of all signs and symptoms

Prompt and efficient care of the patient before transport

Control at the scene

Extrication of the patient and preparation for transport

Sane and supervised transport

Orderly transfer of the patient to a medical facility

Communication with everyone involved

Proper reporting and record keeping

Vehicle and equipment care

If police or other authorities have not assumed control of the situation at an accident scene, the EMT's attitude and leadership will be crucial in gaining control and support from relatives and bystanders. Such people are usually responsive to direction and want to help; but they must be told briefly and clearly exactly what they should or should not do. A calm, decisive manner will create the spirit of effective teamwork necessary for efficient action.

The EMT will often be confronted with situations that tax his ability to remain calm and to perform effectively. Great fortitude is necessary if one is to witness horrifying events and yet exhibit self-control and respond effectively to the suffering of others. Such an attribute can be developed only through training, experience in dealing with all degrees of physical and mental distress, and especially through an unswerving dedication to serve humanity. Even the most experienced physician or combat-hardened medical corpsman may find it difficult at times to submerge personal reactions and proceed without hesitation to release patients from life-endangering situations, administer life-support measures to the mutilated, or recover the remains of those mangled in violent highway accidents, aircraft disasters, or explosions. The EMT

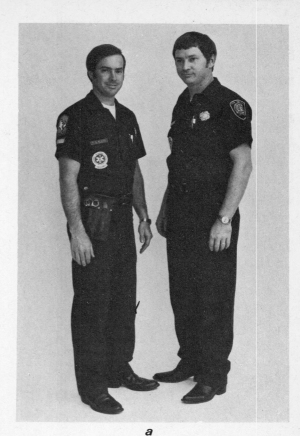

a

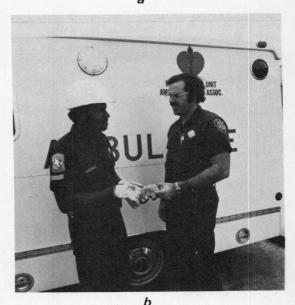

b

3

Figure 1.1 *a–b*

The EMT uniform identifies its wearers as members of the Emergency Medical Services team. *a,* These EMTs reflect the pride and confidence that their calling and responsibility give them. *b,* For special duties, special apparel is needed. Here one member of the team is equipped with a hard hat and protective gloves.

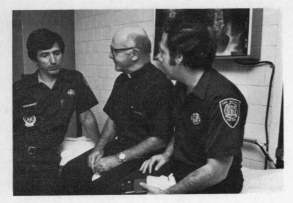

Figure 1.2

Two EMTs have a thoughtful discussion with the chaplain after a patient has died en route to the hospital.

4

must be prepared to face these situations with equanimity and to fulfill his responsibility as a member of the medical team.

Capabilities of the Emergency Medical Technician

Certain capabilities are necessary for the Emergency Medical Technician to carry out his responsibilities. These can be divided into three main categories. The most important is the care of life-threatening conditions.

The EMT must be able to:

Establish and maintain a patent airway
Administer intermittent positive-pressure ventilation
Give cardiopulmonary resuscitation
Control accessible bleeding
Treat shock
Care for cases of poisoning

There are, in addition, conditions which while not life-threatening must be cared for before transport to medical facilities. The EMT must be able to:

Dress and bandage wounds
Splint fractures
Give obstetrical assistance
Care for newborn infants, including premature ones.

Finally, there are important capabilities of a

non-medical nature. The EMT is expected to be competent in:

Emergency and defensive driving
Maintenance and use of supplies
Verbal and written communication
Controlling the scene of illness or injury
Executing proper rescue and extrication
Coping with medico-legal problems

Response to Emotional Reactions

A high percentage of patients attended by the EMT will be rational and cooperative, and much of their concern can be relieved by calm and efficient care. The EMT will often believe that a given condition does not constitute an emergency, but neither actions nor words should reflect such an opinion. Although a doctor may later agree and dismiss the case, the doctor is qualified to do so; the EMT is not. For both ethical and medico-legal reasons, it is incumbent on the medical profession that a doctor examine all patients received and judge the degree of medical needs of every "emergency" patient. The EMT must realize that even the most subtle symptoms may be early signs of catastrophe and that symptoms of many illnesses may be similar to those of alcoholism, drug abuse or withdrawal, hysteria, or other conditions. A patient's complaints must be accepted at face value; and the EMT must care for the injury or illness to the best of his ability until he is relieved of further responsibility by a physician or a member of the staff of a medical facility.

Personality traits are influenced by many factors. Members of some nationalities are highly emotional and demonstrative even for what may seem trivial causes, whereas those of some other groups are stoical and undemonstrative even in the face of serious injury or illness. Social and economic background, dependence on others, immaturity, senility, mental disorders, alcoholism, drug addiction, reaction to medication, nutritional status, and chronic disease may substantially influence a person's reactions to acute injury or unexpected illness.

Although the EMT cannot be expected to know the underlying factors that might trigger abnormal emotional responses, he must quickly and calmly appraise the actions of the patient and of relatives and bystanders and gain the confidence and cooperation of all involved. Courtesy, proper tone of voice, sincere concern, and efficient action in examination and the administration of care will go far to allay anxiety, fear, and insecurity. Reassurance rather than abrupt dismissal, chiding, or accusation will engender confidence and gain cooperation.

The patient should be given the opportunity to express his fears and concerns, many of which may be relieved on the spot. His concern may be for the safety or well-being of others involved in the accident or it may be related to damage and loss of personal property. The EMT's response to such concerns must be discreet and diplomatic, with special consideration given to the time and place when disclosure of the death or critical injury of loved ones might be most appropriate.

Some patients, especially children and confused or aged persons, may be terrified or feel rejected by separation from family members; other patients may prefer to relieve family members of the stress of witnessing their disability or pain. The extent to which relatives participate in patient care, including accompanying the patient to the hospital, must be decided on the basis of the best interests of the patient.

The care of handicapped patients often presents special problems. This is particularly true of the deaf, the deaf-mute, and the blind. The deaf person who does not have a functioning hearing aid will have difficulty in understanding questions about his symptoms. The deaf-mute will be able to respond only in writing to the average person. Unless obtaining information is pertinent at the scene, obvious problems requiring care should be attended to and the patient placated by efficient action, with questioning left until after transfer to a medical facility where relatives or others may act as interpreters.

The blind, of course, can respond to questions. These patients require a careful explanation of what is occurring, of the actions to be taken and the qualifications of those performing these actions. While the majority of the blind are very self-reliant and stable, they may under-

standably become panicky if not properly informed.

Attention to religious customs or needs may be of great importance, not only to the patient but also to his family. Convictions against administration of drugs or blood or the desire to keep religious medals may produce fear and concern. The need for religious counsel, baptism, or last rites, if death is imminent at the scene, must be respected.

In case of death, the body of the deceased must be handled with respect and dignity. Exposure of the body must be minimized, and it must be recognized that changing its position or location at the scene or transporting it from the scene may not be permitted except by the coroner or other authorities.

Relationship with Hospital Emergency Departments

There is no better way in which the EMT can learn to appreciate the extent to which his care influences full recovery or aids in reducing the degree of lasting disability than to observe the continuation of care by staff members of the emergency areas of a hospital. The extent to which he gains this knowledge is dependent upon his sincerity of purpose, his eagerness to improve his practices and skills, and his willingness to accept advice and constructive criticism. On demonstration of these attributes, the EMT can enjoy a close working relationship with hospital staff members.

5

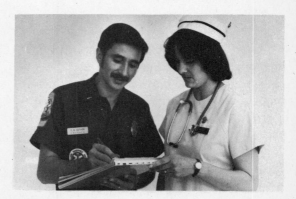

Figure 1.3

A nurse gives information to an EMT which will aid him in completing his report form.

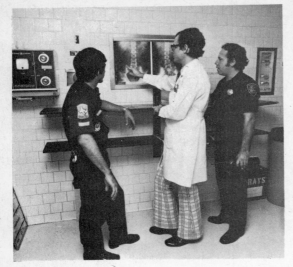

Figure 1.4

A physician explains to EMTs the X rays of a patient they have transported to the Emergency Department. Under teaching conditions like this, learning is accelerated and skills are improved with increased understanding.

While the physician is responsible for the actions of members of his staff, and may not be in a position to permit the EMT to participate actively in all procedures, much can be learned through direct observation, instruction, demonstration, and assisting to the extent permissible. This experience serves to emphasize the importance and benefits of proper initial emergency care and efficient transportation, as well as the consequences of delay, inadequate care, or misjudgment.

As an observer, the EMT will become familiar with equipment and its use, the functions of staff members, and the policies and procedures in all emergency areas of the hospital. He will become more expert through observing methods of resuscitation, handling of the unconscious, management of the mentally disturbed and unruly, the delivery of babies, and care of the newborn infant and mother. In addition, he will keep abreast of medical advances and of the design and use of new equipment.

It is rare that a physician is present at the scene of injury or onset of unexpected illness to give on-the-spot direction to the EMT. In addition to the physician's role as instructor in the didactic subjects of this textbook, it is in the emergency areas of the hospital that he can most effectively train Emergency Medical Technicians in the practical aspects of care by demonstration of techniques of actual patient care. In this way the EMT can become more proficient in the use of medical terminology and in interpretation of signs and symptoms of injury and disease. The physician also becomes familiar with the EMT's capabilities. Such familiarity can make radio communication more effective between the physician and the EMT at the scene and during transport when communication by voice can enable the physician to recommend emergency measures which may mean the difference between survival and death.

The EMT will find the staffs of emergency areas of the hospital eager and willing to improve his skills and efficiency, not only during his initial training but throughout his career. A close rapport among all concerned will assure optimal care and afford the EMT the opportunity to discuss his problems, benefit by experience, and better fulfill his role as a member of the emergency medical care team.

In the structure of emergency medical service systems throughout the country, there is a recognized difference between first aid training and the approved Emergency Medical Technician-Ambulance training course.

First aid training incorporates the basic measures the general public should learn so they may recognize the many hazards encountered during their ordinary daily activity and may give aid to the ill or injured until professionals can assume this responsibility. Ideally, first aid training should begin at the fifth grade level.

Certain segments of the public who are exposed more frequently than others to the ill or injured, either because of occupation or domestic circumstances, should be trained to a higher level. Among these are firefighters, law enforcement officers, lifeguards, industrial safety personnel, and members of the families of patients with chronic diseases. Training given these people must be the responsibility of the American National Red Cross, the American Heart Association, and other similar agencies with available lay instructors.

Professional emergency medical care can be

administered at the scene of an accident or illness and during transport to a medical facility by trained Emergency Medical Technicians, whether they are volunteers, employees of private ambulance companies, or participants in a municipal operation. Training people to give emergency medical care at this level should be under the direction of and, for the most part, conducted by physicians. This is the case in most states today.

The National Registry of Emergency Medical Technicians

The National Registry of Emergency Medical Technicians is the nationally recognized agency for certifying EMTs and documenting their level of competence according to recommended standards.

The National Registry, cognizant of the responsibility of such certification, has established standards that serve as a prerequisite for all seeking examination and subsequent national registration. The foremost of these requirements is the successful completion of an approved EMT-Ambulance course, such as the one developed by the Department of Transportation program, or its equivalent.

The American National Red Cross Advanced First Aid and Emergency Care course does not fulfill the training requirements for examination and entry into the National Registry, regardless of the additional instruction called for by Red Cross and D.O.T. agreement.

The National Registry of Emergency Technicians was formed in June, 1970, in response to the recommendation of the President's Committee on Highway Safety "that there be a national accreditation agency to establish standards."

The purposes of the Registry are:

1. To promote and improve delivery of emergency medical services by
   a. Assisting in the development and evaluation of educational programs to train Emergency Medical Technicians
   b. Establishing qualifications for eligibility to apply for registration
   c. Preparing and conducting examinations designed to assure the competence of Emergency Medical Technicians
   d. Establishing a system for re-registration every two years
   e. Establishing procedures for revocation of certificates or registration for cause
   f. Maintaining a directory of Registered Emergency Medical Technicians
2. To develop guidelines and programs to assist individuals who have completed the program to raise their level of competence, thereby assuring the provision of improved Emergency Medical Services
3. To do any and all things necessary or desirable for the attainment of the purposes stated above

The basic shoulder patch for the Emergency Medical Technician has been copyrighted and registered with the federal government. Bars to attest both the type of activity and the level of knowledge and skill of the EMT are available.

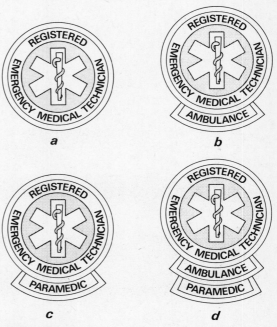

Figure 1.5 *a–d*

a, The basic shoulder patch of an Emergency Medical Technician is shown. *b,* A bar on the basic patch identifies the EMT as a member of a team assigned to an ambulance. *c,* Successful completion of an advanced training course is also signified by a special bar on the basic patch. *d,* The patch illustrated here could be worn by an EMT who has completed advanced training and who is a member of an ambulance team.

7

CHAPTER 2

Legal Responsibilities

GOAL I. Know the legal responsibilities of the Emergency Medical Technician.

OBJECTIVES

A. Define the legal status of someone who acts as a Good Samaritan.
B. Define implied consent.
C. Define informed consent by the emergency patient.
D. Describe the legal duty of the Emergency Medical Technician at the scene of an accident.
E. Describe the legal liability of the Emergency Medical Technician.

Possible legal implications involved in rendering emergency care and transportation to the sick or injured are always a subject of concern to those who provide such services. Because much misconception surrounds this field, the Emergency Medical Technician should have a knowledge of the general principles which govern his actions. The laws of states or districts differ widely; therefore only general principles can be discussed here. A further complication is that the laws vary according to the type of person providing emergency care and thus alter individual responsibility.

The material contained in this chapter is intended to serve only as a guide. The EMT should attempt to ascertain the variances or additions to these general principles which are applicable in his particular area and to know the responsibilities and restrictions which the law places on him.

The Types of Suits

An EMT responding to an emergency situation can become involved in a wide variety of potentially difficult legal situations. Examples of

some of these situations would include an automobile accident en route to the scene of the emergency, injury of passengers in an automobile accident, violation of the motor vehicle act of a state, or possible legal exposure because of emergency care rendered to the patient. Only the last subject will be discussed in this chapter.

The Basis of Legal Responsibility

The law requires that in particular circumstances an individual must act or behave toward others in a certain definable way. Under given circumstances, the individual has a duty to act or to refrain from acting. The manner in which the individual must act or behave is called a standard of care.

Standards of care are established in many ways, among them being local custom, statutes, ordinances, case law, and administrative orders. In most instances the precise standard of care against which an individual's conduct will be measured is decided by a judge. A jury or other fact finder, considering the facts of the particular case, then decides if the standard has been violated.

The basis of legal responsibility is in the main

the result of the doctrine of negligence. Legal negligence results in civil liability in those instances where the actions or behavior of an individual who had a duty to act did not conform to the required standard of care and there was resulting injury.

Duty to Act

The duty to act depends in great part on the law of the particular jurisdiction, the training and medical knowledge of the person answering the call, and the nature of that person's employment. The mere volunteer, a passerby, has under common law no legal responsibility to render aid or assistance at the scene of an emergency situation. However, the ambulance service of a local fire department or of the local hospital may have a responsibility both to respond and to render emergency care. In many states, fire departments and law enforcement agencies are said to have a duty to citizens within a given district to respond; therefore, an Emergency Medical Technician employed by such an agency would have a corresponding duty to act.

On the other hand, a passerby who may have no initial responsibility to render first aid assistance, does have a responsibility, if he chooses to render aid, not to abandon the patient after having started aid. One reason for this responsibility is that if other people pass by and see someone giving assistance at the scene of the accident, they might tend not to stop and render assistance themselves under the belief that the situation was under control. Abandoning a patient under these circumstances could prevent his receiving aid from someone else.

Standard of Care

The required standard of care may be considered technically a fluid concept; that is, the standard applicable to individual conduct is to be determined in each instance, depending upon the particular circumstances. Because of this fluidity, it is impossible to state separate principles which are applicable in all situations. Elements which make up a standard of care include the points discussed below.

The type of individual and community conduct. The conduct of an individual is to be judged in comparison with other hypothetical persons of similar training and experience. For example, the conduct of an Emergency Medical Technician employed by a fire department ambulance service is to be judged in comparison with the expected conduct of Emergency Medical Technicians from other reasonably well-trained fire department ambulance services. EMTs are not to be held to the same standards as physicians or other more highly trained individuals. Further, their conduct must be evaluated in the light of the given emergency situation, taking into consideration the general confusion, the needs of others, and the type of equipment available. Therefore, an important element of the standard of care required is the prevailing custom of the community—that is, a determination of how a reasonably prudent person with similar experience and training would act under similar circumstances, with similar equipment, and in the same place.

Standards imposed by force of law. In addition to local customs, standards of care may be imposed by statutes, ordinances, case law, or administrative orders. In many jurisdictions, violation of one of these types of standards is said to create "presumptive negligence." In these situations, negligence is assumed to exist if a violation of such a standard is shown. The defendant is presumed guilty until he introduces sufficient evidence to show that the standard was not violated or that mitigating circumstances existed which would permit a deviation from the legal standard. The defendant technically need not disprove negligence to counter this assumption, but the burden of proof does shift until such counter evidence has been introduced. Therefore, anyone rendering emergency care should familiarize himself with the particular legal standards which may exist in his state.

Professional or institutional standards. In addition to the standards imposed by the force of of law, professional or institutional standards may be admitted as evidence for the consideration of juries in determining the adequacy of an EMT's conduct. Professional standards, generally speaking, include published recommenda-

10

tions of organizations and societies involved in emergency work. Institutional standards include specific rules of procedure of the ambulance service or of the organization of which the EMT is a part.

These standards do not automatically have the force of law behind them. The judge must rule on which standards or recommendations are admissible into evidence, and the fact finder (usually the jury) must follow what the judge considers admissible when the standard of care in a particular situation is to be determined.

Two words of caution are important. First, the Emergency Medical Technician should familiarize himself with published recommendations of standards from his organization. Second, if an EMT is involved in formulating standards for his particular agency, he should attempt to make sure that these standards are realistic and that they do not impose an unreasonable burden on the EMT. Optimum care should at all times be striven for, but it is not desirable that institutional standards demand optimum care.

Consent

Consent law presents many particular problems. It is a long-established legal right that an individual is entitled to secure his person and to be free from intentional touching or interference by another without his consent. Intentional touching, without consent, is said to constitute a battery.

However, not every touching results in possible exposure to legal action. People often enter situations in which a reasonable man could expect touching. Therefore, bumping in crowds at sporting events does not present legal exposure. An individual's consent is said to be implied from the fact that he voluntarily entered the situation.

This type of implied consent is particularly applicable to emergency situations. Just as a person voluntarily entering a crowd implies consent for bumping, emergency situations create a similar implication that the patient consents to receive emergency care and to be transported to a medical facility.

Therefore, there are two types of consents: actual consent and implied consent. It must be remembered that an actual consent must be obtained if possible. For a consent to be effective, it must also be a knowing consent or, as it is technically called, an informed consent. It is required that the person understand the nature and extent of any procedure to which he is agreeing and that he have sufficient mental and physical capacity to make such a judgment.

Obtaining the patient's consent is more important than obtaining a signature on a printed document. A consent form is useful, and in many situations it is recommended; but it must be recognized that its only usefulness is as evidence the patient was informed of what was about to take place and that he willingly agreed to permit these activities.

Oral consent is valid and binding, but it can be difficult to prove its existence. A consent form can prove that oral consent was given in a conversation between the EMT and a patient, but it does not eliminate the need for the conversation.

Implied consent. There are many situations in which formal consent or the execution of a consent form is not needed. The most significant of these situations is an emergency situation. The law assumes that an individual who is in need of immediate emergency care to prevent his death or permanent impairment of his physical condition would consent to the rendering of such care and to being transported to the medical facility. However, for such a doctrine to be applicable, there must be a bona fide emergency.

An emergency situation is difficult to define. Generally speaking it includes situations in which there is a significant risk of death, of permanent physical impairment, or significant deterioration of condition. It also includes situations in which the patient is unconscious, delusional, or otherwise physically incapable of giving a knowing consent. In these situations, the EMT can proceed to render the required care.

However, even in these situations, it may be possible to obtain consent of someone other than the patient. The law in most instances recognizes the right of a spouse, close relative,

11

or next of kin to render consent for an injured person unable to consent for himself. In these situations it is desirable to obtain the consent of such an individual even when a bona fide emergency situation exists.

Minor's consent. The law recognizes that a minor may not have sufficient wisdom, maturity, and judgment to give valid consent for certain procedures. In these situations, the right to consent for the minor is given to the parents, or to individuals who are so close to the minor as to be treated as the equivalent of parents.

Not all consents given by minors are invalid. The determination depends upon the age and maturity of the individual. It is much more likely that consent given by a seventeen-year-old would be held adequate than a consent given by a four-year-old. Furthermore, many states have passed minor-consent laws which permit individuals who have not reached their legal maturity the right to give a binding consent. In many states, emancipation, marriage, or pregnancy causes the minor to be treated as an adult for the purposes of consent to medical treatment.

These principles merely determine who has the right to consent, not whether a consent is needed. If a bona fide emergency exists, the consent of a minor is implied. However, since the parents possess the primary right to consent, their consent should be obtained if possible.

Consent of the mentally ill. A person who is mentally incompetent is not capable of giving an informed consent. However, this disability exists in the main only if the individual has been judged incompetent. In those situations another individual, either a guardian or a conservator, usually possesses the primary right to consent for the patient. Such situations are similar to those involving minors.

Because of the very nature of the situations in which an EMT is likely to participate, there are many instances in which the patient may appear delusional or confused. This fact should be taken into consideration in determining whether a knowing or informed consent can be obtained. The doctrine of implied consent for bona fide emergency situations is fully applicable in these instances.

The Right to Refuse Treatment

An adult, competent individual has the legal right to refuse treatment. This legal right can create a great dilemma for emergency care personnel. Just as a consent to treatment must be informed, the refusal to consent to treatment must also be informed. Many emergency patients are delusional or confused. Under these circumstances, the refusal of treatment cannot be assumed to be a knowing refusal. On the other hand, competent adults who, for religious reasons, refuse specific kinds of treatment are generally within their legal prerogatives. Emergency care personnel must determine, as best they can, whether the patient's mental condition is impaired. Furthermore, if a parent refuses to give consent for the treatment of a minor, the EMT must also make a judgment as to the emotional effect on the parent of the emergency situation.

Guiding principles. Attention should be given to the requirements of consent law. However, the potential legal exposure should not be overstated. Very few reported cases have imposed liability on an EMT for failure to obtain the necessary consent. The primary purpose of these activities must be remembered, namely, to render emergency care to those in need. Failure to render treatment to an individual creates greater exposure to legal liability. Except in clear-cut situations, it is probably desirable to err on the side of rendering treatment rather than of withholding it. In most instances the law is on the side of emergency care personnel.

Immunities

There are many situations in which the law exempts a person from potential liability under certain circumstances.

Governmental immunities. The doctrine of governmental immunity stems from the ancient concept that a sovereign cannot be sued. This concept, once reserved for the king, is applicable to some extent to governmental employees. For some time this common law principle has been slowly eroding. However, many states retain

12

some limited form of the doctrine. The extent of the immunity granted, if any, is governed by a specific state statute. The EMT should ascertain what protection, and its extent, is granted in his particular area of activity.

Good Samaritan laws. Most states have, in recent years, passed Good Samaritan laws. The intent of these laws is to assure that someone who voluntarily undertakes to help an injured person at the scene of an accident is not chargeable with any fault or responsibility at law for errors or omissions in the care that he renders.

The Good Samaritan laws grant an immunity, but not an absolute one by any means. The provisions of these laws differ widely from state to state. Most of these statutes provide that immunity is not granted when gross negligence or willful and wanton misconduct results in an injury to the individual. Some states limit the Good Samaritan application to physicians or dentists who are passersby. Almost all states limit its application to services rendered at the scene of an accident, not those rendered in transit to a medical facility. This doctrine may afford some protection, but better protection is provided by rendering quality care.

EMT and Paramedic statutes. Some states have adopted specific statutes which grant special privileges to the more highly trained Emergency Medical Technicians. These statutes frequently authorize the performance of certain specified medical procedures and further grant a partial immunity to such personnel and to physicians or nurses who give emergency instructions to EMTs or Paramedics via radio or other methods of communication. Frequently, these personnel are required to obtain a license or certification. Certain training programs are typically required of them.

Exemption from the Medical Practice Act. Nearly every state exempts emergency treatment from the licensure requirements of the Medical Practice Act for the nonprofessional. Since many first aid procedures might be construed to be performance of a medical act, the EMT is protected in these situations. However, this exemption does not necessarily apply to the professionals—those individuals whose jobs require them to render emergency care on a regular and continuing basis. Furthermore, the requirement of a specific licensure or specific certification by state law would affect this exemption.

The effect of licensure or certification. In those states which require licensure or certification by a specified state agency, these licensing requirements are frequently interpreted as necessary conditions to the rendering of emergency care on a regular and continuing basis. Furthermore, the possession of a license or certification by an individual obligates the individual to conform to the standard of care of other licensed or certified emergency personnel. In those states which do not require licensure or certification, if an EMT is certified by a nationally recognized certifying organization, he will in all probability be held to the same standard of care expected of other certified EMTs.

Private Ambulance Services

The primary distinction between an ambulance service attached to a governmental agency and one which is commercial or voluntary lies in the duty to respond. A fire department ambulance service, being a part of a municipal governmental agency, may have a duty to respond to a call within its jurisdiction. A commercial or voluntary ambulance service may not be so obligated.

However, once a response has been made by any type of ambulance service, the principles of duty and the standards of care are equally applicable to both types of emergency personnel. The doctrine of governmental immunity may afford some minimal protection for public ambulance units. Commercial or voluntary services, however, rely mainly on adequate liability insurance and competently trained personnel to avoid legal exposure.

The best defense to legal exposure is a job well done.

Reporting Requirements

Society through its government has formulated a policy to protect its people by health

13

regulations and statutes. Because certain individuals are in a better position to observe and gather information about diseases and injuries, an obligation to report to certain agencies may be imposed. Some of these reporting obligations may be applicable to Emergency Medical Technicians. These reporting requirements include situations described in the following paragraphs.

Child abuse. All states and the District of Columbia have enacted laws to protect abused children. Most states have a reporting obligation for certain individuals, whose definition may range from "physicians" to "any person." An EMT should be aware of the requirements of the law of his state. Such statutes frequently grant immunity from liability for libel, slander, or defamation to the person obligated to report, if the report is made in good faith.

A further discussion of child abuse is included in Chapter 37, Pediatric Emergencies and Special Problems.

Injury during the commission of a felony. Many states have laws requiring the reporting of an injury likely to have occurred during the performance of a criminal act, or of other specific injuries such as gunshot or knife wounds or poisonings. In some instances, drug-related injuries must be reported. These requirements may affect the EMT. However, it should be stressed that the United States Supreme Court has held that drug addiction, as contrasted to drug possession or sale, is an illness, not a crime. Hence, an injury as a result of a drug overdose

may not be within the definition of an injury resulting from a felonious act.

Some states, by statute, specifically establish confidentiality and excuse certain specified individuals from reporting drug cases, either to a government agency or to a minor's parents, if in the discretion of those individuals, withholding reporting is necessary for the proper treatment of the individual.

Other reporting obligations. Other reporting requirements may include attempted suicides, dog bites, communicable diseases, assault, and rape. In addition, many states require anyone in attendance at a birth in a place other than a licensed medical facility either to report the birth or to report it when certain physical conditions are present.

Conclusion

It must again be emphasized that only general legal principles can be stated here since state laws differ widely. It must also be stressed that although the medico-legal responsibility must be taken seriously, it should not intimidate the EMT and prevent him from duly performing his job. In very few cases has liability been imposed on the EMT because of his conduct. The exposure for not performing might be at least as great as for performing. The best legal defense is, in all instances, proper training, continuing education, and skillful rendering of the required emergency care.

II

Anatomy, Diagnostic Signs, and Triage

CHAPTER 3

General and Topographic Anatomy

GOAL I. Know the general and topographic anatomy of the body.

OBJECTIVES

A. Name the major parts of the body.
B. Identify the bony and soft-tissue landmarks.
C. Identify the quadrants of the abdomen.
D. Describe the major organs associated with the divisions or landmarks in the body.

GOAL II. Comprehend the use of general and topographic anatomy in providing emergency care.

OBJECTIVES

A. Describe the relationship of the parts of the body, one to the other, using topographic terminology.
B. Describe the relationship of injured structures to uninjured structures.
C. Identify the arterial pressure points.

The surface of the body has many definite features. These landmarks serve as guides to structures that lie beneath them, giving clues to the anatomy of the body through its external features, its topography. A sharp awareness of the superficial landmarks of the body, or the topographic anatomy, will allow the well-trained examiner to evaluate the magnitude of an injury quickly and to anticipate possible complications. Inspection is the simplest component of the primary and secondary survey of injured persons. It requires no special skill, dexterity, or strength on the part of the examiner. It causes no pain or risk of further injury to the patient. Much information regarding the extent of injury can be obtained by a thorough inspection. The importance of this inspection cannot be over-emphasized; more facts are missed by not looking at a patient thoroughly than are missed by not knowing a specific anatomic relation.

All medical personnel should be familiar with the language of topographic anatomy so that specific information may be transmitted with a minimum of confusion. Picture the body in a standard position, which is always standing erect, facing the examiner with the arms at the sides, palms forward. When the terms right and left are used they refer to the patient's right and left (Fig. 3.1). The principal regions of the body are the head, neck, thorax (chest), abdomen, and the extremities (arms and legs).

The surface at the front of the body, facing the examiner, is the anterior surface; that behind is the posterior surface. An imaginary straight vertical line drawn from mid-forehead through the nose and the umbilicus to the floor is termed the midline. Areas pointing away from this line are termed lateral and areas pointing toward

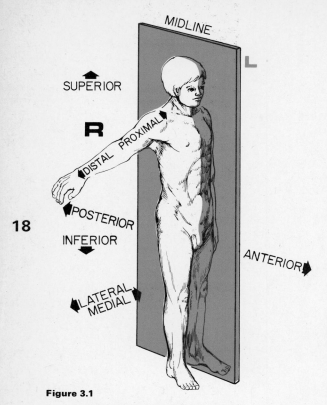

Figure 3.1

General terms of anatomy are shown.

If one keeps these terms in mind and recalls the description of the standard anatomic position, he will be able to describe the location of an injury so that another examiner will know immediately where to look and what to expect. Inspection of the patient may be carried out in any fashion the examiner chooses. It should be systematic, thorough, and performed in exactly the same sequence for all patients. If a routine is developed it will help the examiner avoid the oversight of a major but perhaps subtle sign whose presence might be critical. Examination should begin at the head, proceed through the neck, thorax, abdomen, pelvis, and the extremities. The usefulness for the examiner of comparing a given injured region with the corresponding uninjured location on the opposite side cannot be over-emphasized.

The Head

The head may be divided into the cranium and the face. An imaginary horizontal plane passing across the top of the ears and eyes may be considered to separate the superior (top) and inferior (bottom) portions of the head. The area above this imaginary plane is the cranium. It contains the brain, which connects with the spinal cord through a large opening at the base of the skull and in the center of the upper neck. The most posterior portion of the cranium is the occiput. On each side, the lateral and more anterior portions of the cranium are called the temples or temporal regions; more posteriorly are the parietal regions. One can feel the pulse of the temporal artery just anterior to the ear (Fig. 3.2).

Below the plane lie the ears, eyes, nose, mouth, cheeks, and jowls, which make up the face. The cheekbones are prominent below the eyes. The mandible (jawbone) is also obvious. The most obvious landmarks of the face are of course the eyes, ears, nose, and mouth. Gross injuries of these structures are not difficult to recognize.

Viewing from the side, one observes that the eyeball is recessed. It is protected superiorly and inferiorly by bony ridges and medially by the bridge of the nose. These ridges protect the eye but will obviously receive the greatest force

this line are termed medial, e.g., the medial and lateral surfaces of the knee, elbow, or ankle. Toward the head is the superior end; toward the feet is the inferior end. The nose, for example, is superior to the mouth, while the umbilicus is inferior to the neck.

The other terms which should be familiar are proximal and distal. Proximal refers to a location on an extremity which is nearer to the trunk. It also refers to any location on the trunk which is nearer to the midline or to the point of reference named. Distal is the opposite and refers to a location on an extremity which is nearer to the free end. Similarly it refers to any location on the trunk which is farther from the midline or from the point of reference named.

In general, arms and legs are taken to mean the upper and lower extremities. Specifically, the upper portion of the leg from the hip joint to the knee is the thigh. The lower portion from the knee to the ankle is the leg. The upper arm from the shoulder to the elbow is the arm. The lower portion from the elbow to the wrist is the forearm.

of any impact. A bruise, laceration, or abrasion in these locations must always be viewed, therefore, as a possible manifestation of a significant underlying fracture. Frequently, a fracture of the maxilla (the upper jaw), the bone just below the eyeball, will trap one or more of the muscles which control motion of the eye. If this occurs, the affected eye will often be looking down and its motion in other directions will be limited. This type of fracture is called a "blow out" fracture of the orbit.

Only the proximal one-third of the nose, the bridge, is formed by bone. The remainder is a cartilaginous framework. Any injury of the proximal third is therefore cause to suspect an underlying fracture, while an abrasion on the tip of the nose usually is a minimal injury. Bleeding or discharge from the nose after an injury of the head should always be investigated further. A nasal discharge of clear cerebrospinal fluid is an indication of a fracture of the anterior portion of the skull. A bloody discharge from the ear similarly suggests a fracture of the skull involving the temporal bone.

Unlike the nose, the exposed portion of the ear is composed entirely of cartilage covered by skin. Injuries of this appendage are usually quite obvious. Certain landmarks about the ear should be familiar. Immediately anterior to the notch at the middle of the anterior border of the exposed ear is the easily palpable temporal artery. If one holds a finger gently on the temporal artery at this site and then opens the

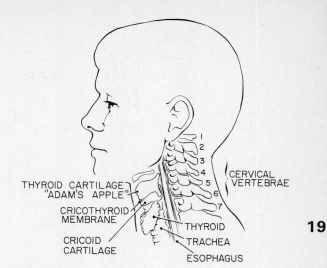

Figure 3.3

Landmarks in the neck are prominent.

19

mouth, he will immediately appreciate that the articulation of the mandible with the undersurface of the skull, the temporo-mandibular joint, lies at this location. The tragus, or small rounded fleshy protuberance immediately at the front of the ear canal, lies just over the area where the temporal artery may be palpated. The pinna is the name given to the ear itself. The lobes are the dependent fleshy portions at the bottom of each ear.

If the mandible is dislocated, the patient often will come to the hospital with his mouth fixed open. He will be unable to close it. There may be point tenderness at the temporo-mandibular joint.

One fingerbreadth posterior to the tip of the lobe of the ear is a prominent, hard, bony mass called the mastoid process. In patients who have suffered a posterior skull fracture, an ecchymosis or purplish-blue discoloration (bruise) may appear in this region some hours after the injury. This is a subtle finding, often overlooked or misdiagnosed as a simple bruise.

The Neck

The neck contains many anatomical structures, including the cervical or upper esophagus and the trachea (windpipe). The first seven vertebrae form the cervical spine (Fig. 3.3). The carotid arteries may be found at either side of

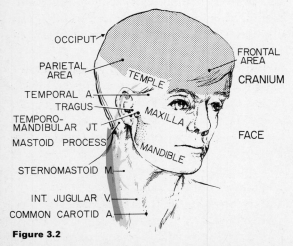

Figure 3.2

The major divisions and areas of the head are shown.

the trachea together with the jugular veins and several nerves.

Several useful landmarks are present in the neck. Most obvious is the firm prominence in the center of the anterior surface known as the "Adam's apple." Specifically, this prominence represents the upper part of the thyroid cartilage. It is more prominent in men than women. Approximately three-quarters of an inch inferior to the upper border of this prominence is a marked soft-tissue depression about one-quarter of an inch wide, which separates the thyroid cartilage from a second, somewhat less noticeable, cartilage—the cricoid cartilage. This latter cartilage is palpable as a firm ridge one-eighth to one-quarter of an inch thick. The thyroid and cricoid cartilages together form the framework of the larynx (voice box).

The soft-tissue depression represents the area of the crico-thyroid membrane, which is a heavy fascial sheet connecting the two cartilages. The crico-thyroid membrane is covered at this point only by skin. The location of the depression separating these two cartilages is important. In a patient with acute upper airway obstruction superior to the upper border of the larynx, insertion of two or three number 14-gauge needles through the crico-thyroid membrane into the trachea as an emergency procedure may be lifesaving. It is at this area that emergency crico-thyroidotomy is performed to assure an airway.

Moving inferiorly from the larynx, several additional firm ridges are palpable in the trachea. These ridges are the cartilages of the trachea. The trachea connects the larynx with the main bronchi (airways) of the lungs.

On either side of the lower larynx and the upper trachea lies the thyroid gland. Unless it is enlarged, this gland is usually not easily palpable.

With the head in extension, pulsations of the carotid arteries are easily palpable two to three fingersbreadth lateral to the larynx. Lying immediately adjacent to these arteries are the internal jugular veins and important nerves. Obviously, injuries which involve these areas of the neck may cause rapid, fatal bleeding.

Posteriorly, there is a series of bony prominences in the midline of the neck which become

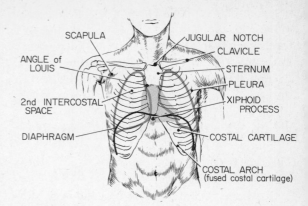

Figure 3.4

The major bony landmarks of the chest are easily palpable.

more obvious as they progress down the spine. They are the spines of the cervical vertebrae. They are most easily palpable when the neck is in extreme flexion. At the base of the neck posteriorly, the most prominent spine is usually that of the seventh cervical vertebra. Ordinarily, the larynx lies just anterior to the fifth and sixth cervical vertebrae.

The Thorax

The thorax (chest) is the cavity which contains the heart, lungs, esophagus, and the great vessels (the aorta and the two venae cavae). It is formed by the twelve thoracic vertebrae and twelve pairs of ribs. The clavicle (collarbone) overlies its upper boundaries in front and articulates with the scapula (shoulder blade), which lies in the muscular tissue of the thoracic wall posteriorly. Pleura lines the chest cavity, arches high in a dome behind each clavicle superiorly, and inferiorly covers the upper surface of the diaphragm—the lower boundary of the thorax (Fig. 3.4. See also Fig. 5.7).

The dimensions of the thorax are defined by the bony rib cage and its attachments. Anteriorly, in the midline of the chest, is the sternum (breastbone). The superior border of the sternum forms the easily palpable jugular notch. The inferior end of the sternum forms a narrow cartilaginous tip, which is called the xiphoid process. In the midline of the upper back, one can palpate the spines of the twelve thoracic vertebrae. Ten of these vertebrae are connected anteriorly to the sternum or to the costal arch by the first through the tenth ribs. Ribs eleven and twelve do not connect to the sternum or the arch and are therefore called floating ribs. Articulation between the ribs and the sternum or the arch is formed by means of an interposed costal cartilage. Inferiorly, the cartilages themselves become longer and form the palpable costal arch which is the definite boundary of the lower border of the thorax and the upper border of the abdomen. The arch itself is made up of the fused costal cartilages of the fifth through the tenth ribs. The jugular notch of the sternum lies at the level of the second thoracic vertebra. The xiphoid tip lies approximately at the level of the ninth thoracic vertebra.

On the male chest the nipples lie at the level of the interspace between the fourth and fifth ribs. In the female, breasts obviously vary in size and consequently nipple position varies. The center of the breast, however, still lies at the interspace between the fourth and fifth ribs.

Posteriorly, the scapula overlies the thoracic wall and is contained within heavy muscles. When the patient is erect, the two scapulae should lie at approximately the same level with their inferior tips at about the seventh thoracic vertebra. If one scapula lies noticeably higher, this may be an indication of neuro-muscular or bony injury.

The diaphragm is a muscular dome forming the undersurface of the thorax, separating the chest and abdominal cavities. Anteriorly it is attached to the costal arch; posteriorly it is attached through ligaments to the first two or three of the lumbar vertebrae, which lie inferior to the thoracic vertebrae. It moves up and down with normal breathing for a distance of one or two intercostal spaces. Injuries of the lower portion of the lung and the diaphragm from penetrating wounds obviously depend on its position at the time the injury is sustained.

Within the thoracic cage, the most prominent structures are the heart and lungs. The heart lies within the pericardial sac immediately under the sternum and immediately above the mid-portion of the diaphragm. It extends from the second to the sixth ribs anteriorly and from the fifth to the eighth thoracic vertebrae posteriorly. Ordinarily it lies from the midline to the left midclavicular line in the fifth intercostal space. Diseased hearts may be larger or smaller.

The major landmarks in the chest that are palpable are obviously the ribs. Most of these can be easily felt. The first rib is not palpable on either side, since it is hidden under and behind the clavicle which joins the sternum. Both clavicle and sternum are easily felt. Just inferior to the junction of the clavicle and sternum is a prominence on the breastbone. This prominence always lies opposite the space between the second and third ribs (second intercostal space). Orientation for counting ribs can be made from this prominence and the palpable interspace opposite it. The bony sternal prominence is called the "angle of Louis."

The major blood vessels traveling to and from the heart lie deep within the chest. On the right side of the spinal column the superior and inferior venae cavae carry blood to the heart. Just beneath the upper one-third of the sternum the arch of the aorta and pulmonary artery rise to distribute blood respectively to the body and to the lungs. The arch of the aorta passes to the left and lies alongside the left side of the spinal column as it descends deep within the chest and into the abdomen. The esophagus lies behind the trachea and directly on the spinal column as it passes through the chest into the abdomen.

All the space within the chest not occupied by the heart, the great vessels, and the esophagus is occupied by the lungs. Anteriorly, the lungs extend down to the surface of the diaphragm at the level of the xiphoid process. Posteriorly, the lungs continue in contact with the surface of the diaphragm down to the level of the twelfth thoracic vertebra. An anteriorly penetrating wound entering below the level of the xiphoid process might still damage the lungs posteriorly and the diaphragm.

The Abdomen

The abdomen is the second major body cavity. It is bounded superiorly by the diaphragm, inferiorly by a plane extending from the symphysis pubis through the sacrum, an-

21

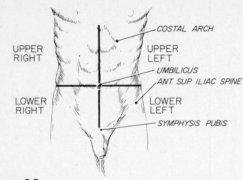

Figure 3.5

The quadrants are the easiest system of identifying abdominal areas.

22

teriorly by the anterior abdominal wall, and posteriorly by the posterior abdominal wall. It contains the major organs of digestion and excretion. There are several methods of referring to the various portions of the abdomen. The simplest and most common uses abdominal quadrants. In this system the abdomen is divided into four equal parts by two lines which intersect at right angles at the umbilicus (the navel). The quadrants thus formed are right upper, right lower, left upper, and left lower (Fig. 3.5). Pain or injury in a given quadrant usually arises from or involves the organs in that quadrant. With the use of this simple means of designation, one may identify quickly and clearly organs that are injured or diseased or that may require emergency attention.

In the right upper quadrant the major organs are the liver, gallbladder, and a portion of the colon. The greater portion of the liver lies in this quadrant almost entirely under the protection of ribs seven through twelve. It extends through the entire antero-posterior depth of the abdomen. Injuries in this area are frequently associated with injuries of the liver. Tenderness without injury in the right upper quadrant is usually a result of gallbladder disease.

In the left upper quadrant the principal organs are the stomach, the spleen, a portion of the transverse and descending colon, and a small portion of the liver. The stomach and the spleen are almost entirely under the protection of the left rib cage. The spleen lies lateral and posterior in this quadrant, under the diaphragm

and immediately beneath the eighth to eleventh ribs. This organ is frequently injured, especially in association with fractures of these ribs. Tenderness or pain in the left upper quadrant often points to a ruptured spleen.

In the right lower quadrant the principal organs are the cecum and ascending colon. The appendix is a small tubular structure attached to the lower border of the cecum. Appendicitis is the most frequent cause of tenderness and pain in this region. In the left lower quadrant the principal organs are the descending colon and the recto-sigmoid colon.

Many organs lie in one or more quadrants. The small bowel, for instance, encircles the umbilicus and parts of it occupy all four quadrants. The large bowel arises laterally in the right lower quadrant and completely encircles the abdomen in one sweep, coming to lie in all four quadrants also. The urinary bladder lies just behind the junction of the pubic bones at the middle of the abdomen; therefore, it lies in both lower quadrants. The pancreas lies transversely on the posterior body wall behind the abdominal cavity and therefore is in both upper quadrants. The kidneys lie in the same plane as the pancreas behind the abdominal cavity. They lie completely above the level of the umbilicus, extending from the eleventh thoracic vertebra to the third lumbar vertebra. They are approximately four to six inches long and lie in an angle formed by the spinal column and the lower ribs, the costo-vertebral angle. They are each attached to the bladder by tubular structures called ureters, which lie in the same plane behind the abdominal cavity. These tubes pass on either side of the spinal column along the posterior wall of the abdomen into the pelvis to enter the bladder.

Posteriorly, one does not usually refer to quadrants. The posterior portions of the iliac crest and the midline spines of the five lumbar vertebrae are the predominant landmarks of reference.

Properly speaking, organs that lie in the lowest portions of the abdominal cavity are not in it but are in the pelvic cavity. This cavity is bounded by the sacrum behind and the pubis in front. It lies between the most inferior portions of the pelvic bone. In this cavity the female genitalia (the uterus, ovaries, and fallopian tubes) and the rectum and urinary bladder are situated. The cavity is continuous with the abdominal cavity.

In the abdomen the chief topographic landmarks are the costal arches, the umbilicus, the anterior superior iliac spines, and the pubic symphysis. The costal arches are the fused cartilages of the fifth through the tenth ribs. They form the superior arching boundary of the abdomen. The umbilicus, a constant structure, is in the same horizontal plane as the fourth lumbar vertebra and the superior edge of the iliac crest. It overlies the division of the aorta into the two common iliac arteries. The anterior superior iliac spines are the hard bony prominences at the front on each side of the lower abdomen just below the plane of the umbilicus. At the center of the lowermost portion of the abdomen, one can feel another hard bony prominence, the symphysis pubis. The bladder lies just behind this bone. Injuries of the bladder frequently accompany fractures which involve the pelvis.

The Pelvis

The pelvis is a closed bony ring consisting of the sacrum in the midline posteriorly, two iliac bones laterally, two ischial bones inferiorly, and two pubic bones anteriorly. The latter three bones, ilium, ischium, and pubis, are fused to form a single bone, commonly called the innominate bone. Gentle pressure on each anterior superior iliac spine in a patient suspected of having a pelvic fracture will usually elicit pain and help to localize the fracture site.

Stretched between the symphysis pubis and the anterior superior iliac spine on either side of the lower abdomen is a palpable tough band of tissue, the inguinal ligament. Deep to this ligament pass the femoral nerve, artery, and vein, and muscles to the lower extremity. The femoral artery is easily palpable just distal to the midpoint of the ligament. The femoral nerve lies immediately lateral to the artery and the femoral vein lies just medial to the artery.

Posteriorly, the pelvis presents a flattened appearance mainly because of the configuration of the sacrum. In the sitting position, a bony prominence is easily felt in the middle of each buttock. These prominences are the ischial tuberosities. The sciatic nerve carrying major motor and sensory innervation to the foot and leg passes lateral to the tuberosity as it enters the thigh. Fractures of the pelvis in this region or a posterior hip dislocation may be revealed by pressure on this nerve.

In the male, inspection of the pelvis must always include inspection of the penis. Pelvic injuries can result in a fixed painful erection of the penis known as priapism. Occasionally, priapism is seen after spinal injuries; it may provide a clue in planning the moving of the patient.

The Lower Extremity

The lower extremity consists of the hip, thigh, knee, leg, ankle, and foot. Strictly speaking, the hip is a joint where the femur articulates with the innominate bone. Just distal to this joint is a bony prominence present on each femur called the greater trochanter. In examination, the position of this prominence should always be compared with that on the opposite side. Changes in the relative positions of these prominences are clues to underlying fractures or dislocations. The hip joint itself is superior and medial to the greater trochanter and about one inch lateral and one inch inferior to the pulsations of the femoral artery at the inguinal ligament.

The thigh extends from the hip joint to the knee. The supporting bone is the femur. Few landmarks are present in the thigh, but fractures of the femur are usually displaced and angulated and can be localized without great difficulty. Particularly powerful muscles attach to the femur. They can act to drive fractured segments of bone through the skin after an injury. Careful determination of the position of fragments of fractured bone must be made to avoid converting a closed fracture into an open one.

At the knee the patella (kneecap) is obvious. This bone is an integral part of and lies within the tendon of the quadriceps femoris muscle which extends the leg. A fracture of the patella will frequently interrupt this tendon and the patient will be unable to extend his leg at the knee. One may also be able to palpate a gap in the patella itself. Normally the patella rides smoothly in a groove on the anterior surface of the distal femur. This groove lies between the rounded condyles which make up the distal end of the femur and the articular surface of the knee joint. When the patella is dislocated it is usually displaced laterally out of its groove to slide over the top of the lateral condyle. In such instances the leg is fixed in flexion at the knee and the pain is extreme. The actual joint line of the knee is usually one inch inferior to the lower margin of the patella. It can easily be appreciated by palpating on either side of the patellar tendon with the knee flexed at forty-five degrees.

The leg is the portion of the lower extremity extending from the knee joint to the ankle joint. The bones of the leg are the tibia and the fibula. The broad tibial head forms the lower surface of the knee joint. Just inferior to the knee joint, the front of the leg is made up of the broad flat tibial plateau. One may palpate the entire extent of the tibia throughout the leg just under the skin on the medial surface; this is the familiar shinbone.

At the postero-lateral corner of the knee, two fingersbreadth below the joint line is the head of the fibula. This bone is most easily palpated with the knee flexed at ninety degrees. Passing immediately distally around this bony prominence is the peroneal nerve. This nerve controls dorsiflexion and eversion at the ankle and sensation over the top of the foot on the lateral surface. Injury of the fibula in this region should always prompt comparison of the function of the nerve with that on the opposite side of the patient's body. Injuries of the tibia, because of its subcutaneous location, are generally obvious.

The ankle is easily located by the prominent distal ends of both tibia and fibula. These are usually visible even in patients with large or fat legs. These knobs are called, respectively, the medial malleolus and lateral malleolus. They form the socket of the ankle joint. The socket receives the talus, which in turn articulates with the calcaneus (heelbone) and the astragalus to

form the main supporting structure of the foot which completes the extremity.

The calcaneus is palpable through the skin of the heel of the foot. The extremity is completed by the tarsal (ankle) bones, five metatarsal bones which form the substance of the foot, the five toes formed of phalanges, and occasional sesamoid bones.

Inspection of the lower extremity may give many clues to an injury. Some fractures are quite obvious. Noting the relative position of bilateral structures suggests other injuries at the hip joint or more distal in the extremity. In an injury in the lower extremity, if the patellae are at the same level on either side, localization of the lesion is probably below the knee. If they are not, the injury may be above. Most patients with hip fractures have a shortened leg which is flexed and externally rotated. In these patients the patella may be above the one on the opposite side and facing outward. A dislocated hip may cause the extremity to shorten, flex, and internally rotate, in which case the patella may face its neighbor. Careful inspection will allow the examiner to make all these observations.

The Shoulder

The shoulder girdle is composed of the clavicle anteriorly and scapula posteriorly. Injury of these structures may be noted simply as "pain in the shoulder." The clavicle is attached medially to the sternum at the sterno-clavicular joint. It is palpable throughout its entire length from the sternum to its attachment to the scapula at the acromio-clavicular joint. Each of these joints may be dislocated and may be palpated. Fractures of the clavicle are easily palpable and usually visible.

The scapula is a broad flat bone overlying the posterior wall of the thorax and articulating with the clavicle. The scapula bears the surface of articulation for the arm with the shoulder. Injury of this bone is extremely uncommon because of its protected situation. It ordinarily is not palpable, although a transverse ridge running across the upper portion of each scapula, called the spine of the scapula, may frequently be palpated under the skin of the back.

The external appearance of the shoulder as a unit is that of a gently rounded area without significantly noticeable prominences. The very top of the shoulder corresponds to the acromio-clavicular (A-C) joint. This joint lies three fingersbreadth from the lateral surface of the arm. Three fingersbreadth anterior and inferior to the A-C joint is the bony prominence of the coracoid process of the scapula. This process serves as the site of attachment for muscles of the upper extremity and muscles which pass between the shoulder and the chest wall. The most lateral structure of the shoulder is the rounded head of the humerus, the bone of the arm, which accounts for the rounded appearance of the shoulder in general. If the humeral head is dislocated from its socket on the scapula, it is no longer laterally located and the configuration of the shoulder changes from a rounded to a squared-off appearance. Conversely, a fracture just distal to the head of the humerus, which is very common, does not displace the head and will not change this rounded configuration.

The Upper Extremity

By definition, the uppper extremity extends from the shoulder to the fingertips. It is composed of the arm, elbow, forearm, wrist, hand, and fingers. The arm extends from the shoulder to the elbow and the supporting bone is the humerus. Injuries involving the humerus frequently are interpreted as injuries of the shoulder and appear as such. Combinations of fractures with dislocation are seen and appear initially as dislocations. In most of these injuries the patient usually complains of shoulder pain but maintains his forearm flexed at the elbow and the extremity held close to the body. Injuries of the upper extremity may result in crippling damage of any of the major nerves supplying the hand and forearm. These are the radial, median, and ulnar nerves.

The arm offers few specific landmarks. Injuries and fractures in the humerus are customarily obvious and are not difficult to diagnose. One must recall that the radial nerve, carrying sensation to the greater portion of the back of the hand and motor function controlling

extension of the hand at the wrist, passes very close around the shaft of the humerus in its midportion. Fractures in this region demand careful evaluation of the function of this nerve.

The elbow presents several bony landmarks. The medial and lateral epicondyles of the humerus form the medial and lateral borders of the upper surface of the elbow joint. They are easy to palpate at the distal end of the humerus with the elbow flexed. A third prominence is the most posterior portion of the elbow at its apex, called the olecranon process of the ulna. These three prominences describe an equal-sided triangle when the elbow is flexed at ninety degrees. In injuries above the elbow these relationships are routinely disturbed and may easily be appreciated by comparison with the opposite side.

Immediately posterior to the medial epicondyle of the humerus is a groove in which the ulnar nerve passes. This groove can be easily felt by extending the elbow fully. The ulnar nerve is extremely important in hand function, controlling sensation over the fifth and fourth fingers on the dorsum of the hand, abduction of these fingers, and inversion of the hand as a whole. The ulnar nerve is easily damaged in elbow injuries. When one strikes his "funny bone" he is actually striking the ulnar nerve at this point in the elbow and he can easily appreciate a tingling in the fourth and fifth fingers.

The median nerve may also be injured above the elbow. This nerve lies near the anterior surface of the elbow approximately in the midline. It is more protected in this area by adjacent muscles than is the ulnar nerve.

At the wrist, a bony prominence is easily felt on the medial (little finger or ulnar) side. This is the end of the ulna and is called the ulnar styloid process. A similar, less obvious, bony process is present on the lateral (thumb, or radial) side of the wrist. This is the radial styloid process and represents the end of the radius. Simultaneous palpation of these distal tips will reveal that the radial styloid process usually lies about one centimeter distal to that of the ulna. With displaced wrist fractures this relationship may be reversed, or the processes may lie at the same level.

If one forms a large claw with the hand, as

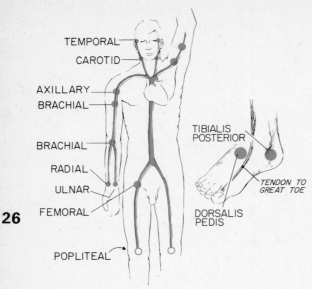

Figure 3.6

The several points where a pulse may be felt are shown. At these areas, major arteries lie close to the skin or over bony prominences.

though attempting to grasp a tennis ball, one may see two tendons on the anterior surface of the wrist at the base of the hand. Between these tendons lies the median nerve carrying the fibers for sensation for much of the palm of the hand and for specialized motions of the thumb. This nerve is frequently damaged at this point after injuries of the wrist.

The hand articulates with the forearm through the eight carpal bones. The palm of the hand is formed by five metacarpal bones and the thumb and fingers by the phalanges.

Arterial Pressure Points

At any point where an artery passes over a bony prominence or lies close to the skin it can be compressed to help control bleeding beyond that point. Theoretically this principle can be applied to every artery in the body. There are many areas where arteries can be specifically palpated and where pressure may be used to con-

trol hemorrhage. Ordinarily the best control of hemorrhage is local pressure exerted on the bleeding vessel at the site of injury. Infrequently, however, pressure on a major feeding artery may be required, and it is proper that the EMT have a knowledge of such points (Fig. 3.6).

Anterior to the upper portion of the ear, just over the temporo-mandibular joints lie the superficial temporal arteries which supply the scalp. Anterior to the angle of the mandible, on the inner surface of the lower jaw on either side, one may palpate the external maxillary arteries which contribute much of the blood supply to the face. The carotid arteries may be compressed anteriorly against the transverse processes of the sixth cervical vertebra behind. At the inner surface of the arm the brachial artery may be palpated approximately four fingersbreadth above the elbow. Pressure here may control circulation in the forearm. Similarly, arterial pulsation may be felt in both the radial and ulnar arteries at the wrist—at the bases of the thumb and little finger, respectively.

The femoral artery may be palpated and compressed as it issues from beneath the inguinal ligament in the groin. At this point it lies just over the ramus of the pubis and compression may be exerted on the artery against this bone. In the popliteal fossa, a triangular space at the back of the knee joint, one may palpate the popliteal artery lying in the medial area of this space. Determination of pulsation in this artery is an intrinsic part of the examination of every wound of the lower extremity.

Just posterior to the medial malleolus is the posterior tibial artery. It is always palpable just under the skin and may easily be compressed. On the anterior surface of the foot just lateral to the major extensor tendon of the great toe is the dorsalis pedis artery. This artery is not as constantly present as the posterior tibial artery, but its pulsations, when present, may easily be palpated and it also may easily be compressed (Fig. 3.6.).

CHAPTER 4

Interpretation of Diagnostic Signs and Triage

GOAL I. Know the normal diagnostic and vital signs and understand how they can change because of disease or injury.

OBJECTIVES

A. List the normal diagnostic signs.
B. Identify abnormalities in diagnostic signs.
C. Describe the relationship of changes in vital signs to patient problems.

GOAL II. Know how to observe normal diagnostic signs.

OBJECTIVES

A. Describe the procedures for determining and recording all vital diagnostic data.
B. Explain the importance of accuracy in measuring and recording diagnostic data.

GOAL III. Know the meaning of triage and its application to injured patients.

OBJECTIVES

A. Explain the importance of discriminating among various types of injury to determine the sequence of treatment.
B. Describe the principles of triage.

A rapid but accurate examination of an injured or critically ill patient is essential for adequate emergency medical care. Exact knowledge of the nature of an injury or illness is not necessary since the pulse, respiration, blood pressure, body temperature, skin color, status of the pupils of the eyes, state of consciousness, ability to move, and reaction to pain usually indicate what emergency action must be taken. These are the basic vital diagnostic signs that can be observed quickly, with a minimum of equipment. Together with observations of the patient's injuries and condition, they form the basis for diagnosis.

Pulse

The pulse is the pressure wave generated by the heartbeat and propagated along the arteries. The usual pulse rate in adults is 60 to 80 beats per minute; a usual pulse rate in children is 80 to 100 beats per minute. The pulse is palpable at

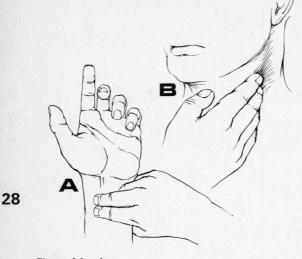

Figure 4.1 a—b

a, Radial and, *b,* carotid pulses are usually easily palpated.

28

any area where an artery passes over a bony prominence or lies close to the skin.

Commonly, the place to feel for the pulse is at the base of the thumb over the wrist (Fig. 4.1 *a*). Here, the radial artery is rather superficial. However, the palpation of the radial pulse may often be difficult in an emergency situation and not always accurate. The carotid artery in the neck is a good place to feel for the pulse; one must palpate gently under the anterior border of the sternomastoid muscle (Fig. 4.1 *b*). One should always palpate carotid pulses with the patient supine or sitting. The femoral arteries in each groin are the most superficial major arteries in the body. If a pulse is not palpable at the wrist or neck, it can usually be felt over the femoral vessels. If no peripheral pulse can be felt anywhere, listen directly over the heart with the ear or a stethoscope to determine the presence and rate of the heartbeat.

Changes in the rate and volume of the pulse are important findings in emergency care. The pulse rate is easily checked and reflects the rapidity of the heartbeat. The volume of the pulse describes the sensation the beat itself gives to the palpating finger. Normally the pulse beat is a strong, easily felt impulse reflecting a full blood volume. A rapid, weak pulse is usually the result of shock from loss of blood; a rapid, bound-

ing (very strong) pulse is present in fright and hypertension. The absence of a pulse means that the specific artery being felt is blocked or injured, or that the heart has stopped functioning Changes in the pulse directly reflect changes in heart rate in response to injury or alarm, changes (cardiac arrest), or that death has occurred. in circulating blood volume, or changes in the vascular bed. They occur almost instantaneously. The pulse should be taken immediately and then periodically during emergency treatmento to note any changes. The pulse rates must be recorded as they are taken and the character of the pulse described (weak or strong).

Respiration

Normal breathing is easy, without pain and without effort. The rate can vary widely. Usually it lies between twelve and twenty breaths per minute, but well-trained athletes may breathe only six to eight times per minute; rarely does the rate exceed twenty breaths per minute. Respirations should not be unusually shallow nor should they be unusually deep. A record should be made of the initial rate and character of the respiration and any change observed.

Rapid, shallow respirations are seen in shock. Deep, gasping, labored breathing may indicate airway obstruction, heart disease, or pulmonary disease. In respiratory depression or respiratory arrest, there will be little or no movement of the abdomen and chest with respiration and little airflow at the nose and mouth. Severe metabolic disturbances, such as acidosis or alkalosis may produce characteristic breathing patterns.

Frothy sputum with blood at the nose and mouth accompanied by coughing following an injury indicates lung damage. Fractured ribs can tear the lung; foreign bodies (e.g., bullets, knives) can penetrate and lacerate it. In each instance bleeding within the lung may appear as coughed-up pink froth. Frothy pink or bloody sputum is also an indication of pulmonary edema, which can accompany acute cardiac failure or severe lung contusion.

Occasionally one can deduce much from the smell of the breath. Obviously the intoxicated person may smell of alcohol. Those in severe diabetic acidosis frequently have a sweet or fruity odor of the breath. Any particularly obvious odor should be noted and recorded.

Blood Pressure

Blood pressure is the pressure that the circulating blood exerts against the walls of the arteries. Since in the normal person the arterial system is a closed system attached to a pump and completely filled with blood, changes in blood pressure indicate changes in the volume of blood, in the capacity of the vessels, or in the ability of the heart to pump. Changes in blood pressure, like those in the pulse, can be rapid. They are not as rapid as pulse changes, however, because normal protective mechanisms exist to maintain blood pressure in spite of injury or disease. Blood pressure can fall markedly in states of shock, after severe hemorrhage, or after a heart attack. Lowered blood pressure means that there is insufficient pressure in the arterial system to supply blood to all of the organs of the body. Some of these organs may thus be severely damaged. The causes of the low blood pressure must be rapidly ascertained and treated (see Chapter 9, Shock).

If blood pressure is abnormally high, damage or rupture of the vessels in the arterial circuit may occur. It is equally important that the cause of this state be ascertained and treated. The treatment of elevated blood pressure may require hospitalization. This therapy is complex and not usually a function of the EMT; on the other hand, treatment of low blood pressure from bleeding requires emergency control of the hemorrhage.

Blood pressure in a patient can change rapidly during transit from the scene of an accident to the hospital. It is important for the attending doctor to know what the blood pressure was as soon after the emergency situation started as possible. This information will allow him to judge the severity and significance of any change when blood pressure is recorded at the hospital. Therefore, as part of the initial care of a patient, the EMT should check blood pressure, record it and the time it was taken.

Blood pressure is recorded at systolic and

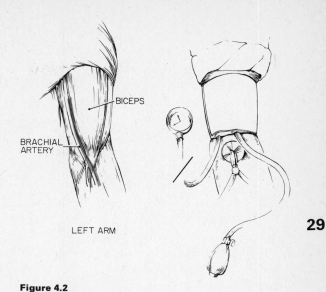

Figure 4.2

The proper location for and application of the sphygmomanometer is shown.

29

diastolic levels. Systolic pressure is the level present during contraction of the heart. Diastolic pressure is the level present during relaxation of the heart. Systolic pressure is the maximum pressure under which the arteries function. Diastolic pressure is the minimum pressure constantly present in the vessels. Usually these pressures change in a parallel fashion. Both rise or fall. Occasionally, a rise in the systolic pressure with a stable or falling diastolic pressure may indicate brain damage in a patient with a head injury. Systolic and diastolic pressures that approach one another as the former falls and the latter rises are indicative of cardiac tamponade.

Blood pressure is determined by an apparatus known as a sphygmomanometer, which is used with the stethoscope (Fig. 4.2). To determine blood pressure, the cuff of the sphygmomanometer is fastened about either arm above the elbow and is inflated with the rubber bulb until the mercury column or the needle of the dial stops moving with the pulse. This point is usually between 150 and 200 millimeters of mercury. The stethoscope diaphragm or bell is placed over the brachial artery which lies medially at the front of the elbow in the antecubital fossa. Air is slowly released from the bulb as the observer watches the mercury column fall or aneroid dial return to zero. The point on the gauge at which the first sounds of the pulse are heard through the stethoscope is the systolic pressure. The level on the gauge at which the sounds disappear is the diastolic pressure. The pressure reading is in millimeters (mm) of mercury (Hg).

Blood pressure levels vary with age and sex. A useful rule of thumb for normal systolic pressure in the male is 100 plus the age of the patient, up to a level of 140–150 mm Hg. Normal diastolic pressure in the male is 65–90 mm Hg. Both pressures are 8–10 mm Hg lower in the female.

One of the most useful instruments the EMT will have is the stethoscope. It is required in the determination of blood pressure and is also used to detect heart, breath, and bowel sounds. The technique of blood pressure measurement has been described. Detection of heart sounds is made by listening over the heart, detection of breath sounds by listening in the interspaces between the ribs over each side of the chest. In the abdomen, one listens in all four quadrants.

When the stethoscope is being used correctly, the earpieces fit into the ears comfortably and exclude all outside noises. It should be worn with the earpieces pointing forward. The principal mistakes made in wearing a stethoscope are selecting one that is too small or too tight or putting it on backwards. Always be sure the stethoscope is picking up sounds before applying it to the chest or pulse.

Temperature

Normal body temperature is 98.6° Fahrenheit (37.0° Centigrade). The skin is largely responsible for regulation of this temperature, by radiation of heat from skin blood vessels and the evaporation of water as sweat.

Changes in temperature occur as a result of illness or injury. A cool, clammy (damp) skin is indicative of a general response of the sympathetic nervous system to trauma or to blood loss (shock). It can be seen also in heat exhaustion. As a result of nervous stimulation, sweat glands are hyperactive and skin blood vessels are contracted, resulting in cold, pale, wet or clammy

skin. A patient with these symptoms should be covered to conserve body heat. These signs are sometimes the first signs of shock and they must be recognized as such. Exposure to cold usually produces a cool dry skin. A dry hot skin may be caused by fever in illness or may be the result of exposure to excessive heat, as in sunstroke. Immediate cooling measures may be necessary in this patient.

Temperature may be taken orally by placing a thermometer beneath the tongue. It should be left with the mouth closed for three minutes. In a child or uncooperative patient, the thermometer can be placed in the axilla (armpit), keeping the arm at the patient's side. A much longer period of time, ten minutes, should be allowed for the thermometer to register temperature if it is placed in the axilla than if it is placed under the tongue. Axillary temperatures are notoriously inaccurate and are seldom used. Rectal temperature is very accurate and will be taken at the hospital on the patient's arrival. It is routinely one-half to one degree above oral temperature. A rectal thermometer is used to measure rectal temperature and is left in place at least one minute.

Skin Color

Skin color depends primarily on the presence of circulating blood in subcutaneous blood vessels. In deeply pigmented people, skin color depends primarily on the pigment. The presence of pigment may obscure skin color changes resulting from injury. In patients with deeply pigmented skin, color changes may be apparent in the fingernail beds, in the sclerae of the eyes, or under the tongue. In lightly pigmented patients where changes may be seen more easily, colors of medical importance are red, white, and blue.

A red color may be present with high blood pressure, certain stages of carbon monoxide poisoning, and sunstroke. The person who has severe high blood pressure may sometimes be plethoric (he will have a dark reddish-purple skin color and all the visible vessels will be full). The person with carbon monoxide poisoning is usually cherry red, as is the sunstroke patient. A person in an advanced stage of carbon monoxide

30

poisoning may be blue, however, because of lack of oxygen in his blood.

A pale, white, ashen, or grayish skin is indicative of insufficient circulation and is seen in patients in shock or suffering from a heart attack or in certain stages of fright. Here there is literally not enough blood circulating in the skin.

A bluish color, cyanosis, results from poor oxygenation of the circulating blood. As a result, blood is very dark red and overlying tissue appears blue. Cyanosis is seen in patients with heart failure or airway obstruction and in some instances of poisoning.

Chronic illness may also produce color changes such as the yellow color, jaundice, seen in liver disease. Here a specific substance, bilirubin, normally present in the liver and the gastrointestinal tract, is deposited in the skin.

Assessment of the patient's color leads to a decision concerning his immediate treatment. Oxygen may be necessary; arrest of hemorrhage may be necessary; resuscitation may be required. A glance at the patient is often sufficient to let the EMT decide this first priority.

Pupils of the Eye

The pupils of the eye, when normal, are regular in outline and usually of the same size. In examination of the pupils the presence of contact lenses or prostheses (false eyes) must be considered.

Changes and variation in size of one or both pupils are important signs in emergency care. Constricted (smaller) pupils (Fig. 4.3) may be present in the patient who is a drug addict or who has a disease that may affect the central nervous system. Dilated (enlarged) pupils (Fig. 4.3)

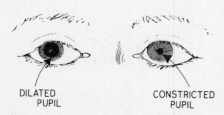

DILATED PUPIL   CONSTRICTED PUPIL

Figure 4.3

Normal pupillary diameter is 2 to 3 mm. Pupils may be dilated or constricted for many different reasons. Usually, pupil size is equal and pupils react together.

indicate a relaxed or unconscious state; such dilation usually occurs rapidly (thirty-five seconds) after cardiac arrest. Head injury or prior drug use, however, may cause the pupils to remain constricted even in patients with cardiac arrest.

Variation in size of the pupils is seen in patients with head injuries or strokes. In a small percentage of normal people, anisocoria (unequal pupil size) is found. The incidence is so small that in the injured patient, pupil variation is regarded as a reliable sign of head injury. Failure of the pupils to react (contract) when a light is shined into the eyes may indicate disease, poisoning, drug overdose, or injury. Ordinarily pupils contract promptly when a light is shined through them. This is a normal protective reaction of the eye. In death, the pupils are widely dilated and fail to respond to light at all.

The state of the pupils should be noted as soon as is convenient. Pupillary change indicates progressive damage within the head or nervous system and may signify the need for an emergency operation after arrival at the hospital. These changes usually reflect central nervous system dysfunction very rapidly. In the patient with central nervous system damage, saving his life or the possibility of avoiding permanent damage may depend on a rapid head operation. Changes that occur in pupil size point to consideration of such an operation.

State of Consciousness

Normally, a person is alert, oriented, and responsive to vocal or physical stimuli. Any change from that state is indicative of illness or injury. Recording such a change is extremely important in emergency care. Changes in the state of consciousness may vary from mild confusion in an alcoholic or mental patient to deep coma as a result of head injury or poisoning. The state of consciousness of an individual is probably the single most reliable sign in assessing the status of his nervous system.

It is extremely important to note the state of consciousness of an injured person at once and to discover and note whether he was rendered unconscious immediately. All subsequent changes

31

in his state of consciousness must be noted. Progressive development of coma or increasing difficulty in rousing a patient are signs that indicate the need for urgent medical attention. They should be recognized at once and recorded. Rapid loss of consciousness may point to a serious head injury which will require an immediate operation. Similarly it may mean that a very large overdose of drug has been taken and the patient will shortly require full resuscitation.

Ability to Move

32   The inability of a conscious patient to move voluntarily is known as paralysis. It may be a result of illness or injury. Paralysis of one side of the body, including the face, may occur as a result of an intracerebral hemorrhage or clot (stroke). Some drugs used over long periods of time also may cause paralysis.

Inability to move the arms and legs after an accident may indicate injury of the spinal cord in the neck. Inability to move the legs while the arms remain normal may indicate a spinal injury below the neck. Paralysis is a particularly important sign and its presence and onset with regard to an injury must be noted. The patient who has a completely severed spinal cord is paralyzed below the level of the injury, immediately and permanently. The person who has a spinal injury in which the cord is gradually compressed experiences the onset of paralysis gradually.

Reaction by vocal response or body movement to painful physical stimulation is a normal function. Changes in these reactions may result from a loss of sensation following injury or illness.

Reaction to Pain

The loss of voluntary movement of the extremities after an injury is usually accompanied by loss of sensation in these extremities. Occasionally, however, movement is retained and the patient complains of numbness or tingling in the extremities. *It is extremely important that this fact be recognized as a sign of probable injury of the spinal cord so that mishandling does not aggravate the condition.*

Severe pain in an extremity with loss of cutaneous sensation may be the result of an occlusion of the main artery of that extremity. In such a case the pulse in the extremity is absent. The ability to move the extremity is usually retained, although it is often held immobile because of pain accompanying any motion.

Frequently, patients suffering from hysteria, violent shock, or excessive drug or alcohol use may feel no pain from an injury for several hours. Concomitant paralysis is usually not seen. Generally, other signs will also support a diagnosis of hysteria or other such reaction.

Interpretation of Diagnostic Signs

After arriving at the emergency scene the EMT will learn most from quick visual observation. Sound judgments as to appropriate action can usually follow a good general survey. Observation should include noting the type of accident, the vehicles involved, the number of patients, the nature of the terrain, and the type of buildings, if any, being used to house the critically ill or injured.

As soon as the ambulance has stopped, the EMT should dismount with the jump kit, field bag, or equipment satchel containing the equipment necessary for lifesaving care and begin a survey. *All involved patients must be surveyed initally.* In the meantime, the driver should park the ambulance, keeping a traffic lane open if possible, set up warning devices if police are not present to do this, and then assist in the survey. A large number of patients may be examined in very short time, using the signs described in this chapter. Until the entire group has been surveyed, the EMT should stop to treat only those with life-threatening problems (massive bleeding externally or obvious difficulty breathing).

During such a survey a definite step-by-step outline of action must be followed (Fig. 4.4). An approach to the patient or patients which is not carefully planned or is disorganized will result in unnecessary loss of time in emergency care and create confusion at the scene. A record of initial observation can be started and should accompany each patient.

The EMT must remain calm no matter what

LIFESAVING SURVEY OF ACCIDENT VICTIM

(The following should be done simultaneously)

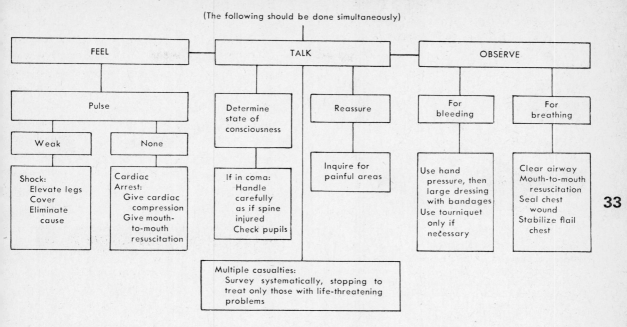

33

SURVEY FOR ADDITIONAL INJURIES NOT ENDANGERING LIFE

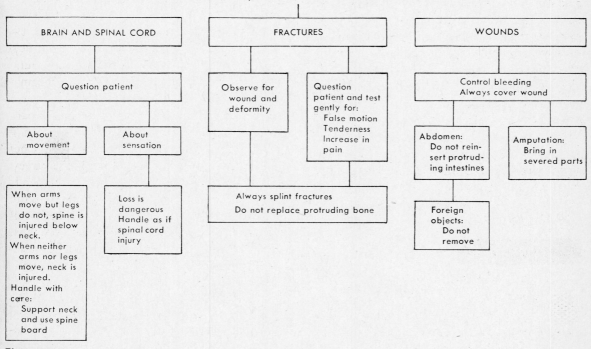

Figure 4.4

   Two charts detail how and what the EMT should survey to determine the condition of an emergency patient. The chart on top is a lifesaving survey for the most serious, life-threatening conditions. The one on bottom is for injuries which do not immediately endanger the life of the patient. (These surveys were developed by Sam W. Banks, M.D., and J. D. Farrington, M.D.)

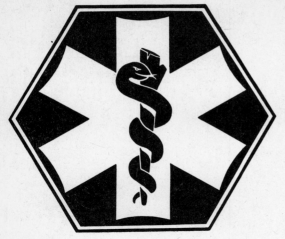

Figure 4.5

   Many persons wear this symbol for emergency medical identification. It is a warning device which can alert medical personnel or laymen that the person wearing it has a medical condition requiring special treatment or that he is allergic to certain medications or takes medication which can cause certain reactions. If a patient is unconscious or unable to communicate, search clothing, body, wallet, or purse to try to find the symbol. It is usually worn as a bracelet or necklace.

the situation. This attitude will instill confidence in the patient and others as to his knowledge and ability to handle the situation.

   During this survey the EMT has only to talk, feel, and observe; no equipment is needed. Inquiry must be made not only about painful areas but about any medical condition that might influence care at the scene, during transport, and at the medical facility. If the patient is unconscious, his wallet, clothes, and wrist or neck should be checked for an Emergency Medical Identification card or tag (Fig. 4.5). This symbol bears a warning on its back if the patient has epilepsy, diabetes, or other serious illness or if he should not be given certain medications because he is allergic to them. The EMT should also seek information from relatives or bystanders. Such questioning is to be carried out during the survey while care is being rendered to those with life-threatening conditions at the same time.

Triage

   Upon completion of the survey and the necessary steps for immediate care, the EMT must examine each patient more thoroughly in preparation for transportation. A head-to-toe general survey must be made to establish the priorities of care and transportation. In addition, less obvious injuries which might be affected by movement or be aggravated during transport must be identified.

   The term given to this initial examination and selection of patients and the determination of how to handle them is *triage*. It is a French word meaning "picking, sorting, or choice." It is the responsibility of the EMT who first arrives on the scene to institute a screening procedure and sort out the pieces of a disaster so that the best care can be given to each individual.

   As soon as or before this action has been taken, the dispatch center should be contacted for additional help if it is needed. The senior EMT on the scene should request what he needs to supplement personnel or equipment.

   Patients with certain conditions or injuries have priority for transportation and treatment over others. An outline of these conditions is as follows:

1. *Highest priority (must be transported first and treated immediately)*
   Airway and breathing difficulties
   Cardiac arrest
   Uncontrolled or suspected severe bleeding
   Shock
   Open chest or abdominal wounds
   Severe head injuries
   Several medical problems: poisoning, diabetes with complications, cardiac disease
2. *Second priority (transportation and treatment may be deferred)*
   Burns
   Major or multiple fractures
   Back injuries with or without spinal damage
3. *Lowest priority (to be transported or treated last)*
   Minor fractures or other injuries of a minor nature
   Obviously mortal wounds where death appears reasonably certain
   Obviously dead (D.O.A.—"Dead on Arrival")

A separate category of triage should also be noted, as it supersedes all the others. Patients who have undergone radiation contamination and are themselves carrying radiating particles must be decontaminated as an initial step. They should not be allowed to contaminate other patients, ambulances, or the hospital. A discussion of radiation injury and management is contained in Chapter 42, Radiation Exposure.

Leadership is paramount during the action. Someone must be in command to guide what is being done and to utilize any help that arrives. This is the duty of the senior EMT or the medical officer accompanying him. The senior EMT usually must decide how and in what order the patients are to be transported. The assignment of a priority to an injury in the process of triage determines who goes first. Available transport vehicles and local conditions determine how the patients are carried.

The following actions are routine duties at an accident site.

1. Further accidents or hazards must be prevented by cautious parking of the ambulance, placing warning devices to divert traffic, and removing patients from the road. Situations threatening their lives and the lives of the ambulance personnel as well—spilled gasoline and chemicals, escaping gas, downed power lines, spreading fire, flooding water, or structures threatening to collapse—must be recognized and avoided.
2. Bystanders must be restrained from crowding or mishandling the patients.
3. The assistance of volunteers for specific tasks as needed must be obtained.

4. Relatives must be reassured; question and inform them away from the patient.
5. Avoid assuming the functions of police or other authorities when they are present. *Do not permit their actions to interfere with care of patients.*

During loading for transportation, emergency care continues. Examination has determined which patients should be transported immediately and which can receive care at the scene and be allowed to wait. The types of transportation and selection of the roads to be used will be determined by the men and equipment available.

Finally, it is necessary to have a brief written summary of the initial observations of the injury and vital signs ready to accompany each patient so that the attendants at the hospital will know where to start treatment. For example, if a patient is unconscious on arrival at the hospital, the doctors must know if he was unconscious at the site of the accident.

Remember the importance of communication with the hospital. Information concerning the condition and number of patients being transported is necessary to give the hospital authorities an idea of the scope of the situation. A decision must be made about the proper speed of the ambulance to be used with a particular patient, remembering that excessive speed in transportation is rarely necessary and usually dangerous. From the time of the initial call, through arrival at the scene, giving emergency care, moving and transporting the patient and leaving him at the hospital, a well-trained, efficient, smooth-working emergency care team will conserve time and save lives.

III

Basic Life Support

CHAPTER 5

The Respiratory System

GOAL I. Know the structures that make up the respiratory system.

OBJECTIVES

A. Define the boundaries of the thoracic cavity.
B. Describe the contents of the thoracic cavity.
C. Name and locate the organs of the body which are involved in normal respiration.
D. Describe the upper and lower airways.
E. Describe the purpose of the respiratory system.
F. Describe how the circulating blood is involved in the respiratory system.
G. Name and locate the major parts of the lung.
H. Locate and describe the larynx.
I. Locate and describe the trachea.

GOAL II. Understand the mechanics of respiration.

OBJECTIVES

A. Describe the thoracic cage.
B. Describe the mechanism by which air moves in and out of the lungs.
C. Describe the pleura.
D. Describe how breathing is controlled.

The thorax is one of the two major body cavities. It is bounded by the rib cage anteriorly and posteriorly, by the diaphragm inferiorly, and the clavicles superiorly. It contains the lungs in each half, or hemithorax. Between the lungs in a space called the mediastinum lie the heart, the great arteries and veins, the esophagus, and many nerves.

The respiratory system consists of all the organs of the body contributing to normal respiration or breathing. Strictly speaking, it includes the nose, mouth, upper throat, larynx, trachea, and bronchi, which are all air passages or airways. It includes the lungs, where oxygen is passed into the blood and carbon dioxide is given off to be exhaled. Finally, it includes the diaphragm and the muscles of the chest wall, which permit normal respiratory movements. In this text, the term *airway* refers to the upper airway or the passages above the larynx (voice box). The lower airway includes the larynx, trachea, major bronchi, and air passages within the lungs. When one "clears the airway," one removes obstructing material or tissue from the nose, mouth, or throat.

All living cells of the body are engaged in a series of chemical processes by which the energy for life is extracted from food. The name given to the sum total of these processes is metabolism. In the course of metabolism each cell uses oxygen and produces carbon dioxide as a waste substance. Cells not able to participate in metabolic processes are dead or dying.

Each living cell in the body requires a constant supply of oxygen; some cells are more dependent on a constant oxygen supply than others. Cells in the brain and nervous system may die after four to six minutes without oxygen. These cells can never be replaced and permanent changes result from this damage. Other cells in the body are not so critically dependent on an oxygen supply because they can withstand periods without oxygen and still reproduce themselves entirely. The respiratory system by which oxygen is delivered to body tissues and carbon dioxide removed is thus a very important part of the body. Normally, air that we breath contains about 21 percent oxygen and 79 percent nitrogen.

Blood that has passed through the body has given up its oxygen to the tissues and absorbed carbon dioxide produced by tissue metabolism. It is collected in the right atrium of the heart. It is pumped into the lung by the right ventricle. It passes in the lung into a fine network of pulmonary capillaries which are in close contact with air in the alveoli (air sacs) of the lung. In these sacs, the blood gives up its carbon dioxide and absorbs new oxygen. This refreshed blood passes into ever larger vessels and is collected from the lungs into the left atrium of the heart. It is passed into the strong left ventricle and

pumped throughout the body to carry oxygen to all tissues.

The capillaries in the lung are located in the walls of the tiny alveoli. The walls of capillaries and alveoli are extremely thin. Air in the alveoli and blood in the capillaries are thus separated by the finest imaginable layers. Oxygen and carbon dioxide can move between the alveoli and capillaries rapidly. Figure 5.1 is a schematic representation of the exchange of gases and nutrients in tissues. Oxygen passes from the lung across capillaries into the blood. It passes from the blood across capillaries into body tissue. In the reverse of this process, carbon dioxide is passed from tissue in the body across capillaries into the blood; it passes from the blood across capillaries and enters the air sacs in the lung. It is then dispersed in the exhaled air from the lung.

The Airways

The upper part of the air passage is made up of the nose, mouth, and the throat. The nose and the mouth lead to the pharynx (throat). At the bottom of the throat are two passageways: the esophagus behind and the trachea in front. Food and liquids entering the pharynx pass into the esophagus, which carries them to the stomach. Air and other gases enter the trachea to go to the lungs (Fig. 5.2).

Guarding the opening of the trachea is a thin, leaf-shaped valve called the epiglottis (Fig. 5.3). This valve opens to allow passage of air into the trachea but closes whenever food or liquids are present in the pharynx. The body is unable to tolerate any solid or liquid material passing into the trachea.

Air moves past the epiglottis into the larynx and the trachea. The first part of the trachea (windpipe) is the larynx (voice box), which consists of a rather complicated arrangement of tiny bones, cartilages, muscles, and two vocal cords. The "Adam's apple," prominent in the neck, is the front portion of the larynx, or the thyroid cartilage (Fig. 5.3). Tiny muscles open and close the vocal cords.

Sounds are created as air is forced past the vocal cords, making them vibrate. These vibrations make the sound. The pitch of the sound

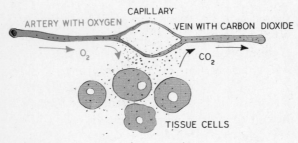

Figure 5.1

The exchange of oxygen and carbon dioxide between blood vessels, capillaries, and tissue cells is diagrammed. The capillary is no larger than a single blood cell. Oxygen (O_2) passes from the blood through capillaries to tissue cells. In the reverse process, carbon dioxide (CO_2) passes from tissue cells through capillaries to the blood.

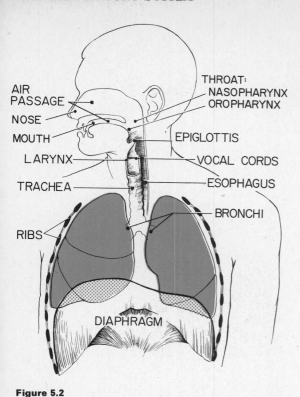

Figure 5.2

The respiratory system includes airways, lungs, and muscles.

changes as the cords open and close. You can feel these vibrations if you place your fingers lightly on the larnyx (Adam's apple) as you speak or sing. Words and other understandable sounds are formed by the tongue and muscles of the mouth.

Immediately beneath the thyroid cartilage is the palpable cricoid cartilage. Between these two prominences lies the crico-thyroid membrane,

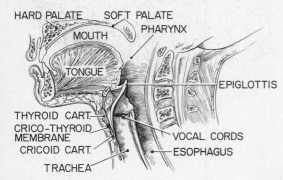

Figure 5.3

This view of the throat shows the relationship of the esophagus, the trachea, the pharynx, and the epiglottis.

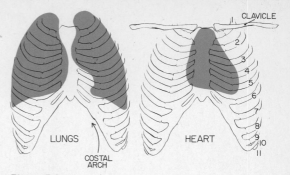

Figure 5.4

The lungs and heart lie within the chest.

which can be felt as a depression in the midline of the neck just inferior to the thyroid cartilage. At this point only the membrane itself and the skin separate the airway from the outside. This is the site for crico-thyroidotomy with a knife, large-bore needles, or a cricothyrotome to relieve acute upper airway obstruction.

Below the voice box is the windpipe, or trachea; it is approximately five inches long. It is a semi-rigid tube made up of partial rings of cartilage that are completed behind by strong connective tissue. The cartilaginous rings keep the trachea from collapsing when air is moved in and out of the lungs.

There are two lungs, one on each side of the thoracic cage (Fig. 5.4). The lungs are suspended within the thoracic cage by the trachea, by the arteries and veins running to and from the heart, and by the pulmonary ligaments.

The trachea ends by dividing into smaller tubes, called the right and left bronchi, which enter the lungs. Each major bronchus immediately branches within the lung into smaller and smaller airways. Within the right lung, three major tubes are formed; within the left, only two. The airways finally end in millions of tiny air sacs called alveoli (Fig. 5.5). Healthy lungs contain about 700 million alveoli. The surface area of these alveoli is equal to that of one-fourth of a basketball court. In these alveoli, oxygen is given to the blood and carbon dioxide is given off by the blood to be exhaled.

Mechanics of Breathing

Lungs have no way of filling themselves with air since they contain no muscular tissue which

41

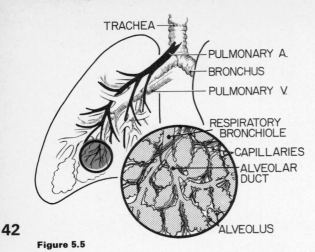

TRACHEA

PULMONARY A.

BRONCHUS

PULMONARY V.

RESPIRATORY
BRONCHIOLE

CAPILLARIES

ALVEOLAR
DUCT

ALVEOLUS

Figure 5.5

Within the lung, millions of air sacs (alveoli) lie at the end of the air passages. In the diagram above, an alveolus is shown in the circle, which is an enlargement of a small area.

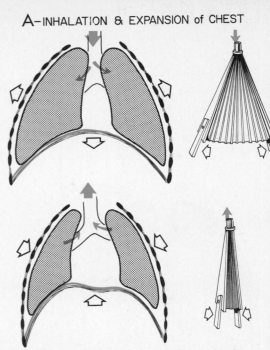

A—INHALATION & EXPANSION of CHEST

B— EXHALATION & CONTRACTION of CHEST

Figure 5.6 a–b

a, Inhaling and, *b,* exhaling can be compared to the action of a bellows, with movement of air in and out of the enclosed thoracic space.

42

would allow them to move. Movement of the thoracic cage and the diaphragm permits air to enter the lungs through the trachea. The thoracic cage is a semi-rigid bony cage enclosed by muscle and skin. The diaphragm is a muscular partition separating the chest and abdominal cavities.

The chest cage can be compared to a bellows. The ribs maintain the shape of the chest bellows. The opening of the chest bellows is through the trachea. Air moves through the trachea to and from the interior of the lung to fill and empty the air sacs (Figs. 5.6 *a–b*). When a bellows is opened, the volume it can hold is increased, causing a slight vacuum. Normally, the pressure within the chest cavity is slightly less than atmospheric pressure. Opening the chest bellows lowers the air pressure in the thorax still further and causes the higher air pressure outside to drive air through the trachea, filling the lung (Fig. 5.6 *a*). When the air pressure inside equals the pressure outside, air stops moving. Air will move from a higher-pressure area to a lower-pressure area until the pressures in both areas are equal. Therefore, as the bellows is closed during expiration, the pressure inside becomes higher than that outside and air is expelled (Fig. 5.6 *b*).

The active, muscular part of breathing is described as follows.

During inspiration (inhaling), the diaphragm and rib muscles contract. When the diaphragm contracts, it moves downward and enlarges the thoracic cavity from top to bottom. When the rib muscles contract, they raise the ribs. These actions combine to enlarge the chest cavity (bellows) in all dimensions. The action is identical to that of opening a bellows. Air rushes into the lungs. Take a deep breath to see how the chest increases in size.

During expiration (exhaling), the diaphragm and the rib muscles relax. As these muscles relax, the chest cavity is decreased in size in all dimensions. As the chest cavity decreases in size, the air in the lungs is pressed into a smaller space, the pressure is increased, and air is pushed out through the trachea. Decrease in size of the chest cavity after relaxation is accomplished largely by action of elastic tissue in the lung, which stretches during inhalation and recoils after relaxation of the muscular chest wall. There is also an inherent tendency for the chest wall to assume a normal resting position, which aids in exhalation.

It is important to remember that there is only one normal opening into the chest cavity. It is through the trachea.

The lungs hang free within the chest cavity, but there is a very definite mechanism to insure that they follow the motions of the chest wall and expand and contract with it. Covering each lung is a layer of very smooth, glistening, slippery tissue called pleura (Fig. 5.7). One layer of

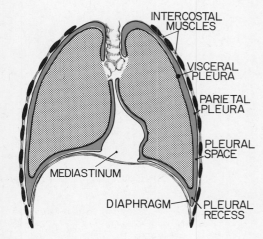

INTERCOSTAL MUSCLES

VISCERAL PLEURA

PARIETAL PLEURA

PLEURAL SPACE

MEDIASTINUM

DIAPHRAGM — PLEURAL RECESS

Figure 5.7

    The pleura lining the chest wall and covering the lung is an essential part of the mechanism for breathing. The pleural space is not an actual space until blood or air leaks into it, causing the pleural surfaces to separate.

this sac lines the inside of the chest cavity and the other layer covers the lungs. These two layers are called parietal pleura (lining the chest wall) and visceral pleura (covering the lung). Between these two layers is the "pleural space," which is not a space in the usual sense because these layers are everywhere in contact. In fact, the layers are tightly sealed one against the other by a thin film of fluid. When the chest wall expands, the lung is pulled with it and made to expand by the suction exerted through these closely applied pleural surfaces. The pleural space is called a potential space because normally there is no space and the lung entirely fills the chest cavity.

The "space" between the pleural surfaces can easily be developed into an actual space and the surfaces separated by blood from a bleeding lung or chest wall, or by air from a torn lung or a hole in the chest. If the surfaces are separated, the mechanism for normal expansion of the lungs is lost. If enough blood or air collects, the lung can even be compressed to the extent that it cannot expand enough on inspiration and not enough oxygen can be taken in to maintain life. Patients with this type of injury may die from lack of oxygen.

The smooth, lubricated pleural surfaces allow the lungs to move perfectly freely in the chest when one is breathing. But if the pleura are injured or become diseased, they no longer have a friction-free, lubricated surface. Then, as the lungs move in breathing, the surfaces rub together, causing friction and pain. This condition is called pleurisy.

43

Control of Breathing

The brain controls breathing. When the brain needs more oxygen, it sends stimuli along nerves to muscles of the chest and diaphragm, causing them to work faster and more forcefully. Breathing is involuntary, but it can be controlled up to a point. Thus, when you want to hold your breath, you can override automatic impulses from the brain for a short while. Similarly, if you want to breathe more rapidly or more deeply, you can do so as long as you consciously think about it. The brain is acutely, but automatically, conscious of the levels of oxygen and carbon dioxide in the body. It responds to these levels in controlling respiration. If the levels become sufficiently abnormal, the brain will automatically control respiration. This is why you cannot hold your breath indefinitely or breathe rapidly and deeply indefinitely. There are direct nervous connections from the brain to the lung through which this control is exerted.

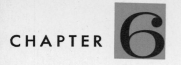

Injuries of the Chest

GOAL I. Know the types of severe chest injuries and how to recognize them.

OBJECTIVES

A. Identify the two classes of chest injuries.
B. Define the significant terms associated with chest injuries.
C. Describe how chest injuries may occur and explain why they are of major importance.
D. List the important signs of a chest injury.

GOAL II. Understand how to treat severe chest injuries.

OBJECTIVES

A. Describe the general principles of care for chest injuries.
B. Describe the management of various types of closed chest injuries.
C. Describe the management of various types of open chest injuries.

Injuries of the chest are of major importance to the EMT because of the likelihood of internal bleeding and a direct injury of the heart or lungs. Chest injuries may be the result of automobile accidents, gunshot wounds, stab wounds, falls, blows, or compression injuries. Any injury of the chest may be serious. Unless properly treated, it may be rapidly fatal. The body has no capacity to store oxygen. Any injury which seriously interferes with the constant replenishment of oxygen through normal breathing must be treated without delay to prevent permanent damage of those cells which are critically dependent upon a constant oxygen supply. Specifically, cells in the brain and other elements of the nervous system require a rich supply of oxygen continuously and may die within minutes if it is not forthcoming.

Classification of Chest Injuries

Chest injuries may be divided generally into two categories: open or closed.

Open chest injuries are those in which the chest wall has been penetrated, as by a knife or a bullet. Open chest injuries may also be associated with severe rib fractures where the broken end of the rib has lacerated the chest wall and the skin. These injuries may be concurrent with contusions or lacerations of the heart, lungs, or major blood vessels.

In closed chest injuries the skin is not broken. Major damage resulting from fractured ribs or from contusion may exist, however, within the chest. There may be lacerations of the heart or lungs. Serious closed injuries include compression injuries of the chest and severe contusions, such as might result from the blunt trauma of hitting a steering wheel, being struck by a falling object, or being buried in a cave-in.

Signs of Chest Injuries

The important signs of chest injuries, either

open or closed, are as shown in the list below:

1. Pain at the site of the injury
2. Pleuritic pain (pain which is aggravated by or occurs with breathing) localized around the site of an injury
3. Dyspnea (shortness of breath or difficulty in breathing)
4. Failure of one or both sides of the chest to expand normally with an inspiration
5. Hemoptysis (the coughing up of blood)
6. A rapid weak pulse and low blood pressure
7. Cyanosis of the lips, the fingertips, or fingernails

Any change in the normal breathing pattern is a particularly important sign to observe. An uninjured person breathes from six to twenty times a minute without difficulty and without pain, depending on his physical fitness. Pain in the chest at the site of an obvious fracture or an obvious bruise indicates injury of the chest wall and may indicate injury of the lung underneath it. Pain which is aggravated by breathing or which occurs when the patient inhales indicates irritation of the pleural surfaces of the lung or the chest wall. Irritation can be a result of the laceration of these surfaces by fractured ribs or it can be the result of some severe disease processes.

The depth of respiration and the difficulty in taking a breath are reliable indicators of respiratory distress. Difficulty in breathing is generally considered under the heading of dyspnea. It may result from several causes. In the injured patient it can come from the fact that the chest cannot expand properly, or that the patient has lost normal nervous control of his breathing, or that the airway is obstructed, or that the lung is itself being compressed from within the chest by accumulated blood or air.

The observation that the chest wall fails to expand when the patient is inspiring is extremely important. It is an indication of loss of the ability of the muscles of the chest to act appropriately. Such muscular dysfunction may result from direct injury of the chest wall itself, from a severe injury of the nerves controlling the chest wall, or from a severe brain injury.

Hemoptysis (coughing up of blood) usually indicates that the lung has been lacerated. In such lacerations, blood can enter the bronchial passages within the lungs and is promptly coughed up as the patient tries to clear the passages.

A rapid, weak pulse and low blood pressure are the signs of shock. Shock may result from the fact that blood is being insufficiently oxygenated by a lung which cannot expand to receive inspired air and oxygenate the blood passing through it. It can also result from the fact that bleeding from the lacerated chest wall can be severe and the blood loss itself causes shock.

Cyanosis (blue color around the lips, the fingernails, or fingertips) indicates that blood is being insufficiently oxygenated. This finding in a patient with severe injuries points to the fact that he is unable to bring adequate oxygen to the blood through his lungs, and consequently the existence of a chest injury ought to be suspected.

General Principles of Care of Chest Injuries

The various types of chest injuries almost uniformly require the same initial care. Emergency care is directly related to the ability of the patient to breathe, and initial attention is given there. The upper airway must be cleared and maintained; the use of oxygen and artificial ventilation must be instituted promptly. The overriding first consideration is to achieve as normal a respiration as possible for the patient, using supplemental oxygen when necessary.

Open chest wounds must be covered. If ribs are broken, the patient should be made comfortable and quiet so that the possibility of further damage of the lungs, heart, or chest wall is minimized. Fractured ribs may be splinted by the use of external supports. Rarely do fractured ribs require the application of adhesive taping to the chest wall since the tape itself limits the ability of the chest to expand and thus interferes with proper resuscitation. Bleeding from the chest wall should be controlled by direct pressure. Embedded or protruding foreign objects, knives and the like, should be bandaged in place and left alone. These generally require removal in an operation at the hospital.

Chest wounds usually require expert treatment in a hospital setting; prompt transporta-

46

tion to an Emergency Department is of paramount importance. Sometimes the patient will be in such extreme circumstances that immediate transportation to the hospital, trying to maintain normal breathing and control bleeding en route are the only things that the EMT should attempt to do.

Types of Chest Injuries and their Emergency Care

Rib fractures. Rib fractures are usually caused by direct blows or compression injuries of the chest. The upper four ribs are rarely fractured because they are protected by the shoulder girdle (scapula and clavicle). The fifth through the ninth ribs are those commonly fractured. The lower two ribs (eleven and twelve) are harder to fracture because they are attached only to the thoracic vertebrae and have greater freedom of movement.

The common finding in all patients with fractured ribs is pain localized at the site of the fracture. By asking the patient to place his hand on the exact area of the pain, the EMT can often determine the location of the injury. There may or may not be a rib deformity or chest wall contusion or laceration of the area. Deep breathing, coughing, or movement is usually quite painful. The patient generally wishes to remain still and may often lean toward the injured side with his hand over the fractured area to immobilize the chest and to ease the local pain.

Simple rib fractures ordinarily are not bound, strapped, or taped. If a patient has multiple fractures and is considerably more comfortable with his chest immobilized, the best bandage is a swathe in which the arm is strapped to the chest to limit motion on that side (Fig. 6.1). Immobilization of both arms may be necessary if the fractures are bilateral. The use of wide strips of adhesive plaster to immobilize the chest wall has been popular in the past. It does contribute to lessening the patient's discomfort. However, much more important is the fact that a tight bandage of adhesive plaster applied to the skin of the chest acts like an unyielding corset and hinders whatever expansion of the injured chest the patient can achieve. It is better to assist his respiration than to try to render him more com-

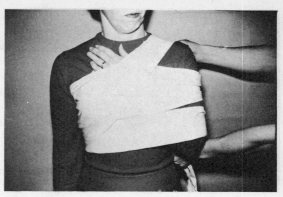

Figure 6.1

A swathe is the best bandage in the case of multiple rib fractures. It will immobilize the injuries more satisfactorily and make the patient more comfortable than a sling.

47

fortable by not allowing the chest to expand.

Occasionally the end of a fractured rib may puncture or lacerate the lung (Fig. 6.2). In such an instance some degree of pneumothorax or hemothorax usually occurs (Fig. 6.3). These two conditions are common results of chest injuries and are discussed below.

Flail chest. When three or more ribs are broken, each in two places, the segment of the chest wall lying between the breaks will collapse rather than participate in the normal expansion of the chest wall each time the patient attempts to inhale. When the patient exhales, this segment will protrude while the rest of the chest wall contracts. This motion of the segment is called paradoxical motion because it is opposite to the normal motion of the chest wall. The portion of

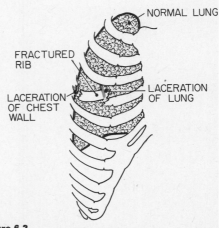

NORMAL LUNG

FRACTURED RIB

LACERATION OF CHEST WALL

LACERATION OF LUNG

Figure 6.2

Fracture of a rib may be associated with a laceration of the skin or lung.

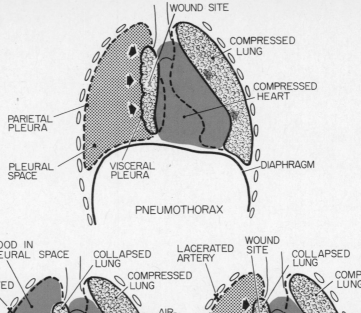

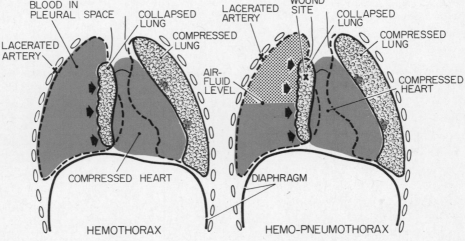

Figure 6.3

A pneumothorax is a collection of air in the pleural space between visceral and parietal pleural surfaces. It can result from an opening into the space through the skin or the lung. Collapse of the affected lung occurs and function of the heart and remaining lung is hampered.

A hemothorax is a collection of blood in the pleural space between the visceral and parietal pleural surfaces. It results from bleeding into the chest.

A hemothorax may occur alone or in conjunction with a pneumothorax. In the latter case, the injury is called a hemo-pneumothorax.

the chest wall lying between the fractures is called the "flail segment" (Fig. 6.4 *a*). There are several terms used to describe this injury. The proper one is flail chest. Other common terms are crushed chest or stove-in chest.

This is a particularly serious injury. Obviously the lung immediately underneath the flail segment does not expand properly when the patient inhales and that amount of lung volume is lost for the patient. Much more important, however, is the fact that the amount of force exerted on the chest wall to cause a series of ribs to fracture in several places and produce a flail segment almost always produces severe contusion damage of the lung itself underneath the flail segment. The injury of the lung may be far more severe than the surface derangements make it appear. The condition can be relatively easily diagnosed through observation. The EMT can see that the chest does not rise properly despite the patient's most desperate efforts to inhale deeply. In some patients rapid signs of hypoxia ensue.

A patient with a flail chest can frequently breathe more comfortably if the fractured ribs are splinted (Fig. 6.4 *b*). If breathing is inad-

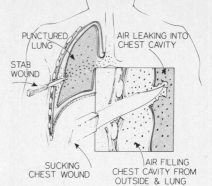

Figure 6.4 *a–b*

A flail chest results when several ribs are fractured in two or more places. *a,* The segment lying between the fractures is the flail segment, which moves paradoxically with the patient's respiration. *b,* This segment can be stabilized immediately by external pressure, but the chest should not be taped circumferentially.

Figure 6.5

49

A knife has punctured the chest wall and lung, allowing air to leak into the chest cavity from the outside and from within the lung. A sucking chest wound has been created.

equate and especially if cyanosis is present, respiration must be assisted with an artificial ventilatory device. This is the most effective way of getting air into the lungs. Its use should be instituted promptly since these patients may die rapidly if oxygen is not supplied. If a ventilation unit is not available, mouth-to-mouth or mouth-to-nose respiration must be given until the patient arrives at the hospital. The EMT must direct his efforts to assisting respiration. These patients should be transported with highest priority as rapidly as possible to the hospital.

The patient will require several weeks of treatment, often in specialized hospital wards using mechanical respirators, before he recovers.

Penetrating injuries. Stab and gunshot wounds are examples of penetrating chest injuries (Fig. 6.5). These will customarily produce varying degrees of hemothorax and pneumothorax. Occasionally they will cause a rib fracture. Sucking chest wounds are very frequently created by these injuries and these wounds must be made airtight promptly by appropriate dressings (Fig. 6.6).

Penetrating wounds must be regarded as able to injure any structure within the thoracic cavity. A grave danger obviously exists of direct laceration or other injury of the heart or the great blood vessels in the chest. In instances such as this, bleeding, which may be massive, is usually into the chest cavity itself and very rarely visible outside the body. The patient, in

addition to having the expected signs of respiratory distress associated with the injury, may be in shock from blood loss. He may require artificial respiration as well as vigorous resuscitation from shock. Rapid transportation to the Emergency Department is mandatory.

When one is dealing with a patient who has sustained a penetrating wound of the chest from a gunshot it is well to examine the chest carefully for both entrance and exit wounds. Such an examination will be carried out at the hospital but it markedly facilitates evaluation of the patient in the Emergency Department if this in-

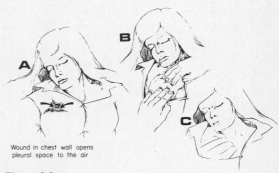

Wound in chest wall opens pleural space to the air

Figure 6.6 *a–c*

a, A sucking chest wound allows free passage of air from the outside to the pleural space of the lung. *b,* Hemoptysis (bleeding from the mouth from coughed-up blood) indicates lung injury. Such a wound should be sealed promptly. *c,* The final bandaging can go over the seal which prevents air from entering the chest through the wound.

formation can be delivered along with the patient.

Compression injuries. In a certain group of patients, injuries of the chest have resulted from circumferential sudden compression of the chest and accompanying rapid increase in intrathoracic pressure. Multiple fractures of ribs can occur and a flail chest may result. Traumatic asphyxia, discussed in a later section, can also be an associated phenomenon seen from the sudden application of high pressure on the chest.

Injuries of the back of the chest. Injuries of the back of the chest other than fractures of the ribs are usually muscle strains and severe open lacerations. Pain and tenderness locally at the site of the wound are common. A close examination should be made for impaled or embedded objects in these wounds but they should not be removed. Impaled objects may be cut off some few inches from the skin if necessary for more comfortable transportation to the Emergency Department. In these patients one should always check for an injury of the spine (Chapter 20, Fractures and Dislocations of the Spine).Observe the patient en route to the Emergency Department to be certain that the airway is maintained. Transportation may be more comfortable with the patient in a prone position but the desirability of this posture varies from patient to patient. An uncommon injury of the back of the chest is a fracture of the scapula, or shoulder blade. This bone is literally buried in a very heavy muscle mass. Accordingly, its fracture indicates that a particularly severe blow has been sustained by the patient. One should bear this possibility in mind if a bad contusion, hemorrhage, or laceration over the shoulder blade is observed.

Results of Chest Injuries

It is convenient to discuss the results of chest injuries as a general section. Many of the injuries described above have similar results. The causes may be different but the results are nonetheless the same. The commonest of the results of chest injuries are considered below.

Pneumothorax. Pneumothorax means the presence of air within the chest cavity but outside the lung (Fig. 6.3). In this condition the lung has been separated from the chest wall and is said to be collapsed. The volume of the lung is diminished and the amount of air that can be inhaled into the lung to exchange oxygen and carbon dioxide with the blood is reduced. Hypoxia ensues; and, as the degree of pneumothorax increases, respiratory distress becomes evident.

Pneumothorax can result from air entering the chest directly through a sucking wound open to the outside. In an intact chest it can also result from air leaking out from a lung which has been lacerated by a fractured rib. In pneumothorax the normal mechanism by which the lung expands—that is, capillary adhesion to the inside of the chest wall—is lost, and the affected, or collapsed, lung cannot expand with inhalation.

Spontaneous pneumothorax. In some people congenitally weak areas exist in the surface of the lungs. Occasionally such a weak area will rupture, allowing air to leak into the chest cavity. Usually such an event is not related to any injury and commonly it occurs while the patient is sitting quietly. The patient experiences a sudden sharp chest pain and increasing difficulty in breathing. The affected lung undergoes collapse and loses its ability to expand normally. All degrees of this condition exist, from the patient who notices no particular discomfort or difficulty in breathing to the patient who requires emergency transportation to the hospital because of respiratory distress. In the latter instance the EMT will not be called upon to make a diagnosis but will be called upon to administer respiratory support while transporting the patient rapidly to the Emergency Department.

Tension pneumothorax. In a patient who develops a spontaneous pneumothorax, and in whom the leak in the lung fails to seal when the lung collapses, a tension pneumothorax may develop (Fig. 6.7). This condition is one in which air continuously leaks out of the lung into the chest cavity with every breath the patient takes. With each breath the affected lung collapses more until it is completely reduced to a very small ball two or three inches in diameter. At this point, pressure in the affected side of the chest cavity begins to rise and the collapsed lung is pressed against the heart and the lung on the

50

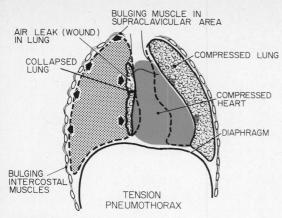

AIR LEAK (WOUND) IN LUNG

BULGING MUSCLE IN SUPRACLAVICULAR AREA

COLLAPSED LUNG

COMPRESSED LUNG

COMPRESSED HEART

DIAPHRAGM

BULGING INTERCOSTAL MUSCLES

TENSION PNEUMOTHORAX

Figure 6.7

A tension pneumothorax occurs when air collects in the pleural space between the visceral and parietal pleural surfaces and cannot leak to the outside. As the air leak into the chest continues, pressure in the chest rises sharply and rapidly and the remaining lung and heart are severely compressed. This condition is a true emergency.

opposite side. The remaining lung in turn is now mechanically compressed. As pressure in the chest cavity rises, it may exceed the normal pressure of blood in veins returning to the heart. Blood can then no longer travel back to the heart to be pumped out; death can rapidly ensue.

Tension pneumothorax is not limited to the closed chest injury. A patient with a fractured rib who has sustained a sucking chest wound may have also sustained a severe lung laceration. If the external wound is effectively bandaged, and the lung continues to leak, a tension pneumothorax may develop. The condition cannot exist in a patient without an intact or well-sealed chest wall.

The signs of tension pneumothorax are severe progressive respiratory distress, a weak pulse, hypotension, bulging of the tissue in the chest wall between the ribs and above the clavicle, and distention of the veins in the neck. The diagnosis is best made by a doctor who can immediately relieve the tension in the chest by simply passing a large bore, no. 13 or 14 gauge, hypodermic needle through the chest wall into the chest cavity. If this is done by the EMT the needle should be left in position and supported there until the patient is transported to the Emergency Department. The patient will re-

quire respiratory support, although relief of the tension within the chest may frequently allow a prompt return of normal or near normal respiration. For the patient with a bandaged chest wound and a tension pneumothorax, simple release of the dressing is often effective.

It must be emphasized that tension pneumothorax is one of the very few true minute-by-minute emergencies. Prompt treatment of this patient may be lifesaving. In some patients with severe tension pneumothorax, death may occur in a matter of a very few minutes from the onset of the process.

Hemothorax. Hemothorax means the presence of blood in the chest cavity outside the lung (Fig. 6.3). It may be seen in open or closed chest injuries. It frequently accompanies a pneumothorax. The bleeding may come from lacerated vessels in the chest wall, from lacerated major vessels within the chest cavity itself or, relatively rarely, from a lacerated lung. If the bleeding in the chest is severe, the patient may show the signs of shock from blood loss alone. Shock (Chapter 9) is manifested by pallor, apprehension, a cold clammy skin, chills, a rapid, weak pulse, and thirst.

Hemothorax, like pneumothorax, fills up the chest with something other than the lung. Once again, normal lung expansion cannot occur and the lung is compressed so that its volume is lost. Less air can be inhaled and there may be significantly less blood to carry the reduced amount of oxygen available to the patient. This patient requires immediate attention to assisting his respiration, the administration of oxygen if needed, and the control of obvious external bleeding by means of pressure dressings. He must then be transported promptly to the Emergency Department.

Sucking chest wounds. In open chest injuries air may enter the chest cavity through the wound when the patient inhales and the chest expands in the normal respiratory cycle (Fig. 6.6). Ordinarily the pressure inside the chest cavity is maintained at somewhat less than atmospheric pressure. Inhalation significantly reduces this pressure. When the chest cavity has been opened, air moves through the wound in the same manner as it moves through the nose and mouth dur-

51

ing normal respiration. However, when this occurs, the air remains outside the lung in the
pleural space. The conditions of a pneumothorax are created and the lung is compromised
in its function. Air is passed back through the
wound to the outside when the patient exhales
and thoracic pressure rises. Such open chest
wounds are called sucking chest wounds because there is a sucking sound at the wound each
time the patient breathes, caused by the passage
of air through the wound. As an initial emergency step it is imperative that these wounds be
blocked up and closed with an airtight dressing
(Fig. 6.6). Almost any material may be used.
Aluminum foil, vaseline gauze, plastic wrap
(Saran), or a rolled-up 8 × 10 dressing held in
place by a pressure dressing may suffice. The aim
of this dressing is to seal the wound. A large
enough cover must be used so that the dressing
itself will not be sucked into the chest cavity. In
the recent Viet Nam war, one Marine covered
such a wound in his own chest with a pair of
rolled-up socks.

Subcutaneous emphysema. If a lung laceration
from a fractured rib has allowed air to escape
into the tissues of the chest wall, this condition
can be detected by a crackling sensation under
the fingertips as one feels over the area of the
fracture; sometimes the crackling can be heard.
The name given to this finding is subcutaneous
emphysema. In very severe instances it can involve the entire chest, neck, and face. It is an
indication that air is being forced out of the
lung into the tissues. It confirms the presence of
fractured ribs and a lacerated lung. Once found,
it indicates that the patient should be promptly
transported to the hospital for further observation and evaluation.

Traumatic asphyxia. Traumatic asphyxia is a
term given to a group of symptoms and signs
that result from very severe sudden compression
of the chest. Such injuries often cause a caved-in
chest wall with fractures of the ribs and sternum.
The sudden pressure on the heart forces blood
back from the right side of the heart into the
veins of the neck, head, and shoulders. Further,
the sudden compression may cause rupture of
air sacs within the lung and severe pulmonary
damage. Signs of traumatic asphyxia are:

1. Severe shock
2. Cyanosis of the head, neck, and shoulders
3. Bloodshot eyes
4. Protruding eyes
5. Swollen and cyanotic tongue and lips
6. Possible chest deformities
7. Vomitus with blood
8. Respiratory distress

Emergency care for this patient consists in
preventing further shock by controlling bleeding
and giving vigorous respiratory resuscitation,
including artificial ventilation and the administration of oxygen. Careful observation is mandatory. The patient should be placed in the position
most comfortable to him and transported
rapidly to the Emergency Department. This patient may require artificial ventilation throughout his transportation to keep him alive until he
reaches a place where definitive care can be
given. The condition shares many of the signs of
traumatic emphysema but is more severe.

Pulmonary contusion. This particular condition is almost uniformly associated with blunt
injuries of the chest such as are seen in automobile accidents and severe falls. It has only
recently become well appreciated. In flail chests
it accounts for much the greater part of the
severity of the injury rather than the anatomically deranged movement of the chest wall itself.
A pulmonary contusion is a bruise of the lung.
It behaves much the same way as bruises of any
other tissues in the body behave. It means that
the blood vessels in the lung are injured and a
considerable amount of blood has been lost into
the lung. Depending on the size of the pulmonary contusion, the person who has sustained
one may or may not be in respiratory distress.
Ordinarily pulmonary contusions do not concern the EMT as they are diagnosed after the
patient has come to the hospital and they develop over the first forty-eight hours of the
hospital stay. Some pulmonary contusions are,
however, so severe initially that the patient is in
respiratory distress almost from the moment he
has sustained the injury. An example of this
condition would be the frail, elderly patient who
sustains a bad fall and injures his chest, for
example on a stair railing or on the edge of a

52

table or chair. Emergency treatment for these injuries is respiratory support and may include the administration of oxygen. If the pulmonary contusion is associated with several rib fractures, artificial ventilation may be required.

Myocardial contusion. Similarly, blunt injuries of the chest may produce myocardial contusions which are bruises of the heart muscle itself. Such injuries may not be detectable until fairly sophisticated laboratory and electrocardiographic studies have been made on these patients. Ordinarily a severe myocardial contusion results in a disturbance of the electrical conduction system which controls the heart rate. In such circumstances the heart is said to be irritable. The signs of such injuries are extra heartbeats which are interspersed irregularly into the normal pulse. Such a patient will have an irregular pulse with occasional pauses and occasional beats coming very close together. There is no treatment the EMT can administer for this condition. He should, however, note the pulse and its character. Early signs of myocardial contusion require rapid transportation of this patient to the Emergency Department.

Pericardial tamponade. Pericardial tamponade is a condition in which blood or other fluid is present in the pericardial sac outside the heart exerting an unusual pressure on the heart itself. In patients with chest injuries it almost always results from gunshot wounds or stab wounds of the heart which have opened one of its chambers so that blood leaks out each time the heart beats. The pericardial sac within which the heart lies is a very tough, fibrous membrane and cannot expand suddenly. When blood leaks out of the heart, it is caught within this unyielding sac; and, as it accumulates within the pericardial cavity, it compresses the heart so that its chambers can no longer accommodate blood normally returned to them through the veins. This intrapericardial pressure must be relieved or death very rapidly ensues.

The signs of the condition are very soft and faint heart tones (hard to hear even with a stethoscope), a weak pulse, blood pressure readings in which the upper and lower pressures come closer and closer together as one takes successive blood pressures, and congested and distended veins in the upper part of the body. As an emergency measure this patient may require very vigorous respiratory support with ventilatory assistance, oxygen, and rapid intravenous administration of fluids. He may require an emergency operation immediately after his arrival at the hospital.

Observation of or suspicion of pericardial tamponade would be indication for the EMT to transport that patient to the Emergency Department as soon as possible. He should, if he can, call ahead to advise the hospital of the type of patient and his status.

Lacerations of the great vessels. There are several large blood vessels in the chest: the superior vena cava, the inferior vena cava, the main pulmonary artery with its right and left branches, four main pulmonary veins entering the left atrium, and the aorta with its major vessels distributing blood throughout the body. Injuries of any of these vessels may be accompanied by massive, rapidly fatal hemorrhage. Any patient who is in shock and who has evidence of a chest wound or injury may likely have an injury of one of these vessels. This fact ought to be recalled by the EMT in assigning priority of transport to the Emergency Department. Frequently the loss of blood is not obvious as it remains within the chest cavity.

Emergency treatment includes pulmonary resuscitation with ventilatory support and oxygen as necessary and the rapid infusion intravenously of saline solutions. Here particularly, rapid transport to the hospital may be lifesaving. A matter of minutes for some of these patients has been the difference between life and death.

Dyspnea

The state of difficult or labored breathing is called dyspnea. It is a serious condition and may be a terrifying one. Dyspnea can be the result of several causes.

1. There may be an obstruction to the flow of air in the trachea and the bronchial tubes such as occurs in many instances of trauma, aspirated vomitus or blood, or foreign bodies caught in the throat or windpipe.

2. Air may not pass easily into or out of the air sacs in the lung, as in patients suffering from asthma or other allergic reactions.
3. A lung may be collapsed and unable to expand, as is seen with spontaneous or traumatic pneumothorax or hemothorax.
4. The air sacs in the lungs themselves may have become inelastic and no longer be re-responsive to the normal motions of breathing (emphysema).
5. The lungs may be filled with fluid backed up in them because the heart muscle has failed and is no longer able to circulate the amount of blood presented to it.

Dyspnea occurring suddenly may terrify a patient. He may exhaust himself simply laboring to breathe. It is mandatory that the EMT have a clear and calm approach to this condition. Some persons experiencing dyspnea need only reassurance by a self-possessed professional person to help them relax and breathe more easily. The proper approach to this problem is stepwise and should proceed as follows:

1. Make certain that the airway is clear of blood, vomitus, or foreign materials.
2. If the patient is conscious, support his tongue so that it does not obstruct the airway.
3. Have oxygen ready to administer by mask.
4. Assist the patient to find a comfortable position for breathing; this may be a semi-sitting posture. With the patient whose dyspnea is on the basis of cardiac failure, it may even be in a straight sitting-up position.
5. Be prepared to aid the patient to control vomiting.
6. Try to find out the possible causes of the attack if an injury is not immediately apparent, such as asthma, heart disease, allergy, or aspiration of foreign material.
7. Be prepared, once all the support that can be given has been rendered, to transport this patient expeditiously to the Emergency Department.

Many of the traumatic causes of dyspnea have been discussed in the foregoing paragraphs.

Dyspnea can also occur as a result of asthma or allergic reactions, or as a manifestation of very severe chronic lung disease. These conditions will be discussed under Dyspnea (Chapter 33) in the section on Medical Emergencies.

Emphysema. Emphysema is a term given to the changes in the lung which occur as a result of long-standing, chronic, mild obstruction of the bronchi. It is a condition in which there is a progressive loss of elasticity of the lungs. Gradual overexpansion of the alveoli and the smaller bronchial tubes and air sacs occurs as they fill with air. Emphysema can be suspected in a patient who has a huge, disproportionately broad, barrel chest and difficulty in breathing.

Traumatic emphysema. Traumatic emphysema may come to the attention of emergency personnel either as part of traumatic asphyxia or by itself.

The most common cause of traumatic emphysema is a severe compression injury of the chest resulting in rib fractures. Laceration of the lungs by displaced rib fragments from these fractures can result in pneumothorax or hemothorax which can limit respiration. If, however, such a violent compression of the chest takes place at a moment when the glottis is closed and air cannot be expelled from the lung through the trachea and the upper airway during the instant of compression, pressure within the chest may rise excessively high. The small alveoli (air sacs) and the small air passageways may become suddenly vastly overexpanded, cannot function normally, and may rupture. In this situation expansion of these air sacs has occurred within moments, while in chronic emphysema such expansion may take years to develop.

As the sudden compression passes, the ribs and chest wall may spring back to their normal position, and muscular motion of the chest may return to normal. The overdistended alveoli have, however, been injured and the ruptured ones will leak air. Leaking of air from a lacerated lung may continue and the symptoms of a tension pneumothorax may develop in this patient. He must be suspected of having sustained a severe injury and should be transported to the hospital as soon as possible.

54

CHAPTER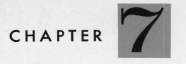

The Circulatory System

GOAL I.   Know the parts of the circulatory, or cardiovascular, system and understand their functions.

OBJECTIVES

A. List the component portions of the cardiovascular system.
B. Describe the functions of the parts of the cardiovascular system.
C. Name, in order, the types of vessels through which blood cells pass from the heart until they return to the heart.

GOAL II.   Know the component cells in the blood and their functions.

OBJECTIVES

A. Identify the components of normal blood.
B. Describe the functions of each of the types of cells and components in blood.

GOAL III.   Know the means by which oxygen and food reach the cells of the body.

OBJECTIVES

A. Describe the exchange of nutrients and oxygen in the tissues.
B. Describe the exchange of oxygen and carbon dioxide in the lungs.

GOAL IV.   Know normal blood volumes and understand how the body adjusts to changes in these volumes or in the circulatory system to maintain its function.

OBJECTIVES

A. Define the terms *pulse*, *blood pressure*, and *venous pressure* and identify the normal reading for each.
B. State the approximate volume of blood for infants, children, and adults.
C. Describe how the circulatory system adjusts to changes imposed on it.

The circulatory, or cardiovascular, system is a complex arrangement of tubes called arteries, arterioles, capillaries, venules, and veins. Through these tubes, blood is circulated throughout the entire body under pressure generated by a two-sided pump, the heart (Figs. 7.1, 7.2). Blood flows outward from the left ventricle of the heart through large arteries. The arteries gradually become smaller (arterioles) until the blood finally passes into and through small capillaries. Capillaries are fine, hair-like vessels in which individual red blood

55

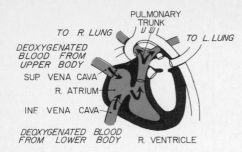

Figure 7.1

The right-sided, or lower-pressure, pump of the heart circulates blood from the body to the lungs.

cells can come into close contact with the individual cells of the body. Blood passes through the capillaries into small veins (venules) which unite and become larger the nearer they approach the heart. They deliver blood to the right side of the heart, which pumps it to the lungs where it passes through a capillary system again. It is then returned to the left side of the heart, completing the circuit. The system is entirely closed, with two sets of capillaries connecting arterioles and venules within the lungs and in the tissues of the rest of the body.

Blood

Blood is a red, sticky fluid composed of plasma, red blood cells (erythrocytes), white blood cells (leukocytes), and platelets. Plasma carries the cells and transports nutrients to all tissues. It also transports waste products to the organs of excretion. Red cells give color to the blood and carry oxygen. White cells play a role in the body's defense against infection. Platelets are essential in the formation of blood clots, which are necessary to stop bleeding.

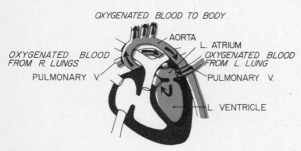

Figure 7.2

The left-sided, or higher-pressure, pump of the heart circulates blood from the lungs to the body.

Blood under pressure will gush or spurt from an artery and is bright red; from a vein or capillary it will flow in a steady stream or ooze and is dark bluish-red. Clotting normally takes six to ten minutes.

The Heart

The heart is a hollow muscular organ approximately the size of a man's clenched fist. A wall (septum) divides the heart down the middle into right and left sides. Each side of the heart is divided again into an upper chamber (atrium) and a lower chamber (ventricle).

The heart is two paired pumps. The right side collects blood from the veins of the body into the right atrium and pumps it into the lungs from the right ventricle (Fig. 7.1). The left side receives oxygenated blood from the lungs into the left atrium and pumps this fresh blood through the arteries to all parts of the body from the left ventricle (Fig. 7.2).

There are two openings in each heart chamber, guarded by one-way valves. The valves prevent the back-flow of blood and keep it moving through the arteries and veins in the proper direction. When one valve is open, the other is shut. Normally blood moves in only one direction through its entire circuit.

When a ventricle (lower chamber) contracts, the valve to the artery opens and the valve between the ventricle and the atrium (upper chamber) closes. Blood is forced from the ventricle out into the artery (pulmonary artery, or aorta). At the end of the contraction, the ventricle relaxes. The valve to the artery closes, the valve to the atrium opens, and blood flows from the atrium to fill the ventricle. When the ventricle is stimulated to contract, the cycle then repeats itself.

The contraction of the heart muscle is called systole; the relaxation of the heart while the ventricles fill with blood is called diastole. Thus we have systolic pressure and diastolic pressure.

The complete cycle which a blood cell makes in the circulatory system is shown in Figure 7.3. In the normal average individual the heartbeat may range from as low as 50 to as high as 95 or 100 beats per minute. At each beat, seventy to

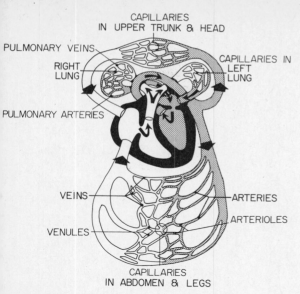

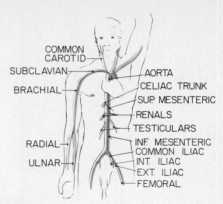

Figure 7.4

57

The major named arteries of the body distribute oxygenated blood from the heart to the principal organs or regions of the body. The name of the artery corresponds to the organ or region served.

Figure 7.3

This sketch is a schematic representation of the circulatory system, including heart, arteries, veins, and interconnecting capillaries. The capillaries are the smallest vessels which connect arterioles with venules. In the capillaries, an exchange of nutrients and waste products between tissues and blood occurs.

eighty milliliters of blood are ejected from the heart. In one minute the entire blood volume of six liters is circulated within the vessels.

Arteries

The aorta is the major artery leaving the left side of the heart; it carries freshly oxygenated blood to the body. This blood vessel is found just in front of the spine in the chest and abdominal cavities. The aorta has many branches supplying the head and neck, arms, and abdominal and chest organs before it terminates in the lower abdomen by dividing into the two main arteries which lead to the lower extremities (Fig. 7.4). Each of these several arteries divides into smaller and smaller branches, finally forming the thin-walled tiny capillaries.

Capillaries and Cells

In the body there are billions of cells and capillaries. Oxygen and other nutrients pass from the blood cells and plasma in the capillaries to the cells of the tissues of the body through the very thin wall of the capillary. Car-

bon dioxide and other waste products pass in a reverse direction from the tissue cells to the blood to be carried away. Blood in arteries is bright red because it is rich in oxygen; blood in the veins is bluish-red in color because it is low in oxygen. Capillaries connect directly at one end with the arterioles and at the other with venules.

Veins

Blood from the capillary system returns to the heart through the veins. Capillaries form small venules which join to form larger veins. The veins of the entire body ultimately join to form two major veins, the superior vena cava and the inferior vena cava (Fig. 7.5).

Blood returning from the head, neck, shoulders, and upper extremities passes through the superior vena cava. Blood from the abdomen, pelvis, and lower extremities passes through the inferior vena cava. Both the superior and inferior vena cava empty into the right atrium at the right side of the heart. The right ventricle receives blood from the right atrium and pumps it into the lungs through the pulmonary arteries.

Circulation in the Lungs

The general plan of circulation through the lungs is essentially the same as that in the rest of the body. Blood vessels from the right side

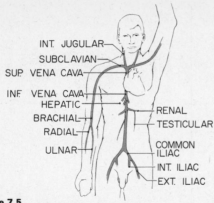

Figure 7.5

The major veins of the body are named to correspond with the regions of the body that they drain. Blood is returned by them to the heart, which pumps it through the lungs for oxygenation.

of the heart branch and rebranch, finally forming capillaries. The capillaries are closely related to the alveoli (air sacs) of the lungs, and an exchange of oxygen and carbon dioxide occurs between the alveoli and the blood in the capillaries (Fig. 5.1). The oxygenated blood from the lungs then returns to the heart and enters the left atrium, from which it passes to the left ventricle and is pumped into the cycle again.

The Pulse

The pulse, which is felt most easily at the neck, wrist, or groin, is created by the forceful pumping of blood out of the heart chambers by the heart muscle into the major arteries. This pulse

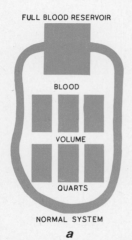

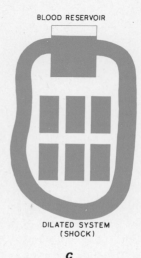

Figure 7.6 a–c

This is a schematic representation of the volume of blood in the body under varying circumstances. *a*, The normal blood volume in an adult is six liters. *b*, When bleeding occurs, the blood volume in the veins and arteries is decreased and the blood vessels constrict. If severe bleeding causes the volume of blood in circulation to be reduced rapidly, the patient may go into shock. *c*, If the walls of the blood vessels become relaxed, the peripheral vascular system enlarges and holds more blood, thereby reducing the amount of blood in circulation as effectively as if bleeding to outside the body had occurred. It is possible, therefore, for shock to be produced in a patient without loss of blood from the body.

is present throughout the entire arterial system but it can be felt most easily where the larger arteries are near the skin. The carotid artery pulse can be felt in the neck below the angle of the jaw; the radial artery pulse is felt at the wrist just at the base of the thumb; the femoral artery pulse is felt in the groin.

Blood Pressure

Blood pressure is the pressure which the blood exerts against the walls of the arteries as it passes through them. The intermittent forceful ejection of blood from the left ventricle of the heart into the aorta is transmitted through the arteries as a repeated pressure wave, which serves to keep the blood moving through the body. The high and low points of the wave can be measured with a sphygmomanometer and expressed numerically in millimeters of mercury. The high point is called the systolic pressure and the low point is called the diastolic pressure.

The pressure wave and the flow of blood in an artery can be stopped by putting pressure on the artery. The pressure applied must be greater than the pressure of the blood flowing through the artery. Several factors control arterial blood pressure. These include the blood volume itself, the state of the arteries and arterioles (dilated or constricted), and the capacity of the muscle of the heart to contract normally.

The pressure of the blood in veins (venous pressure) is much less than that of the blood in arteries. This low pressure aids in the return of blood to the heart. However, if the pressure in the veins falls below normal, insufficient blood is returned to the heart and a failure in the circulatory system occurs. Two factors control the pressure of the venous blood: blood volume (the amount of blood within the circulatory system) and the capacity of the veins.

The average adult has approximately six liters of blood in his arteries and veins. Children have less, varying with their age and size, and newborn infants have only 300 milliliters. The loss of equal amounts of blood may be negligible for an adult but fatal for a baby.

In all healthy people the circulatory system is adjusted and constantly readjusted automatically so that 100 percent of the capacity of the arteries, veins, and capillaries holds just 100 percent of the blood. The size of the arteries and veins is controlled by the nervous system according to the amount of blood available and

many other factors in order to keep the blood pressure normal at all times (Fig. 7.6).

Loss of normal blood pressure is an indication that the blood cannot circulate efficiently to every organ in the body. There may be many reasons for the loss of blood pressure. The end result of the loss in each case is the same: organs are no longer adequately perfused or supplied with oxygen and food and they may die. The state of inadequate perfusion is called shock.

When a patient loses a small amount of blood, arteries, veins, and the heart automatically adjust to the smaller new volume. The adjustment occurs in an effort to maintain adequate pressure throughout the circulatory system, thereby maintaining circulation for every organ. The adjustment occurs very rapidly after the loss, within minutes. Specifically, the vessels contract to provide a smaller bed for the reduced volume of blood to fill, and the heart pumps more rapidly to circulate the remaining blood more efficiently. The reciprocal relationship of pulse and blood pressure (as the latter declines the former rises to compensate) is almost always seen in developing shock.

If the loss of blood be too great however, the system fails and the patient goes into shock. The change in the size of arteries and veins is brought about by muscles in their walls. These muscles can contract or relax in response to changes in blood volume, heat, cold, fright, an injury, or an infection; the contraction or relaxation of the muscle fiber causes changes in the diameter of the artery or vein. These muscles do not act as pumps; they only change the diameter of the vessels and hence their volume. A normal process of continuous adjustment is maintained by the mechanisms of the autonomic nervous system. If the muscles of the arteries and veins contract, the vessel diameters decrease and the system holds less fluid. But if these muscles relax, then the vessels dilate and the system can hold a larger volume of blood. Massive dilation of the vessels can produce a system far too large for the normal volume of blood available and once again shock occurs and

59

all organs, being poorly perfused, are at risk.

Finally, shock can be a manifestation that the muscle of the heart is incapable of pumping sufficiently to maintain circulation. This condi- tion is seen in the patient with a myocardial infarction (heart attack) and direct damage of the heart itself.

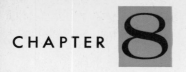

CHAPTER

Bleeding and Control of Bleeding

Direct pressure on a bleeding point is the most effective way of controlling hemorrhage. Bleeding and hemorrhage mean the same thing, namely, that blood is escaping from arteries or veins. Bleeding may be external or internal. In either case it is dangerous. The average adult has six liters of blood in his body. The loss of one liter of blood in an adult or 500 milliliters of blood in a child is very dangerous. In an infant the loss of even 25 to 30 ml of blood can result in signs of shock. Hemorrhage initially results in weakness and ultimately, if uncontrolled, results in shock and death.

Blood is transported within the circulatory system through blood vessels (Chapter 7, The Circulatory System). Accidents and some diseases will disrupt these vessel walls, resulting in bleeding. Characteristically, blood from an artery spurts and is usually bright red. Blood from a vein generally comes in a slow and steady flow and its color is much darker. Bleeding from abraded and open, minute capillaries is a continuous steady ooze (Fig. 8.1). The rapidity of bleeding is very important. The average adult may comfortably lose a pint (500 ml) of blood donated in a blood donor center and taken over fifteen or twenty minutes. During the course of the loss of this blood his body adapts to its

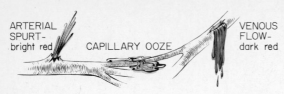

ARTERIAL SPURT- bright red

CAPILLARY OOZE

VENOUS FLOW- dark red

Figure 8.1

A capillary loop connecting an arteriole and a venule is shown. Bleeding from the arterial side and the venous side of the vascular system is typical and recognizable, as is the ooze from lacerated capillaries.

62

being withdrawn quite well. If larger amounts are withdrawn or if this amount is withdrawn much more suddenly, the patient may develop the signs and symptoms of shock and may go on to develop permanent vascular changes or to die.

External Bleeding

External bleeding is a hemorrhage that can be seen coming from a wound. Some examples of external bleeding are: bleeding from open fractures (where the bone protrudes through the skin), bleeding from wounds, and nosebleeds. In most instances bleeding usually stops naturally in six to ten minutes because the body is provided with many mechanisms of defense, among which are those that arrest bleeding. If a finger is cut, blood will gush from the lacerated vessels. These vessels react by constricting at the cut ends, which will diminish the hemorrhage. A clot then forms at the cut end of the vessel and the bleeding stops as the clot increases in size and plugs the hole. Body tissues and tissue juice activate the clotting mechanism within blood and a clot rapidly forms to seal the injured portion of the vessel. Normally, blood within an artery or vein is protected from contact with other body tissues by the blood vessel wall. When blood escapes from the artery or vein and this protection is gone, blood clots.

In some patients who have undergone a severe injury, the damaged blood vessels may be so large that clots physically cannot occlude them. Sometimes only a portion of the vessel wall may be torn and thus it cannot retract and constrict. In these cases bleeding must be

stopped by external means. Blood loss may occasionally be so rapid that if one waits for the bleeding to stop, the patient may bleed to death before normal protective processes can be activated. It is imperative that the EMT know how to control bleeding. In general, after securing an airway and being certain the patient can breathe, the second order of concern for the EMT is the control of hemorrhage.

Controlling External Bleeding

The control of bleeding is often very simple. Almost all instances of external bleeding can be controlled by applying local pressure. Pressure stops the physical flow of blood and permits normal blood coagulation to occur.

There are several ways, however, to control bleeding when it is external (Fig. 8.2 *a–f*).

1. Direct pressure may be exerted over the wound by a finger or hand or by the application of a pressure dressing.
2. A pressure point of the major artery lying proximal to the wound may be found and pressure may be applied at that point to occlude blood flow in that artery.
3. A tourniquet may be applied proximal to the wound on an affected extremity.
4. A splint may be applied.
5. A pressurized air splint may be used.
6. Military Anti-Shock Trousers (MAST) may be used.

Local Pressure. Bleeding is nearly always stopped when pressure is applied directly over a wound (Fig. 8.2 *a*). The initial application of pressure may be done with a finger or hand. A pressure dressing is preferred. It is a sterile dressing made up of gauze pads with a universal dressing (9 × 36 inches) applied above them at the point where pressure is needed. The actual pressure is then generated by wrapping the wound circumferentially and firmly with clean, roller, self-adhering bandages. The entire mass of the sterile dressing should be covered above and below the wound by the bandage stretched sufficiently tight to arrest the hemorrhage. If sterile pads are not immediately available, a handkerchief, a sanitary napkin, a clean cloth,

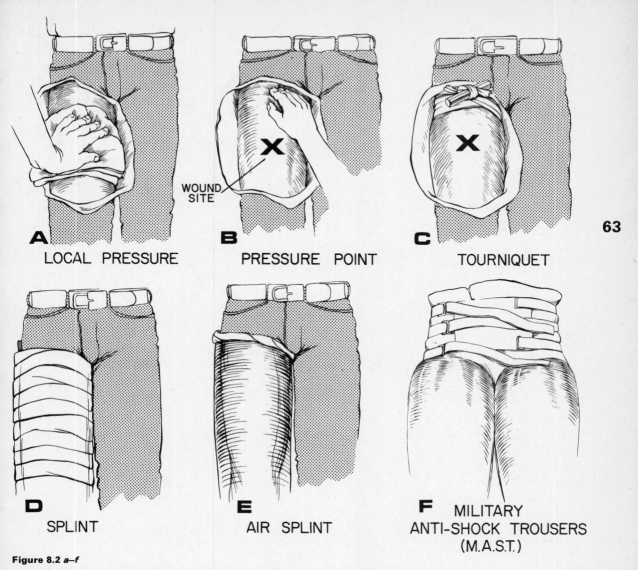

A LOCAL PRESSURE

B PRESSURE POINT

WOUND SITE

C TOURNIQUET

D SPLINT

E AIR SPLINT

F MILITARY ANTI-SHOCK TROUSERS (M.A.S.T.)

Figure 8.2 a–f

The major means of controlling visible bleeding and internal soft-tissue bleeding are shown.

or the bare hand can be used to apply pressure. A dressing should not be removed once it has been placed until the patient is evaluated by the physician in the Emergency Department. If bleeding continues after the dressing has been applied, not enough pressure has been generated. In such instances, use the hand to apply more pressure on the wound through the dressing, or tighten the bandage, or add additional pads. Any of these methods should stop the bleeding.

Pressure-point control. In instances where pressure dressings are not available at all,

pressure-point control can sometimes be used to stop hemorrhage in an emergency (Fig. 8.2 *b*). Pressure points have been discussed in Chapter 3, General and Topographic Anatomy. These points lie proximal to areas of bleeding and indicate places where the major arteries feeding a wound lie close to the surface. Such pressure points may be found in the arm, in the leg, in the groin, and in the neck.

One can practice feeling for the pulse on the inner half of the arm midway between the elbow and the armpit. If this main artery is effectively compressed against the underlying bone, the

64

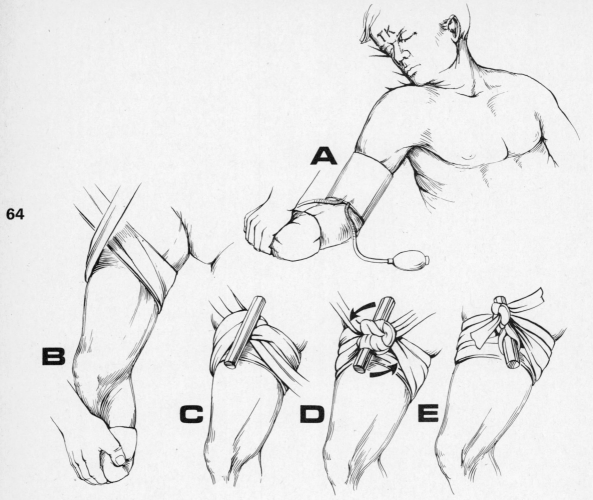

Figure 8.3 *a–e*

The proper application of a tourniquet is shown. It is a simple procedure which is described in the text. The fact that a tourniquet has been applied to a patient must always be indicated by marking TK and the time on the patient's body or on a tag accompanying him. The preferable place is the patient's forehead. Once control of bleeding has been achieved, the tourniquet must be firmly fastened in place.

flow of blood below the point of pressure will be reduced. Practice feeling for the pulse in the groin. At this point one can compress the main femoral artery against the pelvis. Pressure-point control of bleeding is not as satisfactory as direct-pressure control exerted on the wound itself because rarely is the bleeding vessel supplied by a single major compressible artery. Bleeding from a wound which has been controlled by proximal-point pressure will not entirely cease but will probably be significantly slowed so that local pressure, however little, may be made more effective.

Tourniquet. The use of a tourniquet in instances of bleeding is rarely if ever necessary. Tourniquets are not recommended for general use because they have sometimes caused more damage in injured extremities than existed from the injury itself. They crush a considerable amount of tissue underneath them; they have caused permanent damage of nerves and blood vessels; and if they are left on for any appreciable length of time, they may result in the loss of the extremity. Nevertheless, a properly applied tourniquet may be lifesaving for a person whose bleeding from a major vessel is uncontrollable in any other way. Specifically, the tourniquet is useful in the patient who has sustained a traumatic amputation, either partial or complete, or in the patient for whom local pressure has failed. If a tourniquet must be used it should be correctly applied (Figs. 8.2 *c* & 8.3).

1. A triangular bandage should be folded until it is 3 or 4 inches wide and about six or eight layers thick. A rubber tube, blood pressure cuff, or a long handkerchief may also be used.
2. This long 4-inch bandage should be wrapped twice around the extremity at a point proximal to the bleeding but as far distal on the extremity as possible.
3. Tie one knot in the bandage. Place a stick or a metal rod on top of the flat knot and tie the ends of the bandage over the stick in a square knot.
4. The stick can then be used as a handle to twist the bandage to tighten the tourniquet until the bleeding has stopped. Once the bleeding has ceased, make no more turns with the stick. Secure the stick or rod in place and make the wrapping neat and smooth.

   The technique of using a rod passed through a bandage to achieve pressure or generate traction is called the Spanish Windlass. It is also used for the application of traction splints.
5. Occasionally, a blood pressure cuff can serve as an effective tourniquet (Fig. 8.3 *a*).

Precautions in using a tourniquet. Certain precautions must be observed.

1. It is important that as wide a bandage as possible be used and that it be tightened securely. If a blood pressure cuff is used, the same precautions must be observed.
2. Never use wire or any other material that will cut into the skin.
3. Do not loosen the tourniquet until a doctor evaluates the patient.
4. Never cover a tourniquet with a bandage. Leave it open and in full view. Always signify that the patient has had a tourniquet applied by writing TK on his forehead and on the tag attached to his person. This

should be written indelibly so that the script may not be inadvertently wiped away. The time that the tourniquet was applied should also be indicated on the tag. and forehead. In addition, be sure to point out to the medical staff that the person has had a tourniquet applied.
5. Never place a tourniquet below the knee or elbow, because in certain areas in the extremities, nerves lie close to the skin and may be injured by the compression.

Splints. Much bleeding from injured extremities is caused because muscles are lacerated by sharp ends of broken bones or because vessels lying in the bone that is fractured continue to bleed. So long as the fracture has not been controlled, continued laceration and further damage of partially clotted vessels can occur. This continued irritation results in further bleeding. Often the application of a splint to a badly fractured and lacerated extremity will allow very prompt control of the hemorrhage associated with the injury (Fig. 8.2 *d*). In general, the EMT should remember that injuries are not isolated phenomena to be treated separately. Hemorrhage accompanies nearly all severe injuries and the treatment of the underlying injury may aid markedly in controlling the hemorrhage.

Pressure pants and pressure splints. Available on many ambulances throughout the United States now are air pressure splints and on some, pressure pants (Military Anti-Shock Trousers, commonly referred to as MAST trousers) (Figs. 8.2 *f* & 8.4). These devices can aid in controlling severe soft-tissue hemorrhage when massive lacerations of muscles and soft tissues and multiple fractures have occurred. The application of such a splint is described in General Principles of Splinting and Bandaging (Chapter 17). The principle underlying the use of air splinting in the control of hemorrhage is that a pressure bandage may be applied to an entire extremity rather than to a single laceration or a given area on the extremity. The use of such a splint for the control of hemorrhage is appropriate in the patient with extensive lacerations involving one entire extremity (Fig. 8.2 *e*).

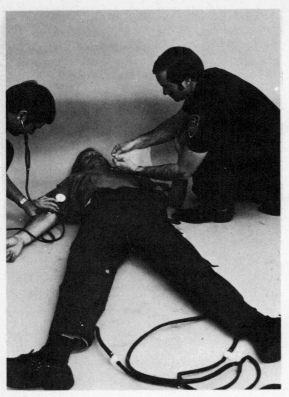

Figure 8.4

Military Anti-Shock Trousers, commonly called MAST trousers, have been placed on the patient shown above, but they are not yet inflated. Bleeding over an entire extremity or area of the body can be controlled through the use of pressure trousers on a patient with a number of lacerations or fractures. MAST trousers are, in effect, large-size air splints. They can also be used to give considerable stability to fractures or dislocations that would otherwise be difficult to manage.

66

Frequently hemorrhage is a severe or fatal accompaniment of bad fractures of the pelvis or fractures of one or both hip joints. Bleeding cannot be observed externally in these patients because it can occur behind the peritoneum and into the tissues of both hips. In such instances, the application of pressure pants will allow counterpressure to be delivered over the entire lower half of the body (Fig. 8.2 *f*). The effectiveness of this particular mode of emergency care can be measured by the return of the blood pressure to a normal level when fluid is administered and by the increasing stability of the patient. The use of pressure pants will also allow the EMT to stabilize to some degree fractures of the pelvis and bad fractures of both hips.

Whenever air pressure splints or MAST trousers are used and it is necessary to transport the patient either in a helicopter or in areas where temperature changes may be marked, the EMT must remember that the volume of air within the splint changes when the external temperature and air pressure change. In helicopters and unpressurized airplanes, external pressure drops with increasing height, and the air in the splint expands. Accordingly the splint will become much tighter than it was when applied. Similarly, cold makes air within the splint contract; if an emergency requires the use of such a splint in very cold areas, the pressure within the splint must be adjusted as the patient comes into a warmer room or into a warm transporting vehicle, for the air in the splint will then expand and the splint will become tighter.

Epistaxis

Nosebleeds (epistaxes) are common emergencies. The amount of blood that a person can lose in a nosebleed may be enough to cause shock. The blood seen coming from the nose may represent only a small amount of the total loss since blood from these bleeding vessels often goes down into the throat and into the stomach as the patient swallows it. A person who swallows enough blood may become nauseated and may vomit up dark clots. Bleeding from the nose can be caused by the following conditions:

1. A fractured skull
2. Facial injuries, including those caused by the direct blow of a fist
3. Sinusitis, infections, or other abnormalities of the inside of the nose
4. High blood pressure
5. Bleeding diseases

Bleeding from the nose or ears following a head injury may mean that there is a skull fracture. If a fractured skull is suspected, do not try to stop this particular bleeding. In general, you will be unable to do so. If successful, you may increase pressure on the brain as the blood leaking out through the ear or nose now collects within the head. This patient should be treated for a skull or head injury, as discussed in Injuries of the Skull and Brain (Chapter 22).

Nosebleeds resulting from all other remaining causes should be initially treated at the scene. The following techniques are successful in stopping most nosebleeds:

1. Apply pressure by pinching the nostrils or by placing a bandage between the upper lip and the gum and pressing against it with the fingers. The patient can sometimes apply enough pressure to stop the bleeding by stretching his upper lip tight against the bandage.
2. Keep the patient in a sitting position whenever possible so that blood which trickles down the back of his throat will not automatically be aspirated into his lungs.
3. Keep the patient quiet. This rule is particularly important if he suffers from high blood pressure or is anxious. Anxiety will tend to increase blood pressure and the nosebleed will worsen.
4. Applying ice over the nose may also be helpful.

The EMT must understand that the person with a prolonged nosebleed or one who is subject to nosebleeds should be taken to the hospital and be seen by a physician. Most nosebleeds arise from injuries of the mucosa overlying the nasal septum, which is anterior in the nose. Accordingly the measures we have listed above are frequently successful in stopping such bleeds. A few nosebleeds, however, arise posteriorly in the nasopharynx and cannot be stopped by normal emergency methods. This kind of nosebleed may require the application of a nasopharyngeal pack, which has to be done in the hospital by the doctor.

Internal Bleeding

Internal bleeding is usually not visible but it can be very serious and the patient may die of shock. Bleeding from the mouth or rectum or blood in the urine may indicate serious internal injury. Nonmenstrual bleeding from the vagina is also significant. Bleeding, however slight, from any body orifice may be serious, as it usually indicates some internal source of a hemorrhage. Examples of internal bleeding are these:

1. Bleeding from a stomach ulcer
2. Bleeding from a closed fracture of any bone
3. Bleeding from a lacerated liver or spleen

The signs which may point to internal bleeding are those which indicate the development of shock:

1. The pulse becomes weak or rapid.
2. The skin becomes cold and clammy.
3. The eyes are dull; the pupils may be dilated and slow to respond to light.
4. The blood pressure falls.
5. The patient is usually thirsty and almost invariably anxious with a feeling of impending doom.
6. The patient may be nauseated and may vomit.

A person with a bleeding stomach ulcer may lose a large amount of blood internally very quickly. Fractured ribs may result in severe internal hemorrhage into the chest. Occasionally with injuries such as this the patient may cough up bright red blood from an injured lung. He may vomit bright red blood or dark blood the color and consistency of coffee grounds from hemorrhage within the stomach.

A person who has suffered severe blunt abdominal trauma with a laceration of the liver or spleen may lose a considerable quantity of blood into the abdominal cavity. Ordinarily, in addition to the signs and symptoms of shock, this patient will have a tender abdomen which progressively enlarges.

A person with a fracture of the shaft of the femur can easily lose a liter of blood or more into the tissues of the thigh with little or no immediate external indication of such blood loss; but swelling is frequently seen with closed fractures of major bones, largely as a result of the accumulation of blood around the ends of the fractured bones.

Control of Internal Bleeding

The control of internal bleeding depends upon the location of the bleeding site and the cause of the hemorrhage.

67

Within the chest cavity, internal bleeding may come from blood vessels in the chest wall or from the major arteries and veins within the chest. Control of this bleeding requires opening of the chest cavity and direct suture of the bleeding vessel. The EMT can recognize the possibility of this type of injury and arrange immediate transport of this patient to the hospital. Operation is usually required for definitive treatment.

Within the abdomen, blunt abdominal injuries commonly result in bleeding, which may be massive, from the liver or spleen. Control of these injuries requires operation with repair of the liver or removal of the spleen and suture of any other major bleeding vessel found. Patients having the signs of an abdominal injury with associated signs of shock should be transported to the hospital as first priority patients.

Internal bleeding from any of a number of diseases is manifested either as hematemesis (the vomiting of bright red blood), or hemoptysis (the coughing up of bright red blood), or melena (the passage of dark black stools of the consistency of tar), or hematochezia (the passage of bright red blood from the rectum), or the vomiting of coffee-ground–like material from the stomach. All such patients are high risk. They may continue to bleed or bleed again massively at any moment. These conditions should all be recognized by the EMT, as they require prompt transportation of the patient to the hospital. Diagnosis of the exact source of bleeding is frequently facilitated if the doctor can see

the patient while the bleeding is taking place.

The control of internal bleeding into the extremities can be managed on the scene in a number of ways. First, simple splinting of an injured extremity may allow complete control. This splinting may progress to the use of single-extremity air splints or MAST trousers. Effectiveness of the control of such hemorrhage is monitored by observing the patient's general status, his vital signs, and the ability to restore his blood pressure with an infusion of saline solution.

The principles for treating any patient with suspected internal bleeding at any site are these:

1. Treat the patient for shock from loss of blood.
2. Anticipate that he will vomit. Give him nothing by mouth and keep him lying down, preferably on his side, with a loosened collar and belt. Make him as comfortable as possible and reassure him.
3. Treat obvious internal bleeding into an arm or leg by applying a splint and local pressure or a pressure splint.
4. Give oxygen. As blood is lost, the tissues of the body are deprived of their needed oxygen supply. Inhalation of oxygen on the way to the hospital may be lifesaving.
5. Transport the patient promptly but gently and as efficiently as possible to the Emergency Department.

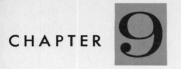

Shock

GOAL I.   Recognize the characteristics and understand the physiology of shock.

OBJECTIVES

A. Recognize the signs and symptoms of shock.
B. Describe the physiology of shock.

GOAL II. Understand the procedures for the treatment of patients in shock.

OBJECTIVES

A. Describe the principles of general care for patients in shock.
B. Describe the procedures for preventing shock.
C. List the steps in administering intravenous fluids.
D. Explain the role of intravenous fluid therapy in the treatment of shock.

The term *shock* has a variety of meanings, physiological and otherwise. It is used to denote the receiving of any amount of electric current by an individual. Some people refer to a sudden hemorrhage or clot in the brain as a shock or, more commonly, a stroke. Generally, in medicine shock means a state of collapse of the cardiovascular system.

The cardiovascular system is that part of the body which provides circulation of the blood to all the cells. Through this system oxygen and food are brought to each cell and waste products are removed. Some areas, such as the brain, the peripheral nervous system, and the heart, require a constant flow of blood to live. These organs, especially the nervous system, cannot tolerate any suspension of blood flow for more than four or five minutes or their component cells will die.

One can look upon the cardiovascular system as consisting of two parts: a container and the contents of the container. The container consists of the heart and its system of blood vessels: arteries, veins, innumerable small arterioles, venules, and capillaries. These are the tubes which extend to every cell in the body. Within the container is the blood.

In an artery and at the arterial ends of the capillaries, the tubes have distinct muscular walls. The tubes can open and close as directed. The system of fine capillaries which pass between cells linking the arterioles to the venules can also be opened or closed. The opening or closing of these vessels is entirely automatic and is under the control of the autonomic nervous system (sympathetic and parasympathetic). Stimuli that cause the opening or the closing of these vessels include fright, heat, cold, the specific need of an organ for oxygen, or the specific need of an organ for disposal of waste. A person can exert no voluntary control over this system. Never are all the vessels fully opened or fully closed in a normal individual.

The second part of this system is the blood within the container. Normally there is just enough blood to fill the system absolutely full;

in an average adult this is six liters. The heart is a muscular pump which serves to circulate the blood within the system. If it pumps six liters a minute through a system that can hold just six liters, every part of the system receives a regular supply of blood every minute. A condition in which this system fails to provide sufficient circulation to every part of the body is what is called shock.

The term *perfusion* is used to signify the circulation of blood within an organ. An organ is perfused if blood is entering it through the arteries and leaving it through the veins. Perfusion of an organ or perfusion of the whole body by blood keeps the component cells of the body healthy. The body depends on adequate perfusion of its organs by blood to bring food to the organs and to dispose of waste products generated by the organs in the course of normal daily living and metabolism. In states of shock, the perfusion of organ systems fails.

Certain organs of the body are more susceptible than others to lack of adequate perfusion. The brain and peripheral nervous system cannot lose perfusion for more than a few minutes without permanent damage of their cells. Damage in the kidney results after inadequate perfusion for a period of thirty to forty-five minutes. The heart requires constant perfusion or it will not function properly. If skeletal muscle is subjected to loss of perfusion for two hours, it can be permanently damaged. The gastrointestinal tract can exist with impaired perfusion for a number of hours. No part of the body can exist without adequate perfusion for an indefinite period of time. Permanent injury of the patient results when the organ system which is most sensitive to the lack of adequate perfusion is damaged. This system is the central and peripheral nervous system.

There are three major causes of shock:

1. The heart can be damaged so that it fails to act properly as a pump.
2. Blood can be lost so that the volume of fluid within the vascular container is insufficient.
3. The blood vessels constituting the container can dilate so that the blood within them, even though it is a normal volume, is still insufficient to fill the system completely and provide efficient circulation.

In all instances, the results of shock are exactly the same. There is insufficient perfusion of blood through the tissues of the body to provide adequate food and oxygen to them. All normal bodily processes are affected. When a person is in shock, his vital functions slow down. If the conditions causing shock are not promptly arrested and reversed, death soon follows.

Types and Causes of Shock

Shock may accompany many different emergency situations. Ordinarily they can all be related to one of the three major causes.

Common types of shock are:

1. Hemorrhagic shock (blood loss)
2. Respiratory shock (inadequate oxygen supply)
3. Neurogenic shock (loss of vascular control by the nervous system)
4. Psychogenic shock (fainting)
5. Cardiogenic shock (inadequate functioning of the heart)
6. Septic shock (severe infection)
7. Anaphylactic shock (allergic reaction)
8. Metabolic shock (loss of body fluid)

Hemorrhagic shock. Shock following trauma is commonly a result of blood loss. External bleeding may be seen in patients who have suffered severe lacerations or fractures; internal bleeding follows rupture of the liver or the spleen or the great vessels within the abdomen or the chest. Hemorrhagic shock is also seen in patients with severe burns and extremely severe contusions where there may not be actual hemorrhage but where a considerable amount of intravascular fluid (plasma and blood) is lost into the muscular tissues of the body. Burns in particular produce extensive and alarming losses of plasma (the colorless part of the blood) and other body fluids into the tissues that have been burned.

70

Crush injuries also may result in the loss of both blood and plasma into the injured tissues from damaged blood vessels. If dehydration (loss of body water) is present before the injury, the state of shock will be aggravated. This particular situation has been commonly seen in personnel wounded in military actions in the tropics where there is constant exposure to the sun and much sweating. In all the instances enumerated above, the common factor is that there is insufficient blood within the vascular container to provide adequate circulation to all the organs of the body. This whole range of conditions is called hemorrhagic shock, or sometimes hypovolemic shock (*hypo* meaning "small" and *volemic* meaning "volume").

Respiratory shock. A sucking chest wound, a flail chest, an obstructed airway, or a pneumothorax all may result in the patient's being unable to breathe an adequate amount of oxygen. This condition may produce what is called respiratory shock. If the patient has a broken neck with a spinal cord injury, paralysis of his chest muscles can result. Since he can then breathe only with his diaphragm he may not be able to breathe deeply enough to take in enough oxygen for his immediate needs.

Inadequate breathing can produce shock as rapidly as hemorrhage. In this instance, shock is produced because an insufficient amount of oxygen exists in the blood. The volume of blood, the volume of the vascular container, and the action of the heart are all normal, but the supply of oxygen carried in the blood is not normal. Without oxygen the organs in the body cannot survive and their functions gradually deteriorate.

Neurogenic shock. Paralysis of the peripheral nerves after spinal cord injuries may cause neurogenic shock. In the patient who is in neurogenic shock, the muscles of the blood vessels are temporarily or permanently paralyzed. In these states of muscle paralysis, vessels throughout the body generally dilate; more blood than the normal volume is then required to fill them. Normally the muscles in these blood vessels are under the control of the autonomic nervous system. This system can be severely damaged by spinal or neck injuries. Blood vessels are constantly under some degree of constriction. If the controlling nervous system is injured, vessels are released from this effect; under no control at all, they dilate widely. The available six liters of blood can then no longer fill the vascular system, which has become a much larger container. The entire system fails, perfusion of all organs becomes inadequate, and shock ensues.

Psychogenic shock. Psychogenic shock or, more commonly, simple fainting is a sudden reaction of the nervous system which allows momentary vascular dilation. The result is a temporary reduction of blood supply to the brain because blood momentarily pools in the dilated vessels in other parts of the body. When the blood supply of the brain is suddenly and sharply reduced, the brain ceases to function and fainting ensues. Fear, bad news, sometimes good news, the sight of an injury or blood, the prospect of medical treatment, severe pain or anxiety are among the many precipitating causes of this condition. If one is not feeling well, is tired or worried, or even if he is obliged to stand quietly in a stuffy room, he may be more susceptible to fainting. Once fainting has occurred and the patient has collapsed and fallen, circulation in the brain is restored and the episode passes promptly. In this type of shock, the major concern is the occurrence of any injury sustained during the fainting spell, such as striking the head.

Cardiogenic shock. Cardiogenic shock implies shock caused by inadequate functioning of the heart. Circulation of the blood throughout the vascular bed requires the constant action of a normal and vigorous heart muscle. Many types of disease cause the destruction or inflammation of this muscle. Within certain limits the heart can adapt to these injuries; but if too much muscular impairment occurs, as follows some heart attacks, the heart no longer functions well. It is the beating of the heart which moves blood through the vessels at distinct pressures (blood pressure). This pressure is necessary to force blood through the entire system. Shock from cardiac origin develops when the heart muscle can no longer impart sufficient pressure.

71

Septic shock. In some patients who are afflicted with severe bacterial infections, toxins (poisons) are liberated by the bacteria into the bloodstream and produce a state of shock which is called septic shock. This condition results from widespread dilation of the small vessels of the vascular system and from loss of plasma through injured vessel walls. The toxins formed by the bacteria directly attack small blood vessel walls, rendering them leaky so that blood and plasma are lost from the capillaries into the tissues. The muscular walls of arterioles are also damaged so that they can no longer contract on direct stimulation.

This type of shock then is rather complex. There is an insufficient volume of fluid because much of the blood has leaked out of the vascular system into the tissues, while at the same time there is a larger than normal blood vessel bed to contain the smaller than normal volume of intravascular blood. The development of this type of shock rarely concerns the EMT. It is almost always seen as a complication in the course of prolonged hospitalization for some serious illness, injury, or operation.

Anaphylactic shock. Anaphylactic shock occurs when an individual who has become sensitized to some substance by previous contact to it reacts violently to another dose or contact. It is the most severe form of an allergic reaction. Substances which most often cause allergic reactions may be grouped as follows.

1. *Injections*—The injection of sera such as tetanus antitoxin or drugs such as penicillin may cause severe reactions.
2. *Ingestion*—Eating foods such as fish, shellfish, or berries, or taking medications or drugs such as oral penicillin can cause slower but equally severe reactions if one is sensitive to any of them.
3. *Insect stings*—Stings of the bee, wasp, yellow jacket, or hornet can cause very rapid and severe generalized anaphylactic reactions.
4. *Inhalation*—The inhalation of dusts or pollens or materials to which a patient is particularly sensitive may similarly cause rapid and severe reactions.

Anaphylactic shock is a very special kind of reaction and very complex. It is frequently encountered, however, and the EMT should know its signs and immediate treatment.

Metabolic shock. Occasionally in severe, untreated illnesses a state of shock may occur because of profound fluid loss from vomiting, diarrhea, excess urination, or severe disturbance of the body fluid and acid-base balance by diseases such as diabetes. Patients who develop shock in the course of this type of chronic disease are desperately ill and may have reached the end stage of that particular disease.

General Signs and Symptoms of Shock

Certain signs and symptoms are common to all types of shock. Anaphylactic shock presents some very special signs which are discussed separately for added emphasis.

The common indications of shock are these:

1. Restlessness and anxiety may precede all other signs.
2. The pulse becomes weak and rapid.
3. The skin becomes cold and clammy.
4. Sweating is profuse.
5. The face may become pale and later cyanotic (blue).
6. Respirations may be shallow, labored, rapid, or possibly irregular or gasping, especially if a chest injury has occurred.
7. The eyes become dull or lusterless, with dilated pupils.
8. The patient is thirsty.
9. The patient may feel nauseated or may vomit.
10. The blood pressure falls gradually and steadily. In general, although some people normally have a systolic blood pressure of only 90 to 100 mm Hg, it is best to assume that any injured patient whose blood pressure is 100 mm Hg or less is developing shock.
11. In cases of rapidly developing transient shock the patient may faint.

Anaphylactic reactions occur in minutes or even seconds following contact with the sub-

72

stances which cause allergic reactions. Obvious disturbances in the skin, respiratory system, and circulation result.

The major signs of an anaphylactic reaction are these:

1. *Skin*—There is flushing, itching, or a burning sensation, especially of the face and upper chest; hives may spread over large areas of the body; edema (swelling), especially of the face and tongue, may occur. A specific swelling of the lips may be seen. Cyanosis may become rapidly visible about the lips.
2. *Respiratory system*—There is a tightness or pain in the chest with an irritating and persistent cough. Wheezing and difficulty in breathing develop. Fluid is lost into the bronchi and the patient tries to cough it up. The smaller bronchi constrict and the passage of air is increasingly difficult; hence wheezing results.
3. *Circulation*—There will be a perceptible drop in blood pressure, a weak or imperceptible pulse, pallor, and dizziness. Faintness and even coma may follow.

General Care and Treatment of Shock

Any patient who exhibits any of the foregoing signs or symptoms should be vigorously treated for shock as soon as the EMT determines its existence. It is important to recognize the probable cause of shock because treatment is adjusted accordingly. However, many specific principles of initial treatment can be applied to all patients in shock. These principles are listed below.

1. Secure and maintain a clear airway and give oxygen as needed. Do this first, before doing anything else.
2. Control all obvious bleeding by gentle, firm compression.
3. Elevate the lower extremities about twelve inches if injuries to them do not make this inadvisable or impossible.
4. Splint fractures. By so doing, bleeding is lessened and pain and discomfort which

would further aggravate shock are minimized.
5. Avoid rough and excessive handling.
6. Prevent the loss of body heat by putting blankets under and over the patient.
7. In general, keep an injured patient supine; remember, however, that some patients in shock after a severe heart attack or with lung disease cannot breathe as well supine as sitting up or in a semi-sitting position. With such a patient, use the most comfortable position for him.
8. Record accurately the patient's initial pulse, blood pressure, and other vital signs and maintain a record of them at five-minute intervals until he is delivered to the Emergency Department.
9. Do not feed the patient or give him anything to drink.

It is important to check the patient's breathing. Lack of oxygen may rapidly cause shock. Inadequate ventilation may be either the primary cause or a contributing factor in shock. It may be the result of an easily removed obstruction of the throat. Establish and maintain an open airway and be sure that breathing is adequate. Oxygen should be given to all patients in shock. A few assisted breaths with a ventilatory apparatus, with or without added oxygen, will usually raise the patient's blood oxygen to an acceptable level.

An oxygen-adding device can provide oxygen on demand to a patient (conscious or unconscious) who is having difficulty breathing. Disposable plastic masks, with or without a breathing bag, may be used to administer the oxygen. Unless oxygen is humidified, inhalation should be limited, to avoid drying the mouth, nasal passages, and throat. If the patient is unable to use his respiratory muscles after his airway is cleared, artificial respiration by either a ventilatory apparatus or a mouth-to-mouth technique may be lifesaving. In some instances the EMT must employ all his knowledge of artificial breathing and cardiac compression to save the patient.

All obvious bleeding must be controlled. This is best done with sterile gauze compresses placed

73

over the bleeding sites and bandaged with local pressure. Bandaging will minimize the loss of blood. Sufficient pressure must be applied to stop any bleeding. The use of tourniquets is a last resort.

Elevating the lower extremities of the patient allows the blood in the legs to be returned to the heart more readily. This is a simple way, after a severe hemorrhage, of supplying as much blood to the heart as possible. Do not attempt it if the patient has fractures of his legs unless they are well splinted. It may well aggravate any unsplinted fracture and cause severe soft-tissue damage.

Fractures should be splinted. This splinting is not a definitive treatment for the fracture but it minimizes the amount of damage that the broken ends of bone can do to adjacent soft tissue. Hemorrhage may thus be minimized around a fracture site. Splinting makes movement of the patient much easier and renders the patient much more comfortable in general. Severe soft-tissue injuries may well be handled best by splinting and occasionally by the use of air splints for compression.

Rough or excessive handling of the patient is to be avoided. An attendant should ride with the patient, keeping him quiet and reassuring him. Transportation should be carried out at a safe speed.

Prevent the loss of body heat, but generally do not add more heat. It is better that the patient be slightly cool than toasting warm. The use of external heat, such as hot water bottles or heating pads, may be harmful to the patient in shock; use them only in cold weather to prevent chilling and be careful to observe all precautions concerning the use of external heat.

Do not give any liquids to the patient in shock. Especially if the patient is vomiting, has an obvious abdominal injury, or is unable to swallow, the rule is specifically *Nothing by Mouth*. In general this is a very good rule to follow for all patients in shock. Nothing should be given orally until the patient has been seen in the Emergency Department by the doctor. Alcoholic drinks are never given to treat shock; other stimulants such as ammonia or coffee have little or no value in the treatment of shock. The intense thirst that

frequently accompanies shock may be allayed by allowing the patient to chew or suck on a moist sponge. It may be alleviated by the use of IV (intravenous) fluids.

Treatment for Specific Types of Shock

Hemorrhagic shock. The treatment of hemorrhagic shock as an emergency includes the control of obvious bleeding as a first step after one is sure that the patient can breathe properly. The EMT must be aware that continued bleeding will result from failure to apply pressure to obvious wounds, from failure to splint fractures, and from rough handling.

Elevate the lower extremities by raising the legs from the hips, keeping the knees straight (Fig. 9.1). This will increase the blood supply returning to the heart and aid in combating shock. A litter may be placed with the patient's head lower if moving the legs is contraindicated (Fig. 9.1). Remember that in this position the entire weight of the abdominal organs falls on the diaphragm and that a patient may be unable to breathe easily and require assisted ventilation. Elevate no more than twelve inches.

The presence of internal hemorrhage can be appreciated if blood is passed from the mouth or rectum. Nothing can be done locally to control

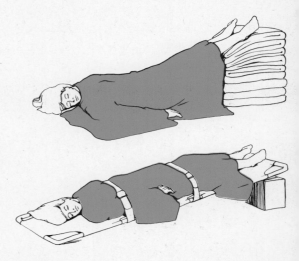

Figure 9.1

Often a slight elevation of the feet and legs or placing the patient in a litter in a head-down position will help alleviate shock. Feet should not be raised higher than twelve inches.

this bleeding; but the EMT must give general support, insure that the patient does not aspirate any vomitus into his lungs, and institute all the general methods for the treatment of shock.

Intravenous administration of fluids should be started promptly, preferably with a balanced salt solution. Ringer's lactate or Plasma-Lyte is usual. If these solutions are not available, 5 percent dextrose in water (D_5W) may be used. The rapid infusion of fluid may counteract shock promptly.

Ventilatory support should be part of this treatment and may include artificial respiration and use of supplemental oxygen while the patient is being transported to the hospital.

Finally, this patient must be taken to the Emergency Department for definitive care as rapidly as possible.

Respiratory shock. The proper management of shock as a result of inadequate respiration involves, first, securing and maintaining an airway. The mouth and the throat down to the larynx must be cleared of mucus, vomitus, foreign material, or anything obstructing the passage. Artificial ventilation using ventilatory aids or mouth-to-mouth resuscitation may be employed. Supplemental oxygen should be given where possible. These patients generally fall into the category of those having severe medical emergencies and they must be treated as rapidly as are patients who have obviously severe chest injuries or other malformations. Prompt transportation to the Emergency Department for them is mandatory.

Neurogenic shock. Shock that accompanies severe spinal cord injuries or that arises from a neurogenic cause is best treated by a combination of all the known supportive measures. The patient who has suffered this kind of injury will ordinarily require hospitalization for a long time. Emergency treatment for him should be directed at obtaining and maintaining a proper airway, supporting blood pressure with intravenous infusions of saline solution, and conserving body heat with blankets. He may not be losing blood but his vascular capacity may have become considerably larger than the volume of blood which it contains. Under these circumstances the correct initial step is to fill up the

reservoir with fluid to maintain proper perfusion of all the organs of the body. Keep him as warm as possible since his body's control of temperature is lost with such an injury. Prompt transportation to the hospital is mandatory since this patient may require care in special wards to survive.

Psychogenic shock. Usually a simple fainting spell will pass very quickly. If the attack has caused the patient to fall, the EMT must be alert for any injuries sustained in the fall. These might include fractures of the long bones or of any bones where the patient may have struck—most particularly fractures of the skull—or cerebral concussions or contusions. In the absence of any such injuries the patient recovers promptly. As soon as the patient has fallen or collapsed, the blood supply to the brain is improved and consciousness usually quickly returns. If it does not or if the patient is confused after such an attack one must suspect a head injury, particularly if he has sustained a fall during the fainting spell. In such an instance prompt transportation to the Emergency Department is necessary with a recording of the initial observations and the length of time the patient was unconscious.

Cardiogenic shock. The patient in shock as a result of a heart attack or severe lung disease specifically does **not** require a transfusion of blood or fluid or elevation of his legs. In this patient, shock is a result of the inability of the heart to handle the blood volume the patient already has. If severe lung disease is associated with this condition, oxygenation of the blood passing through the lungs is normally poor and the states of shock and hypoxia aggravate one another. This patient is often able to breathe better in a sitting position and may tell the EMT so. He should be permitted to sit up if he wishes.

Usually these patients do not have injuries but have had and may still be having chest pain. The pulse is commonly irregular and may be weak. The blood pressure is low. Cyanosis is frequently present about the lips and underneath the fingernails. They may very well be anxious. Occasionally patients who have had heart attacks vomit.

These patients should be treated by placing

them in the position in which they can breathe most easily, by administering oxygen, by assisting ventilation when necessary, and by transporting them rapidly to the Emergency Department. Reassurance and a calm demeanor are required in treating them.

In many places distant electrocardiographic services are available so that electrode leads may be placed on the patient and an electrocardiogram may be monitored at a central Emergency Department. If this capability exists for the EMT, the leads should be placed as directed and the EMT may very well be able to receive instructions from the Emergency Department with regard to diagnosis and further proper treatment of the patient en route.

Septic shock. The proper treatment of septic shock requires complex hospital management. If this condition is suspected, the patient must be transported to the hospital as quickly as possible while being given all the general support available. Intravenous fluid administration and oxygen during transportation are both advisable. Respiratory support may be necessary. Septic shock does not ordinarily concern the EMT as it occurs usually during a long hospitalization and in the course of prolonged and debilitating illnesses. Occasionally the EMT may be faced with this condition and he must recognize that the presence of uncontrolled infection in a patient may produce shock.

Anaphylactic shock. The only really effective treatment for acute allegeric reactions is immediate injection, intravenously, of medication to combat the agent causing the reaction. In general the injection of one single-dose vial of epinephrine intravenously will alleviate the immediate signs of these reactions; such an injection usually must be repeated four or five times as the signs and symptoms recur or worsen. Frequently a drug that is a specific counteragent for the compound causing the reaction can be given. Such treatment usually must be given by a doctor at a medical facility. Therefore, prompt transportation to that facility, while giving all the general support possible, is necessary. The EMT should also attempt to discover or identify what caused the reaction—drugs, insect bites, or food—and how it was received, whether by

mouth or by injection (needle or insect sting).

The severity of such reactions varies greatly. The symptoms may range from mild itching and burning of the skin to a generalized edema, profound coma, and death. Because the EMT often cannot know at once how severe any reaction will be, immediate transportation to a medical facility is important. Supportive measures must be carried out en route.

Metabolic shock. When this condition occurs it usually is the result of illness which has been present for a long while, associated with loss of fluid through vomiting, diarrhea, or urination. With inadequate food and fluid intake to cover the loss of body water, the patient may have literally dried up. Transport this patient to the hospital as promptly as possible, again giving all the support necessary, including intravenous fluid and oxygen during the period of transportation. Try to ascertain the presence of contributory illness, such as diabetes, severe enteritis, and the like.

Intravenous Therapy Administered by the EMT

It is not new for emergency personnel to be responsible for giving intravenous (IV) therapy. Most Emergency Medical Technicians have transported patients who were receiving blood, blood plasma as a blood-volume expander, or intravenous electrolyte solution. What currently is becoming accepted is that most EMTs are being qualified in the technique of starting intravenous fluid therapy, and will under certain circumstances actually carry out the entire procedure of giving these solutions. Ordinarily the EMT will not be responsible for starting IV fluids on children under fourteen. This is the usual age limit in defining the pediatric patient. Intravenous treatment in these patients is difficult because children are not able to cooperate well and their veins are small. Never will the EMT be expected to start IV fluids on an infant. He may, however, be required to transport both infants and children with prior IV fluids running. Under these circumstances he is responsible for the proper maintenance of the system.

There are two important terms to understand

in intravenous therapy. The first is *infusion*. This term implies the administration of fluids other than blood or blood products. These are salt solutions (normal saline, Plasma-Lyte, Ringer's lactate) or sugar solutions (D_5W—5 percent dextrose in water). Solutions so administered expand the blood volume for a very short period of time and then pass out of the intravascular space into the tissues of the body.

Dextran is a solution of a compound whose molecular weight is considerably higher than any of the compounds used in standard salt or sugar solutions. This material stays within the cardiovascular system for a much longer period of time and acts to expand the blood volume much more effectively than intravenous salt or sugar solutions do. It was developed as an artificial blood-volume expander for use in World War II when blood and plasma were not available. It has many side effects, one of which is to alter blood cell membranes so that it is virtually impossible to cross-match the patient for blood after he has received dextran. Use of dextran should be extremely limited and administered only under direct order of a physician.

The second term is *transfusion*. This term applies to the administration of whole blood, packed red cells, cellular products of blood, or other blood products. Ordinarily the EMT will not use these preparations. He will sometimes, however, have to care for a patient receiving blood during transportation. In such instances the EMT must be alert to the signs of a transfusion reaction. These reactions include the sudden development of fever, chills, hives, or itching while a patient is receiving blood.

The administration of cell-free blood products such as plasma or albumin is almost never associated with the development of reactions and can fall under the category of infusions. Almost uniformly, the EMT will be involved with infusions and seldom with transfusions.

Should reactions occur while the patient is under the care of the EMT, the transfusion should be stopped. A careful note should be made of the patient's reaction (fever, hives, chills, or itching) and the container of blood cells or blood products preserved along with all the tubing to be turned over to the receiving

Emergency Department.

In general, the EMT will first learn intravenous therapy technique in the Emergency Department or by assisting a doctor with the administration of fluids to a patient who is being transported from one hospital to another. In these instances the intravenous unit will have already been connected to the patient before the transfer occurs. In other situations or any emergencies, a doctor may request assistance in setting up and administering intravenous fluids before, during, or after an episode of transportation.

In the near future, all EMTs will be trained in this technique. Advance training will be carried out and proper certification will be required. In certain specific situations, most probably occurring in mass disasters or when there is an extremely long transportation period, the EMT may have to carry out the entire procedure alone. Certain basic safety rules and precautions must be observed. While not every technique of intravenous therapy can be covered here, the summary which follows is an introduction to the proper procedures involved.

Equipment needed. Intravenous therapy requires a certain amount of material and supplies (Fig. 9.2). Fluids such as 5 percent or 10 percent glucose (dextrose) in distilled water, 5 percent or 10 percent glucose in normal salt solution, normal salt solution, lactated Ringer's solution, Plasma-Lyte, dextran, other synthetic blood-volume expanders, and whole blood are given intravenously to replace lost blood or plasma or lost body fluids. Additional materials required to effect the therapy properly are tourniquets, arm support boards, the actual IV administration sets, the necessary equipment to cleanse and sterilize the venipuncture site, paper towels, scissors, and adhesive tape. Pens and labels are necessary to identify the containers adequately. A record book is required for recording the essential data on the fluids administered.

Administration of intravenous fluids. The administration of intravenous fluids, other than blood, is commonly a resuscitative measure that can easily be performed by the EMT. The technique of intravenous fluid administration can be learned by practicing on other students or on the

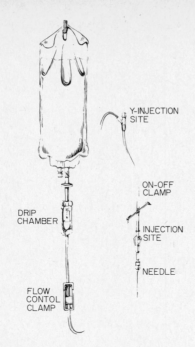

Y-INJECTION
SITE

ON-OFF
CLAMP

DRIP
CHAMBER

INJECTION
SITE

NEEDLE

FLOW
CONTOL
CLAMP

Figure 9.2

The standard intravenous fluid set now used is a plastic bag with attached tubing which allows injection of medicine and addition of other fluids.

78

arm of a mannequin under professional supervision.

The initial replacement transfusion of blood lost by hemorrhage should normally be done in the Emergency Department of a hospital. However, other infusion solutions designed to supply food (glucose) and body salts (electrolytes) can be administered at the site of the accident and during transportation to the hospital.

A most important initial step is to select the proper fluid. Intravenous fluid administration must be ordered by a physician. This can be done through a radio contact if a physician is not present at the scene of an accident.

Those who are permitted to administer intravenous fluids must carefully check the labels of the containers to be certain that the correct fluid ordered by the doctor is being administered and that the expiration date on the bottle of fluid has not passed. The container should be checked for cracks, seal leaks, and content contamination. The fluid should be crystal clear and colorless. If the EMT administers intravenous infusions, an ambulance log must be maintained to include the name of the patient, the type of fluid given, the time the infusion is begun, and the name of the physician authorizing the use of this particular fluid.

Technique of administering intravenous fluids. The following steps are recommended for starting an intravenous infusion:

1. Select the solution ordered by the physician and complete the necessary safety checks.
2. Open a sterile infusion set, which normally should include the following items:
   A drip chamber
   Size 17-, 18-, or 20-gauge needles
   A skin disinfectant
   Adhesive tape 1 inch wide, to be torn into strips four or five inches long
   An armboard
   Bandages
   A tourniquet (rubber tubing)

   There are many types of intravenous infusion equipment sets. Sets may be either permanent or disposable. A permanent set is assembled and sterilized in the sterile supply center of the hospital, and after being used is returned there for repacking and resterilizing. The disposable set, commercially prepared by several companies, is discarded after one use. In general, disposable sets are standard equipment across the country.
3. Using sterile technique, cleanse the top of the solution container, insert the infusion set into the inlet at the top of the bottle, and allow the solution to fill the plastic tubing to expel all the air bubbles. When fully prepared, the set should resemble the one shown in Figure 9.2.
4. Select a vein of an uninjured extremity for venipuncture. When possible, it is convenient to use veins on the anterior surface of the elbow. These vessels lie in what is termed the antecubital fossa and are ordinarily large and easily punctured (Fig. 9.3 *a*).
5. Apply a tourniquet or a blood pressure cuff two to three inches above the selected vein (Fig. 9.3 *a*) tight enough to restrict venous flow toward the heart but not so

tight that the arterial pulse will be cut off (40 mm Hg in the blood pressure cuff).

6. Attach a sterile needle to the plastic tubing adapter, open the clamp and allow some fluid to run through the needle to remove all the air. Reclamp the tubing and cleanse the venipuncture site with skin disinfectant. It is best to select the largest caliber needle that one can insert comfortably, usually 18-gauge.

7. With the thumb apply traction on the skin below the site of the venipuncture. Align the needle along the vein. With the needle bevel in an "up" position, pierce the skin at a 15-degree angle directly over the vein (Fig. 9.3 b). Continue to insert the needle slowly until you feel a "give" and blood appears in the needle adapter (Fig. 9.3 c). Lower the needle so that it is parallel to the vein walls and carefully thread the needle at least one-half its length into the vein (Fig. 9.3 d).

8. Release the tourniquet with one hand, being careful to maintain a grip on the needle with the other. Open the clamp and allow the intravenous solution to drip. A free-flowing drip in the chamber indicates that the needle is in the vein properly. Secure the needle in place with several strips of adhesive tape over the hub of the needle. The tubing should have some slack which should also be secured to prevent any dislodgment of the needle (Fig. 9.3 e).

9. Carefully monitor the drip chamber and adjust the screw clamp to achieve the infusion rate prescribed by the physician. Ordinarily twenty drops in a standard drip chamber equal 1 milliliter. An infusion rate of 125 ml/hr is just over 2 ml/minute or 40 drops/minute.

Transfusions. In blood transfusions a disposable, sterile, blood-recipient set with a filter chamber and a drip chamber is used. These units are separately packaged and labeled. The filter chamber prevents the transmission of clots to the patient. The same technique of venipuncture is used as in the administration of other fluids. With transfusions it is even more impor-

tant to select the largest caliber needle available.

Complications. All patients receiving intravenous fluid must be checked frequently. Swelling around the site of the injection indicates the needle may not be in the vein and that the fluid is running into the tissue around it (infiltration). The EMT should monitor the flow carefully. A change in the rate of flow or its cessation requires correction of blocks in the tubing or the needle.

There are occasional reactions when the patient is receiving whole blood. Signs of a reaction that require stopping a transfusion and checking with the physician are as follows:

Mild reaction
  Itching of the skin and hives

 Major or severe reaction
   Difficulty in breathing
   Chills or fever
   Nausea
   Extremely rapid and weak pulse
   Low blood pressure
   Abdominal cramps
   Flushing of the face
   Back pains
   Symptoms of shock

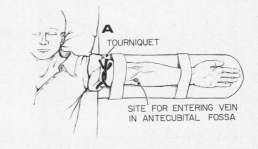

A
TOURNIQUET

SITE FOR ENTERING VEIN IN ANTECUBITAL FOSSA

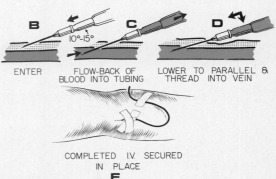

B
10°-15°
ENTER

C
FLOW-BACK OF BLOOD INTO TUBING

D
LOWER TO PARALLEL & THREAD INTO VEIN

COMPLETED I.V. SECURED IN PLACE
E

Figure 9.3 *a—e*

Selection of a vein and insertion of a needle for intravenous fluid therapy are shown.

These signs are also common following severe injuries. When they occur in a trauma victim who is receiving a transfusion, his vital signs must also be carefully monitored to try to find some clue to the cause of the particular signs and symptoms. Ordinarily such complications are not seen with straight infusions of fluid, plasma, or albumin. If such signs occur it is best to stop a transfusion and replace it with a balanced salt solution. Remember to turn blood bottle and tubing over to the receiving hospital so that the occurrence of the reaction may be documented.

CHAPTER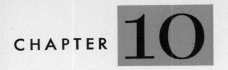

Basic Life Support

GOAL I.   Understand the reasons for basic life support.

OBJECTIVES

A. Define basic life support.
B. Describe the general state of a patient needing basic life support.
C. Describe the circumstances under which CPR is terminated.

GOAL II.   Know the procedures of artificial ventilation.

OBJECTIVES

A. Describe the steps in beginning artificial ventilation.
B. Describe the head-tilt maneuver.
C. List the steps in the jaw-thrust maneuver.
D. Recognize and describe the care of the patient with an airway obstruction.
E. Describe care of the airway in a patient with spinal injuries.
F. Describe mouth-to-mouth ventilation and its problems.
G. Describe the special cases where mouth-to-mouth techniques are not appropriate.

GOAL III. Know the procedures for instituting artificial circulation.

OBJECTIVES

A. Describe the technique of closed-chest compression.
B. Describe resuscitation techniques by two persons and by one person.
C. Describe the differences in resuscitation techniques for children.
D. Describe the precordial thump.

GOAL IV. Know the adjunctive equipment available for basic life support and how to use it.

OBJECTIVES

A. List the indications for and advantages of the use of supplemental oxygen in CPR.
B. List the risks of oxygen therapy.
C. Describe mouth-to-mask breathing techniques.
D. Describe bag-valve-mask breathing techniques.
E. List the types of artificial airways and their uses.
F. Describe the techniques of oropharyngeal and nasopharyngeal suctioning.

Oxygen, which is present in the atmosphere in a concentration of about 21 percent, is essential for the life of all cells. The brain, the principal organ for conscious living, starts to die if deprived of oxygen for as little as four minutes. In the delivery of oxygen from the atmosphere to the brain cells, there are two necessary components, breathing and circulation. Breathing (taking in oxygen through the body's air passages) and the circulation of oxygen-enriched blood are both required. Any profound disturbance of the airway, the breathing, or the circulation can promptly produce brain death.

82

Essentials

Basic life support is an emergency lifesaving procedure that consists of recognizing and correcting failure of the respiratory or cardiovascular systems. Basic life support includes the ABC steps of cardiopulmonary resuscitation: Airway, **B**reathing, and **C**irculation. Prompt application

of basic life support is indicated for

A—**A**irway obstruction
B—**B**reathing (respiratory) arrest
C—**C**irculatory, or cardiac (heart), arrest (Fig. 10.1)

Correct application of the steps of cardiopulmonary resuscitation can maintain life until the patient recovers sufficiently to be transported to a medical facility or until advanced life support can be delivered to the patient.

Basic life support is distinct from advanced life support. The latter consists of the use of adjunctive equipment, cardiac monitoring, defibrillation, the maintenance of an intravenous fluid lifeline, and the infusion of appropriate drugs.

Urgency

There must be a maximum sense of urgency in starting basic life support. The outstanding

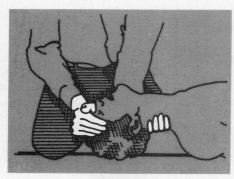

AIRWAY

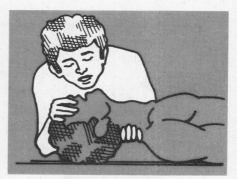

BREATHING

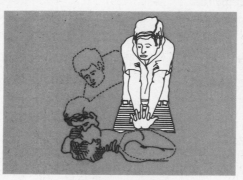

CIRCULATION

Figure 10.1

The ABC steps of cardiopulmonary resuscitation—Airway, Breathing, Circulation—are the essential components of basic life support.

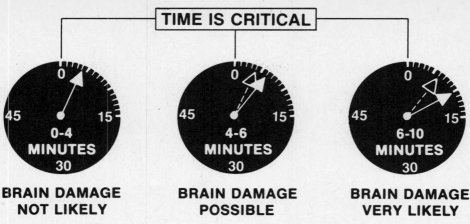

TIME IS CRITICAL

0-4 MINUTES	4-6 MINUTES	6-10 MINUTES
BRAIN DAMAGE NOT LIKELY	**BRAIN DAMAGE POSSIBLE**	**BRAIN DAMAGE VERY LIKELY**

83

Figure 10.2

Time is critical. Deprived of oxygen for four to six minutes, brain damage is likely to occur. After six minutes without oxygen, brain damage is extremely likely.

advantage of cardiopulmonary resuscitation (CPR) is that it permits the earliest possible treatment of airway obstruction, respiratory arrest, or cardiac arrest by properly trained persons. Optimally, only seconds should intervene between recognizing the need and starting the treatment. The inadequacy or absence of breathing or circulation must be determined immediately.

If breathing alone is inadequate or absent, opening the airway or giving rescue breathing may be all that is necessary. If circulation is also absent, artificial circulation must be instituted in combination with the artificial respiration. If breathing stops before the heart stops, enough oxygen will be available in the lungs to maintain life for several minutes. But if heart arrest occurs first, delivery of oxygen to the brain ceases immediately. Brain damage is possible if the brain is deprived of oxygen for four to six minutes. Beyond six minutes without oxygen, brain damage is very likely (Fig. 10.2). Speed is essential in determining the need for and instituting the procedures of basic life support.

Beginning and Terminating Basic Life Support

CPR is most effective when started immediately after cardiac arrest. If there is any question of the exact duration of the arrest, the patient should be given the benefit of the doubt and re-

suscitation started at once. CPR is not indicated, however, for a patient who is known to be in the terminal stages of an incurable condition.

When resuscitation is indicated and started in the absence of a physician, it should be continued until one of the following events occurs:

1. Until effective spontaneous circulation and ventilation are restored
2. Until resuscitation efforts are transferred to another responsible person who continues basic life support
3. Until a physician assumes responsibility
4. Until the EMT is exhausted and unable to continue resuscitation efforts

Unconsciousness

An unconscious patient must be carefully checked to see which steps of basic life support are needed. Unconsciousness is established by observing the responses of the patient to verbal or painful stimuli. In addition, to exclude the possibility of spinal injuries, the EMT should also ask witnesses if the patient had a fall, or look for evidence of an accident or a fall. If no evidence of such injuries is present, he may institute life support without great concern for spinal damage. Conversely, if he suspects spinal injuries, he must take care to protect the spinal cord. Unconscious states, spinal injuries, and head injuries are each treated in separate chapters in this text.

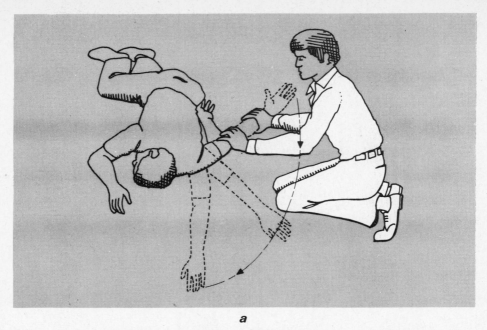

a

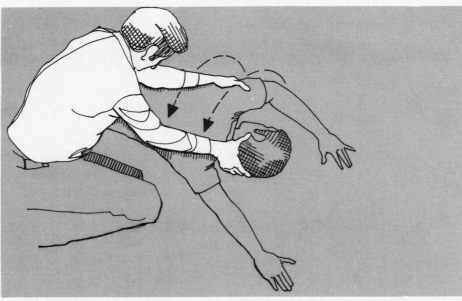

b

Positioning the patient. For cardiopulmonary resuscitation to be effective, the patient must be horizontal, supine, and on a firm surface; for, even flawlessly performed, external heart compression will produce no blood flow to the brain if the body is in a vertical position. Airway management and rescue breathing are also more easily achieved when the patient is supine.

It is imperative, therefore, to position the un-

conscious patient supine and horizontal as quickly as possible in situations where he is found vertical. If the patient is lying crumpled up or face down, it will be necessary to reposition him. Considerable caution must be taken, particularly if a neck or back injury is suspected. The patient must be rolled as a single unit of head, neck, and back. Elevating the lower extremities about twelve inches while keeping the

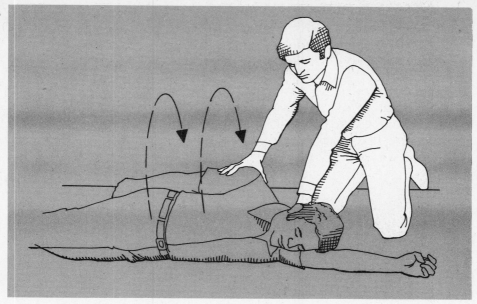

c

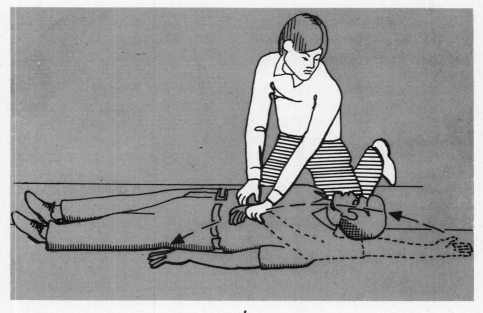

d

Figure 10.3 *a–d*

The steps for properly rolling the patient into a supine position are shown. (*a*) The EMT brings the patient's nearer arm above his head. (*b*) He places one hand behind the back of the patient's head and neck and the other hand on the distant shoulder. (*c*) He rolls the patient toward himself by pulling the shoulder. (*d*) Once the patient is flat, his arm is brought back to his side.

rest of the body horizontal may promote venous blood return and assist artificial circulation if external cardiac compression is required.

The EMT kneels by the patient, but not in contact and sufficiently far away so that when the patient is rolled toward him, the patient does not end up in his lap. He rapidly straightens the patient's legs and moves the patient's nearer arm above his head (Fig. 10.3 *a*). The EMT then places one hand behind the back of the head and neck of the patient and the other hand on the distant shoulder (Fig. 10.3 b). The patient then is pulled toward the EMT by pulling the shoulder, but the head and neck are controlled so that they turn with the rest of the torso as a unit (Fig. 10.3 c). In this way, the head and neck remain in the same vertical plane as the back, and further spinal injury can be prevented. When the patient is flat on his back, the EMT brings his arm back to his side (Fig. 10.3 d). Now airway, breathing, and circulation can be assessed and treated.

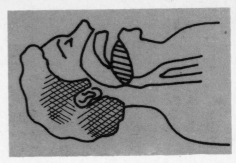

Figure 10.4

   When the patient is unconscious, his tongue can fall back into the pharynx, blocking and obstructing the upper airway.

Artificial Ventilation

   Respiratory inadequacy may result from an obstruction of the airway or from respiratory failure. An obstructed airway is sometimes difficult to recognize until the initial steps of airway management have been attempted. At other times, a partially obstructed airway can be recognized by labored breathing, by excessive respiratory efforts involving the necessary muscles of respiration, and by retraction of the intercostal, supraclavicular, and suprasternal spaces. Respiratory failure or arrest is characterized by minimal or absent respiratory efforts, failure of the chest or upper abdomen to move, and no detectable air movement through the nose or mouth.

   Opening the airway and restoring breathing are the basic steps of artificial ventilation. The steps can be performed quickly under almost any circumstances, without equipment, and without help from another person. They constitute emergency medical care for airway obstruction, respiratory failure, or respiratory arrest.

Opening the Airway

   Immediate opening of the airway is the most important factor in successful artificial ventilation. The airway may be blocked by the patient's own tongue or by foreign material in the mouth or throat.

   Head-tilt maneuver. When consciousness is

lost, muscles relax. The result is that an unconscious patient's tongue can fall back into the pharynx, blocking it and obstructing the upper airway (Fig. 10.4).

   Opening the airway to relieve the obstruction caused by the tongue is accomplished easily and quickly by tilting the patient's head backward as far as possible (Fig. 10.5 a). This procedure is known as the head-tilt maneuver Sometimes this simple maneuver is all that is required to cause the patient to resume breathing spontaneously. For the head tilt to be performed, the patient must be lying on his back. Kneeling close to the patient, the EMT places one hand beneath the patient's neck and the other hand on his forehead. The EMT then lifts the neck with one hand and tilts the head backward by pressure with the other hand on the forehead (Fig. 10.5 b). The hands should not be crossed or reach over the patient's neck. The head-tilt maneuver extends the neck and lifts the tongue away from the back of the throat, relieving any obstruction of the airway caused by the tongue. The neck must then be maintained in the extended position until a more permanent airway is secured.

   Hyperextension of the neck, however, is flatly contraindicated in patients who have suffered a broken neck, as it may cause permanent paralysis. It is imperative to underscore the fact that spinal injuries must be initially sought and treated.

   Jaw-thrust maneuver. The head-tilt method is effective for most patients. If head tilt does not

86

open the air passage adequately, an additional forward movement of the lower jaw—the jaw thrust—may be required. The thrust is a triple maneuver in which the EMT places his fingers behind the angles of the patient's lower jaw. He then

1. Forcefully brings the jaw forward
2. Tilts the head backward
3. Uses his thumbs to pull the lower lip down to allow breathing through the mouth as well as through the nose

The jaw thrust is performed best with the

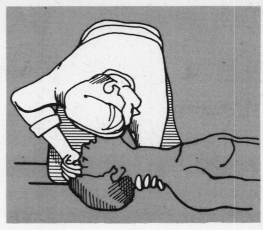

Figure 10.6

Respiration is determined by feeling the movement of air on the cheek, by hearing it, and by seeing the chest and abdomen move with each breath.

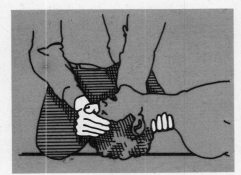

AIRWAY

a

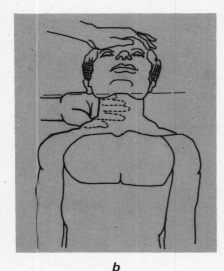

b

Figure 10.5 *a–b*

The head-tilt maneuver is demonstrated. (*a*) One hand beneath lifts the patient's neck. (*b*) The other hand on the forehead tilts the head backward.

EMT in a position at the top of the patient's head.

Once the airway has been opened, the patient may or may not start to breathe again. To assess whether breathing has returned, the EMT must turn his head and place an ear about one inch above the nose and mouth of the patient (Fig. 10.6). Signs of breathing are present if the EMT can feel and hear movement of air and can see the patients chest and abdomen move. Feeling and hearing are far more important than seeing. With airway obstruction it is possible there will be no air movement even though the chest and abdomen rise and fall with the patient's attempts to breathe. Also, observing chest and abdominal movement is difficult in a fully clothed individual. Finally, there may be no chest movement even with normal breathing in patients who have chronic obstructive lung disease.

Artificial Respiration

No equipment is required to give effective artificial ventilation. It should never be delayed while the EMT obtains or applies devices for ventilatory assistance. Artificial ventilation, whether mouth-to-mouth, mouth-to-nose, or mouth-to-stoma, should deliver at least twelve breaths per minute.

87

Mouth-to-mouth. If the patient does not promptly resume adequate spontaneous breathing after the airway is opened, artificial ventilation must be started. Mouth-to-mouth breathing and mouth-to-nose breathing are both types of artificial ventilation. The breath exhaled by the EMT contains about 16 percent oxygen; this content is sufficient to sustain the patient's life.

To perform mouth-to-mouth ventilation, the EMT keeps or places one hand under the patient's neck. With the other hand, he pinches the patient's nostrils together, using the thumb and index finger, while with the heel of his hand he continues to exert pressure on the forehead to maintain the backward tilt of the head (Fig. 10.7 *a*). The EMT then opens his mouth widely, takes a deep breath, makes a tight seal with his mouth around the patient's mouth, and exhales into the patient's mouth (Fig. 10.7 *b*). He then removes his mouth and allows the patient to exhale passively, turning his head slightly to watch the patient's chest fall. The first four breaths must be given in rapid succession without waiting for the patient's lungs to deflate completely between breaths. This succession of breaths creates what is called the "staircase effect."

Adequate ventilation is insured on every breath if the EMT does the following:

1. Sees the chest rise and fall
2. Can feel in his own airway the resistance of the patient's lungs as they expand
3. Hears and feels the air escape during exhalation

When using jaw thrust for mouth-to-mouth ventilation, the EMT must move to the patient's side. He must keep the patient's mouth open with his thumbs and seal the nose by placing his cheek against the nostrils.

Mouth-to-nose. In some cases, mouth-to-nose ventilation is more effective than mouth-to-mouth ventilation. The former is recommended when it is impossible to open the patient's mouth, when it is impossible to ventilate through the mouth because of severe facial injuries, when it is difficult to achieve a tight seal around the mouth in a patient without any teeth, or when,

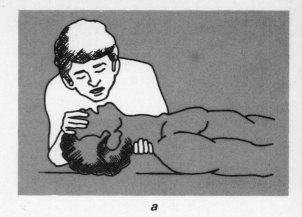

a

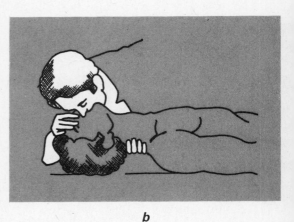

b

Figure 10.7 *a–b*

Mouth-to-mouth ventilation is achieved (*a*) by the EMT's sealing off the patient's nose, and (*b*) by encircling the patient's open mouth with his mouth, and exhaling deeply into it.

for some other reason, the EMT prefers the nasal route.

For the mouth-to-nose technique, the EMT keeps the patient's head tilted back with one hand on the forehead and uses the other hand to lift the patient's lower jaw. This maneuver seals the lips. The EMT then takes a deep breath, seals his lips around the patient's nose, and blows in until he feels the lungs expand. When he removes his mouth, the patient is allowed to exhale passively. The EMT can see the chest fall when the patient exhales. When mouth-to-nose ventilation is used, it may be necessary to open the patient's mouth or separate his lips to allow the air to escape during exhalation because the soft palate may cause nasopharyngeal obstruction.

When using jaw thrust for mouth-to-nose ventilation, the EMT uses his cheek to seal the patient's mouth and does not retract the lower lip with his thumbs.

Mouth-to-stoma. Direct mouth-to-stoma artificial ventilation must be used for persons who have had a laryngectomy. These persons have a permanent stoma (opening) in the neck, which connects the trachea directly to the skin. It may be seen as an opening at the center, in front, at the base of the neck. In many of these patients there will be other openings in the neck, according to the type of operation done and reconstruction attempted. Any opening other than the main mid-line tracheal stoma, however, should be ignored, for it is the only one which can be used to put air into the patient's lungs. In general, any other neck opening will lie on one side or the other but not in the mid-line.

Neither head-tilt nor jaw-thrust maneuvers are required for mouth-to-stoma resuscitation. If the patient has a tube in the tracheal stoma, the EMT blows into the tube. It may be necessary to seal the patient's mouth and nose with a hand to prevent a leak of air up the trachea when blowing into a tracheostomy tube.

Infants and children. Opening the airway and performing artificial ventilation are essentially the same for children as for adults, but there are a few differences. For infants and small children, the EMT should cover both the mouth and nose of the child with his mouth and use small breaths with less volume to inflate the lungs. The tilted position of the head should not be exaggerated, as the neck of an infant is so flexible that forceful backward tilting may dislocate the cervical spine. Infants should receive the smaller-volume breaths every three seconds.

Gastric distention. Artificial ventilation frequently causes distention of the stomach. This event occurs most often in children, but it is also common in adults. It is most likely to occur when excessive pressures are used for inflation or when the airway is obstructed. Slight gastric distention may be disregarded, but marked inflation of the stomach is dangerous because it promotes regurgitation and reduces lung volume by elevating the diaphragm. Obvious gross distention should be relieved promptly whenever possible. Frequently one can do so by exerting moderate pressure on the patient's abdomen between the umbilicus and the rib cage with the flat of the hand. To prevent aspiration of gastric contents during this maneuver, the patient's head and shoulders should be turned to one side and a suction device kept ready for immediate use.

Airway Obstruction

Upper-airway obstruction can cause unconsciousness and cardiopulmonary arrest, or it can be a result of the arrest itself. Either event can be fatal.

Sudden airway obstruction by a foreign body in an adult usually occurs during eating; in a child it occurs during eating or at play (sucking small objects).

There can be other causes of airway obstruction. A patient who becomes unconscious can develop airway obstruction because the tongue falls back into the pharynx, blocking it and obstructing the upper airway. Regurgitation of stomach contents into the pharynx can occur during a cardiopulmonary arrest or during resuscitative attempts and thereby block the airway. Also, head and facial injuries may result in blood clots that obstruct the upper airway, particularly if the patient is unconscious.

Recognition of Foreign Body Obstruction

Early recognition of airway obstruction is the key to successful management of it. The EMT must learn to differentiate between primary airway obstruction and other conditions resulting in respiratory failure or arrest, such as fainting, stroke, or heart attack.

The EMT can be faced with two situations in which upper-airway obstruction is present:

1. The patient may be conscious when discovered but become unconscious.

2. The patient may be unconscious when discovered.

Conscious patient. Sudden upper-airway obstruction is usually recognized when a patient who is eating or has just finished eating is suddenly unable to speak or cough, grasps at his throat, appears cyanotic, or shows exaggerated breathing efforts. Air movement is either absent or not detectable.

Patient becomes unconscious. Initially the patient will remain conscious but if the obstruction is not removed within a short period of time, the oxygen in the lungs will be used up because the obstructed airway prevents the entry of air into the lungs. Unconsciousness and death will follow.

Patient found unconscious. When a patient is discovered unconscious, the cause is initially unknown. The unconsciousness may have been caused by airway obstruction or cardiopulmonary arrest. Any patient discovered unconscious must be managed as a cardiopulmonary arrest, and management of an obstructed airway dealt with only as it becomes apparent during the correct sequence of resuscitative maneuvers.

Maneuvers to Relieve Upper-Airway Obstruction

Back blows. A series of back blows should be delivered in rapid succession. These consist of sharp blows delivered with the hand over the patient's spine between the shoulder blades. The technique should be applied whether the patient is sitting, standing, or lying down.

With patient sitting or standing

1. The EMT positions himself at the side and slightly behind the patient.
2. He delivers sharp blows with the hand to the patient's spine between the shoulder blades.
3. The other hand may be placed in front of the patient's chest to support him.

With patient lying down

1. The EMT kneels down and rolls the patient

toward him so that the patient's chest rests against the EMT's knees.
2. He delivers sharp blows with the hand to the patient's spine between the shoulder blades (Fig. 10.8).

The technique should be modified for an infant or small child by holding it head down, supported on the EMT's forearm, while the back blows are delivered (Fig. 10.9).

Manual thrusts. A rapid series of thrusts is delivered to the upper abdomen (abdominal thrust/Heimlich Maneuver) or lower chest (chest thrust).

Abdominal thrust, with patient sitting or standing

1. The EMT stands behind the patient and wraps his arms about the patient's waist.
2. He grasps one fist with his other hand and places the thumb side of his fist against the patient's abdomen, between the xiphoid and umbilicus (navel).
3. He presses the fist into the patient's abdomen with a quick upward thrust (Fig. 10.10).

Abdominal thrust with patient lying down

The EMT should modify the technique as follows:

1. He positions the patient supine and kneels close to the patient's hips.
2. He places the heel of one hand against the patient's abdomen, between the xiphoid and umbilicus. The second hand is placed on top of the first.
3. He presses the hand into the patient's abdomen with a quick upward thrust (Fig. 10.11).

Instead of performing this maneuver from the patient's side, the EMT may straddle either the hips or one leg of the patient.

Chest thrust. When the patient is markedly larger in the abdomen and the EMT is unable to wrap his arms fully about it, as in advanced pregnancy or gross obesity, an alternate technique—chest thrust—can be applied.

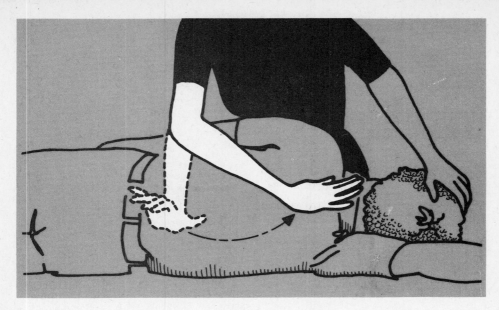

Figure 10.8

A series of sharp back blows delivered rapidly with the heel of the hand to the patient's spine between the shoulder blades will often dislodge an obstruction in the airway of an adult. The patient may be sitting, standing, or on his side.

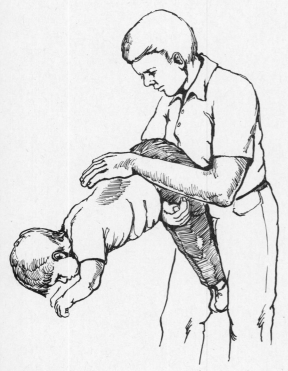

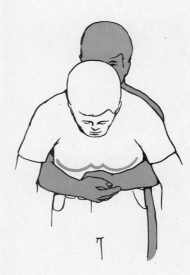

Figure 10.9

A child may be turned head down over an adult's arm and struck several times between the shoulder blades. The head must be lower than the body so the object can fall out of the airway.

Figure 10.10

The abdominal thrust with the patient sitting or standing is shown. The EMT stands behind the patient and wraps his arms around the patient's waist, grasps one fist with the other hand, and places the thumb side of the fist against the patient's abdomen, between the xiphoid and the umbilicus. The fist is pressed into the patient's abdomen with a quick *upward* thrust.

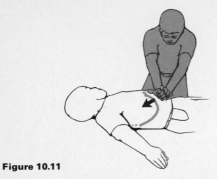

Figure 10.11

The abdominal thrust with the patient supine is shown. The EMT positions the patient flat and kneels close to or astride his hips. The EMT places the heel of one hand against the patient's abdomen, between the xiphoid and the umbilicus. With the other hand resting on top of the first, the EMT presses into the patient's abdomen with a quick *upward* thrust.

92

Chest thrust with patient sitting or standing

1. The EMT wraps his hands under the patient's arms to encircle the patient's lower chest.
2. He graps one fist with his other hand, with the thumb side of the fist on the lower sternum but clear of the xiphoid process.
3. He presses his fist into the patient's chest with a quick backward thrust (Fig. 10.12).

Chest thrust with patient lying down

1. The EMT positions the patient supine, with the EMT's knees close to the patient.

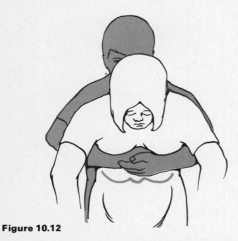

Figure 10.12

The chest thrust with the patient sitting or standing is shown. The EMT stands behind and encircles the patient's lower chest with his arms. He grasps one fist with his other hand, with the thumb side of the fist on the lower sternum but clear of the xiphoid process. He presses his fist into the patient's chest with a quick *backward* thrust.

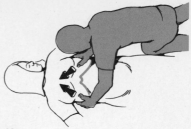

Figure 10.13

The chest thrust with patient lying supine is shown. The EMT positions the patient flat on the back and kneels close to or astride the patient. The EMT places one hand on either side of the patient's lower chest with the heels of the hands in line with the axillae and the fingers wrapped around the side of the patient's chest. With the hands in this position, the EMT squeezes the patient's chest with a quick *downward* thrust of the arms and an *upward* thrust of the hands.

2. He places one hand on either side of the patient's lower chest, with the heels of the hands in line with the axillae (armpits) and the fingers wrapped about the side of the patient's chest.
3. He squeezes the patient's chest with a quick downward thrust of the arms and an inward thrust of the hands (Fig. 10.13).

Combined use of back blows and manual thrusts. Back blows produce an instantaneous increase in pressure in the respiratory passages which may result in either partial or complete dislodgement of a foreign body. The manual thrusts produce a lower, though more sustained, increase in pressure in the respiratory passages and may further assist in the dislodgement of the foreign body. The combination of these two techniques appears to be a more effective method of clearing upper-airway obstruction than the single use of one or the other.

Manual removal of foreign body. If at any time the foreign body causing the airway obstruction appears in the mouth or is believed to be in the mouth, it should be removed by the EMT with his fingers.

Back blows and manual thrusts may dislodge the foreign body but not expel it, for when unconsciousness occurs, the patient's jaw muscles relax. The EMT should turn the patient's head away from him, open the patient's mouth with the cross-finger technique, and clear the airway obstruction with finger probes (Fig. 10.14).

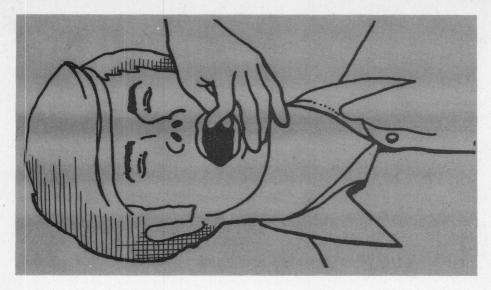

Figure 10.14

The cross-finger technique is performed by crossing the thumb under the index finger. The thumb is then placed against the lower teeth and the index finger against the upper teeth. As the fingers are spread apart, the patient's jaw will be forced open.

Cross-finger technique for opening the mouth

1. The thumb is crossed under the index finger.
2. The thumb and index finger are braced against the patient's lower and upper teeth respectively.
3. As the fingers are pushed apart, the patient's jaw is forced open.

Finger probes

1. Hold the patient's jaws open with the cross-finger technique.
2. Use the index finger of the other hand as a hook to sweep down the inside of the patient's upper cheek to the base of the tongue.
3. The index finger is then used as a hook to attempt to dislodge the impacted foreign body up into the mouth.
4. When the foreign body comes within reach, grasp and remove it.

Care should be taken when finger probes are attempted that a dislodged foreign body is not pushed back into the airway.

A summary of the maneuvers in proper sequence is given in Table 10.1.

Artificial Circulation

A disturbance of the regular rhythm of the heart may prevent adequate cardiac contraction, resulting in failure to generate blood flow and produce a pulse. The absence of a strong palpable central pulse, such as the carotid pulse in the neck, indicates no blood flow and hence cardiac arrest.

After determining unconsciousness, turning the patient if necessary, opening the airway, and giving four quick breaths, the EMT must assess the status of the patient's circulation. Cardiac arrest (lack of effective circulation) is determined by the absence of a palpable pulse in a large artery. The carotid pulse is such an artery; it is close to the heart, large in diameter, and palpable in the neck. It is found most easily by locating the larynx at the front of the neck and then sliding two fingers toward either side of the neck. The pulse is felt in the groove between the larynx and the sternomastoid muscle with the pulp of the index and the middle fingers (Fig. 10.15). Light pressure is sufficient. Excessive pressure should not be applied because it can obstruct the circulation, dislodge blood clots, or produce marked cardiac slowing.

TABLE 10.1

**Sequence of Maneuvers in Attempt to Clear
Airway Obstruction**

In the Conscious Patient
1. Give 4 back blows
2. Perform 8 manual thrusts
3. Alternate each until the airway is clear or the patient becomes unconscious

If the Patient Becomes Unconscious
1. Place him supine
2. Open the airway and attempt to ventilate
3. If unsuccessful
   a. Give 4 back blows
   b. Perform 8 manual thrusts
   c. Turn the head, open the jaw using the cross-finger technique and probe with the fingers to clear the airway
4. Reposition the head and attempt to ventilate
5. If unsuccessful, repeat no. 3 and no. 4
   If the foreign body appears, or is suspected to be in the mouth, interrupt the sequence and remove it.

When the Patient is Found Unconscious
1. Shake and shout*
2. Establish the airway, check for breathing, and attempt to ventilate. In cases of suspected neck injury, open the airway by the modified jaw thrust instead of the head tilt
3. If unable to ventilate, reposition the head and attempt again to ventilate†
4. If attempts to ventilate remain unsuccessful and the EMT suspects the pharynx contains regurgitated stomach contents or blood clots, turn the patient's head, neck, and torso as a unit, open his mouth with cross-finger technique, sweep out the pharynx with two fingers of the other hand, and attempt to ventilate
5. If unsuccessful
   a. Give 4 back blows
   b. Perform 8 manual thrusts
   c. Turn the head again, open mouth using cross-finger technique and probe with fingers to clear airway†
6. Reposition the head and attempt to ventilate†
7. If unsuccessful, repeat nos. 5 and 6
8. When successful ventilation has been achieved, assess the carotid pulse, and perform external cardiac compression if necessary

---

* If neck injury is present or suspected, do not shake the patient.

† If neck injury is present or suspected, do not turn or reposition the head except as a unit of head, neck, and torso.

The hand on the forehead which had previously been maintaining backward head tilt can be left in position to maintain the airway, but it is not necessary to continue to pinch off the nostrils. The hand previously placed beneath the neck is used for locating the carotid pulse.

If the pulse is present but breathing is absent,

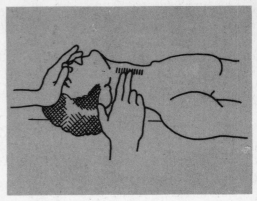

Figure 10.15

The carotid pulse is felt in the groove between the larynx and the sternomastoid muscle.

the EMT should breathe for the patient once every five seconds until adequate spontaneous breathing resumes.

If the pulse is absent, the EMT should start external cardiac compression, which adds artificial circulation to the already initiated artificial ventilation.

External Cardiac Compression

The heart lies slightly to the left of the middle of the chest between the sternum and the spine (Fig. 10.16). Rhythmic pressure and relaxation applied to the lower one-half of the sternum compresses the heart and produces an artificial circulation. In a patient with cardiac arrest, the carotid artery flow resulting from external cardiac compression is only about one-quarter to one-third normal. **External cardiac compression must always be accompanied by artificial ventilation.**

The patient must be on a firm, flat surface. This may be the ground, the floor, or a spineboard on a wheeled litter. If the patient is in bed, put him on the floor. Chest compression must not be delayed to seek a spineboard or other support.

Technique of external cardiac compression. The EMT kneels close to the patient's side with one knee at the level of the head and the other knee at the level of the upper chest. He places the heel of one hand on the lower half of the sternum. Great care must be exercised **not** to

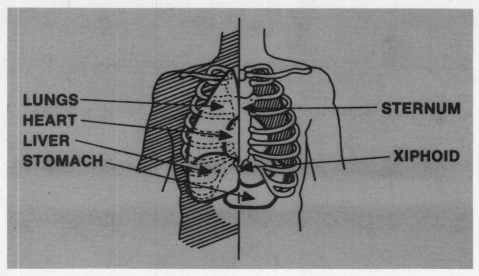

Figure 10.16

The heart lies slightly to the left of the middle of the chest between the sternum and spine, with the lungs on either side and with the liver and stomach below.

place the hand on the lower tip of the sternum (xiphoid process), which extends downward over the upper abdomen (Fig. 10.17), or beside the sternum onto the ribs. Correct positioning of the hands is achieved in the following manner. The index and middle fingers of the hand nearer the patient's feet are slid along the edge of the ribcage until the fingers reach the notch in the center chest (Fig. 10.18 *a*). The middle finger is pushed as high as possible into the notch and the index finger is then laid on the lower portion of the sternum with the two fingers touching each other (Fig. 10.18 *b*).

The heel of the second hand is then placed on the lower half of the sternum (Fig. 10.18 *c*) with the heel of the hand touching the index finger of

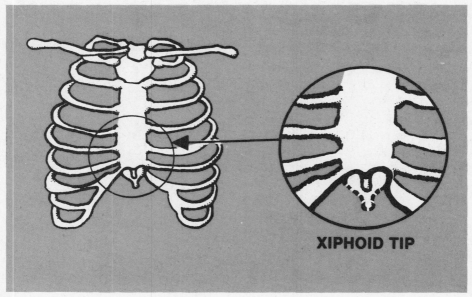

Figure 10.17

The xiphoid process is at the lower tip of the sternum and extends downward over the upper abdomen.

96

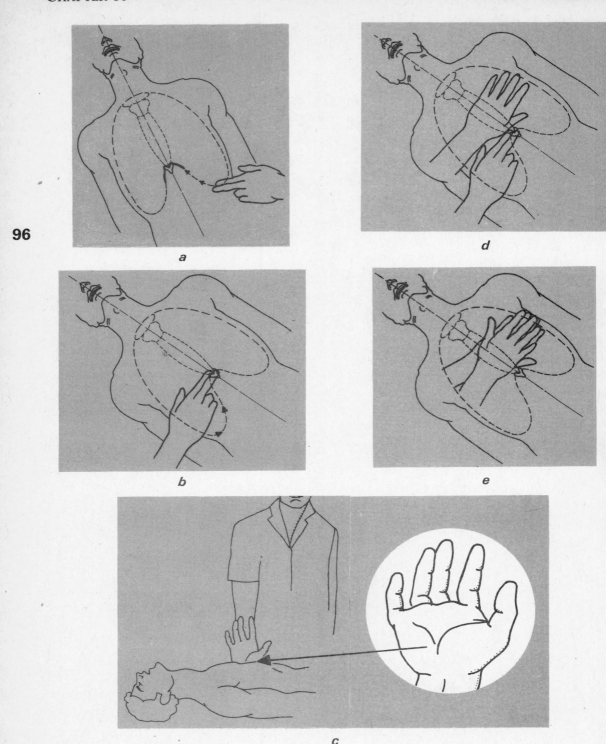

Figure 10.18 *a–e*

The correct hand position for cardiac compression is shown. (*a*) The index and middle fingers of the EMT's hand nearer the patient's feet are slid along the center of the patient's ribcage to the notch in the center of the chest. (*b*) The middle finger is pushed high into the notch, and the index finger laid on the lower portion of the sternum. (*c*) The heel of the second hand is then placed on the lower half of the sternum, (*d*) touching the index finger of the first hand. (*e*) The first hand is then removed from the notch and applied over and parallel to the hand on the patient's lower sternum.

the first hand (Fig. 10.18 *d*). The first hand is then removed from the notch in the center of the ribcage and applied over and parallel to the hand now resting on the patient's lower sternum (Fig. 10.18 *e*). **Only the heel of one hand is in contact with the lower half of the sternum.**

The technique may be improved or made more comfortable for the EMT if the fingers of the lower hand are interlocked with the fingers of the upper and pulled slightly away from the chest wall.

Pressure is then exerted vertically downward through both arms to depress the adult sternum one and one-half to two inches. A rocking motion allows pressure to be delivered vertically downward from the shoulders while the arms are kept straight (Fig. 10.19). Vertical pressure downward produces a compression, which should be immediately followed by a period of relaxation. Compression and relaxation should be of the same duration. The heel of the EMT's hand should not be removed from the chest during relaxation, but pressure on the sternum should be completely released so it can return to its normal resting position between compressions. Compression and relaxation must be rhythmic. The EMT must not jab downward; neither should his hands bounce or come away from the patient's chest (Fig. 10.20).

Resuscitation. When two EMTs are performing CPR, one giving cardiac compression and

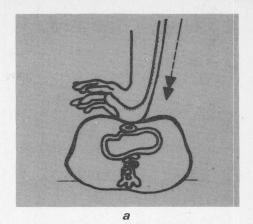

a

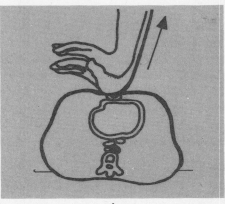

b

Figure 10.20 *a–b*

Compression and relaxation should be rhythmic and of equal duration. The heel of the hand should not be removed from the sternum, but pressure on the sternum should be released so it can return to its normal resting position between compressions.

the other artificial ventilation, the compression rate should be 60 per minute, with a single breath given after each fifth compression (ratio 5:1). To help maintain a compression rate of 60 per minute, the EMT delivering the compressions can count: "One thousand and one, one thousand and two, one thousand and three," etc., as approximately one second is required to say this phrase. Two EMTs can provide more effective CPR than a single EMT because ventilation can be delivered without any pause in compression; and, since cardiac compression is not interrupted, blood flow is never allowed to fall to zero.

With two EMTs, CPR should be performed with an EMT on each side of the patient (Fig. 10.21). They can then switch positions when

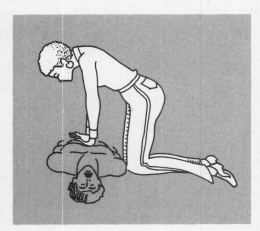

Figure 10.19

External cardiac compression is produced by vertical downward pressure through both arms to depress the adult sternum one and one-half to two inches.

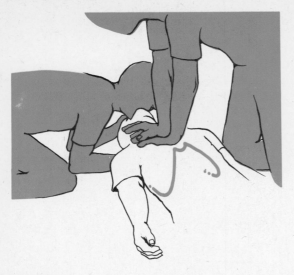

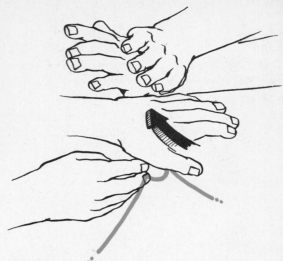

98

Figure 10.21

  When two EMTs are performing CPR, one is on each side of the patient. Here, one EMT is performing mouth-to-mouth ventilation while the other is delivering external cardiac compression.

Figure 10.22

  When switching positions, the new compressor carefully locates the correct hand position with his index and middle fingers and then sweeps the first compressor's hands away.

necessary without interrupting the 5:1 rhythm. A switch can be smoothly accomplished if the EMT who is performing the compressions changes from counting and says instead: "Switch, on, three, next, time". After the next ventilation, the EMT at the patient's head swings his body to face the other EMT and places the middle and index fingers of the hand which is toward the patient's feet into the notch of the ribcage and on the lower half of the sternum. With the other hand, he pushes the compressor's hand up toward the patient's head following the count of three (Fig. 10.22). The new compressor then positions his hands to continue this activity without any interruption. The new ventilator interposes the next breath after the count of five (Fig. 10.23).

  When performing CPR on a litter in an ambulance, both EMTs must perform on the same side of the patient (Fig. 10.24). They switch positions using the following technique. The EMT performing the ventilation rapidly moves behind the compressor and assumes the role of the compressor. The original compressor moves to the patient's head to continue ventilation.

  Because of the interruptions for lung inflation, the single rescuer must perform each series of 15 chest compressions at the faster rate of 80 com-

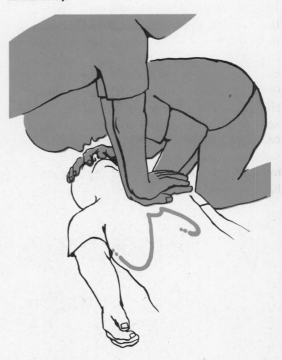

Figure 10.23

  The switch of EMTs is completed. The new ventilator is giving mouth-to-mouth ventilation while the other EMT is performing external cardiac compression.

pressions per minute in order to achieve an actual compression rate of 60 per minute. After

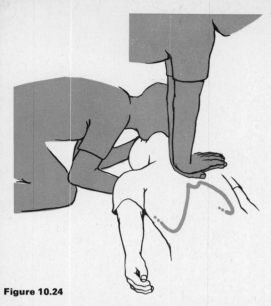

Figure 10.24

In an ambulance, two EMTs perform CPR on the same side of the patient.

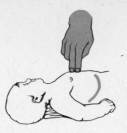

Figure 10.26

For external cardiac compression on an infant, use only two fingers, which are placed in the middle of the sternum (mid-nipple line). A folded sheet beneath the shoulders provides support.

99

15 compressions, the EMT delivers two ventilations (ratio 15:2). The 15 compressions are delivered in eleven to twelve seconds, followed by two full, rapid ventilations (with minimal exhalation time) delivered in four to five seconds. Using this technique, 60 cardiac compressions can be provided per minute.

Infants and Children. With a few exceptions, cardiac compression is similar for children. For small children, the heel of one hand depresses the middle one-third of the sternum, while the other hand maintains head tilt (Fig. 10.25). For in-

fants, the tips of the index and middle fingers depress the sternum in the mid-nipple line (Fig. 10.26). The ventricles of infants and small children lie higher in the chest and the external pressure should be exerted over the mid-sternum. The danger of lacerating the liver is greater in children because of the pliability of the chest and the higher position of the liver under the lower sternum and xiphoid. Infants require one-half to three-fourths of an inch compression of the sternum; young children require three-fourths to one and one-half inches. The compression rate should be 80 to 100 per minute, with breaths delivered as quickly as possible after each five compressions.

In infants and small children, a backward tilt of the head lifts the back, requiring an additional firm support beneath the back for external cardiac compression. It can be provided by the EMT himself if he will slip one hand beneath the child's back while using the other hand to compress the chest. A folded sheet or baby blanket or similar article can also be placed beneath the shoulders to provide the necessary support (Fig. 10.26).

An alternate two-person technique for small infants consists of one EMT providing ventilation while the other encircles the infant's chest with his two hands. The tips of the fingers should be beside each other on the spine, and the thumbs used to compress the midsternum. The EMT's hands must not compress the sides of the infant's chest wall.

Effectiveness of CPR. The reaction of the pupils to light should be checked periodically during CPR, since constriction provides a good indication of the delivery of oxygenated blood

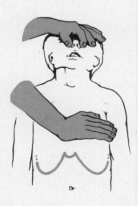

Figure 10.25

External cardiac compression for a small child is shown. The heel of one hand is placed over the middle one-third of the sternum. The other hand maintains head tilt.

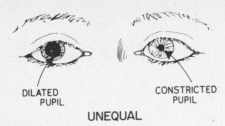

Figure 10.27

A constricted pupil and a dilated pupil are shown.

100

to the patient's brain. Pupils that constrict when exposed to light indicate adequate oxygenation and blood flow in the brain. If the pupils remain widely dilated and do not react to light, serious brain damage may be imminent or may have occurred (Fig. 10.27). Dilated but reactive pupils are a less ominous sign. Normal pupillary reactions may be altered in the elderly and frequently are altered in any individual by the administration of drugs.

The carotid pulse should be palpated periodically during CPR to check the effectiveness of external cardiac compression or the return of a spontaneous effective heartbeat. Palpation should be done after the first minute of CPR and every few minutes thereafter. Pupils and pulse should be checked by the EMT performing the ventilation, particularly just before a change of persons giving CPR.

CPR interruption. Do not interrupt CPR for more than five seconds for any reason, except when it is necessary to move a patient up or down a stairway where it may be difficult to continue effective resuscitation. Under these circumstances, it is best to perform CPR at the head or foot of the stairs, then interrupt at a given signal and move quickly to the next level, where effective activity is resumed. These interruptions should not exceed fifteen seconds each. Do not move the patient to a more convenient site until he is stable and ready for transportation or until arrangements have been made for uninterrupted CPR during the movement.

Witnessed Cardiac Arrest

If the EMT is present and witnesses a cardiac arrest, the steps of the CPR should be modified. At this time, the heart is still oxygenated and

may respond to an external stimulus, the precordial thump.

Precordial thump. If the patient does not respond to verbal or painful stimuli, the EMT simultaneously tilts back the patient's head and palpates the carotid pulse. If the pulse is absent, the EMT raises his fist about eight to twelve inches above the patient's sternum and thumps the mid-sternum strongly with the fleshy part of the fist, once and only once (Fig. 10.28). Follow with four quick breaths of artificial ventilation and recheck the pulse. If the pulse cannot be detected, continue with standard CPR techniques by either one or two EMTs. The EMT should not continue to apply precordial thumps after the first and only initial attempt. Standard CPR techniques have been proved to be successful, and time should not be wasted in employing techniques which have not yet been as thoroughly investigated.

Adjunctive Equipment

The preceding portion of this chapter presented management of the patient with a respira-

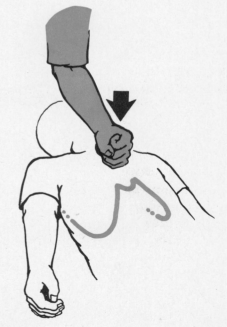

Figure 10.28

A precordial thump is delivered to the center of the patient's sternum with the fleshy part of the EMT's fist. It is delivered only once.

tory or cardiac arrest, using the mouth and hands without any adjunctive equipment. As adjunctive equipment becomes available, it should be used where appropriate. CPR which is being well managed without adjunctive equipment can be converted to a total disaster when these aids are improperly used.

Oxygen

Oxygen is present in the atmosphere in concentrations of about 21 percent. We inhale this 21-percent oxygen, utilize some 5 percent of it, and exhale about 16 percent. Nature has supplied the atmosphere with more oxygen than we need when our vital organs (heart and lungs) are functioning properly. During cardiopulmonary resuscitation, using mouth-to-mouth breathing, 16-percent oxygen is delivered from the rescuer to the patient. This concentration is sufficient to sustain life for a short period of time. However, because external cardiac compression produces a pumping activity (termed cardiac output) which is only 25 to 30 percent of the action of the normal heart, oxygen delivery by the blood is impaired. The combination of the low oxygen received and the low pumping activity renders the patient grossly oxygen deficient (hypoxic). Hypoxia rapidly damages the vital organs; therefore, the addition of supplemental oxygen as early as possible promotes recovery. Oxygen of 100-percent concentration should be delivered to the patient who has had a cardiopulmonary arrest. Indeed, patients with wet lungs (pulmonary edema) may still be inadequately oxygenated even when 100-percent oxygen is delivered. The adage that a high oxygen concentration given to a patient with chronic obstructive lung disease will cause depressed respiration is not valid in this context. Patients who have a cardiopulmonary arrest are clinically "dead" and need the maximum oxygen concentration that can be delivered.

It is now known that a high oxygen concentration can damage the lungs in adults and children (pulmonary oxygen toxicity) and also damage the eyes in the newborn sufficiently to result in blindness (retrolental fibroplasia). However, pulmonary oxygen toxicity only occurs after the lungs have been exposed for several days to an oxygen concentration in excess of 50 percent. Short-term delivery of a high concentration of oxygen does not cause lung damage, and there is no valid reason to withold a high-oxygen concentration from a patient during and immediately following cardiopulmonary arrest.

Similarly, management of a cardiac arrest in the newborn requires the use of a high oxygen concentration for the following reasons:

1. Pumping activity of the heart is reduced during external cardiac compression.
2. Most newborns arrest because of an oxygen deficiency. This oxygen deficiency may be associated with lung disease which impairs the passage of oxygen from the alveoli into the lung capillaries (Respiratory Distress Syndrome of the Newborn, or RDS).

These two elements prevent large quantities of oxygen from being carried by the blood to the eyes. Resuscitative principles are identical for adult and child, and both should be given oxygen.

Delivery of oxygen. During an arrest, circulation and breathing are absent. Treatment for breathing, utilizing a high oxygen concentration, must have not only an oxygen source, but also a method of delivery.

Pocket mask with oxygen inlet valve (mouth-to-mask system). A pocket mask designed for mouth-to-mask ventilation can be combined with an oxygen inlet which has a one-way valve (Fig. 10.29). The mask allows the EMT to

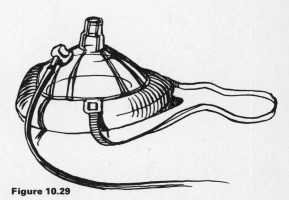

Figure 10.29

A pocket mask with a chimney can be used for mouth-to-mask ventilation. An inlet port for supplemental oxygen is shown.

101

ventilate the patient with supplemental oxygen. while giving breath from his own lungs at the same time.

The major advantage of the mouth-to-mask system is that, unlike the bag-valve-mask system which requires one hand to hold the mask and maintain the airway while the other hand squeezes the bag, the mouth-to-mask system allows both hands to keep open the airway and seal the mask to the face. Rising from the center of the dome of the mask is a chimney with a 15-mm connector. The mask, triangular in shape, has its narrow angle at the apex. The apex of the mask is placed across the bridge of the nose and the base lies in the groove between the lower lip and the chin.

Technique for mouth-to-mask breathing. The technique for using the mouth-to-mask system is described below.

1. The EMT stands behind the patient's head and opens the airway with a backward head tilt.
2. The mask is applied to the face with the apex over the bridge of the nose and the base between the lips and the chin.
3. The index, middle, and ring fingers of each hand grasp the patient's jawbone between the angle and the lobe of the ear (vertical ramus of the mandible), while the thumbs are placed on the dome of the mask. Firm pressure between thumbs and fingers maintains an airtight seal (Fig. 10.30).
4. Simultaneously, the airway is kept open by the upward and forward pull of the fingers behind the jaw.
5. The EMT takes a deep breath and exhales through the open port in the chimney (Fig. 10.31).
6. He then removes his mouth and allows the patient to exhale passively. The timing of each breath is as previously described in mouth-to-mouth technique.

The oxygen concentration delivered to the patient can be increased by the addition of supplemental oxygen through the one-way valve in the inlet nipple. The principle of the system is mouth-to-mask ventilation; therefore, any oxygen delivered to the patient will be

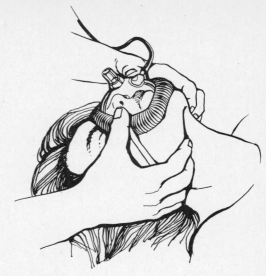

Figure 10.30

The pocket mask is sealed to the face by both hands. The apex of the mask is over the bridge of the nose and the base is between the lips and chin.

diluted with the EMT's exhaled breath. Five liters of oxygen per minute will provide the patient with approximately 50 percent oxygen, and fifteen liters with approximately 55 percent oxygen.

The mask has an elastic head strap and, provided that oxygen is being given and an airway maintained, this system works equally well for a patient who is breathing on his own and does

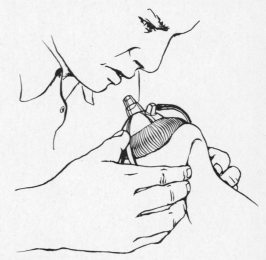

Figure 10.31

The EMT provides ventilation by exhaling into the chimney of the mask. He then turns his head to draw fresh air into his own lungs.

not require the rescuer's assistance—for example, a stroke patient.

The pocket mask may also be used for infants. Reversing the mask, the apex is placed under the infant's chin while the base covers the bridge of the nose and the sides of the face. The EMT exhales small puffs into the open port in the chimney. Again, supplemental oxygen can be given.

Bag-valve-mask system (BVM system). The primary function of the bag-valve-mask system is to deliver high concentrations of supplemental oxygen and simultaneously ventilate the patient (Fig. 10.32).

A bag-valve-mask system should consist of:

A self-refilling bag, without sponge rubber inside (because of difficulty in cleaning, disinfecting, eliminating ethylene oxide, and fragmentation)

A non-jam valve system set at 15 liters per minute oxygen-inlet flow, which cannot be incorrectly reassembled and will not jam at this flow

A transparent plastic facemask with an air-filled or contoured, resilient cuff

No pop-off valve, except in pediatric models

Standard 15 mm/22 mm fittings

A system for delivery of 90 to 100 percent oxygen via an ancillary oxygen inlet, and an oxygen reservoir

A true non-rebreathing valve

The system should be available in adult and pediatric sizes. Bag-valve-mask systems are difficult to use, and the EMT requires considerable training to acquire the skills necessary.

Technique for use of the bag-valve-mask system. The EMT positions himself at the patient's head, where he maintains the neck in extension to keep the airway open. The mask, triangular in shape, is applied over the patient's face with the apex over the bridge of the nose and the base between the lower lip and the chin. To achieve this fitting, the EMT must select the correct mask size. If the mask has an inflatable collar, it should be inflated before use to obtain a better and easier seal between the mask and the face.

The mask is held in position by placing the little, ring, and middle fingers on the jawbone between the chin and the lobe of the ear (horizontal ramus of the mandible), while the index finger is held over the lower portion of the mask and the thumb over the upper portion of the mask. Firm pressure between the fingers on the jaw and those on the mask maintains the seal while the jaw is pulled upward to keep the airway open (Fig. 10.33). With the mask firmly applied to the face and the neck maintained in extension with one hand, the other hand compresses the bag in a rhythmical manner once every five seconds (Fig. 10.34). Lung expansion must be evident by rise of the chest or descent of the diaphragm; otherwise, the oxygen mixture may be escaping, unnoticed, through a leak between mask and face. When this system is used in conjunction with external cardiac compression, the bag should be squeezed between the fifth upstroke and the first downstroke without inter-

103

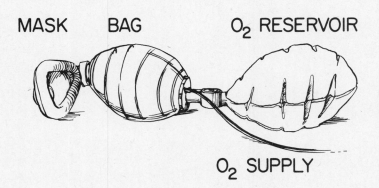

MASK   BAG   O₂ RESERVOIR

O₂ SUPPLY

Figure 10.32

A bag-valve-mask system is shown with all its component parts. Note the oxygen supply, oxygen reservoir, and resuscitation bag, in addition to the mask.

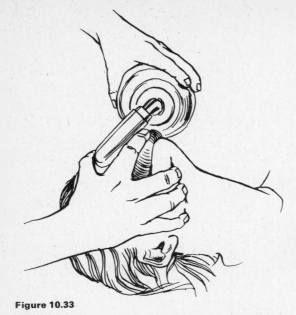

Figure 10.33

The mask of the bag-valve-mask system is shown, supported closely against the face. Three fingers are along the mandible, as shown, and the EMT's thumb is on the upper part of the mask.

rupting the rhythm of external cardiac compression.

Mouth-to-mouth and mouth-to-mask ventilation can provide large breaths, up to four liters if necessary. A bag-valve-mask system can only deliver as much as can be squeezed out with one hand (since the other hand is holding the mask). A liter is the usual volume. Better volumes of ventilation can be achieved by mouth-to-mouth than with a bag-valve-mask system, but supplemental oxygen cannot be

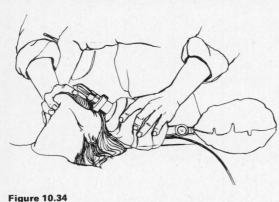

Figure 10.34

The bag-valve-mask system with an oxygen reservoir is shown. Its limitations in terms of volume of inspired gas delivered are apparent since it can deliver only the volume that one hand can displace.

provided with mouth-to-mouth ventilation. The mouth-to-mask system allows for larger volumes than a bag-valve-mask system. Its only drawback is that at 15 liters per minute of oxygen flow, the mouth-to-mask system will deliver only 55 percent oxygen, while the BVM with oxygen reservoir system will deliver more than 90 percent oxygen.

BVM systems should be used only when it is desired to deliver a high-oxygen concentration (above 55 percent) and preferably when an endotracheal tube is in place.

Oropharyngeal and Nasopharyngeal Airways

The primary function of artificial airways is to keep the tongue from blocking the upper airway.

Oropharyngeal airways. An oropharyngeal airway is positioned in the mouth with the curvature of the airway following the contour of the tongue. The flange end should rest against the lips or cheek and the other end in the pharynx. The airway is open in the center or on either side to permit breathing or to allow easy access for suctioning. These airways are manufactured in a variety of sizes for both adults and children.

Oropharyngeal airways should always be used when a bag-valve-mask system is used. These airways should be inserted only in unconscious patients. If introduced into a conscious or stuporous patient, they may promote vomiting or spasm of the vocal cords. If incorrectly placed, instead of maintaining the airway, they can displace the tongue backward into the pharynx, producing airway obstruction.

The technique for insertion of an oropharyngeal airway is described in steps.

1. The EMT opens the patient's mouth using the cross-finger technique described earlier.
2. Holding the airway upside down in his other hand, he inserts it into the patient's mouth, rotating it through 180°, until the flange rests on the lips or teeth (Fig. 10.35). A moistened airway will ease introduction.

An alternative technique is to open the mouth,

Nasopharyngeal airways. A nasopharyngeal airway is positioned in the nasal cavity with the curvature of the airway following the floor of the nose. The flange end rests against the nostril while the other end is in the pharynx. The airway must be well lubricated before it is inserted.

If a patient is conscious but not able to maintain his natural airway, a nasopharyngeal airway should be inserted. A nasopharyngeal airway is not as liable to stimulate vomiting and is usually well tolerated.

The airway is inserted through one nostril until the flange rests against one nostril (Fig. 10.36). If an obstruction is met as the airway is introduced, it should be removed and reinserted into the other nostril.

105

Sequence for use of bag-valve-mask and airway systems. The EMT should adopt the following sequence in giving ventilation:

1. Open the oxygen regulator and check to see that the pressure in the tank is adequate for its use.
2. Connect the plastic oxygen line to the flow-meter nipple, and connect the other end to the manual resuscitator bag (be sure the bag has an oxygen reservoir).
3. Turn on the flow meter to deliver ten liters per minute.
4. Select the correct size mask for the patient and attach the mask to the valve on the resuscitator bag.
5. Open the patient's mouth with the cross-finger technique and insert the oropharyngeal airway.
6. With one hand, maintain the facemask seal and neck extension.
7. With the other hand, ventilate the patient by squeezing the bag.
8. Check to be sure that lung expansion is occurring.

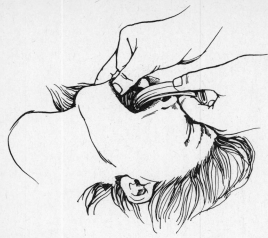

Figure 10.35

The placement of an oropharyngeal airway is shown. The mouth has been opened, using the cross-finger technique. The airway, upside down, is introduced into the mouth; it will be turned 180°, to lie over the tongue with its flange against the teeth.

depress the tongue with a tongue blade, and slide the airway into the mouth.

Any unconscious patient who is breathing spontaneously can have his airway kept open with greater ease if an oropharyngeal airway is in place than through the constant use of head tilt.

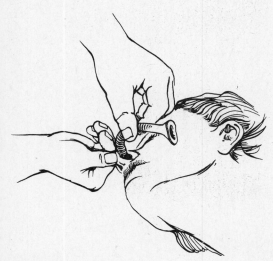

Figure 10.36

The insertion of a tubular nasopharyngeal airway into one nostril is shown. The convex curve of the airway is upward, toward the patient's head. This airway is usually well tolerated even by stuporous or semiconscious individuals, whereas an oropharyngeal airway might cause vomiting.

Suctioning Devices

Portable or fixed suction equipment is essential for resuscitation emergencies.

The portable unit should provide a vacuum pressure and a flow adequate for pharyngeal suction. The unit should be fitted with a wide bore, a thick wall, non-kinking tubing, semi-rigid pharyngeal suction tips, and multiple sterile suction catheters. Also available should be a nonbreakable collection bottle and a supply of water for rinsing tubing, tips, and catheters. The fixed unit should generate an air flow of more than thirty liters per minute and a vacuum of more than 300 mm Hg when the tubing is clamped.

Rigid pharyngeal suction tips (tonsil suction tips) are best for suctioning the pharynx. They are large bore, rigid and do not collapse. A fixed contour allows easy and rapid placement when necessary. They should be used with the greatest caution in awake or semi-awake patients because of the hazard of inducing vomiting. The suction yoke, collection bowl, water for rinsing, and suction tube should be readily accessible to the rescuer at the patient's head.

Suction apparatus should be cleaned and decontaminated after each use. Suction catheters should be sterile and disposable.

Technique for oral or pharyngeal suction. In using pharyngeal suction, the EMT must follow these steps:

1. Inspect the unit to see that all parts are assembled, switch on the suction, clamp the tubing, and see that the pressure dial registers more than 300 mm Hg.
2. Attach a flexible catheter or rigid tonsil sucker.

3. Open the mouth with the cross-finger technique.
4. Insert the catheter into the pharynx. The length for insertion of a flexible catheter is the distance between the mouth and the lobe of the ear. Rigid tonsil suckers are inserted with the convex side along the roof of the mouth until the pharynx is reached (Fig. 10.37).
5. Suction should be applied only after the the catheter is in position and should not exceed fifteen seconds.
6. After reoxygenation, suctioning may be repeated.

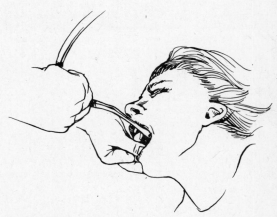

Figure 10.37

Suctioning the oropharynx with a rigid, tonsil suction device is shown.

CHAPTER 11

Oxygen Therapy and Equipment

GOAL I. Know the situations in which oxygen therapy is needed.

OBJECTIVES

A. Define hypoxia and describe its consequences.
B. Match the types and causes of hypoxia.
C. Identify the characteristics of patients needing oxygen therapy.

GOAL II. Understand the procedures and the hazards of oxygen therapy.

OBJECTIVES

A. List the types, functions, and safety features of oxygen-therapy equipment.
B. Point out the hazards of oxygen therapy.
C. Explain the need for humidification of oxygen.

Hypoxia is a condition in which there is a deficiency of oxygen reaching the tissues of the body. It is an extremely serious condition affecting the brain, adrenal glands, heart, kidneys, and liver, in the order named. Table 11.1 lists some of the causes of hypoxia. This chapter includes a discussion of the use of oxygen and the various modes of its delivery in the prevention or relief of hypoxia.

Patients Requiring Oxygen Therapy

Oxygen therapy for hypoxia, from whatever cause, is used in the two major groups of patients described below:

1. Patients who are apneic (have no spontaneous breathing) rapidly develop hypoxia in the vital organs, especially the brain and the heart. Clinical death is imminent if the hypoxia is not corrected within a matter of minutes.
2. Patients who can breathe but who are unable to move a sufficient quantity of air with each breath to insure adequate oxygen delivery to the lungs develop hypoxia, but the onset and degree of tissue damage will depend on the degree of respiratory inadequacy.

Situations Requiring Oxygen Therapy

The most important indication for oxygen therapy is hypoxia. The early signs of hypoxia are tachycardia, nervousness, and irritability. Cyanosis is a late finding.

The ideal time for the correction of hypoxia is when the first symptoms appear, before severe damage has been done to the essential organs of the body. Some common specific situations in which oxygen therapy is indicated include those listed below.

1. *Myocardial infarction*—The cause of hypoxia in myocardial infarction is the slow

TABLE 11.1

CAUSES OF HYPOXIA

Type	Cause	Example of Cause
Hypoxic hypoxia (Decreased oxygen reaching blood in the lungs)	Reduction of inspired oxygen	Fire damp
	Rarefied air	High altitude
	Decreased amount of air in the lungs	Emphysema; asthma; pulmonary edema; paralysis of muscles; drug overdose
	Diseased lungs	Pneumonia; lung collapse
Hemic hypoxia (Decreased oxygen carried in blood)	Reduction of circulating hemoglobin	Anemia
	Decreased function of circulating hemoglobin	Poisoning by carbon monoxide or by various coal tar derivatives
Circulatory hypoxia (Decreased blood flow)	Blood loss	Shock from hemorrhage; burns; trauma
	Abnormal blood routes	Congenital heart disease
	Heart failure	Myocardial infarction
	Arterial obstruction	Arteriosclerosis; blood clot
	Venous obstruction	Heart failure; venous stasis; phlebitis
Cellular hypoxia (Disturbed function of cells)	Destruction of cellular respiratory enzymes	Cyanide poisoning

circulation of blood which carries oxygen to the tissue (circulatory hypoxia). Administration of oxygen will make more oxygen available for circulation and also may help the heart muscle regain some strength, thereby improving circulation.

2. *Pulmonary edema*—In pulmonary edema, fluid within the lung prevents oxygen transfer to the blood (hypoxic hypoxia). In the severe state, 80 to 100 percent oxygen should be administered.

3. *Chronic obstructive lung disease*—Ordinarily, the normal stimulus for breathing is the level of carbon dioxide in the blood. As it rises, the stimulus to breathe rises. Patients with chronic obstructive lung disease have lived with high carbon dioxide levels in the blood for a long time. In many instances the level is so high that the patient has become insensitive to carbon dioxide as a respiratory stimulant. In these patients, a low oxygen level in the blood is the stimulus for breathing. Inspired oxygen concentrations higher than 25 to 30 percent must be given with caution unless the EMT is prepared to breathe for the patient. He may, in his attempt to help, entirely do away with the patient's own respiratory stimulus. These patients have labored respiration with wheezing and may require high pressures to assist their breathing. A good example of such a condition is emphysema (hypoxic hypoxia). Ventilation therapy usually includes administering aerosols to help dilate the bronchi.

4. *Acute drug ingestion*—Respiration in patients who have taken overdoses of drugs may be very depressed, resulting in infrequent, shallow breaths and insufficient oxygen in the lung (hypoxic hypoxia). Artificial ventilation may be required with the use of supplemental oxygen. In these patients the brain is itself depressed, causing diminished respiration.

5. *Pulmonary burns*—Burns of the lungs result from the inhalation of steam, hot fumes, or smoke. They may be severe and acute. They produce local edema and destruction of pulmonary tissue (hypoxic

hypoxia). Treatment should include oxygen administration and artificial ventilation when necessary.

6. *Cerebrovascular accident*—The cause of hypoxia in a patient who has suffered a stroke is poor control of respiration by the brain. The rate and depth of breathing are both decreased (hypoxic hypoxia). Therapy is aimed at assisting or controlling breathing.

7. *Crushed chest*—Often seen following an injury of the chest wall, a crushed chest may result in a "flail chest," a condition characterized by severe local lung damage and insufficient respiration (hypoxic hypoxia). Supplemental oxygen must be given and ventilation assisted until the patient is in the care of a physician.

8. *Shock*—A state of shock often accompanies other injuries in which much blood is lost. The capacity of the cardiovascular system to carry oxygen is reduced (circulatory hypoxia). Supplemental oxygen is needed in the immediate treatment and transportation of these patients.

Hazards of Oxygen Therapy

Even though oxygen does not burn and does not explode, it does support combustion. A small spark becomes a flame in an oxygen-enriched atmosphere; a glowing cigarette can also burst into open flame. Therefore any possible source of a flame must be kept away from an area where oxygen is in use.

In some chronic disease states like emphysema, the normal stimulus to respiration is no longer effective. In these situations where low blood-oxygen level is the primary stimulus for the patient's respiration, the administration of oxygen can cause decreased ventilation to the point of its ceasing altogether. Such patients should not be given oxygen unless they are apneic.

Patients receiving high levels of inspired oxygen may develop atelectasis (areas of lung collapse) or oxygen toxicity (actual destruction of lung tissue). However, in situations involving emergency care and transportation, rarely

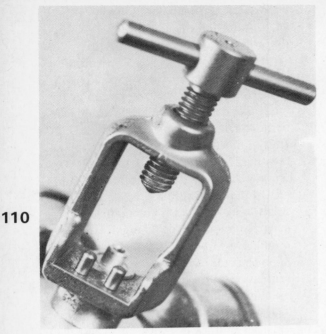

Figure 11.1 *a*

The yoke connector is used with small oxygen cylinders.

110

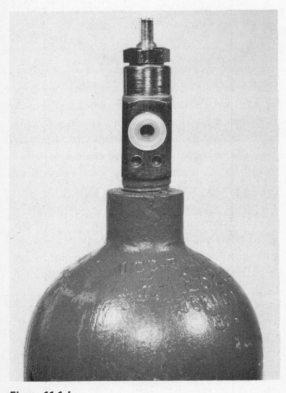

Figure 11.1 *b*

A size E oxygen cylinder is shown with the pin index safety system and gas outlet.

would a patient receive a high enough concentration of oxygen for a sufficient period of time to develop these complications.

Oxygen Sources and Regulators

Sources. In locations other than hospitals and similar facilities, oxygen is usually supplied as a compressed gas in seamless steel cylinders. These cylinders are available in various sizes. The two most frequently used in emergency equipment are the E and M cylinders. The E size contains 650 liters and the M size contains 3,000 liters when each is filled to specified limits with a pressure of 2,000 to 2,200 pounds per square inch (psi).

Cylinders of E size or smaller have outlet valves designed to accept pressure-reducing gauges of the yoke type (Fig. 11.1 *a*). To prevent the attachment of a pressure regulator for a different gas to an oxygen cylinder, the yoke contains a pin-indexing safety attachment (Fig. 11.1 *b*). This system is comprised of a series of pins on the yoke which must be matched with holes on the yoke attachment of the gas cylinder if a satisfactory connection is to be made. The arrangement of the pins and holes varies for different gases according to accepted national standards (Fig. 11.2). Each cylinder of a specific gas has a given pattern and a given number of pins. When two or more different gases are being used, one cannot, for example, attach a cylinder of nitrous oxide to an oxygen line by mistake as it will not fit.

Cylinders larger than E size are equipped with threaded gas-outlet valves (Fig. 11.3). The inside and outside diameters of these threaded outlets vary according to the medical gas contained in the cylinder. Therefore, the gas cylinder will not accept a regulator valve unless it is properly threaded to fit that specific outlet. This safety system for large cylinders is known as the American Standard System (Fig. 11.4). The purpose of these safety devices is to prevent the accidental attachment of a regulator to a wrong supply tank (for example, to acetylene or carbon dioxide instead of oxygen).

Compressed gas cylinders must be handled carefully since their contents are under pressure.

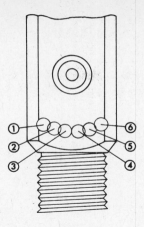

Figure 11.2

The locations of the pin-index safety system holes in a cylinder valve face are shown. Various pairs constitute indexes for different gases.

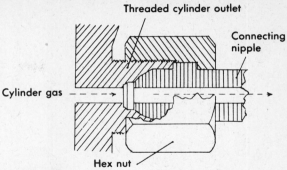

Figure 11.4

The typical American Standard connection is used to attach a reducing valve to a large high-pressure cylinder.

111

Regulators must be firmly attached to the cylinders before they are transported; a loose regulator or a perforation of the tank can cause it to become a deadly missile.

Pressure regulators. The pressure of the gas in an oxygen cylinder is too high to be useful medically. Therefore, regulators must be attached to medical gas cylinders to reduce the pressure to levels suitable for the operation of medical equipment, usually 40–70 psi. Most pressure regulators in medical use today reduce the pressure in a single stage, although multiple-stage regulators do exist. A two-stage regulator will usually initially reduce the pressure to 700 psi and then reduce it further to 40–70 psi in the second stage. After the cylinder pressure is reduced to a workable level, the final attachment for delivery of the gas to the patient is usually through one of these two ways:

1. A quick-connect female fitting that will accept a quick-connect male plug from the pressure hose of a ventilator or resuscitator

2. A flowmeter that will permit the regulated release of gas in liters per minute

Flow regulators. In emergency equipment, where the supply of medical gas is usually in a compressed gas cylinder with a pressure regulator, flowmeters are ordinarily permanently affixed to the pressure regulator. The two types of flowmeters commonly in use are these:

1. Pressure-compensated flowmeters (Fig. 11.5)—Pressure-compensated flowmeters incorporate a float ball within a tapered, calibrated tube. The float rises or falls according to the gas flow within the tube. The flow of gas is regulated by a needle valve placed downstream from the float ball. Back pressure resulting from an obstruction of gas outflow (e.g., kinked tubing)

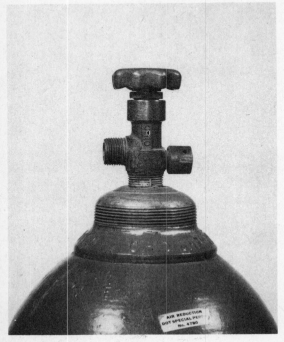

Figure 11.3

A size H oxygen cylinder has a valve with the threaded-connector gas outlet of the American Standard Safety System.

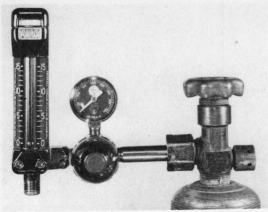

112

Figure 11.5

A pressure-compensated flowmeter attached to a large gas cylinder via threaded connection allows a regulated flow from 0 to 15 liters of oxygen per minute.

will cause the float-ball level to drop, since the float will record only actual, delivered flow. This type of flowmeter is affected by gravity and must always be maintained in an upright position.

2. *Bourdon gauge flowmeter* (*Fig. 11.6*)—The type of flowmeter represented by the Bourdon gauge is very common in emergency use because it is not affected by gravity and may be used in any position. A Bourdon gauge is actually a pressure gauge calibrated to record flowrate. The major disadvantage of this flowmeter is that it does not compensate for back pressure and

will actually record a higher flowrate when any obstruction to gas flow is encountered downstream.

Humidification. Oxygen from a gas cylinder source is extremely dry; for all practical purposes, it is completely free of water vapor. Therefore, in order to prevent drying of the patient's mucous membrane surfaces, humidification is an important component of oxygen administration (Fig. 11.7). Excessive drying of the mucous membranes of the nose, throat, and lung can rapidly cause the accumulation of crusts which in turn can obstruct the airway and interfere with respiration.

Duration of Use of Oxygen Cylinders

Several methods are available for calculating how long an oxygen cylinder can be used before its contents are depleted. It should be emphasized that one must always make arrangements

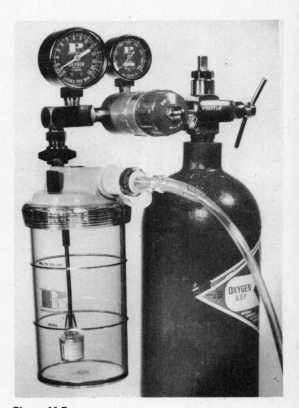

Figure 11.7

An evaporative oxygen humidifier is shown attached to a Bourdon gauge flowmeter/pressure regulator.

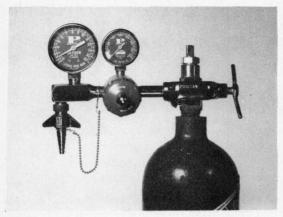

Figure 11.6

A Bourdon gauge flowmeter attached to a small gas cylinder via a yoke attachment allows a regulated flow from 0 to 15 liters of oxygen per minute.

to switch to a fresh cylinder before the one in use has become completely empty. Normally a cylinder is replaced at a certain level above the zero psi reading on the pressure gauge. This level may be called the "safe residual." Knowing the current pressure reading, the current flow in liters per minute, and the safe residual, which is always 200 psi, one can calculate how much useful life remains in any cylinder.

One of the methods of calculating the remaining duration of flow in a cylinder at any time after it has been used is shown in Table 11.2.

Equipment for Oxygen Delivery

Various pieces of equipment for the administration of supplemental oxygen to assist ventilation in the spontaneously breathing patient are described in the following paragraphs.

Nasal cannula. With a nasal cannula (Fig. 11.8a) oxygen is administered to the patient through two small tubular prongs which fit into the nostrils. If the flowmeter is set to read between five and eight liters per minute, it is possible to obtain oxygen concentrations ranging from 35 to 50 percent in inspired air. Since the nasal cannula delivers dry gas directly into the nostrils, humidification is necessary if extensive drying and subsequent damage of the nasal mucous membrane are to be avoided. If pro-

longed oxygen administration by this method is anticipated, an air-evaporative type of humidifier should be attached to the flowmeter (Fig. 11.7). A patient who is a mouth-breather or who has a nasal obstruction derives minimal benefit from this form of oxygen administration.

Simple facemask. Simple oxygen masks (Fig. 11.8b) contain a small-bore inlet port, an elastic strap for a snug fit, and perforations on either side to allow for the escape of excess gases, especially during exhalation. Several sizes of adult facemasks exist. Two smaller sizes (infant and pediatric) are also in common use. All types of these maks are fitted to the face in the same manner, by the use of a soft or inflatable cushion which can be contoured to the face. With flow-rates of six to ten liters per minute, oxygen concentrations of 35 to 60 percent can be obtained in inspired air.

Humidification is possible in a manner similar to that described above for the nasal cannula. With a facemask there may be some mixing of air and oxygen prior to inhalation; however the mixing is minimal with the flowrates usually used and the inspired mixture is still dry. Humidification is advised as tissue dehydration can occur with prolonged use.

Mask and bag. In the mask and bag system (Fig. 11.8c), the mask is similar to the facemask described above. However, in this system the

113

TABLE 11.2

CALCULATING THE DURATION OF CYLINDER FLOW

(In minutes)

Formula: $\dfrac{\text{(Gauge pressure in psi} - \text{Safe residual)} \times \text{Factor}}{\text{Flowrate (liter flow per minute)}} = \begin{array}{c}\text{Duration of flow}\\\text{(in minutes)}\end{array}$

Factors for Various Oxygen Cylinders

D—0.16
E—0.28
G—2.41
H & K—3.14
M—1.56

Safe residual pressure is 200 psi

Example: M cylinder, gauge pressure at 1,200 psi, safe residual is 200 psi, flowmeter set for 5 liters per minute. How long will the cylinder last?

Solution: $\dfrac{(1,200 - 200) \times 1.56}{5} = \dfrac{1,560}{5} = 312$ minutes (or 5 hrs., 12 min.)

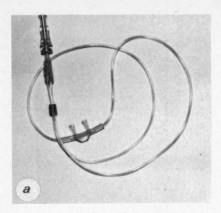

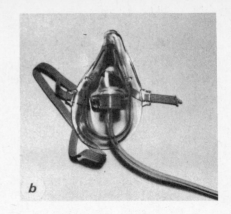

114

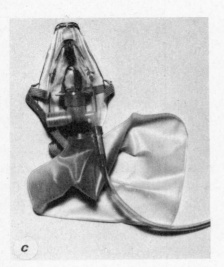

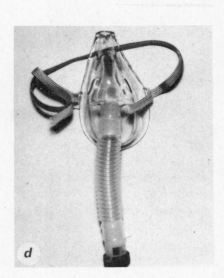

Figure 11.8 *a–d*

Various types of equipment are shown for the administration of oxygen to assist breathing: *a*, nasal cannula; *b*, simple facemask; *c*, mask with bag; *d*, venturi mask.

oxygen inflow fills a bag which is attached to the mask by a one-way valve. This system is occasionally called a non-rebreathing mask and bag. By removing the one-way valves (flapper valves), the system can be converted to a partial-rebreathing mask and bag (Fig. 11.9). Oxygen concentrations in excess of 60 percent in inspired air can be obtained with this system. There is no pre-set flowrate. The gas inflow must be set at whatever level will prevent complete collapse of the bag during inhalation. With infants or children, obviously a smaller gas flow will be needed since the volume inhaled each time will be less.

Flapper valves over the mask perforations serve as one-way ports of exhalation. This modification prevents taking in room air that could mix with and dilute the oxygen concentration. These exhalation valves may be removed if necessary. Again, humidification will be necessary if prolonged administration is anticipated. The humidification system described above is also used with this unit.

Venturi masks. In the venturi system (Figs. 11.8*d* & 11.10), before the oxygen delivery tube reaches the mask it passes through an air-entrainment device that specifically regulates the concentration of delivered oxygen and also the volume of gas delivered to the patient per unit of time. Venturi masks are usually designed to deliver an inspired oxygen concentration of either 24, 28, 35, or 40 percent; however, the stated concentrations are not entirely accurate and

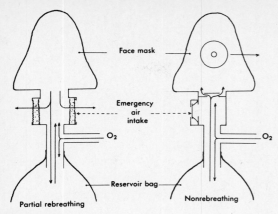

Figure 11.9

A comparison of non-rebreathing and partial-rebreathing bag and mask is shown.

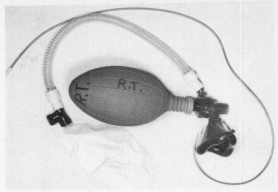

Figure 11.11

A bag-valve-mask resuscitator is shown with modification for administration of a high concentration of oxygen.

115

some variation should be expected. Humidification is recommended with prolonged use to prevent tissue dehydration and drying of secretions.

Bag-valve-mask resuscitator. All types of bag-valve-mask resuscitators (Fig. 11.11) have several common components:

1. An inflatable-deflatable bag
2. A valve that incorporates the exhalation port, the oxygen inflow, and a means of connection between the facemask or the endotracheal tube adapter and the bag
3. A facemask

The total amount of gas contained within the bag of an adult resuscitator is 1,200 to 1,500 cc. The pediatric bag for children contains approximately 700 cc, while the infant-size bag holds about 150 cc. The majority of the bag-valve-

mask resuscitators currently on the market are available with modifications or accessories to permit the delivery of oxygen concentrations approaching 100 percent. Without these modifications, it is difficult to achieve concentrations above 50 percent.

The oxygen inlet of a bag-valve-mask resuscitator is attached to the flowmeter nipple of the oxygen clyinder by a small-bore tube. These resuscitators may be used to assist the ventilation of patients who are breathing spontaneously but not receiving adequate air. The operator using a bag-valve-mask resuscitator for this purpose should deflate the bag simultaneously with the patient's inspiratory efforts, and ultimately attempt to achieve a more normal rate and depth

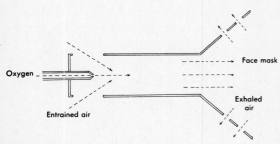

Figure 11.10

A diagrammatic representation of the functions of the venturi mask is shown. As oxygen is delivered, a certain amount of room air is also entrained with each inhalation, providing a given oxygen concentration. The amount of room air taken in is dependent on the size of the ports through which it passes.

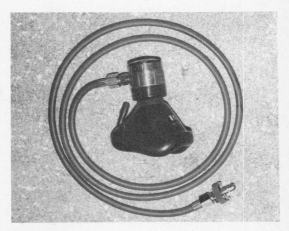

Figure 11.12

A demand-valve resuscitator with high-pressure hose and quick-connect fitting is shown.

of respiration (tidal volume). The function of the unit is subject to the manual control of the operator.

Demand-valve resuscitators. Demand-valve units (Fig. 11.12) are also used as described above. They may be used either to assist ventilation or to control it. A valve is placed in the circuit that connects the oxygen supply source to the patient. The valve can open either in response to the inspiratory effort of the patient or to manual control of the operator, who ventilates the patient by periodically depressing a button on the valve. Federal specifications require that demand-valve resuscitators used in ambulances be equipped with manual control. The EMT should monitor this control at all times.

The unit inflates the lungs until a pre-set pressure limit is reached. Pressures are calibrated in millimeters of mercury (mm Hg) or centimeters of water (cm H_2O). One mm Hg equals 1.36 cm H_2O. The pressure limit is initially pre-set at 10 to 20 cm H_2O or 8 to 15 mm Hg. This limit may have to be increased as necessary to provide an adequate respiratory volume for the patient.

Demand valves are powered by a pressure-source supply, usually a size D or E cylinder of oxygen. These valves will operate effectively in a supply-pressure range of 40 to 80 psi. Since the power source is 100 percent oxygen, the concentration delivered to the patient will be 100 percent. For these units to operate effectively, there must be no pressure leak. Therefore an airtight fit must be obtained between the patient's face and the mask.

The amount of pressure necessary to ventilate a patient adequately will vary according to the size of the patient, his lung volume, and the condition of his lungs. A patient with stiff, diseased lungs or with chronic obstructive lung disease (emphysema) will require a greater pressure to receive a given volume than would be necessary for someone with normal lungs.

Demand-valve resuscitators are not in common use in emergency work in the United States today, but they are commercially available and are in use in many hospitals. It is important that the EMT recognize the unit when he sees it.

Intermittent positive-pressure breathing unit. Another kind of equipment is the intermittent positive-pressure breathing unit, commonly referred to as the IPPB unit. The use of this equipment is beyond the scope of training of the Emergency Medical Technician, and it has been condemned by national committees for use during cardiopulmonary resuscitation. Therefore it will not be further discussed here.

IV

The Musculoskeletal System

CHAPTER 12

The Skin

GOAL I. Know the structure and function of the skin.

OBJECTIVES

A. Identify the layers of the skin.
B. Define the functions of the skin.
C. Identify the organs and structures contained within the skin.

The skin is one of the most important organs of the body and not just a cover for the organs underneath; it is a tough tissue, constantly renewed, which covers the entire body. It serves two main functions: to protect the body in the environment and to maintain nerves which convey information about that environment to the brain.

The protective functions of the skin are numerous, all equally important. Over 70 percent of the body is water, with a delicate balance of substances in solution. Skin is watertight and serves to keep this internal solution intact. Bacteria are everywhere around us; but, unless the skin is broken by an ulcer or laceration, germs usually cannot pass through it. They are routinely found on the skin and deep in its grooves and glands, but rarely beneath it. The skin is a constant protection against outside invaders.

The energy of the body is derived from chemical reactions that must take place within certain temperature ranges. If the temperature is too low, reactions cannot proceed; metabolism ceases and the body dies. If the temperature becomes too high, as with severe fever, metabolism increases. Dangerously high temperatures can result in permanent tissue damage. The major organ for the regulation of the temperature of the body is the skin. It does so through the evaporation of water from its surface in hot weather (sweating) and through the constriction of skin blood vessels in cold weather. Automatically the skin serves to isolate us within our environment, to protect us from that environment, and to assist us in adapting to it.

Information from the environment is carried to the brain through a rich supply of nerves in the skin. Nerves in this organ are adapted to perceive changes in and transmit information about heat, cold, external pressure, pain, and the relative position of a given part of the body in space. Changes in the environment or the surroundings are recognized by the skin. The appropriate sensation notifies us when the atmosphere is hot or cold. Pressure on a portion of the body is recognized by the skin sensory apparatus. Pain may warn us of a dangerous situation. Many pleasurable stimuli are also perceived by the skin.

Layers of the Skin

There are two major layers of the skin: the epidermis and the dermis. A subcutaneous layer of fat lies just under these layers and surrounds the body (Fig. 12.1).

The epidermis, the outer layer, is composed of cells that are especially durable. The outer-

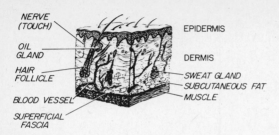

Figure 12.1

The major structures within the skin are shown in this diagram.

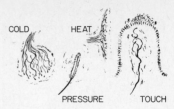

Figure 12.2

Four specialized nerve endings which interpret sensations are found in the skin.

120 most layer of the epidermis is made up of dead, cornified (hardened) cells which are constantly being rubbed off and replaced. This layer is the first mechanism of defense of the body. It is watertight and impervious to bacteria. In the deeper part of the epidermis are cells which constantly reproduce to replace the outer cells being shed or rubbed off. Some of the cells in this deeper layer also contain pigment granules. These cells, together with the blood flowing in the small vessels in the skin, are responsible for skin color.

The deeper layer of skin is the dermis. It is separated from the epidermis by a line of special basal cells. Within the dermis, which is composed of very strong elastic and fibrous tissue, are found many of the special structures of the skin: sweat glands and ducts, sebaceous or oil glands and ducts, hair follicles, blood vessels, and specialized nerve endings (Fig. 12.2).

Sweat glands produce sweat, which is discharged onto the surface of the skin through small pores and ducts. There is one pore for each gland. Sebaceous glands produce an oily substance called sebum. This is discharged along the shafts of the hairs on the head and body and accounts for the natural oiliness of hair and skin. Sebum is important in maintaining the waterproofing of the skin and in keeping it supple so that it does not crack.

Hair follicles are the small organs that produce hair. There is one follicle for each hair in the body, usually connected with a sebaceous gland. All hair grows continuously and is usually either cut off or worn away by clothes. Blood vessels and a complex array of nerves complete the structures contained within the dermis.

Immediately under the skin is the subcutaneous tissue. It is largely fat and serves as an insulator of the body. Characteristic body curves are usually derived from subcutaneous deposits of fat.

Skin is one of the largest and most complex of the body organs, subserving two major functions: protection and perception of external changes.

CHAPTER 13

The Muscular System

GOAL I. Understand the various muscular functions.

OBJECTIVES

A. Identify the locations and describe the characteristics and functions of the voluntary muscles.
B. Identify the locations, and describe the characteristics and functions of the involuntary muscles.
C. Define the term *cardiac muscle* and describe its functions.
D. Explain the function of muscle attachments to bones or other muscles.
E. Describe the process of peristalsis.

Muscle is a special kind of tissue that contracts, or shortens, when stimulated. Several different kinds of muscle exist in the body. Muscle forms the bulk of the tissue of the arms and legs; it is present in almost every blood vessel; the heart is a single large specialized muscle; the gastrointestinal tract is made up largely of muscle. Nearly every system of the body and every organ has some elements of muscle associated with it. All bodily motion is a result of muscle actions. Most often, a given movement is the result of the actions of several muscles working together.

All muscles are supplied with arteries, veins, and nerves (Fig. 13.1). Blood brings oxygen and food to muscles and carries away the waste produced by muscular contractions. Muscles cannot function without a continuous supply of food and a continuous removal of waste. Cramps result when insufficient oxygen or food is carried to muscles or waste is allowed to accumulate. Muscles are under the direct control of the nervous system. Some muscles respond to a willed command, as in the movement of an arm or a leg. Other muscles require constant automatic regulation but their function

cannot be controlled voluntarily; the muscles of the gastrointestinal tract and heart are examples of this type of tissue. Nerves pass directly from the spinal cord or brain to all muscles, connecting them to the central controlling organ of the body. Thus movements and functions are voluntarily or involuntarily coordinated. Without nervous innervation or supply, a voluntary muscle cannot be contracted and an involuntary

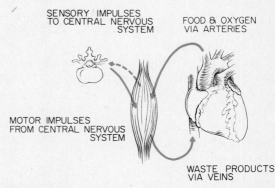

SENSORY IMPULSES
TO CENTRAL NERVOUS
SYSTEM

FOOD & OXYGEN
VIA ARTERIES

MOTOR IMPULSES
FROM CENTRAL NERVOUS
SYSTEM

WASTE PRODUCTS
VIA VEINS

Figure 13.1

All muscles are equipped with arteries to supply them with food and veins to remove waste as they create it. They are also equipped with nerves to receive impulses from the central nervous system or to transmit impulses to the central nervous system.

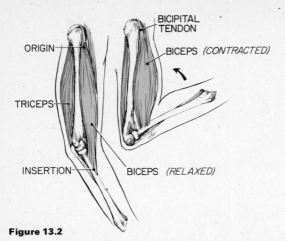

122

Figure 13.2

Relaxation (left sketch) and contraction (right sketch) of the biceps brachii (a skeletal muscle) are shown. Note the origin and insertion points where a tendon connects the muscle to a bone.

muscle assumes an unregulated sustained activity.

There are three major different types of muscle.

1. *Voluntary*. Voluntary muscle is the muscle forming the bulk of the arms and legs. It is also called striated, from its microscopic appearance. It is under direct control of the conscious will. Voluntary muscles whose nerves have been destroyed or damaged will not function.

2. *Involuntary*. Involuntary muscle forms the bulk of the gastrointestinal tract, the bladder and other organs, and the muscular portions of the vascular and bronchial systems. It is also called smooth muscle, from its microscopic appearance. It is under the control of the autonomic nervous system (Chapter 21). The function of this muscle cannot be controlled by conscious will. When it is deprived of its nerve supply, it continues to contract and relax in an unregulated fashion.

3. *Cardiac*. Cardiac muscle is a specially adapted involuntary muscle able to contract and relax continuously. It possesses an unusually good blood supply.

Voluntary Muscles

Voluntary muscles are so called because their actions are under conscious control. They are also called skeletal because they form the great

bulk of the muscles attached to the skeleton; they can be contracted or relaxed at will.

Most of these muscles attach directly to bones by tendons—tough, rope-like cords of fibrous tissue. Usually these attachments are at two definite points. A muscle and its tendon pass between two bony attachments called the origin of the muscle and the insertion of the muscle (Fig. 13.2). When a muscle contracts, a line of force or pull is created between the origin and the insertion, that is, between the two bones to which the muscle is connected. Most voluntary muscles pass over or across joints. Movement can take place because of these joints, the junctures where bones come together. Most voluntary muscles exist in groups or pairs having relatively equal but opposite functions so that when one muscle or group of muscles contracts, the other must relax (Fig. 13.2).

An aponeurosis is a broad fibrous sheet attaching a muscle to another muscle. Ligaments usually attach bones to bones.

Overexertion or overextension may produce an injury in which the muscle or its tendon is torn or stretched. Muscular injury, bruising, or rupture may occur with or without injury of the skin.

Diaphragm. The diaphragm is both an involuntary and a voluntary muscle. It is a large domelike sheet of muscle dividing the thorax and the abdomen. It is attached to the costal arch and the lumbar vertebrae (Fig. 13.3). When one takes a breath the diaphragm flattens and its

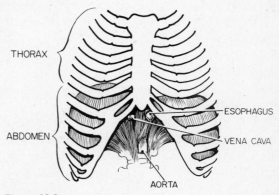

Figure 13.3

The dome-shaped diaphragm is pierced by the great vessels and the esophagus.

center part moves down. The volume of the chest cavity is increased and inspiration can take place. Breathing is an automatic function that continues when we are asleep and at all other times. Automatic control of breathing can however be overridden by conscious will, and a person can breathe faster, slower, or hold his breath. He cannot do so indefinitely, however, and in the end automatic control is resumed. Hence, although the diaphragm looks like voluntary, skeletal muscle and is attached to the skeleton, it behaves like involuntary muscle most of the time.

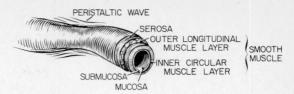

Figure 13.4

Smooth muscle layers or individual fibers allow tubular organs (intestine, blood vessels, or bronchi) to contract or dilate. A peristaltic wave of intestinal contraction is shown.

Involuntary Muscles

Involuntary muscles are so called because they continue to contract rhythmically regardless of the conscious will of the individual. They handle the work of all the internal organs except the heart. Blood vessels constrict or dilate in response to heat or cold, work load or rest, fright, or a number of other stimuli. Smooth muscle fibers in the vessel walls perform this action. We can exert no conscious control over this function. The bronchi and bronchioles (air passages in the lung) dilate or constrict in response to cold or inhaled irritants because of the action of involuntary muscles in their walls.

In the gastrointestinal tract two layers of smooth muscle exist. One is oriented around the bowel; one is oriented longitudinally. Peristalsis, a coordinated wave-like contraction of these involuntary muscles, starts at the stomach and proceeds to the anus, propelling food through the digestive tract (Fig. 13.4). Similarly, when the urge to void urine occurs because the bladder is full, a peristaltic contraction of muscle empties the bladder.

123

Involuntary muscles are constantly responding to changes in their immediate surroundings, although many of the specific stimuli are not perceived consciously by the individual. These stimuli and their muscular reactions keep one automatically in balance with the surroundings.

Cardiac Muscle

The heart is a large muscle made up of a pair of pumps of unequal force, one of lower and one of higher pressure. It must function continuously from birth to death. It is an especially adapted involuntary muscle with a particularly good blood supply and its own regulatory system. It can tolerate interruption of the blood supply only for a very few minutes before severe chest pain and the signs of a "heart attack" develop. Like all other involuntary muscles, it is under automatic control of the autonomic nervous system.

CHAPTER 14

Soft-Tissue Injuries

GOAL I. Know the types of soft-tissue injuries.

125

OBJECTIVES

A. Discriminate between open and closed soft-tissue injuries.
B. Identify the types of open and closed soft-tissue injuries.
C. Describe the development of ecchymoses and hematomas.

GOAL II. Know the appropriate treatment for soft-tissue injuries.

OBJECTIVES

A. Describe the treatment of closed soft-tissue wounds.
B. Describe the treatment of open soft-tissue wounds.
C. Describe the treatment of impaled foreign objects.

Most injuries involve soft tissues, skin, muscles, or fascia. Any such injury may be closed or open. A closed wound is one in which soft-tissue damage occurs beneath the skin but in which there is no break in the surface. An open wound is one in which there is a break in the surface of the skin or in the mucous membrane which lines the major body orifices (mouth, anus, and vagina).

Closed Soft-Tissue Injuries

A blunt object striking against the body with sufficient force crushes the tissue beneath the skin. Within this tissue a contusion (bruise) develops (Fig. 14.1a). It is a closed injury if the skin remains intact. Subsurface damage may extend for varying depths from the skin. The injury is followed by the development of swelling and pain. Small blood vessels in the tissues are usually torn and varying amounts of blood and plasma leak into the tissue. The immediate leak accounts for the swelling and the pain. Excess

blood in the tissue gradually migrates toward the skin and causes a characteristic discoloration, an ecchymosis (black and blue mark).

When considerable amounts of tissue are damaged or torn or when large blood vessels are disrupted at the site of the contusion, a lump

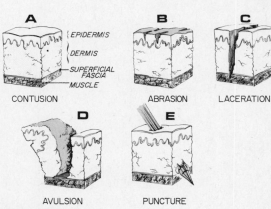

Figure 14.1 *a–e*

The types of soft-tissue injuries are shown. Abrasions usually involve the epidermis but may penetrate deeper. Avulsions raise large flaps of tissue, usually at normal tissue planes. Other injuries may penetrate to any depth.

may develop rather rapidly from a pool of blood collecting within the damaged tissue. This condition is the most severe closed soft-tissue injury and is called a hematoma or, literally, a blood tumor. In cases of bad fractures of the femur or the pelvis, a hematoma may collect about the broken ends of the bones, consisting of several hundred milliliters or more than a liter of blood about each fracture.

Management of Closed Wounds

126 Small bruises require no special emergency attention. With more severe soft-tissue injuries, swelling and bleeding beneath the skin can be extensive and may cause shock. Some control of this bleeding can be achieved by applying local padding and a soft roller bandage for counterpressure. Local applications of cold may help control initial tissue swelling and reduce it to some degree. If the patient has suffered extensive soft-tissue damage, the question of underlying fractures must be raised and such injuries must be sought. Extensive soft-tissue injuries of the extremities may also be treated immediately with the use of air-pressure splints, which provide support for the extremity and a balanced, distributed counterpressure. With soft-tissue injuries associated with fractures, splinting is a first priority.

Open Soft-Tissue Wounds

Open wounds cause obvious bleeding and are subject to direct contamination which may result in their becoming infected. There are four major kinds of open wounds of soft tissue with which the EMT should be familiar.

1. *Abrasions.* An abrasion (sometimes called a mat burn) is a loss of a portion of the outer layer of the skin from its being rubbed or scraped across a hard surface (Fig. 14.1b). Generally it is extremely painful and blood may ooze from injured capillary vessels at the surface.
2. *Lacerations.* A laceration is a cut produced by a knife, razor, or any other object which

may leave a smooth or jagged wound through the skin, the subcutaneous tissues, the underlying muscles, and associated nerves and blood vessels (Fig. 14.1 c).

3. *Avulsion.* An avulsion is an injury in which a whole piece of skin with varying portions of subcutaneous tissue or muscle is torn loose and left hanging as a flap (Fig. 14.1 d). Ordinarily, avulsed flaps of tissues separate at normal planes, for example, between fascia and subcutaneous tissue. Occasionally, avulsed tissue will be torn completely free and will be lying apart from the patient. All avulsed tissue that is torn away from the patient should be collected and taken to the Emergency Department along with the patient. The EMT may encounter persons who have had avulsion injuries of fingers or hands, arms or legs, or who have lost a portion or all of an extremity. This tissue, if it is readily available should be retrieved and transported along with the patient to the hospital. Some success is being realized now in reimplanting avulsed portions of the body.
4. *Puncture wounds.* A puncture wound results from a stab with a knife, nail, ice pick, splinter, or other pointed object, or from a gunshot injury (Fig. 14.1 e). Obvious external bleeding is usually not severe from a puncture wound because it is so small. However, these instruments, particularly bullets, may injure major vessels within body cavities and cause rapid, fatal bleeding within the chest or abdomen. There is no way for the EMT to assess the amount of damage sustained from a puncture wound. Ordinarily this requires an exploratory operation in either the chest, the abdomen, or the extremity involved.

   Extensive damage should always be suspected. Some puncture wounds, especially those in extremities, may traverse the entire limb or body cavity to exit on the opposite side. These are perforating (through-and-through) wounds. The EMT should always seek an exit wound, especially in the case of a gunshot injury.

The Management of Open Wounds

Open soft-tissue wounds are treated with regard to three general rules. The order of the treatment is determined by the extent of the wound itself, the severity of bleeding, and the amount of blood lost. Usually one approaches treatment of these wounds in this order:

1. Control the bleeding.
2. Prevent further contamination.
3. Immobilize the part and keep the patient quiet.

Bleeding is controlled by the application of a pressure dressing directly over the wound. Such an application of pressure may be accomplished with:

1. The bare hand or a dressing held by the hand (Fig. 14.2 *a*).
2. A dressing held by a pressure bandage (Fig. 14.2 *b*).
3. A dressing held by an air splint (Fig. 14.2 *c*).

Uncontrolled bleeding may, in some cases, require the use of pressure points in the body or, in more extreme cases, the use of a tourniquet to stop the hemorrhage. Care should be taken to follow the directions for application of a tourniquet given in Chapter 8.

Frequently the control of bleeding from soft-tissue wounds, whether or not they are associated with a fracture, is markedly improved by splinting the bleeding extremities. If an air splint is used, a considerable amount of gentle pressure may be exerted throughout the entire length of the extremity and bleeding may be controlled more readily than with the use of a local pressure dressing. When bleeding is associated with a soft-tissue wound accompanying a fracture, splinting is absolutely necessary before adequate control of soft-tissue bleeding from the wound can be achieved. Further, splinting of an extremity which has undergone significant soft-tissue injury will allow the patient to be moved much more readily and more comfortably without further damage to an already injured arm or leg. An initial step in controlling soft-tissue bleeding is appropriate splinting and immobilizing of the bleeding extremity.

Contamination of a wound and resultant secondary infection is made less likely if the EMT can use clean, sterile materials for his initial dressing. Every effort should be made to keep foreign matter out of the wound. Hair, cotton.

127

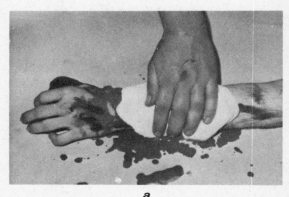

a

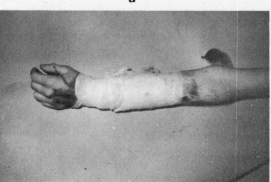

b

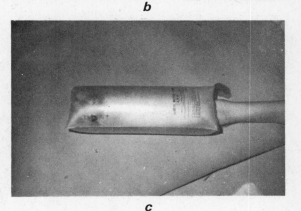

c

Figure 14.2 *a–c*

Three different kinds of pressure to control bleeding are shown. *a*, A simple dressing, preferably sterile, is applied to the laceration with pressure by the hand. If no dressing or cloth is available, the hand alone can be used. *b*, A pressure dressing is held in place by a circular bandage. *c*, A pressure dressing is held in place by an air splint.

clothing, dirt, and fluids all involve the hazard of secondary infection. However, in the initial treatment do not try to remove material embedded in the wound, no matter how dirty it may be. Only the gross matter on the surface around the wound should be removed. The final definitive cleaning of the wound may be a procedure for the surgeon to carry out in the operating room. Much time may be lost in a fruitless attempt to clean a wound that requires operative manipulation for adequate treatment.

Clothing covering a wound must be removed. It is far better to tear or cut away clothing from the wound than to attempt to remove it in a normal manner, as motion may be painful and cause additional tissue damage and contamination. Care should be taken to remove clothing with as little movement of the patient's body as possible. What may seem an insignificant motion to the EMT may cause excruciating pain to the patient.

Impaled Foreign Objects

Occasionally an object such as a knife, splinter of wood, or piece of glass will be seen in a puncture wound (Fig. 14.3 *a*). This is called an impaled foreign object. In addition to local control of bleeding, one must follow three rules in treating a patient who has an impaled foreign object in his body.

1. Do not remove the object. Its removal may cause severe hemorrhage or damage of nerves or muscles lying close to the object. Try to stop any bleeding from the entrance wound by direct pressure but avoid exerting any force on the impaled object itself or on tissue directly adjacent to its cutting edge (Fig. 14.3 *a*).
2. Use a bulky dressing to stabilize the object. The impaled foreign body itself should be incorporated within the dressing so that its motion after the bandage is applied is reduced (Fig. 14.3 *b*).
3. Transport this patient promptly to the Emergency Department with the object

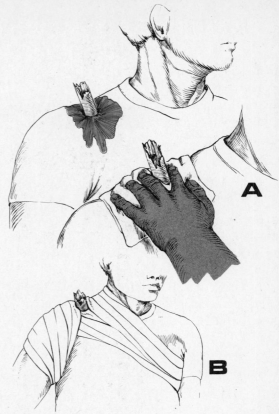

Figure 14.3

An impaled object should be left in place while, *a*, bleeding is controlled with pressure. *b*, A bandage is applied about the object to stabilize it and to maintain pressure while the patient is transported to the hospital where the object may be removed.

still in place. Ordinarily it will require an operation for its removal so that the tissues immediately around the impaled object may be examined directly and treated if they are injured.

If it is necessary to shorten a very long impaled object to allow transportation of the patient, remember that even the slightest movement may cause severe additional pain, hemorrhage, or damage of the tissue around it. Before an object is cut off, it must be made quite secure and any motion transmitted to the patient must be minimal. Pain is a factor aggravating shock in the patient who has undergone severe hemorrhage. It must be avoided whenever possible.

128

15

The Skeletal System

GOAL I. Know the characteristics and functions of the bones and joints of the skeletal system.

OBJECTIVES

A. Define bone.

B. Define joint.

C. Describe the characteristics of each of the following components of the skeletal system: spinal column, skull, thorax, upper extremities, pelvis, and lower extremities.

D. Name the protective functions of the skeletal system.

E. Label the parts in a drawing of the anatomy of the bones and joints.

The skeleton forms the supporting framework of the human body (Fig. 15.1). Normally, it is composed of 206 bones. It gives form to the body, allows bodily motion, and serves several functions. The skeleton affords protection to vital organs shielded by it. The brain lies within the skull; the heart and lungs within the thorax; much of the liver and spleen are protected by the lowermost ribs; and the spinal cord is contained within the spinal canal formed by the vertebrae.

Bones of the skeleton come into contact with one another at joints, where they can be moved by the action of muscles. The skeleton thus serves as a rigid framework for the attachment of muscles and protection of organs and as a moveable framework so that muscular contraction may express purposeful motion. The framework provided by the skeleton allows an erect posture against the pull of gravity and gives recognizable form to the body.

Bones form the skeleton, but not every bone is fully developed at birth. Bones must be rigid and unyielding to fulfill their function but they must also grow and adapt as the human being grows.

Bony growth of a person is usually complete in the late teens. Unless some abnormality is present, there is usually little bone change after this period.

The dual requirements of a tissue that must be at once firm and unyielding but still grow are met by the very special material which makes up bone. Bones are composed of a framework of protein which allows for growth and change in the shape of the bone, and by calcium and phosphorus minerals which are deposited into the framework to make the bone hard and strong. Bones in young children are more flexible than in the adult. Therefore they are less likely to fracture. Bones are just as much living tissue as are muscle and skin; they have a blood supply and their tissue requires oxygen and nutrients. Throughout the lifetime of the individual, calcium and phosphorus are constantly being deposited in bones and withdrawn from them under the control of very complex metabolic systems.

Whenever two or more bones come into contact, they articulate with each other and form a

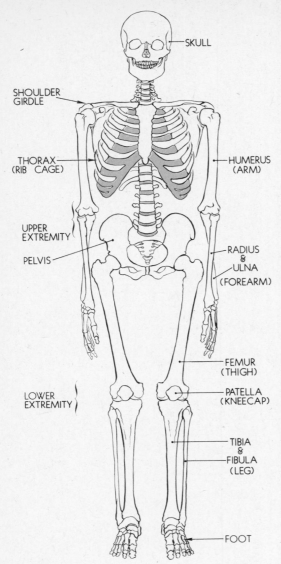

Figure 15.1

The human skeleton forms the frame of the body.

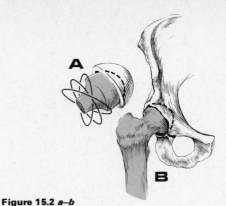

Figure 15.2 a–b

a, Motion in all planes is possible at a ball-and-socket joint, *b,* The hip joint is a typical ball-and-socket joint.

pass around and across joints. The ends of the bones which articulate with each other are covered with a smooth surface of articular cartilage. The moveable joints are lubricated by a yellowish clear fluid called synovial fluid.

Motion within a joint is made possible by the action of muscles which attach to bones. Muscles contract or relax, thereby moving the bones to which they are attached as levers. The actual extent of motion at a given joint is determined by the type of joint, the location and resistance of the ligaments supporting the joint, and the location of the muscles and tendons. There is no motion at a fused joint; the two bones forming the joint have grown together and are immobile.

There are many different types of joints which allow motion in the body. The hip and shoulder joints are ball-and-socket type and have a wide range of motion in all planes (Fig. 15.2). The thumb is of particular interest because of the unusual saddle-shaped joint surface (Fig. 15.3). This joint is quite stable; yet it allows motion in many planes. It can flex, extend, abduct, adduct, and circumduct. Hinge joints allow motion in just one plane; the joint can flex (bend) or extend (straighten) but cannot rotate. Examples of a hinge joint are the knee, elbow, and finger (Fig. 15.4). Still other joints have very little motion because of the arrangement and strength of the connecting ligaments—for example, the sacroiliac joint in the pelvis.

The motion of each joint has certain definite limits. If a joint is forced to move in a manner for which it was not designed or beyond its

joint. Some joints allow motion—for example, the knee, hip or elbow—whereas other bones fuse with one another at joints so that a solid, immobile, bony structure results. The skull is composed of several different bones which fuse as the person grows into adulthood.

A joint consists of the ends of the bones which make up the joint and the surrounding connecting and supporting tissues. In joints that allow motion the bones are held together by a capsule and supporting ligaments, which are bands of tough fibrous tissue. Muscles and their tendons

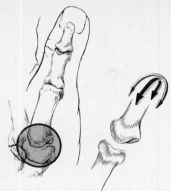

Figure 15.3

The special joint of the metacarpal bone of the thumb and its carpal bone at the wrist, like two saddles fitted together, allows motion in many planes.

limits, one of several events may occur.

1. The bones forming the joint may break.
2. The ligaments connecting the bones forming the joint may stretch or tear.
3. The joint may be displaced (dislocated) so that the ends of the bones will no longer be in proper contact with one another. For example, when a person steps unexpectedly into a hole, he may twist his ankle with a resultant fracture, tear of the ligaments, or dislocation of the ankle joint.

Skull

The skull has two main divisions—the cranium (brain case) and the face (Fig. 15.5). The cranium is composed of a number of broad flat bones which fuse to form the shell which protects the brain.

The face is made up of multiple bones which

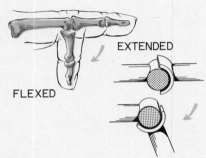

Figure 15.4

The finger joints are hinge joints, which allow motion in only one plane.

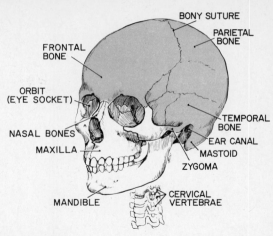

Figure 15.5

The skull includes the flat bones of the cranium, which are fused, and the facial bones. The mandible (lower jaw) is freely moveable.

131

fuse to give shape to the face. Specifically, these are the facial bones, nasal bones, the orbital bones, the maxillae (upper jaw), and the mandible (lower jaw). The mandible completes the bones of the face.

Spinal Column

The spinal column is the central supportive bony structure of the body (Fig. 15.6). It is composed of thirty-three bones, called vertebrae.

The spine is divided into five sections:

1. Cervical spine (neck)
2. Thoracic spine (upper part of the back)
3. Lumbar spine (lower part of the back)
4. Sacral spine (part of the pelvis)
5. Coccygeal spine (coccyx, or tailbone)

The first seven vertebrae form the cervical spine (neck). The next twelve vertebrae make up the thoracic spine (upper back) and twelve pairs of ribs articulate with these vertebrae. The next five vertebrae form the lumbar spine of the lower back. The five sacral vertebrae are fused to form the sacrum. The sacrum joins the two large bones of the pelvis at the sacroiliac joints to form the pelvic girdle. The last four vertebrae form the coccyx (tailbone).

The skull articulates with the first cervical vertebra. The spinal cord, which extends from

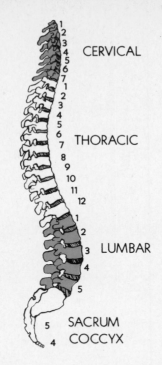

Figure 15.6

The spinal column consists of 33 vertebrae in five definite sections.

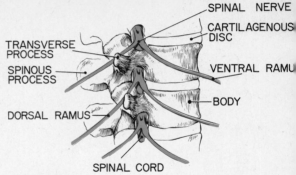

Figure 15.8

The relationship of the spinal nerve roots to the bony spinal column is shown.

132

the brain, is contained and protected by the vertebrae of the spinal column.

The front part of each vertebra is a round, solid block of bone called the body; the back part of each forms an arch (Fig. 15.7). This series of arches forms a tunnel which runs the length of the spine and is called the spinal canal. The spinal canal encloses the spinal cord. Nerves branch off from the spinal cord to form the motor and sensory nerves of the body (Fig. 15.8). The vertebrae are connected by ligaments; between each two vertebrae is an intervertebral

disc which acts as a cushion. The ligaments and discs allow some motion such as turning the head, bending the trunk forward or backward or leaning it to either side, but they also act to limit motion of the vertebrae so that the spinal cord will not be injured. When a fracture of the spine occurs, the protection of the spinal cord and its nerve roots may be lost. Until the fracture is made stable, the possibility of further injury of the spinal cord must be a paramount consideration of the EMT.

Thorax

The thorax (rib cage) is made up of the ribs, twelve thoracic vertebrae, and the sternum (breast bone) (Fig. 15.9). There are twelve pairs of ribs, which are long, slender, curved bones. Each rib is attached to a thoracic vertebra at the back and curves around to form the rib cage. At the front of the rib cage, ribs 1 through 10 connect with the sternum by strips of cartilage. The sternum forms the middle part of the front of the thoracic cage. It is a bone approximately seven inches long and two inches wide. The xiphoid process is the small tip at the bottom of the sternum.

A free pivoting motion of the ribs at their joints with the vertebrae allows expansion of the thorax when one inspires (breathes in). When the ribs pivot upward, the thoracic cavity become larger and air is drawn into the lungs. Movements of the rib cage are discussed in more detail in connection with the respiratory system.

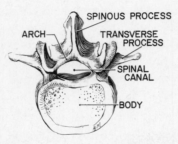

Figure 15.7

The top view of a thoracic vertebra shows the spinal canal.

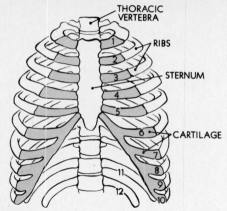

Figure 15.9

In the thoracic cage, twelve pairs of ribs articulate with the vertebrae in the spinal column through small joints. The first ten pairs also articulate with the sternum or the costal arch in front, through heavy cartilages.

Upper Extremity

The shoulder serves as a base of attachment for the upper extremity. It is formed principally by the scapula (shoulder blade), the clavicle (collarbone), and the upper end of the humerus (arm) (Fig. 15.10).

The scapula is a flat, triangular bone which is supported against the rib cage posteriorly by large muscles. The upper and outer part of the scapula forms the socket of the shoulder joint. Muscles also pass from the scapula to the arm, crossing the shoulder joint. Motion of the upper extremity at the shoulder joint is as described for a ball-and-socket joint and can occur in any plane. Since the major attachment of the scapula to the chest is muscular, considerable freedom of

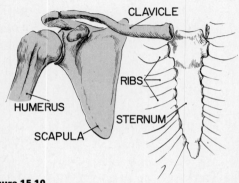

Figure 15.10

The scapula (shoulder blade) and the clavicle (collar bone) form the shoulder girdle. They overlie the thorax.

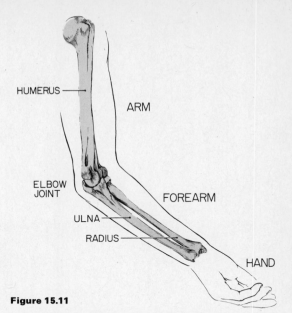

Figure 15.11

The upper extremity and the major bones above the hand are shown.

motion is given this bone as it slides over the chest wall. Such motion may be limited by conscious contractions of the muscles attaching it to the chest.

The clavicle is a long slender bone. One end of the clavicle is attached by ligaments to the top of the sternum while the other end is attached to the scapula near the shoulder joint. The clavicle acts as a support or a prop for the shoulder.

The upper extremity (Fig. 15.11) consists of the shoulder joint (articulation of head of humerus with the scapula); the arm (the humerus); the elbow joint (articulation of the distal end of the humerus with the head of the radius and the upper ulna); the forearm (the radius and ulna); the wrist joint (articulation of the distal end of the radius and ulna with the carpal bones and the carpal bones with the metacarpal bones) (Fig. 15.12); and the hand (the metacarpal bones and phalanges). In the forearm the radius is on the lateral side of the arm, i.e., on the thumb side, and the ulna is on the medial, or inner, side. At the elbow the ulna is larger than the radius, but at the wrist the radius is the larger bone.

Pelvis and Lower Extremities

The pelvis or pelvic girdle is a bony ring (Fig.

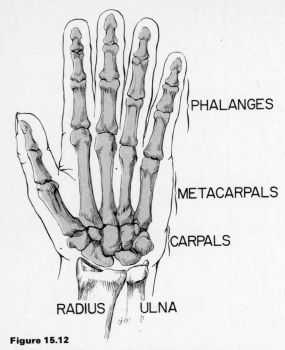

PHALANGES

METACARPALS

CARPALS

RADIUS   ULNA

134

Figure 15.12

The bones of the wrist and hand are shown in articulation with the radius and ulna.

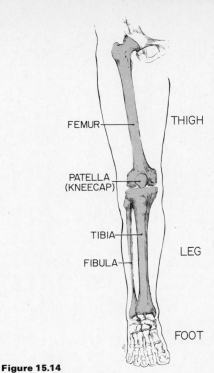

FEMUR   THIGH

PATELLA
(KNEECAP)

TIBIA

FIBULA   LEG

FOOT

Figure 15.14

The femur is the single bone of the thigh. The leg is formed by the fibula and the tibia.

15.13) formed by the sacrum (lower five vertebrae) and the two large wing-like innominate (pelvic) bones. Each of these two bones has three separate components (ilium, ischium, and pubis). The two innominate bones join in front to form the pubic symphysis. The symphysis can be felt at the middle of the lower abdomen. The bladder lies just behind this joint. Posteriorly each innominate bone articulates with

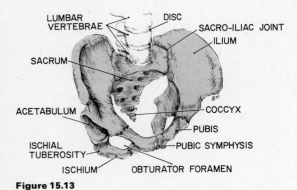

LUMBAR
VERTEBRAE   DISC
                  SACRO-ILIAC JOINT
                  ILIUM
SACRUM

ACETABULUM
                  COCCYX
                  PUBIS
ISCHIAL
TUBEROSITY   PUBIC SYMPHYSIS
  ISCHIUM   OBTURATOR FORAMEN

Figure 15.13

A full-view drawing of the pelvic girdle shows the sacrum joined to the pelvic bones (also called innominate bones). A strong supportive ring is formed. Each of the two pelvic bones consists of a fusion of the iliac, ischial, and pubic bones. They are joined in front at the pubic symphysis.

the sacrum (sacroiliac joint) and is connected by broad, very strong sacroiliac ligaments.

The pelvis is adapted for great strength and support. It contains the sockets of the two hip joints. A hip socket is called an acetabulum. Each socket is made up of the union of the three bones which form each innominate bone, i.e., the ilium, the ischium, and the pubis. The entire weight of the body is transmitted through this bony pelvic ring across the hip joint and into the legs.

The ischial tuberosity forms a bony prominence in each buttock. It is very important in applying traction splints on an injured lower extremity, as weight can be borne by it or force applied to it.

The pelvis surrounds and affords protection to the pelvic cavity, the lowermost portion of the abdominal cavity. Within this cavity lie the bladder, the rectum, and, in the female, the internal sexual organs.

The lower extremity (Fig. 15.14) consists of the hip joint (the articulation of the upper end or head of the femur with the acetabulum of the pelvis); the thigh (femur); the knee joint (the

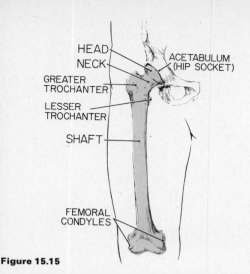

Figure 15.15

The upper half of the lower extremity (the thigh) and its bone are shown.

foot (the tarsal bones, metatarsal bones, and phalanges).

The femur is the longest and one of the strongest bones in the body. It is divided into three separate areas, the head and neck, the shaft, and the femoral condyles (Fig. 15.15). The distal end of the femur, which articulates with the upper end of the tibia, is formed of two large condyles. The patella (kneecap) is a moveable bone in the front of the knee joint. It is located in the large tendon of the quadriceps muscle which crosses the front of the knee joint (Fig. 15.16). The knee joint is the largest joint in the body and the liagments which give it stability are very complex and quite susceptible to injury. The tibia or shinbone of the leg is larger than the fibula throughout most of the anterior length. Because it is located just beneath the anterior skin of the leg it is very susceptible to sustaining an open fracture. At the ankle joint the distal end of the tibia forms the medial malleolus and the distal end of the fibula forms the lateral malleolus. Heavy ligaments support the malleoli with the tarsal bones.

135

articulation of the distal end of the femur with the upper end of the tibia and the patella); the leg (the tibia and fibula); the ankle joint (the articulation of the distal end of the tibia and fibula with the talus or a tarsal bone); and the

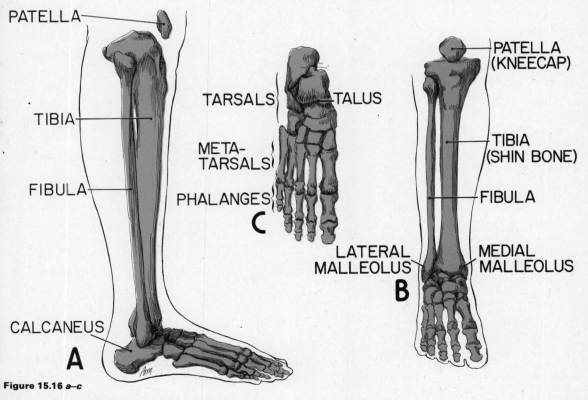

Figure 15.16 a–c

Bones of the leg and foot are shown in three views.

```
```

16

Fractures, Dislocations, and Sprains

GOAL I. Know the characteristics of fractures and dislocations.

OBJECTIVES

A. List the causes of fractures and dislocations.
B. Describe the characteristics of fractures.
C. List the signs of dislocations.
D. Describe the characteristics of dislocations.
E. Identify the differences between open and closed fractures and dislocations.

GOAL II. Know the procedures for evaluating dislocations and fractures.

OBJECTIVES

A. Describe the proper examination of a suspected fracture or dislocation.
B. Explain the importance of evaluation and proper care of fractures and dislocations.

Injuries of the musculoskeletal system (bones, joints, muscles, and tendons) are often seen in emergency care work. The EMT should check every injured patient he treats for the presence of fractures or dislocations. He should learn how to evaluate a patient for a fracture of any bone in the body, and how to manage that injury properly. Proper emergency care will result in decreased pain and shock, a shorter hospital stay, and a better chance for a rapid return of the patient to normal activities.

A fracture is any break in the continuity of a bone. In some fractures the bone may only be cracked. In others, the pieces of the bone may be separated, making the fracture easy to recognize because of the motion of the fragments. In still other instances, the fragments of the broken bone may be bent on one another.

A dislocation is the displacement of the bone ends that form a joint so that the joint surfaces are no longer in proper contact.

A sprain is the partial tearing or stretching of the ligaments around a joint.

The care of a bone injury must include the recognition of all other possible injuries and an evaluation of the general condition of the patient. Occasionally fractures may be the result of causes other than accidents.

Causes of Fractures and Dislocations

Fractures and dislocations may occur as the result of many different factors: trauma, fatigue, or disease. A severe injury may sometimes include both a fracture and the dislocation of a joint. This type of injury is called a fracture-dislocation.

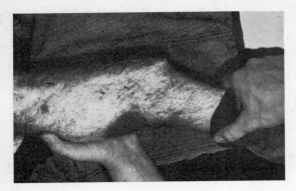

Figure 16.1

A closed fracture of the tibia is demonstrated. Note that the skin is intact.

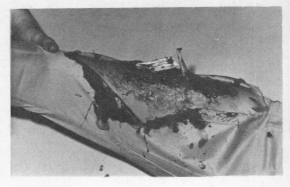

Figure 16.2

An open fracture of the femur shows the skin disrupted and bones protruding.

Various causes of fractures and dislocations are discussed below.

Direct blows. The injury occurs at the site of impact; for example, the patella (kneecap) may be fractured when it strikes against the dashboard in an automobile accident.

Indirect blows. The injury occurs not at the site of direct impact but at a site some distance from the blow; for example, the wrist can be broken when one falls on an outstretched hand, or the hip can be dislocated when the knee strikes a dashboard.

Twisting forces. A strong twisting force may result in a bad sprain, fracture, or dislocation. This type of injury is seen at the ankle in skiing and football accidents. Many knee injuries are produced by twisting forces.

Muscle contractions. Sometimes muscles can contract so powerfully that they actually produce an avulsion fracture; that is, a piece of bone may be pulled away by the muscle-tendon unit.

Fatigue. Bones may fracture when they are subjected to repeated stress, as during a long march.

Pathological conditions. Localized destructive disease processes, such as cancer, can weaken a bone so that only a slight force, sometimes an imperceptible one, will produce a fracture.

Fractures

Certain fractures are easily identified by a localized mass, by pain, or by a laceration in the skin where the bone has penetrated it. Some fractures, however, can be recognized only by an appropriate X-ray examination.

Major classifications. The two major classes of fractures are:

1. *Closed (simple) fractures*—The skin has not been penetrated by the bone ends (Fig. 16.1).

2. *Open (compound) fractures*—The bone has broken through the skin, or there is an accompanying wound which extends from the broken bone through the skin (Fig. 16.2). This wound may be only a small opening over the fracture, or it may allow one or both ends of the broken bone to protrude through the skin.

It is extremely important to determine at once whether the fracture is open or closed. Open fractures are much more serious than closed fractures because of their greater blood loss and because they are contaminated and may become infected.

All open fractures should be treated by covering the bone and the wound with a sterile dressing, by applying local pressure to stop any bleeding, and by appropriate splinting of the extremity, gently correcting any gross deformities. The protruding bone ends should not purposely be pushed or pulled back beneath the skin by traction. The bone ends may be obviously contaminated (covered with grease, dirt, or grass), which will only increase the possibility of infection of the fracture. Proper cleaning in these instances can only be carried out in the hospital. The physician must always be notified should the bone end spontaneously slip back into the wound.

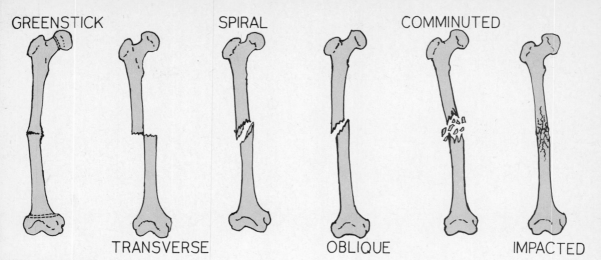

GREENSTICK   SPIRAL   COMMINUTED

TRANSVERSE   OBLIQUE   IMPACTED

139

Figure 16.3 *a–f*

Six types of fractures are shown. *a*, In a greenstick fracture, the bone in children which is soft is not broken completely through. *b*, A transverse fracture divides a long bone across the long axis. *c*, A spiral fracture takes a spiral or winding course. It usually results from a twisting injury. *d*, An oblique fracture cleanly divides a bone at an angle. *e*, A comminuted fracture is characterized by many fragments of bone. *f*, An impacted fracture is one in which the bone ends are driven together.

Other classifications. Fractures may also be classified according to the appearance of the broken bone, as listed below (Fig. 16.3).

1. *Greenstick fracture*—An incomplete fracture which passes only part way through a bone is called a greenstick fracture. It occurs only in a child.

2. *Transverse fracture*—The fracture line is straight across the bone at a right angle to its long axis.

3. *Oblique fracture*—The fracture line crosses the bone at an oblique angle.

4. *Spiral fracture*—The fracture line twists around and through the bone.

5. *Comminuted fracture*—The bone is broken into more than two pieces.

6. *Impacted fracture*—The broken ends of the bone are jammed into each other.

Signs of fractures. A fracture is easily recognized if one sees bone ends penetrating the skin or if there is an obvious deformity of an extremity, but these signs of fractures are not always present. Among the signs and symptoms, which should lead the EMT to suspect a fracture, and to treat the patient accordingly, are the following:

1. *Deformity*—An arm or leg may lie in an unnatural position or be angulated where there is no joint.

2. *Tenderness*—Tenderness is usually sharply localized at the site of the break. The sensitive spot (point tenderness) can be located by gently pressing along the bone with the tip of one finger.

3. *Grating or crepitus*—A sensation can often be felt when the broken ends of the bone rub together. This sign should not intentionally be sought, as it only increases pain for the patient.

4. *Swelling and ecchymosis (discoloration)*—Swelling to some degree is almost always present with fractures. The swelling is either a result of hemorrhage which occurs immediately after the injury or of edema (increased fluid in the tissues), which may not become obvious for several hours. Bleeding associated with a fracture occurs when major blood vessels in the bone and in the soft tissue and muscle near the fracture rupture.

5. *Inability to use the extremity*—A patient who has sustained a severe leg or arm injury usually guards the injured part and will not attempt to walk or use the arm or leg. However, in some cases of incomplete or impacted fractures, function of an extremity may be retained to a remarkable degree. There may, however, be partial or complete loss of motion in the adjacent joints.

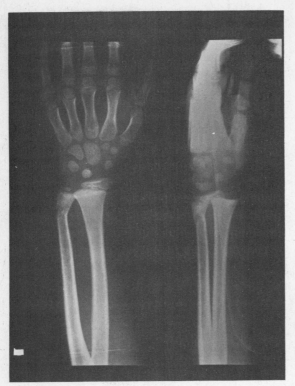

Figure 16.4

A combined fracture of the radius and ulna in a child is shown in these X rays. Left, a partial (greenstick) fracture of the distal ulna produces a deformity. Right, the distal radius has been entirely separated through the epiphysis.

6. *Exposed fragments*—In an open, or compound, fracture, bone fragments may protrude through the skin or be seen in the depths of the wound.

The EMT should be aware that, in children, fractures in long bones can occur at the epiphyseal, or growth, plates. An epiphyseal growth plate is located at both ends of most long bones and is responsible for the longitudinal growth of the bone. Without X-ray films it is essentially impossible to distinguish some fractures of a bone from epiphyseal injuries (Fig. 16.4).

Dislocations

A joint consists of the opposing ends of two bones, covered by cartilage, which are held together by a joint capsule, ligaments, and tendons. The capsule and the ligaments help provide stability in the joint. When there is a dislocated joint, the capsule and ligaments are usually torn and one of the bone ends is dislodged from its normal position (Fig. 16.5). Joints which are frequently dislocated are the shoulder, elbow, fingers, hip, and ankle. Less frequently the EMT may see a dislocated wrist or knee.

The most important symptoms and signs in identifying a dislocation are:

1. A marked deformity of the joint
2. Pain or swelling of the joint
3. Pain on any attempted movement of the joint
4. Complete or nearly complete loss of movement at the joint
5. An immovable (locked) joint, often fixed in a deformed position

Sprains

Sprains are usually produced by twisting or stretching of a joint beyond its normal range of

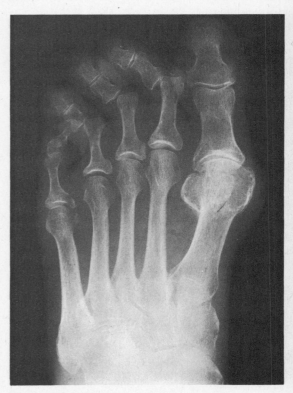

Figure 16.5

In this X-ray photograph, dislocations of the proximal interphalangeal joints of the second, third, and fourth toes can be seen.

140

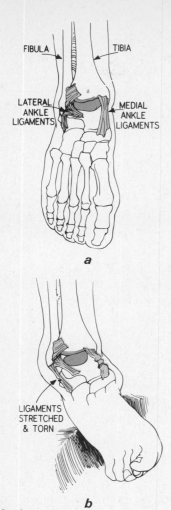

Figure 16.6 *a–b*

A joint sprain is shown. *a*, Note the normal relationship of the foot to the leg and the presence of intact ligaments. *b*, Note the medial shift of the foot on the leg and the subsequent stretching and tearing of the ligaments on the lateral side of the ankle.

motion, resulting in an abnormal stretch of the ligaments around the joint. Sprains vary in severity from slight injuries to those causing serious damage of all the tissues around a joint. Two very common locations of sprains are the ankle and the knee. The ankle injury is usually the result of a sudden inward twisting of the foot and ankle, damaging the lateral ligaments of the ankle (Fig. 16.6).

The damage to ligaments may be only a partial stretch or it may be a complete separation. Dislocation of a joint can occur as a result of complete ligament separation. Because dislocation

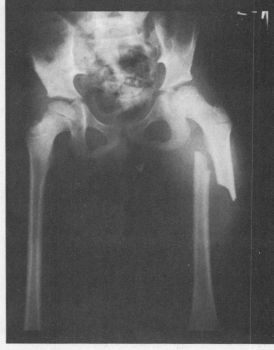

Figure 16.7

A major oblique fracture of the femoral shaft is shown in X ray. There is dislocation of the bone ends. The obvious deformity of the thigh is apparent. In addition, the injured leg will be shorter and immovable.

141

of joints can occur with ligament injuries, they can be mistaken for fractures.

Examination and Treatment of Fractures and Dislocations

When the EMT first evaluates the patient, he should quickly look for any deformity and ask the patient if he has any pain. He should determine whether the patient can move the injured extremity. If there is a fracture or dislocation, movement or even attempted movement is nearly always painful (Fig. 16.7). The patient will usually point to the site of the fracture or dislocation as being the source of pain. Remember that very little motion is possible with a dislocation because of the mechanical block at the injured joint.

The EMT should carefully palpate the extremities and the spine to see if he can find evidence of a fracture or a dislocation. Fractures and dislocations are painful if lightly pressed.

There may be swelling and discoloration at an injury site caused by internal bleeding. The patient's clothing must be removed or cut away to examine any suspicious areas.

If the patient is unconscious, the examination will be more difficult to perform. The EMT must rely on a physical examination of the extremity, noting deformity, swelling, and bleeding. He should always appropriately splint any area in question to try to avoid complications. In managing an unconscious patient who has been involved in an accident, the EMT should always assume that there may be a neck or back injury and should carefully immobilize the patient on a spineboard. The rules given in Chapter 10, Basic Life Support, for moving and resuscitating this patient must be observed.

A fracture of a bone or a dislocation at a joint may damage or lacerate nearby soft-tissue vessels and nerves. Therefore, always examine the patient with a fracture or a dislocation for:

1. Numbness or paralysis below the fracture or the dislocation (from pinching or cutting of the nerves)
2. Loss of the pulse below the fracture or the dislocation (from pressure, pinching, or cutting of the blood vessels)

If the blood vessels are pinched or cut, the extremity may feel cold and the pulse cannot be palpated. When this finding is noted, treatment by the physician is urgently required and an operation to repair the blood vessels may be necessary.

The EMT should be aware that much blood loss can be caused by a fracture, either open or closed. When a bone breaks, there is bleeding from inside the bone as well as from surrounding damaged tissues. Because of excessive blood loss, either to the outside or into the tissue, the patient with a bad fracture can develop hypovolemic shock. Appropriate measures to control bleeding are discussed in Chapter 8, Bleeding and the Control of Bleeding.

The EMT should seek hidden problems as well as note obvious injuries. A careful, complete examination for other injuries must be carried out even when a grotesque injury is obvious. The first complete examination is especially important when a fracture or dislocation is suspected since additional handling should be avoided. Repeated manipulation will produce further hemorrhage and unnecessary pain. The part that is believed to be injured should be immobilized.

17

General Principles of Splinting and Bandaging

143

GOAL I. Understand the general principles of splinting of fractures and dislocations.

Objectives

A. Explain the reasons for splinting fractures.
B. State the general rules of splinting.
C. Name the types of splints and describe the methods of application.

GOAL II. Understand the general principles for dressing and bandaging.

Objectives

A. Explain the main functions of bandages and dressings.
B. Describe the methods used to stop severe bleeding in an extremity.

Proper emergency care rendered a patient with a fracture or dislocation will decrease the length of his hospitalization and speed his recovery, as the chances for developing serious complications will be less. Skilled treatment can be learned only with a thorough understanding of the principles of the care of fractures and with diligent practice.

A splint can be fashioned from any material or appliance which will prevent the movement of a fractured or dislocated extremity. However, the EMT should have available an adequate supply of standard commercial splints (Fig. 17.1). Only occasionally should he be obliged to improvise in applying a splint.

Why Splint a Fracture or Dislocation?

The primary objective of emergency splinting is preventing motion of the fragments of a frac-

tured bone or of the bones at a dislocated joint. The application, before moving the patient, of a splint that will immobilize a fractured spine and protect the spinal cord may prevent months or years of disability and suffering as a result of cord damage.

The use of a splint alleviates pain by minimizing movement at the site of the injury. It can also help prevent:

1. Further damage of muscles, nerves, and blood vessels by the broken ends of bone
2. Laceration of the skin by the broken bones (an open fracture is far more dangerous because of direct contamination and possible infection)
3. A restricted flow of blood as a result of the pressure of bone ends on blood vessels
4. Excessive bleeding into the tissue around the fracture site caused by unstable bone ends

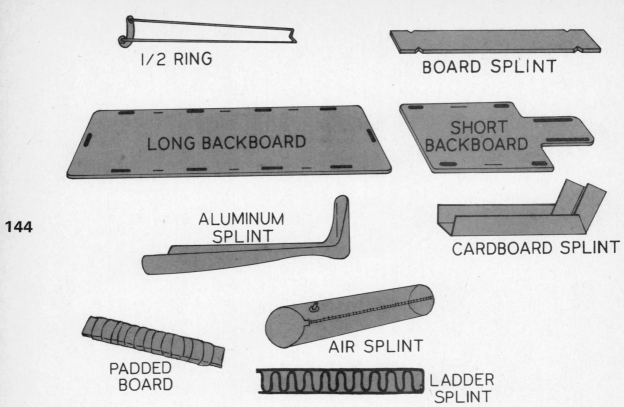

144

Figure 17.1

Many different kinds of commercial splints are available. A selection of these splints should constitute routine equipment on any ambulance.

5. Paralysis of extremities as a result of spinal cord injury from fractured or dislocated vertebrae

General Rules of Splinting

1. The clothing must always be cut away or removed from any suspected fracture or dislocation.
2. Always note and record the circulatory and the neurological status distal to the site of injury.
3. In a fracture or dislocation the splint should immobilize the joint or the bone both above and below the site of the injury.
4. A dislocation or an obvious fracture with a deformity near a joint can be a very serious injury because of possible damage to adjacent nerves and blood vessels. In general, the deformity may be straight-

ened with steady, gentle traction if the maneuver does not significantly increase pain for the patient and if no resistance to the correction is encountered.

5. A severely angulated fracture should be straightened with gentle traction so that the limb can be incorporated into a splint.
6. Cover all wounds with a sterile dressing before applying a splint.
7. Pad the splint to prevent excessive pressure.
8. In neck and spine injuries, correct the deformity only as much as is necessary to eliminate airway obstruction.
9. Do not move or transport a patient before splinting fractures or dislocations.
10. In open fractures, avoid pushing the fragments of bone back beneath the skin. In the event that the bone ends return into the soft tissue during splinting, the physician should be notified of the event

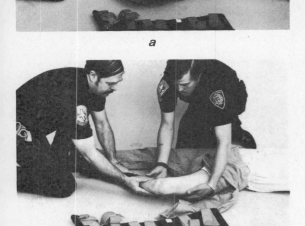

a

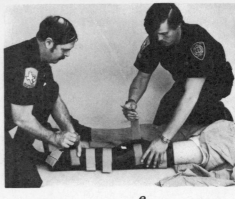

e

Figure 17.2 *a–e*

Steps in the application of a rigid splint are shown. *a*, The trouser leg is cut open to expose the injured area. *b*, One EMT supports the limb; the other begins to apply gentle traction. *c*, One EMT continues to support the limb and apply traction while the other slides the rigid splint under the patient's leg. *d*, Padding is placed to protect the limb from excessive pressure from the splint. Note that one EMT continues to maintain traction on the extremity. *e*, Velcro straps are secured to hold the splint in place, fastened loosely enough that circulation is not impaired.

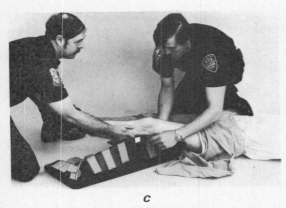

b

upon arrival at the Emergency Department.

11. When in doubt, "Splint."

Types of Splints

Many different materials are used for splints; and splints may be of several types: rigid splints, soft splints (air splint, pillow splint, or sling), or traction splints.

Rigid splint. A rigid splint is made of a firm material, either unbending or flexible, and is applied along the sides, front, or back of an injured extremity. When used correctly, it will prevent motion at the fracture site. Examples of rigid splints include padded wooden, metal, or plastic splints, padded wire ladder splints, and folded cardboard splints.

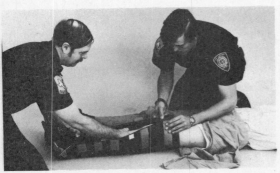

c

The rigid splint can be used for either a fracture or a dislocation. The splint should immobilize the joint above and the joint below the suspected fracture. In immobilizing a dislocation, the splint should be long enough to immobilize the bone above and the bone below the injured joint.

The application of a rigid splint follows these steps (Fig. 17.2):

d

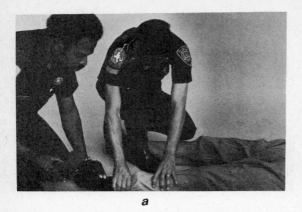

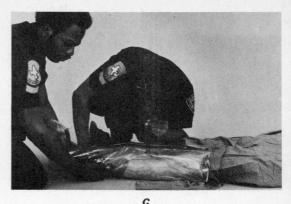

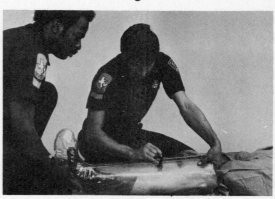

Figure 17.3 a–d

The application of an air splint with a zipper is shown. *a*, The injured area is exposed and a sterile dressing is applied to the open wound. *b*, The splint, with a zipper throughout its length, is positioned around the limb. *c*, With the zipper closed, the air splint is inflated by mouth. A pump should never be used to inflate an air splint. *d*, The EMT tests the pressure exerted by the splint after it has been inflated. He should be able to slip his fingers between the splint and the limb, and the surface of the splint should yield slightly to the pressure of a thumb or finger.

1. One EMT gently supports the limb and applies slight steady traction.
2. The second EMT places the splinting device under, alongside, or on top of the limb.
3. Enough padding should be placed to insure an even pressure and even contact between the limb and the splint everywhere and to protect bony prominences from undue pressure.
4. Apply the bindings to hold the limb to the splint. Be careful not to bind them so tightly that circulation is obstructed.

At times, in the case of a severe dislocation for instance, it may be necessary to improvise when it is impossible to insert a dislocated limb into a commercial or pre-prepared splint. In these instances, other parts of the body may be used as splints. An injured leg can be bound to an un-injured one, thereby gaining support and stability. The torso of the body can be used as a splint for an injured upper extremity.

Soft splints. Some soft splints are air splints which are simply a double-walled tube, usually made of a heavy-duty clear plastic. These splints are available in a variety of sizes and shapes, with or without a zipper which runs the length of the splint. Inflation of the splint should be only by mouth, never by a pump. This type of splint is comfortable to the patient, provides uniform contact, and has the added advantage of applying gentle, diffuse pressure on a bleeding wound.

The method chosen to apply an air splint depends on whether or not the splint has a zipper. If a zipper is present, the opened splint is gently placed around the extremity, zipped up, and inflated (Fig. 17.3). If a non-zipper type is used, follow the procedure outlined below.

146

1. The EMT must pull the splint onto and around one of his own arms, to hold it open. His hand beyond the splint should then grasp the hand or the foot of the injured patient.
2. His other arm should support the patient's injured limb.
3. The EMT then applies gentle traction and slides the splint from his arm onto the patient's injured extremity.
4. He inflates the splint by mouth. A pump must not be used because it can develop too much pressure, overinflate the splint, and cause severe damage of a limb. With an open wound or compound fracture, the air splint should be applied over an appropriate sterile dressing.

Another type of soft splint is a pillow splint which, when wrapped and secured around an injured extremity, is very comfortable and can provide effective immobilization.

Slings are excellent devices for immobilization of the upper extremity. A sling can be combined with the use of a swathe around the body to offer comfortable, effective immobilization for most injuries of the upper extremity (Fig. 17.4).

Traction splints. A traction splint holds a fracture or dislocation immobile and allows a steady longitudinal pull on the extremity. The traction splint is usually called a Thomas splint, after the famous orthopaedic surgeon Sir Hugh Owen Thomas. While the original splint had a full ring at the upper end, most of the commercial splints used today have a hinged half-ring. A half-ring offers more comfort to the patient, and the hinge allows the splint to be used on either the right or the left leg.

When traction is applied through the foot and ankle hitch, counter traction is applied by the padded half-ring which seats against the ischial tuberosity of the patient's pelvis. The traction splint is therefore not suitable for use on the upper extremity, as counter traction cannot be tolerated by the major plexus of nerves and blood vessels in the patient's axilla. The traction splint should be applied by two EMTs working together; it is impossible for one to apply the splint alone.

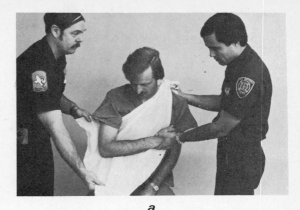

a

147

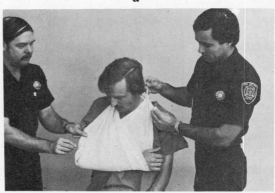

b

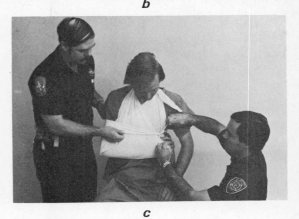

c

Figure 17.4 *a–c*

The application of a sling and swathe bandage is shown. *a,* A sling is applied to the upper extremity as one EMT supports the injured arm in the desired position. *b,* The sling is made secure, especially at the elbow, and adjusted for comfort. *c,* A swathe binds the sling to the torso to immobilize the injured arm.

The technique of application of the traction splint is extremely important and not simple. The EMT team should practice the steps over and over until the sequence and necessary teamwork have become routine. In Figure 17.5 the application of a splint is illustrated.

148

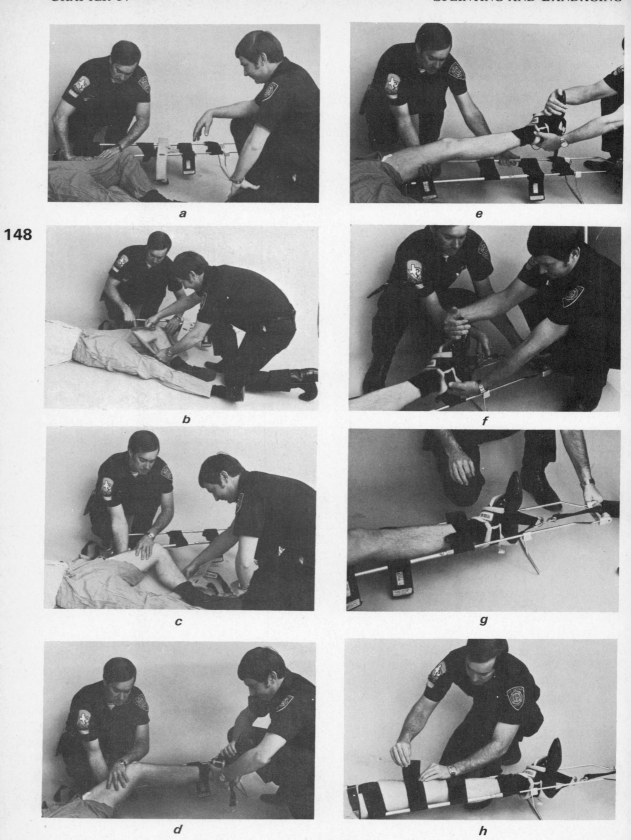

Figure 17.5 *a–h*

Traction on the leg may be applied by either of two methods:

1. *Traction strap*—A traction strap is a length of $\frac{3}{4}$-inch webbing with a buckle. It is passed through the rings of the ankle hitch and then over the end of the Thomas splint. The loop is then tightened to develop and maintain traction. If direct tightening does not apply enough traction, a tongue blade or stick may be placed between the loops of the webbing, twisted, and secured. This tightening and twisting maneuver is known as the Spanish windlass technique.

2. *Commercial rachet*—In a commercial rachet, a strap connects the rings of the ankle hitch and the rachet mechanism on the end of the splint. The knot on the rachet should be turned only by hand to apply traction.

The amount of traction which should be applied is the degree which holds the limb in a secure and corrected position and is comfortable for the patient.

When should a traction splint be used? Traction splints are used primarily and to best advantage in securing fractures of the femur. However, one can also be used to immobilize fractures about the hip or knee or a fracture of the tibia. When a traction splint is not available, hip fractures (femoral neck fractures) can also be immobilized by securing the injured limb to the uninjured limb. A pillow or a folded blanket should first be placed between the patient's legs.

Cautions. Because the traction splint immobilizes the limb by counter traction on the ischium and the groin, care must be used to pad the groin properly and to avoid excessive pressure, especially on the external genitalia.

Commercial padded ankle hitches are preferred to improvised hitches made of rope, cord, or tape. These materials should not be used, for they can be painful and can obstruct the circulation in the foot. A folded triangular bandage may be used as a hitch over a shoe if a commercial hitch is not available; the ankle must always be well-padded.

General Principles in the Application of Dressings and Bandages

Dressings and bandages have three main functions: to stop bleeding, to protect a wound from further damage, and to prevent further contamination and possible infection.

Universal dressings. All ambulances must carry supplies with sterile dressings. Universal dressings, conventional 4×4-inch gauze pads, and an assortment of small adhesive-type dressings will provide coverage for most wounds. A universal dressing is made of thick, absorbent material; it measures 9×36 inches and is packed folded into a compact size (Fig. 17.6). While available commercially, it can be made locally at a reasonable cost. Bandage material is available in 9-inch wide, twenty-yard rolls. When cut into 36-inch long pieces and folded on itself three times from each end, each length becomes a compact dressing which can fit conveniently into a no. 2 paper bag. The end of the bag can be folded and stapled; the package can be sterilized by local hospital personnel and placed in a protective plastic bag with a soft roller bandage. It is an efficient, reasonably priced dressing for

149

Figure 17.5

The proper application of a traction splint by two EMTs is demonstrated. *a*, Place the splint beside the patient and adjust it to the proper length. Open and adjust the Velcro support straps. *b*, Cut open the patient's trouser leg or otherwise expose the injured limb so that it is possible to see exactly what is being done. *c*, One EMT secures the leg from movement while the second EMT fastens the ankle hitch about the patient's ankle and foot. The shoe is customarily left on the foot. *d*, The first EMT lifts and supports the leg at the site of suspected injury while the second EMT applies traction with his hands. *e*, Maintain the traction while sliding the splint into position under the patient's leg and gently applying the ischial strap. *f*, The first EMT maintains the traction with his hands while the second EMT connects the loops of the ankle hitch to the end of the splint. *g*, Adjust the splint and apply traction with the splint. *h*, When proper traction has been applied with the splint, fasten the Velcro support slings so that the limb is closely secured to the splint.

wounds or burns and can serve when necessary as an effective cervical collar or as padding for splints.

Stabilizing dressings. Dressings must remain in place during transport. The stability of the dressing can be provided by soft roller, self-adherent bandages, rolls of gauze, triangular bandages, or adhesive tape. The soft roller bandages are probably easiest to use as they are slightly elastic, the layers adhere to one another, and the end of the roll can be tucked back into the layers (Fig. 17.7). Triangular bandages can hold the dressing in place when the ends of the bandage are tied together. Adhesive tape can hold small bandages in place and help secure other dressings. Elastic bandages should not be used to secure dressings. Sucking chest wounds and abdominal wounds where organs are exposed may require the use of adhesive tape to secure the bandage. Remember, however, that some patients are allergic to ordinary adhesive tape.

A dressing should never interfere with circulation. The EMT should always check the limb

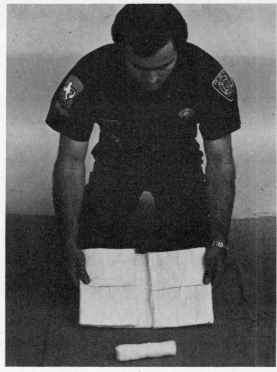

b

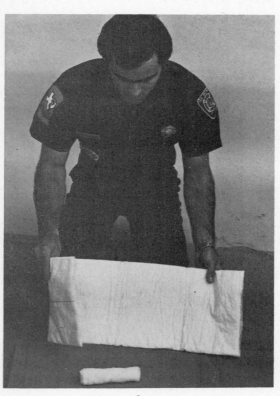

a

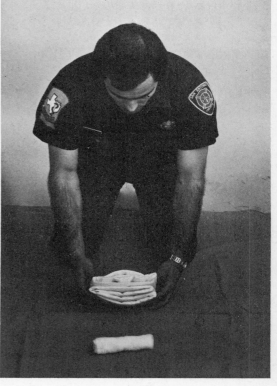

c

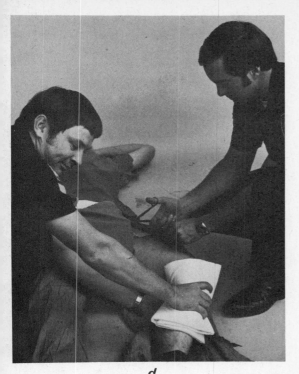

d

distal to a dressing, after applying it, for signs of impaired circulation or loss of skin sensation.

Occlusive dressings. A satisfactory occlusive dressing for sucking chest wounds or abdominal wounds is aluminum foil. The entire roll of foil can be sterilized in its original package, which may be resterilized after each use. Besides being an excellent occlusive and nonadherent dressing, aluminum foil is a valuable multipurpose item of equipment. It can act effectively, for example, as an insulator to conserve body heat when wrapped about a premature infant, when no incubator is available.

Pressure dressings. A pressure dressing is recommended to control bleeding from a wound. The universal dressing is perfect as a pressure dressing because it can be folded or opened to adapt to most wounds.

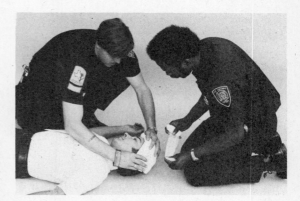

a

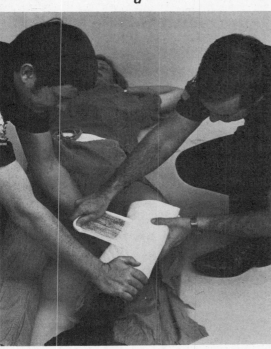

e

Figure 17.6 *a–e (opposite page and above)*

  a, The basic material forming a universal dressing is shown. *b*, Properly folded, the dressing becomes a multi-layer pack. *c*, When it is completely folded, the universal dressing is small and can easily be sterilized and stored. *d*, A universal dressing has been applied on a lower extremity wound. *e*, The dressing is made secure.

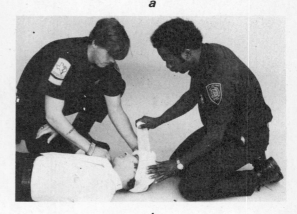

b

Figure 17.7 *a–b*

  Stabilization of a bandage on a scalp wound is shown. *a*, A sterile universal dressing is applied with hand pressure on the wound to stop the bleeding. *b*, The bandage is fixed in place and pressure maintained by the use of a self-adherent roller bandage.

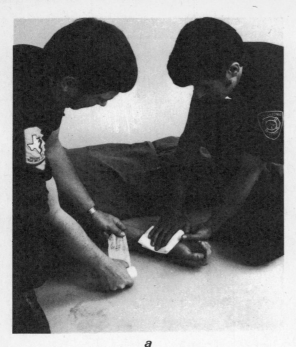
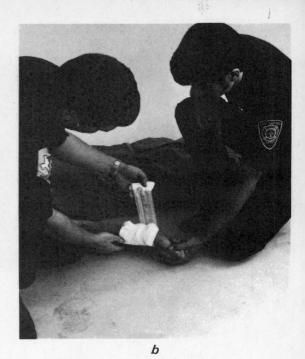

a   b

Figure 17.8 *a–b*

a, Local pressure on a bleeding wound is applied through a dressing. A small, folded, sterile pad is placed over an arm wound. Pressure is maintained by the hand of the EMT. *b,* The pad is secured with a soft, self-adherent roller bandage.

The EMT should then apply hand pressure on the wound, through the dressing, until bleeding has slowed or stopped (Fig. 17.8). Continued pressure is maintained by firmly applying a roller bandage to the injured part. If bleeding continues or recurs, the original dressing and bandage should be left in place and an additional large dressing applied and secured with an additional roller bandage. Elastic bandages should not be used for pressure dressings because of the possibility of complications from unevenly distributed pressure.

At times bleeding will continue through the bandage and the EMT must apply yet another universal dressing and secure it with another firmly applied roller bandage. Hand pressure should also be used. It should be emphasized that the primary purpose of a pressure dressing is to stop bleeding and that in order to do so, sufficient pressure must be applied to exceed the pressure in the bleeding vessels.

Tourniquet

Tourniquets are to be used only as a last resort in the control of bleeding. The only time the use of a tourniquet is justified is when well-applied pressure dressings and hand pressure cannot stop bleeding. The type of injury in which a tourniquet might be used is a complete or partial amputation of a limb. A discussion of the application of a tourniquet and the necessary precautions in using a tourniquet is in Chapter 8, Bleeding and Control of Bleeding.

Fractures and Dislocations of the Shoulder and Upper Extremity

GOAL I. Know the characteristics and management of fractures and dislocations of the upper extremity.

OBJECTIVES

A. Name the mechanisms of injury in fractures and dislocations of the shoulder and upper extremity.
B. Describe the most common signs and symptoms of fractures and dislocations of the shoulder and upper extremity.
C. Describe the management of fractures and dislocations of the upper extremity.

Injuries of the shoulder are those that involve the clavicle, the scapula, and the proximal humerus (Fig. 18.1).

Fractures of the Clavicle

Fractures of the clavicle (collarbone) are most common in children and the mechanism of in-

jury is usually a fall on the outstretched hand, that is, an indirect injury (Fig. 18.2). The patient complains of pain in the shoulder and usually holds his arm against the chest with the opposite hand. Generally there is swelling, tenderness, and deformity in the area and inability to move

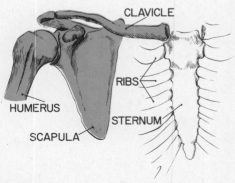

Figure 18.1

The bony structures making up the shoulder joint and the shoulder itself include the scapula, the clavicle, and the proximal humerus.

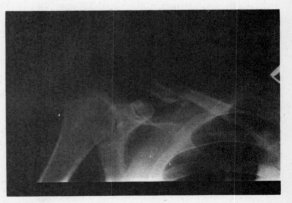

Figure 18.2

In an X-ray view, a fracture of the clavicle (collarbone) is well demonstrated.

the arm because of pain. An injury of the clavicle can be immobilized by the use of a sling.

Fractures of the Scapula

Fractures of the scapula usually occur as the result of a violent direct injury. Blows sustained directly over the scapula in an automobile accident or other traumatic incident can produce a fracture. This injury is usually diagnosed by swelling, pain, and tenderness around the scapula itself. The patient will limit the motion of the affected shoulder. An injury of the scapula can be immobilized by the use of a sling.

154

Dislocations of the Acromioclavicular Joint

Dislocations between the acromion process of the scapula and the outer end of the clavicle are called dislocations of the acromioclavicular joint. These injuries are sometimes called a "knocked down" shoulder. They are commonly sustained in athletic events when a participant falls on the point of the shoulder. These injuries can be immobilized effectively by an arm sling.

Dislocations of the Shoulder Joint

Anterior dislocation of the shoulder is the most common type of major joint dislocation in the body. Dislocations of the shoulder joint (the glenohumeral joint) can be anterior or posterior and are usually sustained through injuries in which the arm is forcibly externally rotated or abducted. This abnormal motion commonly dislocates the humeral head forward and produces the so-called anterior dislocation (Fig. 18.3). The shoulder is grossly deformed, and the patient will try to protect his injured shoulder by holding the dislocated arm with his opposite hand to stabilize it.

It is difficult to immobilize this dislocation as the arm is fixed in a position away from the trunk. To overcome the difficulty that this fixed position of the arm causes, a pillow or a rolled blanket can be placed between the arm and chest. The arm can then be secured against the chest with a sling and swathe or soft roller bandages. At times the patient may be more

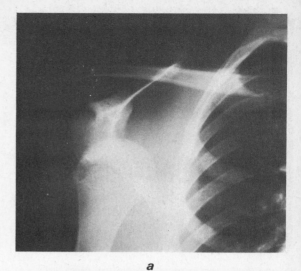

a

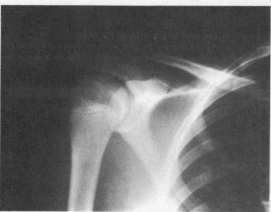

b

Figure 18.3 *a–b*

a, In this X-ray view, the head of the humerus has been dislocated forward. Compare this picture with the following one. *b*, In this view of the same patient, reduction of the dislocated shoulder has been achieved and the humeral head again lies in its normal position.

comfortable if the arm is simply placed in a sling and he is transported in a semi-sitting or sitting position. The patient should be allowed to support the dislocated arm with his uninjured arm during transport if he wishes.

Fractures of the Humerus

Fractures of the proximal end of the humerus. Fractures of the proximal end of the humerus are most often sustained through falls on the outstretched hand, producing an indirect force on the shoulder (Fig. 18.4). They can also be sus-

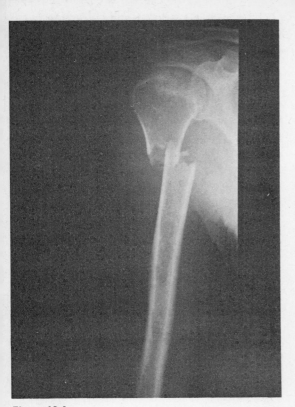

Figure 18.4

 A fracture of the upper humeral shaft, shown here in an X-ray view, is most often sustained as an indirect injury through a fall on an outstretched arm.

tained by a blow directly on the shoulder. These injuries are usually very painful and a marked deformity may be present. They are a common injury in the elderly. Appropriate splinting is provided by the use of a sling and swathe or by binding the arm to the trunk with soft roller bandages.

 Fractures of the shaft of the humerus. Fractures of the humeral shaft can be caused either by a direct blow or by an indirect force, such as a twist or a fall on the outstretched hand (Fig. 18.5).

 These fractures usually present gross deformity, swelling, tenderness, pain, and an inability of the patient to move the arm. Occasionally, because of the close proximity of the radial nerve to the humeral shaft, the nerve is damaged or compressed at the fracture site. The patient is then unable to dorsiflex or extend his wrist and fingers and a characteristic "wrist drop" is seen.

 The fracture can be splinted by an arm sling and swathe. First, support the arm in a sling; then wrap a bandage completely around the chest, enclosing also the injured arm in its sling. A long arm, padded splint fastened to the chest with a swathe is also satisfactory.

 Fractures of the distal humerus. A fracture of the distal humerus just above the elbow joint is called a supracondylar fracture of the humerus

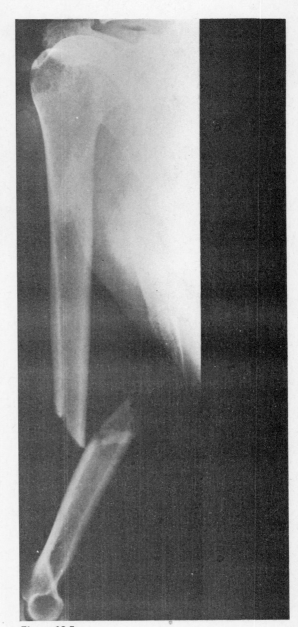

Figure 18.5

 A fracture of the lower humeral shaft with marked displacement of the distal fragment is seen in this X-ray view.

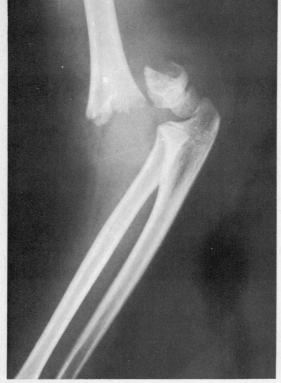

156

Figure 18.6

This X-ray view shows a supracondylar fracture of the humerus in a child. The injury can be accompanied by impaired blood flow in the forearm and hand muscles.

(Fig. 18.6). Fractures of the distal humerus are commonly seen in children. They can produce a grotesque deformity; at times the bone may even protrude through the skin (compound fracture). They are frequently accompanied by nerve and vascular injuries. Supracondylar fractures should be treated with extreme care because of the proximity of the vital neurovascular structures to the bone.

Fractures of the distal humerus can occur in adults also. When these fractures occur in adults, they usually extend into the elbow joint itself. There is severe swelling, instability of the joint, a marked deformity, and an inability to move the elbow. They are extremely serious injuries, associated with nerve and vascular damage as in children.

Fractures of the humerus near the elbow can best be immobilized in adults or children by using a sling and swathe around the chest or a long arm padded splint. The sling should be applied in a comfortable position without much flexion at the elbow, because it can shut off the circulation to the forearm and hand when the elbow is unstable. If flexion of the elbow during immobilization shuts off the circulation, the arm should be immobilized with the elbow straight.

It is particularly important in patients with fractures about the elbow to check the radial pulse and the color and temperature in the fingers for signs of circulatory impairment. The neurological status should also always be assessed by testing for sensory or motor loss in the hand.

Dislocations of the Elbow Joint

The elbow joint is formed by the distal hu-

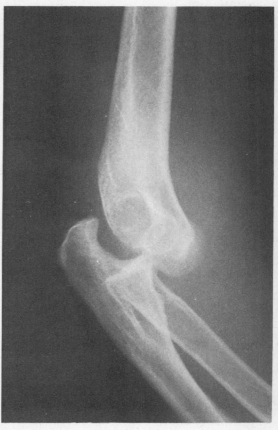

Figure 18.7

In an X-ray view of a dislocation of the elbow joint, the bones are seen to be intact. Physical examination alone would find it difficult to differentiate this injury from a fracture with its associated deformity.

merus and the proximal ends of the ulna and radius. Dislocations of the elbow joint can present grotesque deformities. Without an X ray they are almost impossible to differentiate from fractures of the distal end of the humerus (Fig. 18.7). Dislocations of the elbow are immobilized in the same manner as fractures of the distal end of the humerus.

Fractures of the distal humerus and dislocations of the elbow are usually caused by the same mechanism, a fall on an outstretched hand. In the event of an injury of this kind, the wrist must be closely examined as there may be an associated fracture at this point.

Fractures of the Proximal Ulna and Radius

Fractures of the proximal ulna (the olecranon process) are usually sustained through a direct blow, but fractures of the radial head are usually sustained indirectly through a fall on the outstretched hand (Fig. 18.8). Fractures of the proximal ulna and radius can be splinted by means of an air splint, a folded pillow, a long arm padded splint, or an arm sling and swathe.

Fractures of the Forearm

Fractures of the forearm bones, that is, the shafts of the radius and ulna, are usually produced by an indirect force, such as a fall on the outstretched hand, but also they are often the result of a direct blow on the forearm. Injuries of the radius and ulna usually are produced simultaneously. These fractures can be extremely painful and marked deformity is usually present (Fig. 18.9).

Fractures of the forearm can be immobilized by an air splint or a long arm, rigid, padded splint. The wrist and elbow should be included in the splint. The arm usually is held in a sling to afford greater stability.

Fractures of the Wrist

Fractures of the wrist may include fractures of either the distal radius, distal ulna, both radius and ulna, or the carpal bones of the wrist (Fig.

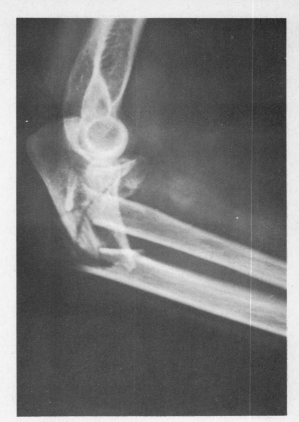

157

Figure 18.8

This X-ray shows a fracture of the olecranon process and the radial head. Notice the severity of the destruction about the elbow joint. Nerve and blood vessel injuries can easily be sustained with these fractures.

18.10). A fracture of the wrist can occur when the patient falls on an outstretched hand and the force of the fall is transmitted to the distal radius and ulna. These fractures, common in elderly patients, usually produce a marked deformity. It is sometimes called the "silver-fork" deformity because the fractured wrist assumes the curve of the side view of a dinner fork, but it is more commonly called a Colles' fracture. Injuries of the wrist may occur in children, and in this group the fracture may pass through the epiphyseal plate, or growth center.

Wrist fractures can be immobilized by the use of a padded-board splint or an air splint. It is not strictly necessary for the splint to include the elbow in fractures of the wrist, but the patient will be more comfortable when it does. The arm should be further supported with a sling.

Fractures of the carpal bones can result from a

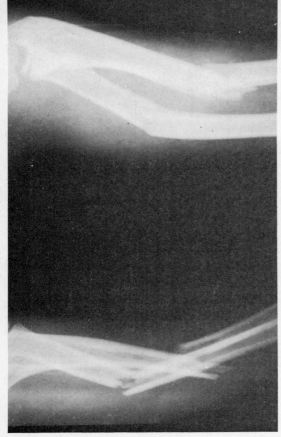

Figure 18.9

In this X-ray picture of a fracture of the radius and ulna in a child, the extreme deformity caused is obvious. These fractures are common in children.

fall onto the outstretched hand and may occur with or without a fracture of the radius and ulna. Deformity may be noted but it is usually minimal. Point tenderness over the wrist is usually noted. Carpal bone fractures should be immobilized in the same manner as described for wrist fractures.

Dislocations of the Wrist

Dislocations of the wrist result from the same causes as fractures of the distal radius, ulna, or carpal bones. It is unusual to see a dislocation of the wrist without an accompanying fracture of either the distal radius and ulna or the carpal bones. Dislocations of the wrist should be gently straightened and splinted in the same manner as

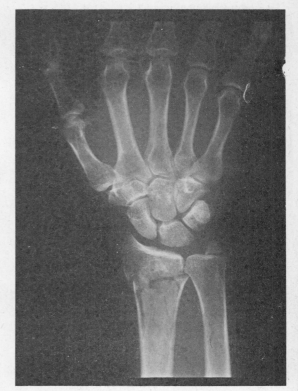

Figure 18.10

An X-ray view of a fractured wrist reveals the injury at the distal radius.

fractures of the distal end of the radius and ulna or fractures of the carpal bones.

Fractures and Dislocations about the Hand and Fingers

Fractures and dislocations of the metacarpal

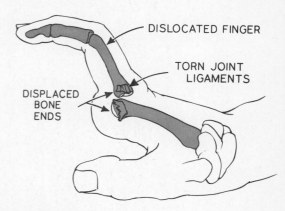

Figure 18.11

A dislocated finger is drawn. Note the displaced joint surfaces and the disrupted ligaments.

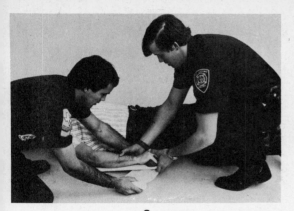

a

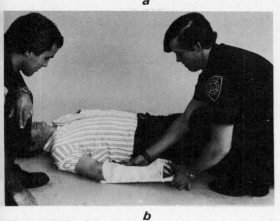

b

Figure 18.12 *a–b*

   When an injured hand is to be splinted, it should be in the position of function. This position can be achieved by, *a*, placing a roll of gauze in the palm. *b*, The hand and wrist are then immobilized with a board splint.

bones or the phalangeal (finger) bones are common (Fig. 18.11). The hand should be splinted in the position of function, with a roll of gauze placed in the palm. An air splint or a padded rigid splint can be used (Fig. 18.12).

Open Injuries of the Upper Extremity

   Open fractures or dislocations of the upper extremity are splinted in the same fashion as closed injuries. However care should be taken not to push the contaminated ends of the bone back beneath the skin. Since these injuries are open, the most important steps of treatment by the EMT consist of protecting the open injury from further contamination by an adequate dressing, controlling the bleeding, and immobilizing the extremity. The very serious complication of an infection occurring after an open fracture must be kept in mind at all times.

159

CHAPTER 19

Fractures and Dislocations of the Hip, Pelvis, and Lower Extremity

161

GOAL I. Know the diagnosis and treatment of fractures and dislocations of the hip, pelvis, and lower extremity.

OBJECTIVES

A. Explain how to diagnose a fracture of the pelvis.
B. Describe the treatment and list the complications of fractures of the pelvis.
C. List the types of dislocations of the hip and their treatment.
D. List the types of fractures of the hip and their treatment.
E. Describe the treatment of fractures of the femur.
F. List the types of injuries of the knee.
G. List the types of fractures of the knee.
H. List the complications of fractures and dislocations of the knee and their treatment.
I. Describe the treatment of fractures of the tibia and fibula.
J. Describe the treatment of fractures of the foot and ankle.

Injuries of the hip joint, pelvis, and the bones of the lower extremity (Fig. 19.1) are sustained usually as a result of very severe trauma, such as an automobile accident. Motorcycle accidents, for instance, are notorious for causing injuries of the lower extremities.

Injuries of the Pelvis

A fracture of the pelvis is commonly sustained as a result of a compression injury in which the pelvis is literally crushed on both sides by a heavy impact. It can also occur as a result of a direct blow on one side of the pelvis. Indirect forces acting on the femur through the hip joint can also fracture the pelvis. It is not uncommon

to see injuries of the pelvis in falls from heights and similar accidents. In an elderly person, minor injuries of the pelvis can occur from a slight fall if the side of the pelvis hits the ground.

Fractures of the pelvis may be associated with blood loss severe enough to cause hypovolemic shock. It is important for the EMT to understand the possibility of shock as a result of the fracture and to take steps to combat it. Open fractures of the pelvis with obvious bleeding are uncommon, and the extent of blood loss in a closed fracture may not be apparent because the hemorrhage is within the pelvis and thus not visible. The patient's vital signs must be surveyed as soon as possible and carefully monitored during transport. An IV infusion should

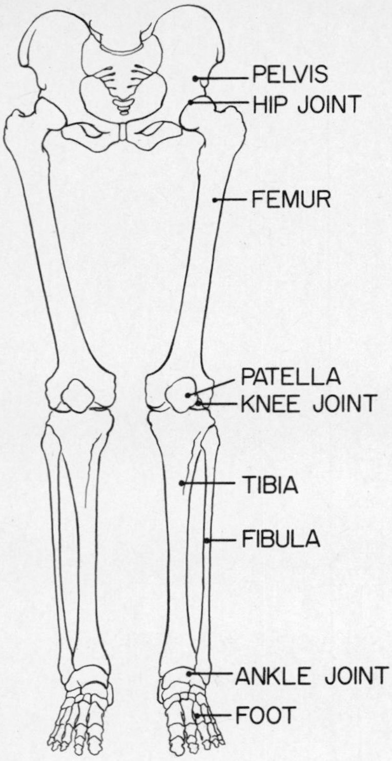

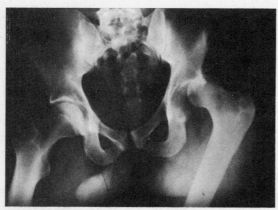

PELVIS
HIP JOINT

FEMUR

PATELLA
KNEE JOINT

TIBIA

FIBULA

ANKLE JOINT
FOOT

Figure 19.1

The joints and bones of the lower extremity are shown.

162

be started for a patient with a suspected pelvic fracture to help combat shock during transport.

The patient usually complains of pain in the pelvis. The most important sign in the diagnosis of these fractures is pain felt when the sides of the pelvis are compressed. Patients with actual or suspected fractures of the pelvis should be trans-

Figure 19.2

In this X-ray view, a posterior dislocation of the hip is shown. The head of the femur no longer lies within the acetabulum.

ported on a long spineboard, as it provides support for the pelvis and makes it possible for X-ray films to be obtained without moving the patient and with a minimum of disturbance. Injuries of the genitourinary system (rupture of the bladder or a laceration of the urethra) are frequently associated with these fractures.

Injuries about the Hip

Dislocations of the hip. Dislocations of the hip joint are primarily anterior or posterior. Posterior dislocations are commonly sustained in vehicular accidents. When a seated person is thrown forward and strikes a knee against the dashboard, the head of the femur is indirectly pushed and displaced from within the acetabulum to a position posterior to it (Fig. 19.2). Anterior dislocations usually occur when an abduction force is applied to legs which are already abducted (spread apart). For example, consider an individual with one foot on a dock and one foot on a boat. If the wind suddenly pushes the boat away from the dock, his legs will unexpectedly and quickly be spread apart more widely and his hip joint may be dislocated anteriorly.

Posterior dislocation may be complicated by a nerve injury. When the head of the femur is forced out of its joint posteriorly, it directly damages the sciatic nerve by pressing on it or stretching it. This nerve is located behind the joint and is responsible for the movement of some of the muscles in the thigh and all of the muscles below the knee. A "foot drop" is characteristic of damage of the sciatic nerve (the patient is unable to raise his toes or his foot). The EMT should always remember to check and record the motor power of muscles below any fracture or dislocation.

A patient with a posterior dislocation of the hip characteristically lies with the hip joint flexed (the knee drawn up) and the thigh in internal rotation and adducted. The flexed thigh of the dislocated hip lies across the midline over the thigh of the normal leg. In a patient with an anterior dislocation of the hip, the position of the limb is almost exactly the opposite of that found in a posterior dislocation. In an anterior dislocation, the thigh is stretched out from the side of the body and is extended (lying flat on the ground), externally rotated, and abducted (away from the midline).

A patient with a dislocation of the hip should be transported with the dislocated limb supported by pillows or rolled blankets and long straps, as it is impossible to apply an effective splint of any type. Transportation should be on a rigid stretcher. The EMT should always notify the physician if the hip is noted to relocate spontaneously during extrication from an accident or during transportation.

Dislocations of the hip are usually sustained in very serious vehicular accidents, and it is not unusual to see associated injuries, such as fractures of the femur, pelvis, or the patella.

Fractures of the hip. Fractures of the hip are those which occur at the upper end of the femur (Fig. 19.3). The fracture may occur in the head of the femur, in the neck of the femur, in the intertrochanteric area (between the greater and lesser trochanters at the point where the shaft of the femur joins the neck of the femur), or in the subtrochanteric area (below the trochanters in the upper shaft).

Fractures of the hip usually occur in elderly patients as a result of a fall sustained while standing or walking, but they may occur in younger individuals who sustain severe trauma, as in vehicular accidents. A fracture of the neck of the femur usually occurs because of a twisting force applied to the femur during the fall. An intertrochanteric fracture usually occurs as a result of a direct force applied when the patient lands on the side of the hip joint. A patient with a fractured hip will usually lie with the leg externally rotated (the foot pointing outward), and the leg may appear to be shortened.

Fractures of the hip are best treated with traction splints. Adequate immobilization can also be obtained by placing pillows or folded blankets between the legs and using cravats, roller bandages, or straps to hold the legs together. Patients with hip fractures may lose significant amounts of blood. Regardless of the age of the patient, the EMT should be aware of the possibility of shock occurring in patients with fractures of the hip.

Fractures of the Femur

Fractures of the femur are those which occur primarily in the shaft of the femur—the area extending from just below the hip joint to just above the femoral condyles at the knee joint. These fractures are ordinarily the result of vehicular accidents. The EMT examining a patient with a fractured femur will have little difficulty in making the diagnosis of this fracture. The patient will lie with the leg in a marked deformity: severely angulated or rotated below the fracture (Fig. 19.4).

Fractures of the femur are often open. Either closed or open, they are associated with the loss of large amounts of blood. It is not unusual for a patient with a fracture of the femur to develop profound shock. The EMT must be extremely careful in the handling of these patients because extra movement and manipulation increase the blood loss. An open fracture of the femur should be treated as any other open fracture, with appropriate pressure dressings applied over the wound. No effort is made to replace protruding bone beneath the skin.

A fracture of the femur should be immobilized with a traction splint. The application of the traction splint is discussed in Chapter 17, General Principles of Splinting and Bandaging. The sequence of actions in the application of this

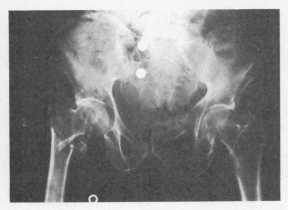

Figure 19.3

A fracture of the hip is one that occurs at the most proximal portion of the femur. In this X-ray view, the fracture is at the intertrochanteric part of the femur (left side of the picture). One can easily see why the fractured leg would appear shorter.

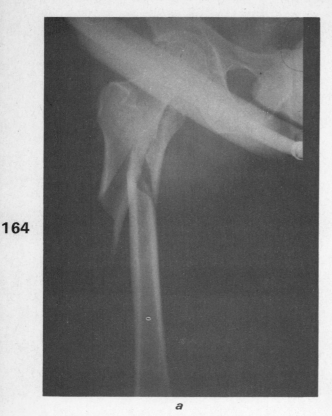

←—⟨⟨⟨⟨

Figure 19.4 *a–b*

Two fractures of the femur are shown in X-ray views. *a*, A comminuted fracture of the proximal femoral shaft may be seen. One can appreciate the extent of muscular damage and bleeding with such an injury. *b*, In a comminuted mid-shaft femoral fracture, the deformity of the thigh is obvious.

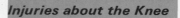

important splint should be reviewed frequently until the EMT is certain he knows every step.

A fracture of the femur can be associated with vascular injuries resulting in impaired circulation in the foot, causing it to become pale, cold, and pulseless. Applying traction, turning the leg from the deformed position, and splinting it in its proper position will usually restore circulation. If signs of returning circulation are not seen after appropriate treatment, immediate transportation to the Emergency Department is necessary as a serious vascular injury may have occurred.

Injuries about the Knee

Several types of injuries can occur about the knee, including sprains, dislocations of the knee joint, dislocations of the patella (knee cap), or fractures of the distal femur, the upper tibia, or the patella (Fig. 19.5).

Ligamentous injury of the knee can occur when abnormal medial or lateral or rotational forces are applied to the knee joint. This injury is commonly seen in a football game when the player is clipped or tackled from the side and his knee is driven inward. Torn ligaments on the

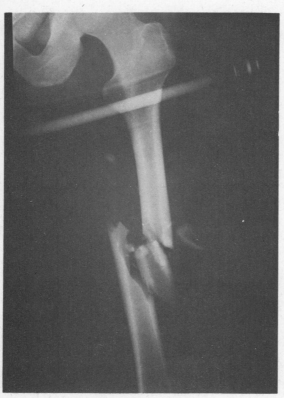

164

a

b

⟩⟩⟩→

Figure 19.5 *a–d*

Four X-ray views are shown of fractures or dislocations about the knee. *a*, In a fracture of the distal femoral shaft, the injury does not involve the knee joint itself. *b*, A dislocation of the knee has resulted in lateral displacement of the tibia. No bone injury can be seen. Extensive destruction of the ligaments supporting the knee must occur for such a dislocation to be seen. The deformity is obvious. *c*, An extensively comminuted fracture of the proximal tibia and fibula has resulted in some damage of the knee joint and some lateral displacement. *d*, Two pieces of a fractured patella are completely separated. While this injury produces much less deformity than a dislocated patella, the emergency treatment for each is the same.

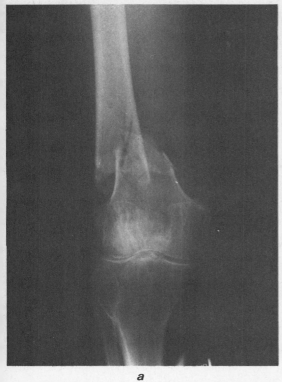

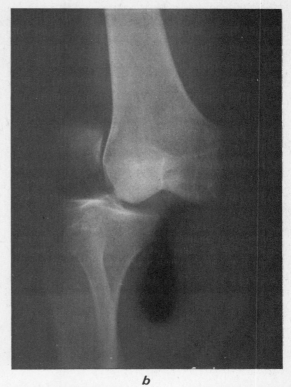

a

b

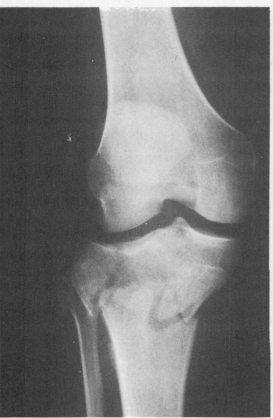

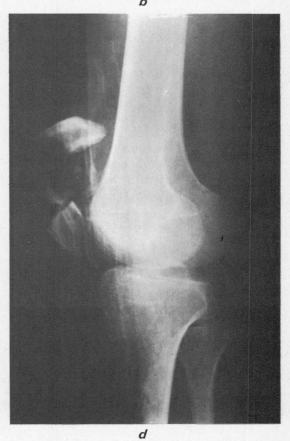

c

d

medial side of the knee are more frequently seen than lateral ligamentous injuries. When an injury of the ligaments of the knee occurs, a deformity may be apparent with the leg bent at an awkward angle away from the knee joint. The EMT should gently straighten the leg and apply a long-leg splint. All suspected ligamentous injuries of the knee should be splinted with a long-leg rigid splint or an air splint.

Dislocation of the knee. A dislocation of the knee joint is a serious injury. It presents a grotesque deformity, as the proximal end of the tibia is completely displaced from its articulation with the femur. In the dislocation of the knee, severe ligamentous damage must have also occurred. However the seriousness of the dislocation is not related to the ligament damage but to the possible injury of the major artery supplying the leg below the knee—the popliteal artery lying behind the knee joint. When a dislocation of the knee is suspected, the EMT should always note the color, temperature, and the presence or absence of pulses in the foot before splinting is accomplished.

The EMT should gently straighten the de-deformity but only to a point that does not produce additional discomfort for the patient. Occasionally, during a gentle straightening maneuver the knee will revert to its normal contour and circulation may be restored. The leg can be immobilized on a traction splint without using any traction, or with a long-leg rigid splint or an air splint. A pillow or blanket splint is also effective and comfortable.

If the pulse does not return after the splint has been applied, the EMT must be certain to notify the personnel at the Emergency Department. If dislocation of the knee joint is suspected and it is noted to relocate upon application of slight traction during immobilization, the EMT must also remember to notify the Emergency Department personnel of this fact.

Fractures about the knee. Fractures about the knee may occur in the distal end of the femur or in the proximal end of the tibia, or at the patella. Fractures about the knee can look like ligamentous injuries or knee joint dislocations. Regardless of the problem, there is usually much pain and swelling and there may be a significant de-

formity. The same possibility of vascular injury exists with fractures about the knee as with knee joint dislocations. The EMT should gently straighten the deformity but never force it; he should splint the leg in a long leg splint, as described for dislocations of the knee.

Dislocation of the patella. The patella (knee cap) may be dislocated from its articulation with the front of the distal femur. Usually the dislocation is to the lateral, or outer, side of the knee and the knee is in a flexed position. The EMT should gently straighten the leg to a point that does not produce additional pain for the patient. Occasionally the patella will relocate itself with the straightening. For transport, the leg should be immobilized in a padded long-leg splint or an air splint.

Fractures of the Shaft of the Tibia or the Fibula

Fractures of the shaft of the tibia (the large leg bone) or the fibula (the smaller leg bone) may

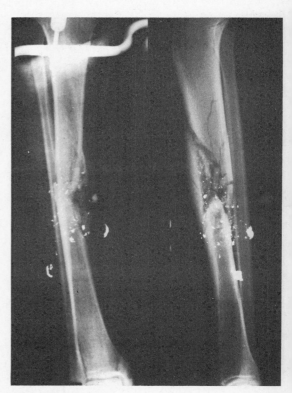

Figure 19.6

This fracture of the mid-shafts of both tibia and fibula is extensively comminuted.

occur any place between the knee joint and the ankle joint (Fig. 19.6). Because the tibia is located just beneath the skin, which offers little soft-tissue resistance, open fractures of the tibia are common. The fibula is well protected with muscle and other soft tissues and therefore fractures of this bone are less likely to be open. Open fractures of the tibia are handled with the same procedures as are other open fractures; sterile pressure dressings are placed over the wound and appropriate splints are used.

These leg fractures may result in severe deformity and cause grotesque degrees of angulation or rotation. Fractures of the tibia and fibula may be immobilized by using a traction splint, a padded long leg rigid splint, or an air splint that extends from the foot to the upper thigh. As with most fractures, the deformities (rotation and angulation) should be gently corrected. The EMT should always remember not to force a deformity straight and never to straighten a deformity if to do so causes additional discomfort for the patient. However, in most instances the extremity should be straightened enough to apply a splint. Usually, circulatory problems in the foot, indicated by paleness, coldness, and

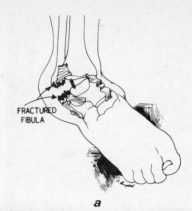

FRACTURED
FIBULA

a

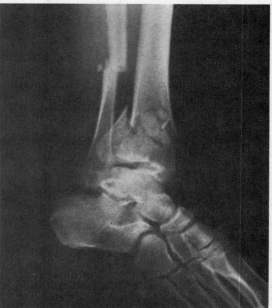

167

Figure 19.8 *a–b*   *b*

a, A common fracture of the ankle is diagrammed. In this instance, the fracture involves the lateral malleolus in the most distal portion of the fibula. The foot is displaced medially. *b,* Both tibia and fibula are fractured just above the ankle joint in this X-ray view. A lateral displacement of the foot has resulted.

the absence of pulses, can be corrected by applying gentle traction, straightening the leg, and immobilizing the extremity. In the event that circulation has not returned, the personnel at the Emergency Department must be promptly informed.

Injuries about the Ankle

Injuries of the ankle are those that occur at the junction of the distal end of the tibia and fibula with the foot (Fig. 19.7). They are commonly

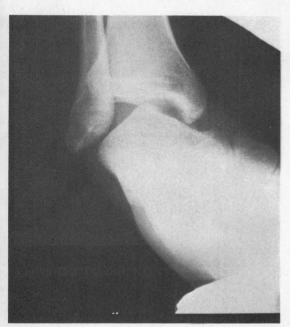

Figure 19.7

A severe medial dislocation of the ankle is shown in X-ray view. Destruction of the lateral ankle ligaments must occur for this deformity to be seen.

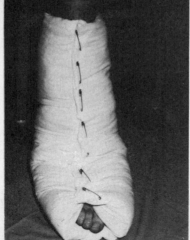

Figure 19.9

A pillow splint is an excellent means of immobilizing the ankle and foot.

168

Fractures of the Foot

Fractures of the foot can involve the tarsal calcaneus (heel bone), the remaining tarsal bones, the metatarsal bones, or the toes (Fig. 19.10). A fracture of the calcaneus usually occurs when the patient falls from a height and lands on the heels. Because the injury often occurs in a fall from a ladder, a tree, or a roof, it is commonly associated with a fracture of the spine. This point is a very important one for the EMT

associated with a deformity or a dislocation of the ankle joint. The injury may consist of fractures of the distal tibia or fibula or ligamentous injury of the ankle, which may allow a dislocation. The injury, which may occur when an individual falls and twists an ankle, is often seen with recreational or athletic activities.

Fractures of the ankle usually involve the most distal end of the tibia (the medial malleolus) or the most distal end of the fibula (the lateral malleolus) (Fig. 19.8). The more severe the injury, the more severe is the fracture or the ligamentous injury and resultant deformity of the ankle.

It will usually be impossible for the EMT to determine whether the exact nature of an ankle injury is primarily a fracture, a dislocation, or a combination of both. As with any dislocation or severe fracture deformity, he should check and record the color, temperature, and pulses distal to the injury. Severe deformities should be gently straightened with traction so that they can then be properly splinted. Ankle injuries can be adequately immobilized with either a padded long-leg or short-leg splint, an air splint, or a pillow splint (Fig. 19.9).

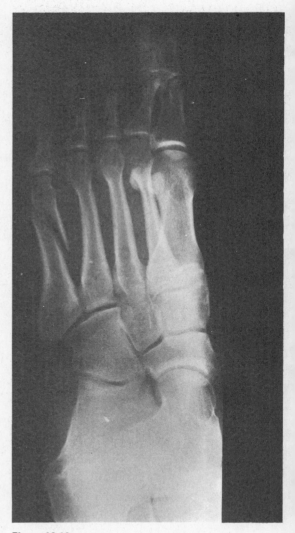

Figure 19.10

A fracture of the fifth metatarsal bone is shown in this X-ray view of the foot.

to remember. Obviously, patients with heel pain associated with back pain should always be transported on a spineboard.

Fractures of the tarsal bones, the metatarsal bones, and the toes may be associated with pain and swelling, but gross deformities, except occasionally for dislocations of the toes, are uncommon. Vascular injuries are unusual. Fractures of the foot can be adequately immobilized with a rigid short-leg splint, an air splint, or a pillow splint.

169

CHAPTER 20

Fractures and Dislocations of the Spine

171

GOAL I.   Understand the anatomy and function of the spine.

OBJECTIVES

A. Describe how the spine is formed and its function.
B. Describe the effects of a fracture or a dislocation of the spine.

GOAL II.   Know the signs and symptoms of spinal injuries.

OBJECTIVES

A. Name the types of trauma most likely to produce spinal injuries.
B. Describe signs and symptoms of spinal injuries and methods of determining their significance.

GOAL III.   Know proper emergency care of spinal injuries.

OBJECTIVES

A. List the rules for proper initial care of a patient with spinal injuries.
B. Identify special problems in resuscitating the spinal injured patient.
C. Describe under what conditions a patient with spinal injury may be repositioned.
D. Describe how to provide emergency care and remove someone safely from the water after sustaining possible injury in a diving accident.

The spine is a segmented column of thirty-three fused and separate bones extending from the base of the skull to the tip of the coccyx (Fig. 20.1). Each segment surrounds and protects the spinal cord and specific nerve roots. Although most spine fractures are simple skeletal injuries which heal well and have an excellent long-term prognosis, fractures and dislocations of the spine are of great importance because they are sometimes associated with damage of the spinal cord or nerve roots, producing paralysis or death. Diagnosis of spine injuries and differentiation between those which threaten nerve function and those which do not can be quite difficult and often require special X-ray studies. Since the EMT at the scene of an accident can never be certain if a suspected spine injury is safe or dangerous, he must consider all spine injuries as potentially dangerous and treat them as such.

If the fracture or dislocation has made the spine unstable, it is no longer able to protect the cord. The patient's movements may cause a shift of the bony segments, which can compress and severely damage the spinal cord and nerve roots

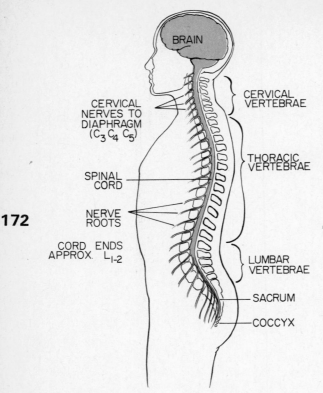

Figure 20.1

A lateral view of the spine shows the spinal cord well protected by its armor of bone in the spinal column.

(Fig. 20.2). Before making any attempt to reposition or move an injured person it is extremely important to consider that a spine fracture or dislocation may be present.

Recognition of a possible spinal injury is one of the major responsibilities of the EMT. A spinal cord injury alone associated with paralysis is rare; usually there is an accompanying fracture or dislocation of the spinal column. Therefore, all accident victims with weakness or numbness of the arms or legs must be assumed to have an unstable and dangerous spine fracture or dislocation.

The types of trauma most likely to produce a spinal fracture are automobile and motorcycle accidents, diving injuries, falls from a height, and cave-ins. Any individual injured in a diving accident should be handled as if he had a cervical spine fracture or dislocation as well as a respiratory problem.

Signs of Spinal Injuries

The signs and symptoms of spinal injuries and the methods of determining their significance are discussed below.

Pain. If the patient is conscious, he will be aware of pain and will be able to direct attention to the area of injury in his back or neck. If the patient is unconscious, this most important and reliable sign is not available. Occasionally, a conscious patient will not complain of pain in the area of a spinal fracture. This finding is especially true if he is lying very still and in a position of relative comfort, or if other more painful injuries distract his attention. In this situation, the next two signs will be useful.

Tenderness. Local tenderness over a portion of the spine is sufficient reason to suspect an injury there. Feel gently on both front and back of the patient at the area of suspected injury. If careful examination causes a complaint of increased pain, the patient should be handled as if he definitely had a spinal injury.

Painful movement. If the patient attempts to move the injured area of his back, pain may increase considerably. Never try to test this increase in pain by moving the patient or repositioning his back. You may cause pressure on the spinal cord and even paralysis. Cautious movements made by the patient without assistance are much less likely to cause cord damage, as the

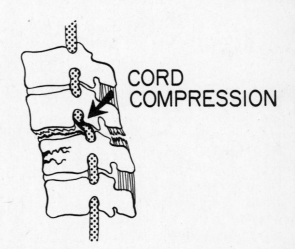

Figure 20.2

If the spine is unstable, even a small shift of bony fragments may damage or even crush the spinal cord.

patient usually will cease even the slightest movement upon experiencing increased pain. Do not encourage him to move if he has pain. Proceed immediately to splint.

Deformity. Only rarely and with very severe injuries can a deformity of the spine be seen. The spine usually does not appear bent. Absence of deformity in no way rules out the possibility of fracture or dislocation of the spine. With the unconscious patient, who cannot communicate, the EMT must rely on any abnormality or bony prominence he can observe. **With or without this indication, the unconscious patient who has been involved in a fall or a car accident should be handled as if he had a spinal injury.**

Lacerations and contusions. Cuts and bruises are reliable signs that strong forces have been applied to the patient's body (Fig. 20.3). Almost all cervical spine fractures or dislocations, including those resulting from diving accidents, will be accompanied by a cut or bruise on the head or face. Patients with serious injuries in other areas of the spine are likely to have bruises over the shoulders, the back, or abdomen. These signs are equally visible in conscious and unconscious patients. However, even if there are no cuts and bruises, a spinal fracture or dislocation cannot be ruled out.

Paralysis and anaesthesia. If the conscious patient has lost muscle function and has areas of numbness in his extremities, there is probably spinal cord damage. He will be unable to move some parts of his body and may have a loss of sensation in some areas. Touch his hands, feet

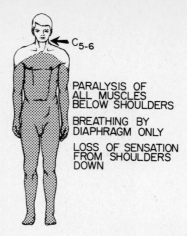

Figure 20.4

The shaded area indicates the region of numbness and paralysis from a spinal cord injury at the level of the fifth and sixth cervical vertebrae.

173

(if shoes are off), arms, and legs. If he cannot feel your touch, proceed as if there were a spinal fracture or dislocation. Muscle function may be tested by judging the force of his grip. Ask him to grasp your hand and evaluate his power to hold on. Ask him to move his feet, very carefully.

Most spinal injuries associated with paralysis occur in the neck and may cause numbness or paralysis of all four extremities as well as impaired breathing (Fig. 20.4). The next most common location for paralyzing spine fractures is at the waist. These injuries may cause numbness or paralysis below the pelvis but breathing and the arms are not affected.

The EMT can follow a simple series of steps for checking signs and symptoms of spinal fractures or dislocations in conscious patients.

1. *Ask* the patient or witness about the accident; get details. Question the patient carefully about areas of pain, numbness, or weakness.
2. *Look* for contusions or abrasions about the face and head or a deformity of the spine.
3. *Feel* for any irregularity, deformity, or tenderness along the spine that may indicate a fracture or dislocation. Check the arms and legs for numbness.
4. *Have the patient move himself*, unassisted, to see if he is paralyzed and to see if motion causes increased pain at a specific location.

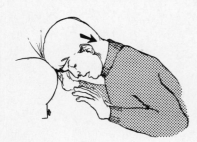

Figure 20.3

Scalp lacerations or bruises are clues that spinal injury may have occurred. Force applied to the forehead can bring about a hyperextension injury, as in an automobile accident when a person's forehead strikes against the dashboard.

With an unconscious patient, the order of these steps is changed.

1. *Look.*
2. *Feel.*
3. *Ask others.*

If unconsciousness has resulted from the type of accident that is known to cause spinal injury— for example, a vehicular or diving accident— assume that the patient has an associated spinal fracture until proven otherwise.

174

Care of Spinal Injuries

Proper initial care for a spinal fracture may save thousands of hours of nursing care and years of disability. The EMT has the opportunity to prevent paralysis or even death. The emergency care of spinal injuries follows the same rules as for all other major injuries.

1. Restore the airway; be sure that breathing is satisfactory.
2. Control serious bleeding by local pressure dressings.
3. Most important, **splint the patient before moving him.**

Effective splinting markedly relieves the patient's pain and stabilizes the injured spine so that nerve damage from the movement of bony fragments is much less likely.

While splinting an injured spine, avoid abnormal or excessive motion. Be sure that the injured person is transported on a long backboard or special stretcher, without bending or twisting the spine in any direction. If the head of an individual with a cervical spine fracture is allowed to move, a single motion may cause paralysis or death.

Specific techniques for splinting and transporting persons with spinal injuries are discussed in Chapter 47, Patient Handling and Extrication.

Protective helmets. In the past several years many persons have been involved in motorbike or snowmobile accidents while wearing protective helmets. A new problem is thus posed in emergency medical care, whether the helmet should be removed or left on the head of the injured person.

If a patient with a potential cervical spine injury is still wearing a helmet at the time the EMT arrives on the scene, he deserves special consideration. If there is any difficulty or increase in pain at the site of injury when the EMT attempts to remove the helmet, or if the patient is unconscious, he should be immobilized on the spineboard with the helmet left in place. It may be necessary to place a rolled blanket under his shoulders to prevent flexion or hyperflexion of the cervical spine. Otherwise, the helmet can be removed, with care, and the patient immobilized on the spineboard in the usual manner.

Opening the airway. The EMT must always be aware of the possibility of a cervical spine injury in a patient who has been in an accident and of the danger of causing permanent paralysis through improper handling. However, this possibility should not interfere with providing an open airway for the patient, as inability to breathe would result in his death at once.

If the patient is found with his head in a twisted position, it may be necessary to straighten it to open the airway; but if there is no obstruction of the airway or any other compelling reason to change the patient's position, it is best to splint the deformed neck or back in the original position of deformity. Straighten the neck only to help open the airway. Do not try to straighten a deformity simply to make splinting easier or more convenient.

To open the airway, the EMT should extend the patient's neck only to the degree necessary. Such extension must be in the midline and must be accomplished with gentle traction (of approximately ten pounds) on the head. If resistance is encountered, the head should be stabilized in the position in which it is found and the tongue lifted forward out of the airway by careful use of either the chin-lift or jaw-forward technique. In an unconscious patient, an artificial airway of either the oropharyngeal or the nasopharyngeal type may then be used.

The head and neck should then be immobilized by a collar or heavy rolled cloth about the neck or by sandbags placed on either side to hold the head in a neutral position

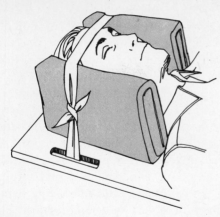

Figure 20.5

A satisfactory head support can be improvised by using two rolled towels or two blankets, even two sandbags. One is placed close to each side of the head, and the supports and the head are made into one unit by a wide cravat or bandage tied across the forehead.

as illustrated in the drawing in Figure 20.5

The EMT should be aware of two specific problems that a patient with a cervical spine fracture and consequent spinal cord injury may develop before he reaches the hospital:

1. Inadequate breathing because of paralyzed chest muscles
2. Neurogenic shock

Impaired breathing. The motor nerves to the diaphragm branch off the spinal cord high in the neck and are rarely injured by fractures or dislocations of the cervical spine. However, the nerves which control the chest wall muscles branch from the spinal cord below the middle part of the neck. If the spinal cord is damaged at this level, these nerves to the chest muscles may be paralyzed along with the muscles of the arms and legs (Fig. 20.4).

A patient with an injured spine whose chest wall muscles have been paralyzed by spinal cord damage can then breathe only with his diaphragm. As one observes the breathing in this patient, it can be noticed that his chest wall moves very little but his abdomen moves in and out slightly with each respiration. Respirations may be weak and rapid so that the patient may seem to be panting. These signs indicate that the diaphragm is the only muscle doing the breathing. When the diaphragm is unable to substitute

adequately for the paralyzed chest muscles, the person with a broken or dislocated cervical spine and spinal cord damage will develop respiratory insufficiency. Watch his breathing and be ready to provide oxygen-enriched air.

The presence of a fracture or dislocation of the cervical spine will make it difficult to assist respiration, regardless of the equipment available. Care must be taken to avoid extending or twisting the neck; however, respiration may be assisted by devices for artificial ventilation (Chapter 10, Basic Life Support). Keep the air passages clear with suction.

Neurogenic shock. There is a special type of shock caused by paralysis of the nerves which control the size of the blood vessels. It is called neurogenic shock. The arteries and veins of a paralyzed person increase in size (dilate), particularly in the lower extremities. The circulatory system may fail because not enough blood is returning to the heart. Refer to Figure 7.6 c to visualize the pooling action when a normal volume of blood is contained in a dilated vascular system.

The treatment of neurogenic shock is simple. Splint the injured spinal column and put the patient in the shock position by elevating the legs with the knees straight. Blood then drains better from the enlarged vessels in the legs and returns to the heart for active circulation. The safest way to put the patient in the shock position is by elevating the lower end of the stretcher, not just the lower part of the patient. Elevate the foot of the stretcher only about twelve inches. Excessive elevation may cause the bowels and other viscera to fall against the underside of the diaphragm and compromise the patient's principal remaining breathing mechanism. Twelve inches of elevation is sufficient to assist blood return and will not significantly impair diaphragmatic action.

Although the preceding discussion has dealt mainly with cervical spine fractures, injuries at lower levels are also common. They are suggested by pain and tenderness in the area of the injury (often at the waist), and occasionally by paralysis of the legs. Patients with spinal cord damage at lower levels of the spine may also develop neurogenic shock. They do not

175

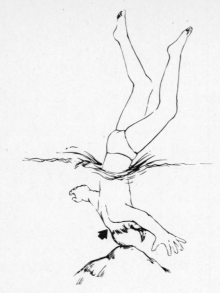

Figure 20.6

A cervical spine injury can result from a dive if the head strikes an underwater object or the bottom of the pool.

have paralysis in the chest muscles and therefore do not have impaired breathing, unless from another injury. Backboards and special stretchers should be used for these patients also. As with cervical spine fractures, fractures in other areas of the spine should be splinted in the position of deformity. Do not attempt to reposition the patient or straighten a deformity simply to make splinting more convenient. However, if repositioning is necessary because of some compelling reason, such as access to the airway, reposition the patient using the same precautions and gentle longitudinal traction recommended for correction of cervical spine fracture deformity.

Diving Injuries

Diving injuries are among the most common causes of cervical spine fractures (Fig. 20.6). If the spinal cord is not damaged when the injury occurs, the patient has an excellent chance of living a normal life. However, if the spinal cord is damaged at the time of the accident or by improper handling of the patient after the accident, paralysis or death may follow. Remember that a cervical spine fracture or disloca-

tion may or may not be accompanied by a spinal cord injury; in any case, the spinal cord must be protected while resuscitation from immersion in the water is being performed (see Fig. 44.2 in the chapter on Water Hazards).

It is unfortunate that patients injured in diving accidents are often carried from the water before the EMT arrives on the scene. Because of improper handling, patients with cervical spine injuries have died or have been paralyzed for life when an uncomplicated fracture was changed to a fracture with spinal cord damage. Patients with cervical spine injuries must always be handled so as to avoid hyperextension (having the head flop backward), severe flexion (having the head bend forward), or bending or twisting of the head to either side (Fig. 20.7). Patients injured in diving accidents should be removed from the water only after the cervical spine has been splinted properly, unless enough persons

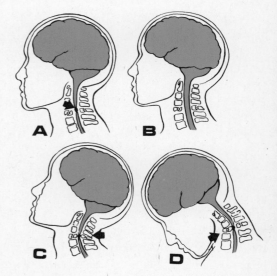

Figure 20.7 a–d

a, Severe damage of the spinal cord often occurs at the moment of injury.

b, Even though the spinal cord may be uninjured or only partially injured, it must be protected from damage that can occur when the patient is moved. The head and neck must be maintained in a stable, neutral position. Extension or flexion may cause the cord to be compressed disastrously, as demonstrated in the next two sketches. Paralysis can result in either case.

c, If the neck is hyperextended (the head falls backward), posterior compression of the spinal cord by fractured vertebrae can occur.

d, If the neck is flexed (the head falls forward), anterior compression of the spinal cord by fractured vertebrae can occur.

are available to help so that the head and neck of the patient can be held immovable at all times.

When the patient is floating face up, supported by the water, little effort is needed to maintain him on the surface in a satisfactory position. Follow these steps:

1. Start mouth-to-mouth ventilation if necessary, or assist the patient's diaphragmatic breathing.
2. Do not hyperextend or flex the patient's neck. When the patient is floating face down, support the head and neck while turning him over, being certain that the head, neck, and trunk move as a single unit with no motion at the site of a suspected cervical fracture. Float the patient onto a long spineboard and secure him to it so board and patient can be lifted from the water without bending the body.
3. After the board has been floated under the patient, continue to protect his head and neck before and while lifting him out of the water head first. Folded towels, a blanket, or a water ski belt applied as a collar may be used to support the head.

The patient should be carried from the water only when there are enough persons to provide proper handling and insure that his head and neck are adequately supported on the board. Each person who is helping must be told exactly what to do. Float the board to the edge of the pool or beach and gently pass the board with the patient on it out of the water. Still on the board or stretcher, he should be lifted into the ambulance, again head first.

177

V

The Head and Nervous System

CHAPTER 21

The Nervous System

GOAL I. Know the structures and understand the function of the nervous system.

OBJECTIVES

A. Identify all the structures of the nervous system and its divisions.
B. Describe the functions of the central nervous system, cerebrum, cerebellum, brain stem, and spinal cord.
C. Describe the functions of the autonomic nervous system.
D. Describe the functions of nerve cells.

The nervous system is composed of the brain, spinal cord, and branches from the spinal cord and brain which are called nerves. The system is divided anatomically into two parts: the central nervous system and the peripheral nervous system.

The central nervous system includes the brain and the spinal cord. The peripheral nervous system includes the nerves, which are either sensory or motor or a combination of both. Sensory nerves are adapted to carry sensations of touch, taste, heat, cold, pain, and the like. Motor nerves are adapted to transmit impulses to muscles, causing them to move.

That part of the nervous system which regulates functions over which there is voluntary control is often called the somatic nervous system.

There is also a subdivision called the autonomic, or involuntary, nervous system. Part of this system lies alongside and is connected with the spinal cord; part originates in the brain. Automatic functions such as digestion, the size of blood vessels, ability to sweat, and all such sensations and responses which cannot be controlled by a voluntary act of conscious will are under the direction of this system.

Central Nervous System

The brain. The brain is the controlling organ of the body (Fig. 21.1). It is the center of consciousness. Functions of the normal brain include perception of ourselves and our surround-

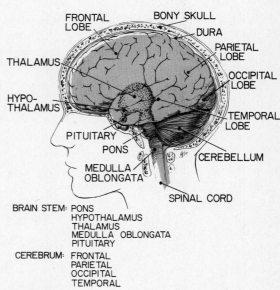

Figure 21.1

The head as shown in cross section contains the brain and its covering membranes and the origin of the spinal cord.

ings, control of our reactions to the environment, emotional responses, judgment, appreciation, and all the nuances that make conscious individuals.

The brain occupies the entire space within the cranium. It is made up of many different types of cells. Each type of cell has a specific function. Some cells in the brain receive sensory impulses or messages; other brain cells are responsible for signaling muscles and organs to act. Still other cells are responsible for transmitting impulses to other areas of the brain and to the spinal cord. The whole might be compared to an exceedingly complex miniaturized switchboard or computer where multiple sets of information can be received and spread through millions of circuits to the consciousness of an individual or to specific effector organs of the individual.

Certain parts of the brain enable us to perform certain functions. For instance, one part of the brain receives sensations; another sends impulses which allow us to move individual muscles at will. Other areas of the brain are responsible for hearing, seeing, thinking, and experiencing emotional responses. It is possible to determine which areas of the brain are damaged by injury or disease by a close assessment of what functions (such as hearing, smelling, moving, or breathing) are lacking, since damage to the controlling mechanisms in the brain results in loss of specific functions. The specialized areas of the brain are connected to each other by a complex network of conducting nerve fibers which carry impulses.

In general, the portions at the very front of the brain are the sites of emotional control. Behind them are the centers that control motion on each side of the body. In the brain, such centers lie on the sides opposite to the areas they govern. Centers in the right cerebrum, for instance, control functions on the left side of the body. Deep within the brain lie areas that control hearing, balance, and speech. The area at the back of the cerebrum controls visual perception.

Underneath the great mass of cerebral tissue lies the smaller cerebellum or little brain (Fig. 21.1). The major function of this area is coordination of all the commands of the brain so that very finely adjusted movements can be

carried out. Without the cerebellum, writing or sewing would be impossible.

Brain stem. Between the spinal cord and the cerebrum and surrounded by the cerebellum lies an area called the brain stem. The term arises from the fact that the brain looks as if it were sitting on this portion of the nervous system as a plant sits on its stem. In evolutionary terms, this is one of the oldest parts of the nervous system. It is one of the most protected parts of the body. Nearly every animal possesses this structure. It is the controlling center for those functions which are absolutely necessary for life. The lowermost area is the medulla oblongata where control of respiration lies. Above this region lie the thalamus, hypothalamus, and other areas where the involuntary muscles and other automatic bodily functions are controlled.

Spinal cord. Ultimately, all the important centers of the brain are connected, by long tracts of nerves, directly with the organs or muscles they control. These tracts join to form the spinal cord, which is therefore a continuation of the brain (Fig. 21.2). It transmits messages between the brain and the peripheral nervous system. These messages are passed along the nerve as electrical impulses, much as messages are passed in a telephone cable. The spinal cord is simply a collection of nerve cells connecting the brain directly with the muscle to be moved or the organ to be stimulated, or connecting the brain with the area from which an impulse or sensation is received.

The Peripheral Nervous System

At each individual spinal bone (vertebra) on each side of the spinal cord, a spinal nerve extends outward (Fig. 21.3). These nerves branch and pass to all parts of the body as the peripheral nervous system. For the upper and lower extremities, certain spinal nerves combine and then subsequently redivide to form two major nerve networks (plexi)—brachial for the upper extremity and lumbosacral for the lower (Fig. 21.2). The extremities are thus excepted from a strict pattern of nervous innervation passing from top to bottom. Within each of these nerves are motor fibers which relay impulses from the

182

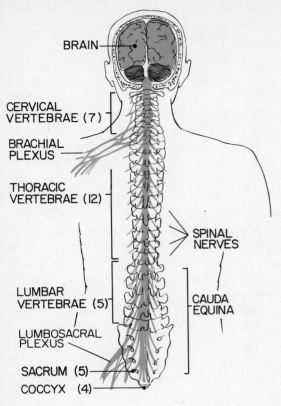

Figure 21.2

A posterior view of the spinal cord shows the spinal nerves and the two major plexi for the upper and lower extremities.

brain to muscles, and sensory fibers which relay sensory impulses from the skin and other organs to the brain.

A significant portion of the autonomic nervous system, called the sympathetic nervous system, lies outside the spinal canal and parallel to the spinal cord, along the thoracic and lumbar vertebrae. This system connects with the spinal cord at each opening where nerves emerge. It maintains constriction of blood vessels, stimulation of sweat glands, and many other automatic functions. Under the control of the parasympathetic system, which issues directly from the brain and from the lowermost end of the spinal cord at the sacrum, are functions which are opposite to those of the sympathetic system and which balance it, such as dilation of blood vessels.

Sensory nerves. The sensory nervous system of the body is quite complex. There are many different types of sensory cells in the nervous system. Some form the retina of the eye; others, the hearing and balancing mechanism in the ear. Other sensory cells are located within the skin, muscles, joints, lungs, and other organs of the body. When a sensory cell is stimulated, it transmits its own special message to the brain. There are special sensory cells which detect heat, cold, position, motion, pressure, and pain

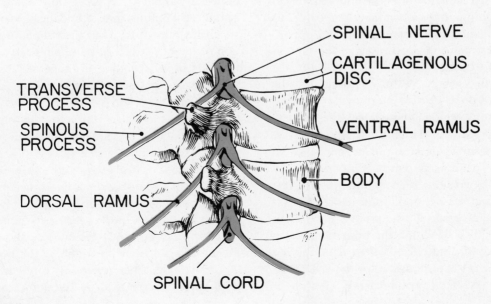

Figure 21.3

The nerve roots of the central nervous system extend to form the peripheral nervous system.

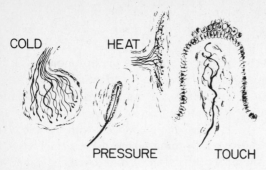

Figure 21.4

The principal sensory receptors of the skin are shown. They include separate organs to distinguish pain, temperature, and pressure.

184

(Fig. 21.4). These sensory impulses constantly tell us what the different parts of our body are doing in relation to our surroundings. By performing this function, they make us aware of our surroundings. The sensations we receive travel to the brain; some go directly. Visual sensations (what we see) reach the brain directly by way of the optic (eye) nerves. Hearing sensations reach the brain by way of the auditory (hearing) nerves. Most other sensations reach the brain by traveling along sensory nerves to the spinal cord, then to the brain.

The brain analyzes, sorts, and stores information about these different sensations. When it makes a decision to do something, the brain sends motor impulses down the spinal cord into the peripheral motor nerves to an appropriate muscle or organ, causing muscular contraction or other reaction.

Connecting nerves. Within the brain and the spinal cord there are also internuncial (connecting) neurons which interconnect the sensory (input) nerves with the motor (output) nerves. These internuncials are not a part of the peripheral nervous system but do act to interconnect its two sides, sensory and motor. They may connect sensory and motor nerves directly in the spinal cord, short-circuiting the brain. They may also lie within the brain connecting many receptor and effector sites. This specific set of neurons is responsible for the vast interconnection of all parts of the nervous system.

Types of Action of the Nervous System

Some of the activities of the nervous system are automatic, some are reflex, and some are performed only after thinking and conscious decision by the brain. Some examples of the types of nervous activities follow.

Automatic action. Breathing is done automatically. To a certain extent a person can breathe rapidly or hold his breath by conscious will. He cannot do these things, however, indefinitely. A complex system of chemical control takes over when a person approaches danger from voluntary breathing control, and respiration returns to normal. This response is one of the most primitive functions of the brain, present at every level of animal development.

Reflex action. A person pulls his hand away from a hot stove before there is time for thought and decision. Usually the hand jerks away from the stove at the same time he realizes it is hot. This action is completed by a circuit involving sensory, short-circuiting internuncial, and motor nerves. It is what is termed a reflex arc. No decisions are made in instituting this reaction.

Conscious action. Driving a car requires thinking. This action requires the appreciation of sensory input from eyes and ears; general sensation of bumps, shocks, and the like; synthesis of this knowledge; and the conscious direction of the car. It is a series of willed or voluntary acts, each depending on a separate decision.

Voluntary control of muscles. The skeletal muscles that move the parts of the body can be voluntarily controlled through the somatic nervous system. They are activated and inactivated in response to one's will.

Involuntary control of muscles. Muscles in the walls of arteries and the intestines, or the muscle of the heart cannot be voluntarily controlled. The action of the heart speeds or slows in response to demands put on it by the body. Sweating is initiated by fright or the need of the body to dissipate heat. Dilation or constriction of blood vessels is automatically and constantly done in response to a number of specific stimuli. All these functions are controlled by the autonomic nervous system, which is made up of the two systems, sympathetic and parasympathetic. The constant balance of these two systems provides the individual with automatic responses to changes in the surrounding environment and keeps him in equilibrium with his surroundings.

Protective Coverings of the Nervous System

The tissue of the brain and spinal cord is soft and easily injured; it is protected by a special set of coverings (Fig. 21.5). The brain and spinal cord are surrounded by three layers of tissue which suspend them within the skull and the spinal canal. Between these tissues and the brain and cord are spaces which are filled with a liquid known as cerebrospinal fluid. It provides nutrition to some of the brain cells and serves as a shock absorber for the brain and spinal cord.

These layers are distinct. The brain and spinal cord are first covered by a tough fibrous outer layer much like leather, which is called the dura mater. Beneath this layer, two filmy layers lie immediately over the brain and cord. They are called the arachnoid and the pia mater. Blood vessels nourishing the brain run in these layers. Cerebrospinal fluid lies underneath the arachnoid and over the pia mater covering the brain and cord. In head injuries where clear cerebrospinal fluid is seen coming from the nose or the

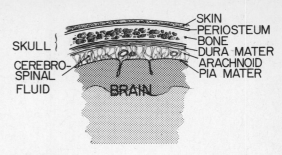

Figure 21.5

The covering membranes of the central nervous system (the meninges) suspend the system within the skull and spinal cord.

185

ear, one can assume that a skull fracture with laceration of the dura exists. Hemorrhage underneath the dura and over the brain is very common in head injuries from damage of blood vessels in this area; often there are subsequent neurologic symptoms from the damaged brain.

A not infrequent, very serious condition is meningitis. The disease can be caused by a variety of organisms—bacterial, viral, or fungal. Ordinarily it is spread by droplet contact in close quarters, as in barracks or day nurseries. It can result in an extreme headache, fever, and stiffness of the neck. The EMT will rarely be called upon to make such a diagnosis but may be required to transport this patient. Precautions listed in Chapter 35, Communicable Disease, must be observed.

The disease should be suspected in patients complaining of these symptoms without a preceding injury and with fever. The disease is commonly seen in children as well as adults.

CHAPTER 22

Injuries of the Skull and Brain

GOAL I. Know the characteristics of head, brain, and spinal injury.

OBJECTIVES

A. Describe the signs of head, brain, and spinal injury.
B. Identify the types of skull fractures.
C. Describe physiological characteristics of brain injury.

GOAL II. Understand the principles of treatment of head and brain injuries.

OBJECTIVES

A. Describe the examination procedures for head and brain injuries.
B. Describe the procedures for treatment of head and brain injuries.

In vehicular accidents, over 70 percent of the injuries sustained involve the skull and the brain. A head injury may be an isolated one or it may be a part of massive multiple trauma. The damage may be a trivial scalp laceration or a severe brain injury which rapidly causes death. Most head injuries lie somewhere between these two extremes. All severe head injuries are potentially life-threatening, whether they are accompanied by immediate unconsciousness or not. For recovery and satisfactory return of normal function, proper treatment is vital as a first step, especially if the patient is unconscious. Care must start at the scene of the accident and should be maintained while the patient is transported to the Emergency Department.

The Unconscious State

The unconscious person is unable to offer complaints. He cannot defend himself and may have lost his normal protective reflexes, such as withdrawing from a painful stimulus or cough-ing when he aspirates secretions into his trachea. The management of the helpless, unconscious patient can follow a straightforward A-B-C-D outline.

A - Airway support. More than any other part of the body, the brain requires a constant, rich supply of oxygen. A person who cannot breathe cannot live for more than a few minutes unless air or oxygen is artificially supplied. A relative lack of oxygen may exist in the blood even when respiration appears adequate or normal. Cyanosis, a bluish-grey color of the skin around the lips or in the nail beds, indicates an extreme depletion of oxygen in the blood. Although most patients who have sustained a brain injury and are unconscious have a relatively low oxygen level in their blood, they are not usually cyanotic. The presence of cyanosis requires immediate action by the EMT to aid respiration because the injured brain is even more sensitive to hypoxia (lack of oxygen) than the normal brain and cannot tolerate it as well.

Almost all patients who require artificial ventilation are unconscious. When the uncon-

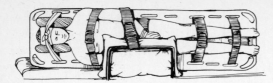

Figure 22.1

A semiprone position improves the patient's breathing and reduces the possibility he may aspirate vomitus. For a suspected neck injury, the head should be firmly maintained in a neutral position to the shoulders. Note that most of the patient's clothing has been removed. A brain injury can cause body temperature to rise, and the patient should not be allowed to overheat.

188 scious state is a result of brain dysfunction alone, the individual is usually breathing; in fact, he may be breathing more deeply or rapidly than normal. An altered breathing pattern in the patient who has sustained a severe injury usually indicates brain damage. In the absence of other significant injuries, one should turn this unconscious patient to a semiprone position (Fig. 22.1), for turning usually improves the patient's breathing. An equally important reason for using this position is that the unconscious patient with a brain injury tends to vomit. When he is flat on his back, he will aspirate the vomitus and thereby compound any airway problem.

When the patient has been in a vehicular accident or has fallen from a height (especially down steps), a cervical or other spinal injury must be suspected. Nevertheless, this patient too can be turned safely if his head is maintained in strict alignment with his body and supported with sandbags or other unyielding materials (Fig. 22.1). Ideally, the patient should be secured to a spineboard. The methods of establishing the airway when a fractured neck is suspected include the insertion of one of the various oro-

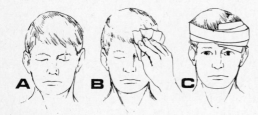

Figure 22.2

The scalp contains many arteries and veins and an injury here will usually bleed freely. Bleeding can usually be controlled by local pressure and a roller bandage wrapped around the head.

pharyngeal or nasopharyngeal airways or bringing the lower jaw forward (jaw-thrust maneuver). These maneuvers are discussed in Chapter 10, Basic Life Support.

B - Bleeding control. Bleeding from the head usually is from vessels within the scalp; bleeding can also develop inside the skull and within the brain itself. The blood supply of the scalp is unique in that blood vessels are sandwiched between two very tough layers of tissue. The surface layer is a thick layer of skin and the bottom is a thin but extremely strong tissue called the galea aponeurotica.

Control of bleeding from the head is usually achieved with local pressure over the bleeding point and the use of a circumferential roller bandage. Bandaging the head should be routine procedure for all patients who have sustained scalp lacerations. The proper application of this bandage will usually stop hemorrhage (Fig. 22.2). If the galea itself is lacerated, the scalp wound tends to gape wide and often bleeds very vigorously. This profuse bleeding can sometimes produce hypovolemic shock.

A rapid method to control bleeding from the scalp is to compress the scalp itself against the skull, using the fingers. However, if the injury has caused a skull fracture with bony fragments lying underneath the scalp laceration, localized compression should be avoided. A pressure dressing should be applied with a self-adhering roller bandage. In those instances where control of bleeding cannot be readily achieved, it may be arising from within the skull; the wound should be covered with a sterile dressing and secured with a roller bandage. The bandage should be reinforced as necessary. The patient should be taken to the Emergency Department at once, for uncontrolled bleeding in addition to a head injury constitutes a serious condition.

C - Cervical spine injury evaluation. Some 10 percent of patients who are unconscious after vehicular accidents or falls may also have suffered neck injuries with spinal cord damage. It is often difficult to determine which patient has sustained a spinal injury. Some methods of determining the presence of this additional injury in the unconscious patient are discussed in the following paragraphs.

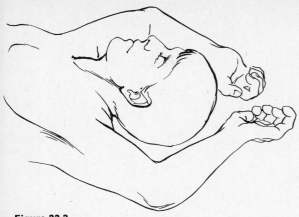

Figure 22.3

A patient with an injury of the lower cervical spinal cord will hold his arms in a "hold up" position. If the arms are brought down and placed alongside the chest, they will revert to the hold-up position automatically when released.

1. Observe the chest and abdomen as the patient breathes. If the abdomen distends when the patient inspires and the chest barely moves, then the diaphragm is performing the principal breathing function because the chest muscles are paralyzed. The diaphragm is controlled by nerves that rise high in the neck, usually above the area of a cervical spine fracture. The chest muscles are controlled at a considerably lower level in the spine by nerves which pass directly to them from the spinal cord in the thorax.

2. Starting at the feet, prick the patient lightly with a pin and observe his face. As the pin approaches the upper chest he may grimace, which will indicate that he has lost sensation below the area where the pricking begins to produce a reaction. The finding is seen in patients with fractures of the cervical spine and spinal cord damage at the level of the fracture.

3. The forearms may lie across the chest or may be elevated alongside the head in the "hold-up" position (Fig. 22.3). Patients who have sustained spinal cord injuries at the level of the lower neck cannot extend their upper extremities (stretch out their arms) because of nerve injury, but the muscles that flex (bend) the elbows and lift the arms can still function.

4. The blood pressure may be below 100 mm Hg systolic without any other signs of hypovolemic shock.

5. The male may have a penile erection.

When a neck or spinal injury is suspected, either from the history or because of any of the above-mentioned findings in the patient who is unconscious, this patient should be treated with all the precautions reviewed in Chapter 20, Fractures and Dislocations of the Spine, and should be transported to the hospital properly supported on a spineboard.

D - Description of the patient. In the unconscious patient, it is most important that the EMT establish a base line for further evaluation of the patient by hospital personnel. Most patients show prompt improvement with proper care, but some do not. Lack of improvement can suggest a developing neurosurgical problem. Thus the observations of the EMT may play a major role in a decision to perform or not perform an operation. Attending physicians must know if loss of consciousness was immediate or if it developed after the patient was first treated. They must know if it developed slowly or speedily. They must know if specific physical signs which would indicate certain injuries were seen. A summary of the observations relating to the neurological state of a patient is contained in what is called a neural observation chart or neural watch chart or sheet. Several such charts have been developed across the nation; they are used to record specific observations on patients at ten- or fifteen-minute intervals. The most important function of these charts is to allow the attending physician to review changing states in a patient's condition and to determine from the changes whether an operation should be considered. A copy of one such neural watch chart is included here (Fig. 22.4). The observations to be included in this chart are considered below. All these data must be observed and recorded on the sheet at specific intervals of time.

First, record the patient's vital signs. A rising blood pressure, especially if the pulse is slow, usually indicates cerebral (brain) hemorrhage. **However, low blood pressure, or shock, is almost never a result of brain damage;** it is usually caused by blood loss from other injuries.

Brain injury tends to cause a rise in body temperature, which itself further damages the

189

UNIT		Time:				
I Vital signs	Blood pressure					
	Pulse					
	Respiration					
	Temperature					
II Conscious and	Oriented					
	Disoriented					
	Restless					
	Combative					
III Speech	Clear					
	Rambling					
	Garbled					
	None					
IV Will awaken to	Name					
	Shaking					
	Light pain					
	Strong pain					
V Non-verbal reaction to pain	Appropriate					
	Inappropriate					
	"Decerebrate"					
	None					
VI Pupils	Size on right					
	Size on left					
	Reacts on right					
	Reacts on left					
VII Ability to move	Right arm					
	Left arm					
	Right leg					
	Left leg					

Figure 22.4

A neural watch sheet is simple to use, and the information recorded on it can be of great significance in charting the progress of the patient's condition and determining treatment for him.

brain. In warm climates be sure that the patient is stripped of heavy clothing and that he is not wrapped in a blanket (Fig. 22.1).

If the patient can talk, note this fact. An oriented person should know his name, age, the date, and where he is. Disoriented speech or a low moan can be recorded as "garbled" speech. If the patient cannot talk, this fact should also be recorded.

If the patient is sleepy, or is actually unconscious, the EMT should see if he can be roused when spoken to or shaken. Pain may be required to rouse him. A pin prick is considered light pain. Pinching the skin with an instrument is regarded as strong pain. Record his reaction as "appropriate," "inappropriate," or "decerebrate." An appropriate response means that the

patient attempts to move away from a painful stimulus or to protect himself. An inappropriate response means that his movements are ineffective against the painful stimulus. A patient in a coma does not respond to pain at all. A decerebrate response means that the extremities stiffen when the patient is stimulated by pain.

The size of the pupil of the eye and ability of the pupil to constrict in reaction to a bright light shined into it are important. A sketch of the pupils may be made by the EMT to indicate any difference in size. He should then check each pupil to see if it contracts upon exposure to light. Changes in pupillary reaction are extremely important observations to record.

Finally, try to estimate the strength of the upper and lower limbs. In a conscious patient, this test is easy to do. In the patient who is unconscious, painful stimuli may be required to make the limbs move. Normal strength is ordinarily marked down as 4 and no movement as 0. The ratings should reflect the EMT's estimate of the patient's capability and his weakness in response to stimuli.

Properly kept, a neural watch sheet should reflect a stable state, an improving state, or a progressively declining one. Only by making repeated observations and recording them as long as the patient is under his care, can the EMT develop a careful record of the patient's changing neurological status.

Specific Head Injuries

Skull fractures. Much too much emphasis has been placed on the presence of a skull fracture in predicting brain damage. The main function of the skull is to protect the brain. If a fracture has occurred, it is an indication that the mechanical force exerted on the head was great, but the fracture alone offers no proof that the brain has been damaged. In fact, serious brain injury is much more common when there is no skull fracture. There may be no external evidence of injury at all, but brain damage may be found to exist.

The diagnosis of a skull fracture is usually made at the hospital by X-ray examination, but the EMT may conclude there is a fracture if the patient's head appears deformed. If the scalp has been lacerated, there may even be a visible crack in the skull. Injuries from bullets or ice picks almost always result in fractures.

An indirect indication of fractures in a hidden area of the skull, such as in its base, is the appearance of a watery clear or watery pink fluid dripping from the nose, from the ear, or from a scalp wound. This is cerebrospinal fluid, formed within the head. Where this fluid is seen, no attempt should be made to pack the wound, the ear, or the nose. The scalp wound should be covered with sterile gauze but should not be bandaged tightly, as such packing will block the escape of cerebrospinal fluid and cause secondary pressure on an already damaged brain. Ecchymosis of the soft tissues under the eyes or

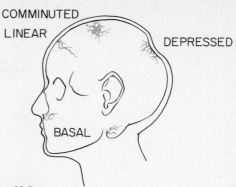

Figure 22.5

Various types of fractures about the head and face are illustrated.

191

behind the ear, especially if the area of impact was elsewhere in the skull, also suggests fractures of the base of the skull.

Skull fractures are either open or closed. They can be further divided as shown in Figure 22.5.

1. Linear—A linear fracture is a thin line crack in the skull.

2. Comminuted—In a comminuted fracture, multiple cracks radiate from the center of impact. The pattern is similar to that seen in a cracked egg.

3. Depressed—In a depressed fracture, a fragment or fragments of bone have been pushed inward against the brain. Such fractures are common in penetrating injuries. Bullets notoriously thrust fragments of the skull deep into the brain. These fragments may come to lie on the brain or to lacerate it, causing extensive damage.

4. Basal—Basal skull fractures usually cannot be seen even with excellent X rays. They can present severe clinical problems, especially if there is an obvious cerebrospinal fluid leak. The appearance of clear cerebrospinal fluid at the ear, the nose, or from a scalp laceration may be the only indication that such a fracture exists.

The emergency care of skull fractures consists of:

1. Controlling and maintaining the airway
2. Controlling bleeding from the edges of the wound
3. Covering open wounds properly

Impaled foreign objects. The brain may be

severely injured by penetrating or impaled objects. Bullets may pass through the skull and enter the brain. Ice picks or knives may likewise be impaled within the brain. **No attempt should be made to remove an impaled foreign object from the head.** The object should be removed only by a physician. Occasionally, and only when proper equipment is available, the protruding end of an object may be cut off to allow easier transportation of the patient. If it is absolutely required that the impaled object be cut, it must first be completely stabilized so that it cannot move and further injure the brain during the cutting. In general, these objects should not be cut but should be stabilized with soft, very bulky dressings, firmly applied.

Injuries of the Brain

Injuries of the brain are relatively common. The brain is very delicate tissue, very delicately supported. When it is injured, the patient may lose consciousness and slip into a deep coma. Occasionally a brain injury may produce paralysis on one side of the body, vomiting, sleepiness, or loss of respiration. Brain tissue is susceptible to the same types of damage as all other tissues in the body:

1. Bruises
2. Pressure damage
3. Lacerations

Concussion. When a person has been struck on the head or hit in the face, a brain concussion can result. There is no universal agreement on the definition of concussion except that it involves a temporary loss of some or all of the ability of the brain to function. No demonstrable damage may have been done to the brain at all. The patient who has sustained a concussion may become totally unconscious and unable to breathe for a short period of time, or he may only be confused and staggering. In general, the concussive state is usually of very short duration and should be terminated by the time the EMT arrives at the scene of the accident. Nevertheless, a neural observation sheet should be initiated for evaluating this patient. Further signs of neurological (nerve) degeneration are very impor-

tant and should be recorded, as they may indicate more severe damage. Most patients who have sustained a concussion have some loss of memory for the events surrounding the accident (amnesia). If the patient cannot remember the events prior to the injury (retrograde amnesia), a more severe concussion is evident.

Contusion. The brain may sustain a contusion or a bruise when any object hits the skull with force. Contusion implies that bleeding from injured blood vessels has occurred. When the brain is brusied, the individual may lose consciousness. Other signs of dysfunction from contusion include paralysis on one side of the body, dilation of one pupil, and alteration of the vital signs. Very severe contusions can produce unconsciousness for prolonged periods of time and may cause paralysis of all four limbs.

Brain tissue itself is easily damaged by the abnormal swelling of the brain after a contusion. Secondary pressure within the skull from a contused brain may damage still more brain tissue and result in a progressive deterioration of neurological or vital signs. The longer the pressure continues, the more permanent the brain damage may be.

Even with severe contusions, however, recovery can occur without the necessity of an intracranial operation (an operation inside the skull). The chances of recovery are directly proportional to the care given from the time the injury was sustained. Patients must receive adequate ventilation, supplemental oxygen when necessary, and all necessary cardiopulmonary resuscitation. They must be transported to the Emergency Department for expert neurosurgical evaluation and care.

Cerebral hematoma. The brain takes up the entire space within the skull. There is very little, if any, room for blood clots. Any severe injury within the skull may cause a collection of blood either between the inner table of the skull and the brain or under the heavy membrane which covers the brain. These collections of blood are called, respectively, epidural and subdural hematomas (Fig. 22.6). Either injury can produce similar clinical signs. The signs are related to the development of pressure on the brain where it is compressed by an expanding mass of blood clot

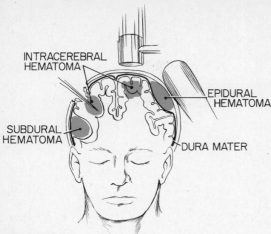

Figure 22.6

Severe blunt or penetrating skull injuries can produce various types of collections of blood (hematomas) within the cranium. Any of these blunt injuries could also result in a basal skull fracture.

within the skull. These hemorrhages usually require an operation to remove the clot. If it is not removed, the patient may die. Occasionally, bleeding occurs within the brain itself, causing pressure to be exerted on the brain around the area of the hemorrhage. Intracerebral bleeding (inside the brain) can occur spontaneously in patients with high blood pressure or abnormal blood vessels. These patients are said to have sustained a stroke.

Care of the patient who may have developed an intracerebral hematoma includes careful observation of his initial neurological status and any changes in it, bandaging of any obvious scalp wound, and prompt transportation to the Emergency Department.

Evaluation and Initial Care

In evaluating the patient who may have sustained brain damage, all the points noted in the discussion of the neural watch sheet are important. Probably more important than evaluating any single point at any one time is the repeated evaluation of this patient over the period of time he is being treated and transported to the hospital. **The single most important observation that the EMT can make concerning the neurological status of any patient is to record the state of his consciousness. If a patient with an apparent head injury becomes progressively more unconscious, he must be transported to the hospital immediately.** This patient has evidence of rapidly developing brain damage and he must be promptly treated.

Suspecting spinal injury. In general, a patient with a serious brain injury must always be suspected of having sustained a neck injury. If the patient is not conscious, and the EMT feels he cannot adequately rule out the possibility of spinal injury, the patient should be treated as if he had a cervical spinal fracture (broken neck).

Importance of initial care. The initial emergency care of patients with brain injuries is extremely important. The ultimate success of weeks of treatment may depend on the first half-hour of care and observation. Proper emergency treatment includes these procedures in the following order of their importance:

1. Correct life-threatening problems.
2. Splint all back and neck injuries.
3. Position the patient properly with regard to his injuries.

The single most important aspect of care for the patient who has sustained a severe injury of the brain or the skull is maintenance of adequate respiration. Even with an aequate artificial airway, the patient may not breathe often enough or deeply enough to provide his body adequate oxygenation. Indeed, he may not breathe at all. Inadequate respiration and resulting shock may be a result of:

1. Brain damage itself, with loss of the stimulus to breathe
2. Paralysis of the muscles of respiration in the chest as a result of cervical spine injury

Positioning the patient. The patient with a head or brain injury should be positioned according to the circumstances of his associated injuries or the requirements for his treatment. Indications for deciding how to position these patients for transportation are discussed below.

1. The ideal position for a patient with an isolated head injury is with the head of the stretcher somewhat elevated. It should not be elevated, however, if secretions are accumulating

193

in the patient's throat. Mucus can cause a secondary airway obstruction in this situation. The patient's head should not be put on a pillow, as this position will flex the neck and produce airway obstruction.

2. When there is bleeding in the mouth and throat, the patient must be positioned on his side or on his face so that blood can drain out of the mouth and not down into the larynx. If the EMT cannot position the patient to allow drainage easily out of the mouth, a suction unit must be used. At times, it will be mandatory to position the patient carefully on his side to maintain his airway.

3. Always recall that these patients vomit easily. In such instances, when the head is elevated, it must quickly be lowered and the patient turned on his side. The vomitus should then be sucked from the throat to prevent aspiration of material into the lungs.

Convulsions. Convulsions can occur after relatively mild head injuries. When convulsing, the patient must be protected from himself. Since the usual severe seizure results in a jerking motion of all the limbs, protecting the patient may not be an easy task. A padded mouth gag should be inserted between the teeth to prevent the patient from biting his tongue and to help maintain his airway. Immobilization of the cervical spine and maintenance of an airway present difficult problems during a convulsion.

If the EMT has radio contact with the Emergency Department or with a physician, he may request permission to use an intravenous anticonvulsant medication. These medications must be administered promptly to control a convulsion. Intramuscular or oral anticonvulsant medications should never be used except by order of a physician and ordinarily never in an acute situation, as they could depress the breathing mechanism of a patient and create a much more serious condition.

Summary of Responsibilities

The EMT has a significant role to play in the management of the patient with a head or brain injury. He can improve the patient's airway, stop obvious bleeding, immobilize the cervical spine when an injury is suspected, provide supplemental oxygen, and properly describe the patient's reactions on a neural watch sheet. It must be remembered that in spite of the seriousness of brain injuries, a very large percentage of these patients survive without the need of an operation if proper initial treatment is given promptly. Considerably more patients survive, if an operation must be performed, because they have been transported to the hospital promptly and safely. In addition to the fact that lives have been saved, many patients have survived with relatively little or no permanent brain dysfunction because of proper emergency treatment.

Although a patient may have sustained a severe head injury, he must be evaluated for all other contributing and associated injuries. The appropriate splinting of extremity fractures should be done, and all other indicated emergency treatment should be concluded prior to his being transported to an Emergency Department. The fact that he has sustained a severe head or brain injury does not mean that he has sustained a fatal injury. It does mean that his chances for survival and resumption of a normal existence are directly related to the quality of the initial care he receives.

194

CHAPTER **23**

The Eye

GOAL I. Know the various structures of the eye and understand their function.

OBJECTIVES

A. Explain the process of "seeing."
B. Name the specific anatomical structures of the eye.
C. Describe the specific functions of the eye structures.
D. Describe pupil reaction and the neurologic significance of this reaction.

The eye is an organ of special sense, adapted for vision. It has a lens system similar to that of a camera. This system focuses an image which special sensory cells in the retina change into an electrical message that is carried by the optic nerve to a special part of the brain. The brain receives the sensory message and interprets it. The entire process is "seeing."

Parts of the Eye

Like a fine camera, the eye has many intricate parts; all are important if the eye is to function properly. For the needs of the EMT in learning to provide emergency care and in understanding vision, the most important parts of the eye will be described (Fig. 23.1).

The eye is globe-shaped and approximately one inch in diameter. The shape of the globe is maintained by the fluid contained within it. This is a clear, viscous or jelly-like fluid called the vitreous humor. When the globe is lacerated, this fluid may leak out.

The front part of the globe is clear and transparent so that light may enter the eye. It is called the cornea. The rest of the globe is made up of a tough tissue called the sclera, which is the white part of the eye. In the visible portion of the eye, the sclera is covered by a layer of smooth

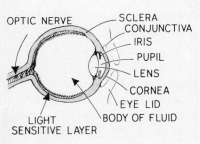

Figure 23.1

The major components of the eye are shown. They include specific apparatus to control the admission of light, to focus an image, to perceive and transmit an image, and to nourish and protect the organ.

mucous membrane called conjunctiva. This layer is reflected over the inside of the eyelids. Thus, when the lids move, two smooth conjunctival surfaces slide over one another. Inflammation of the conjunctiva or irritation of this layer gives the eye a characteristic pink or red color ("pink eye").

There is an adjustable circular muscle behind the cornea with an aperture, again like that of a camera, which regulates the amount of light that enters the eye. This muscle is called the iris; the opening in this muscular curtain is the pupil. Behind the iris is a lens that focuses an image on the light-sensitive layer, the retina. The retina is a layer of cells at the back of the eye that changes the light image into electrical im-

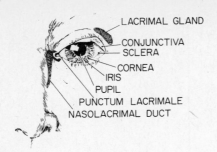

LACRIMAL GLAND
CONJUNCTIVA
SCLERA
CORNEA
IRIS
PUPIL
PUNCTUM LACRIMALE
NASOLACRIMAL DUCT

Figure 23.2

The parts of the eye viewed from the front include pupil, iris, sclera, and cornea. The elements of the lacrimal system are shown.

196

pulses which can be carried by the optic nerve to the brain for interpretation. Between the retina and the sclera is a layer of blood vessels nourishing the eye and especially the retina. This layer is the choroid. The retina and choroid are supported against the sclera by the pressure of the vitreous humor.

The lacrimal system consists of lacrimal (tear) glands and ducts (Fig. 23.2). This system is important in the protection of the eye. Lacrimal glands produce tears which act as a lubricating substance to prevent the eye from drying. The glands that make tears are located beneath the upper eyelid. Tear ducts are located on the inner side of the eye along the lower lid. They drain the tears through a tiny duct into the nose. The opening of this duct in the inner corner of the eyelid forms a small but prominent point called the punctum lacrimale.

Upper and lower eyelids protect the eyes. The inside of the eyelids is the very smooth conjunctival surface which is kept moistened by tears produced by tear glands. The eyelids glide up and down over the eye to protect it from dust and other irritants. The upper eyelid travels over the greater surface of the eye and is moulded by a tough fibrous plate (tarsal plate) which provides

its form. It has a separate muscle (levator palpebrae) to lift it. The eyelids are closed by the contraction of a circular muscle around the eye called the orbicularis oculi.

The pupil of the eye becomes smaller or larger to adjust to various levels of light, just as the aperture of a camera is adjusted. The pupil also adjusts if one is viewing objects close at hand or far away. It becomes larger if the object is distant. Adjustment for light or dark is automatic and almost instantaneous.

When an injured or ill person is evaluated, it is important to look at the pupils of the eyes, especially when a head injury is suspected. Normally, when a light is directed into someone's eyes the pupils constrict (become smaller). When the eyes are in darkness, or are shaded or closed, the pupils dilate (become larger) (Fig. 23.3). The size of the pupils and particularly any difference in size between the two pupils and their reaction to light are important signs which help determine the nature and severity of a head injury. Hence, one often sees a doctor gently lifting the eyelids of an unconscious person to see if the pupils are of the same size and if they constrict when the eyes are open or when a light is shined into them.

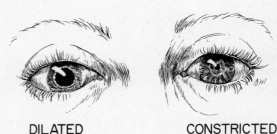

DILATED　　　　　　　　CONSTRICTED

Figure 23.3

Normal pupil diameter is 2 to 3 millimeters. Pupils may be dilated or constricted for many different reasons. Usually, pupil size is equal and the pupils react together.

24

Injuries of the Eye, Face, and Throat

GOAL I. Know the procedures for evaluating and treating injuries of the eye.

OBJECTIVES

A. Understand the diagnosis and treatment of lacerations and contusions of the eye.

B. Describe the treatment for an extruded eyeball.

C. Explain the relationship of eyeglasses and contact lenses to injuries of the eyes.

D. State the significant aspects of treatment of blunt trauma of the eye.

E. Describe the diagnosis and treatment of the types of burns that can affect the eyes.

F. State the condition of the pupils that may lead the EMT to suspect a head injury.

GOAL II. Know the procedures for evaluating and treating injuries of the face and throat.

OBJECTIVES

A. List the possible causes of breathing problems in relationship to face and head injuries.

B. Describe the emergency care of soft-tissue injuries of the scalp, face, and throat.

C. Explain the results of various injuries of the throat and the emergency treatment for them.

D. Describe the treatment of injuries of the nose.

E. State the possible result of injuries of the facial bones and describe emergency treatment for them.

The Eye

The eye is an important sensory organ, and blindness is a very severe physical handicap. Proper initial emergency care of the injured eye not only relieves pain but also helps prevent permanent optical injury and loss of vision.

The eye should never be examined with dirty hands. The examination must be careful, thor- ough, and very gentle. It is easy to aggravate any injury because the eye is very sensitive. Great care must be taken in all eye examinations.

The eyelids may be swollen or lacerated from either blunt or cutting injuries. The conjunctiva frequently becomes bright red (bloodshot) when injured or irritated. The cornea is easily scratched by foreign objects. Normally, an entire circle of the iris should be visible. The pupils

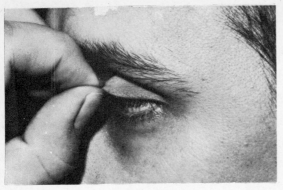

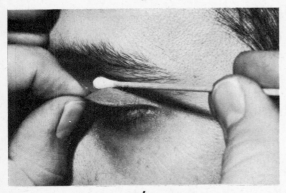

198

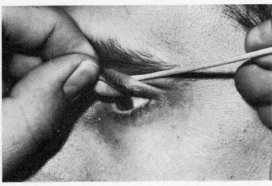

Figure 24.1 *a—c*

To remove an object from under the upper lid, follow the steps shown. *a,* Ask the patient to look down. Then grasp his eyelashes with your thumb and index finger, and gently pull the lid away from the eyeball. *b,* Place a cotton-tipped applicator (or cotton-tipped matchstick) horizontally along the center of the outer surface of the upper lid. *c,* Pull the lid forward and upward, causing it to roll or fold back over the applicator. The undersurface of the lid will be exposed. With practice, this procedure becomes easy to do; and when performed gently, it is not painful.

should be equal in size. Normally, both eyes move together, in the same direction.

Foreign Bodies

Foreign bodies of many sizes and types can enter the eye. They are most commonly found under the upper lid or on the cornea. Foreign bodies irritate the eye, and any such irritation causes tears to flow more freely. Tears may wash away the foreign body. Sometimes it can be washed away by pouring saline solution gently over the eye or by using a squeeze bottle of eye-irrigating solution. Opening the eye under gently running water is also sometimes effective. The first two methods are preferable.

To examine the undersurface of the eyelid for a foreign body, the eyelid must be everted (turned up) (Fig. 24.1).

When there is a foreign body on the underside of the lid, gently remove it with a clean, moist, sterile applicator. The EMT should never attempt to remove a foreign body from the cornea.

Large foreign bodies may become impaled in the eye; they should be removed only by a physician. Cover the eye with a paper cup or a cardboard cone to prevent the object from being driven farther into the eye, and to provide a dressing around the eye. Cover both eyes even though only one is injured. Remember, the eyes move together. This maneuver will keep both eyes quiet and will help prevent motion of the injured one.

A person with eyes covered cannot see and may be easily frightened. This fact is especially true with children, and covering both eyes without warning may be unwise, as the child may become uncooperative and struggle, risking more damage. Calm reassurance, a quiet, matter-of-fact explanation of why both eyes are being temporarily covered, and assistance in moving will be needed.

Burns

Chemical burns, thermal burns, and light burns can affect the eyes.

Chemical burns. Injuries from chemical burns require immediate emergency care to prevent permanent damage. Chemical burns are caused principally by acids or alkalies.

The one and only emergency treatment is to

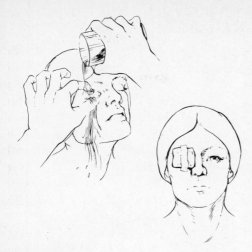

Figure 24.2

Emergency treatment for chemicals in the eye is to flush the eye immediately with large amounts of water. At least five minutes of washing the eye will be necessary. For alkali in the eye, twenty minutes irrigation is not too much. A soft bandage may then be placed over the eye while the patient is transported to the hospital.

dilute the chemical immediately by flushing the eyes with water or with the sterile saline solution carried on ambulances. Use any clean water available. It may be necessary to pour the water into the eyes (Fig. 24.2) or to hold the patient's head under a gently running faucet, or even to have him put his face in a large pan of water and blink his eyes rapidly. The eyes should be irrigated for five to ten minutes at least. If the burn has been caused by an alkali, irrigation should last twenty minutes. One cannot use too much water. Since the pain may make it difficult for the patient to open his eyes, the EMT may have to force the lids open so that the eyes may be washed. A clean dressing should then be applied and the patient taken promptly to the hospital for further care. If eye irrigation can be carried out satisfactorily in the ambulance, it should be done enroute.

Thermal burns. When a person suffers burns of the face from a fire, the eyes usually close rapidly because of the heat; this reaction is a natural reflex to protect the eyeballs. However, the eyelids remain exposed and are frequently burned. The treatment of burned lids requires specialized care. It is best to transport the patient with burned eyelids without further examination of

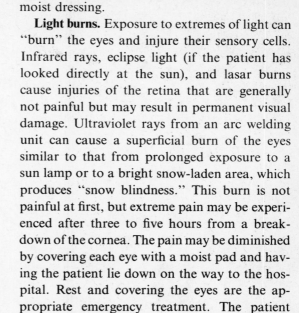

the eye. The eyes may be covered with a sterile, moist dressing.

Light burns. Exposure to extremes of light can "burn" the eyes and injure their sensory cells. Infrared rays, eclipse light (if the patient has looked directly at the sun), and lasar burns cause injuries of the retina that are generally not painful but may result in permanent visual damage. Ultraviolet rays from an arc welding unit can cause a superficial burn of the eyes similar to that from prolonged exposure to a sun lamp or to a bright snow-laden area, which produces "snow blindness." This burn is not painful at first, but extreme pain may be experienced after three to five hours from a breakdown of the cornea. The pain may be diminished by covering each eye with a moist pad and having the patient lie down on the way to the hospital. Rest and covering the eyes are the appropriate emergency treatment. The patient should be seen by a physician as soon as possible.

Lacerations and Contusions

Soft-tissue injuries of the eye may be quite severe. Lacerations of the eyelid may appear to be very serious, but as long as the eyeball itself is not involved, vision will not be impaired. On the other hand, lacerations of the eyeball, either the cornea or sclera, frequently can cause loss of sight.

Lacerated eyelids usually bleed profusely because of their rich blood supply. Direct hand pressure or a pressure dressing will control the bleeding.

The one time that pressure should not be applied to the eye is when there is a laceration of the eyeball itself. The eyeball contains fluid, and if pressure is applied over the eye, the fluid will be forced out. Irreparable damage may be done to the eyeball. A protective dressing should be applied without pressure.

Torn eyelids should be handled very carefully to prevent further injury. Cover them with a loose dressing. Any detached fragment of eyelid skin should be wrapped separately in a moist bandage and taken directly to the hospital, where the surgeon may want to use it to repair the lid.

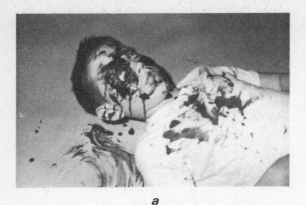

a

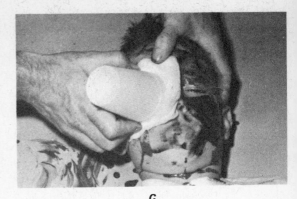

c

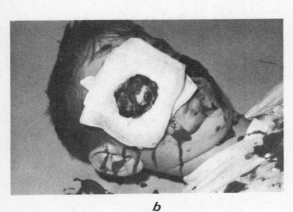

b

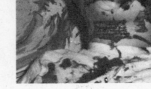

d

Figure 24.3 *a–d*

a, An extruded eye sometimes occurs in an accident. *b*, Pressure should never be applied on the eye. *c*, It may be covered with a paper cup or cone to protect it while the patient is being transported. *d*, Both eyes should be bandaged to help the injured eye remain still. A protective cone should be used when a foreign object is imbedded in the eye.

The care of eyeball lacerations involves three important principles.

1. Cover both eyes with a loose dressing and transport the patient to the hospital quietly on his back.
2. Never exert pressure on a lacerated eyeball.
3. Do not remove a protuding foreign body from the eye. Cover it with a cup or cone, cover the other eye, and carefully and quietly transport the patient on his back to the Emergency Department (Figs. 24.3 & 24.4).

Extruded eyeball. Sometimes one may see an extruded eyeball after a severe injury; it should **not** be pushed back into the socket. The eyes should be gently covered with a moist dressing and a protective cone and the patient trans-ported carefully on his back to the Emergency Department (Fig. 24.3). Detachment of the retina may result from such an injury when the patient is not kept quiet and on his back.

Blunt trauma. Blunt injuries of the eye can cause a hemorrhage within the eye and blood may be seen overlying the iris or the pupil (Fig. 24.4). It is important that the patient be kept still and that the eye be covered with a protective dressing. This patient similarly should be trans-ported immediately to the Emergency Depart-ment.

Head Injuries

Examination of the eyes may lead the EMT to suspect a head injury. Findings such as the fol-

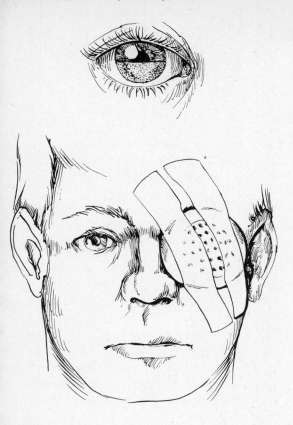

A patient may have an artificial eye. The EMT should inquire about this possibility when it is suspected. An artificial eye will not respond to light and may appear somewhat different but be difficult to tell from a normal eye. No harm is done if it is given the same care.

Many people wear contact lenses. They can be the small hard plastic lenses that are usually tinted, or the large clear soft lenses that are very difficult to see on the eye. Unconscious patients wearing hard lenses should have them removed, for prolonged wearing with the eyes closed can damage the cornea. A suction cup with the end moistened with saline can be used to remove the lenses (Fig. 24.5). Removal should not be attemped if there is a question of an injury of the eye since manipulation can aggravate the condition. The presence of contact lenses should be recorded, to warn hospital personnel.

201

All spectacle lenses made since 1971 are either heat-treated safety glass or plastic. With severe injuries the lenses can break, forcing glass fragments around and into the eye. Large pieces can be removed from outside and inside the eyelids; but any fragments that have penetrated the eye should be left alone since their removal could further damage the eye or cause a loss of some of the vitreous humor. Place a protective shield or cone over the eye and tape to the face.

Figure 24.4

A hemorrhage in the eye has caused blood to overlie the iris and pupil. Proper treatment is to place a protective metal shield over the eye and tape it securely to prevent further injury while the patient is being taken to a hospital.

lowing should alert one to the possibility of a head injury:

1. One pupil is larger than the other.
2. The eyes turn in different directions.
3. One eye does not move.
4. The white of the eye is bright red from hemorrhage.
5. One eye protudes.

These findings must be recorded along with the time of the observation, for they may change later.

One should remember to keep the eyes of an unconscious patient closed, as drying of the tissues can cause permanent injury and blindness. The lids can be covered with a moist bandage or taped closed with clear tape; normal tears will then keep the tissues moist.

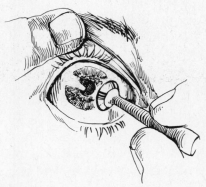

Figure 24.5

Contact lenses may be removed from the eyes of unconscious patients with a small suction cup fashioned for that purpose. The cup should first be moistened with a saline solution.

The Face and Throat

Accident victims often sustain soft-tissue injuries of the scalp, face, and neck as well as fractures of the bones of the face and the jawbone. These injuries may vary greatly in severity; some may be potentially life threatening. When taking care of a person with a head injury, remember that he may also have a neck injury.

Breathing problems and hemorrhage are common in injuries of the head and face. There are many possible causes for these problems.

1. The upper airway may be obstructed by blood clots or loose teeth in the throat.
2. The upper airway may be obstructed because of injuries of the mouth and nose and fractures of the lower jaw.
3. The upper airway may be obstructed because of swelling resulting from soft-tissue injury.
4. The position of the patient's head may cause the airway to be obstructed. When the neck is flexed (the head bent forward), the jaw and tongue drop backward, blocking the airway.
5. The larynx or trachea may be injured directly.
6. Severe brain damage may interfere with the breathing mechanism.

The Face

Soft-tissue wounds. Soft-tissue injuries of the face and scalp are common. Abrasions of the skin cause no serious problems. Contusions usually cause swelling; a contusion of the scalp looks and feels like a lump.

Laceration and avulsion injuries are similarly common. Avulsions are particularly frequent at the scalp, where any sharp blow may separate the scalp from the skull beneath it. The face and scalp are richly supplied with arteries and veins; wounds of these areas usually bleed heavily.

Emergency care of soft-tissue injuries of the face and scalp is identical to the treatment of soft-tissue injuries elsewhere.

1. Control bleeding by local pressure. Be careful not to apply too much pressure on the scalp if bone damage is suspected.
2. Apply a dressing that will help control bleeding. A compression bandage placed around the head above the eyes is useful in helping control bleeding from forehead and scalp.
3. When nerves, tendons, or blood vessels are exposed, cover them with a sterile bandage and keep it moist so they will not dry and sustain severe damage.
4. The local application of ice may aid in controlling swelling of soft tissues and bleeding.

Bleeding can usually be controlled by direct pressure applied over a sterile dressing placed on a wound. The dressing can be held by a bandage or by an assistant. When a laceration extends through the cheek directly into the mouth, it may be necessary to hold a gauze padding against both the inside and the outside of the cheek. Objects penetrating the cheek may have to be removed before it is possible to control the bleeding.

Check for bleeding inside the mouth. Broken teeth and lacerations of the tongue may bleed heavily into the throat. This hemorrhage may not be apparent outside the mouth. It should be specifically sought.

Blood draining into the throat may produce vomiting and airway difficulties. The airway should be maintained by tilting the head and lifting the chin. An artificial airway may be inserted if the patient is unconscious; suction and artificial ventilation are used as necessary (Fig. 24.6).

It may be necessary to turn the patient on his side so that blood or vomitus can drain out rather than obstruct the airway. When there is a possibility of a fracture of the cervical spine, the head must be immobilized before the patient is turned and must be maintained in a stable position while he is on his side. When positioning the patient, take into consideration these factors:

1. If there is a severe skull or brain injury, the patient is best positioned with his head slightly elevated. His feet may also be ele-

202

vated if necessary to treat shock.

2. If a cervical spine fracture is suspected, immobilize the head and neck to prevent bending of the neck.

Check to see if tissue has been lost. Missing pieces of an ear or nose should be sought and taken to the Emergency Department with the patient. Often they can be restored.

When there is a flap (avulsion) of skin, particularly in the scalp, wash as much foreign matter as possible from the wound and replace the flap in its normal position. This frequently will control much of the bleeding caused by the injury. A simple circular bandage will work very well and serve to hold the flap in place (Fig. 22.2).

Injuries of the nose. Injuries of the nose generally produce bleeding. An ice pack applied over the nose, pinching the nostrils together, when it can be tolerated, or packing the nostril with strips of gauze may control bleeding. A roll of gauze packed between the upper teeth and lip will sometimes help exert pressure and control a nosebleed. Objects inhaled in the nose may cause severe pain but should be removed only by a physician.

Facial fractures. Fractures of facial bones commonly result from impact injuries—for example, collision of the patient with a steering wheel or windshield. The fracture may be of the nose, of the circle of bone around the eye, of the checkbone, or of the lower jaw.

Fractures of facial bones are dangerous because bone fragments may cause airway obstruction. Blood clots from a fracture of the cheekbones or the jawbone may block the airway. Fractures and lacerations around the mouth and nose may result in a serious deformity. It is not uncommon to see someone whose entire face is battered. This type of injury almost always results in total airway obstruction caused by a block at the mouth and nose.

Emergency care of facial fractures consists of keeping the patient breathing and stopping the bleeding. The rules for the management of soft-tissue injuries of the face apply also to facial fractures.

Many times fractures of the facial bones are

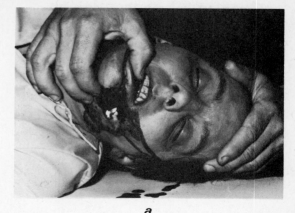

a

203

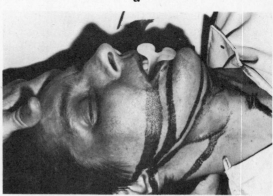

b

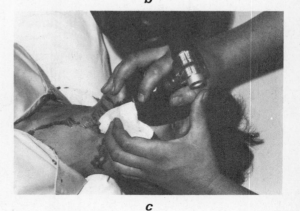

c

Figure 24.6 *a–c*

The initial management of a patient with a severe facial wound is shown. *a*, Secure an open airway. *b*, Use an oropharyngeal or nasopharyngeal artificial airway when needed for an unconscious patient. *c*, Supplemental oxygen or assisted respiration may be required.

not evident on first examination but are found later by the surgeon. Such fractures obviously are of little consequence in initial emergency care. In fractures of the lower jaw, there may be an irregularity of the teeth or loss of teeth, inability to swallow or talk, increased salivation, and bleeding in the mouth.

In all such injuries, extreme caution must be taken that injured soft tissue or the tongue does not drop back into the throat or airway to cause obstruction. One of the most important phases of initial emergency care is to clear the upper respiratory passage of any obstructing material.

The Throat

204

Soft-tissue wounds of the throat may produce severe bleeding. Lacerations may result in arterial bleeding, which may require manual pressure for control. If a large vein is lacerated, pressure should be applied both above and below the point of bleeding to prevent air from entering the circulatory system. Air embolism is not common but may be fatal. The entry of air into the circulatory system is more liable to occur if the patient is sitting up and the injury is higher than the heart.

Deep wounds may penetrate into the pharynx or larynx. An airway must be maintained by preventing blood from blocking the air passage. Suction may be required together with artificial ventilation. Oxygen inhalation may be of value. If there is an impaled object, cut it off if possible, six to eight inches from the skin surface and immobilize it; then transport the patient as rapidly as possible to the hospital. If a neck fracture is suspected, treat this injury initially before doing any of the preceding steps except to control bleeding.

Laryngeal and tracheal injury. The voice box and windpipe may be fractured by any crushing injury. Impact upon a steering wheel, attempted suicide by hanging, a clothesline injury sustained perhaps while riding a bicycle are all means of fracturing the trachea. When this injury occurs, loss of voice, severe and sometimes fatal airway obstruction, and air leakage into the soft tissue of the neck result. The presence of air in soft tissue gives a very characteristic crackling sensation called subcutaneous emphysema. Fracture of the cervical spine (neck) often co-exists.

Emergency care consists of recognition of the injury, administration of supplemental oxygen by face mask, and as little manipulation of the patient as possible. Keeping the patient calm and breathing slowly may be lifesaving. Rapid breathing usually makes the situation worse. Oxygen inhalation should be used wherever this injury is suspected. Positive-pressure ventilation is avoided.

When the patient's airway is totally obstructed, the EMT may be required to perform a cricothyroidotomy with a large-bore, hollow needle. If, however, the patient is able to breathe to a limited degree, avoid all manipulation of the airway and give oxygen.

VI

The Abdomen and Genitourinary System

CHAPTER 25

The Abdomen and Digestive System

GOAL I. Know the structures of the abdominal cavity.

OBJECTIVES

A. Define the boundaries of the abdominal cavity.
B. List the contents of the abdominal and pelvic cavities.
C. List the components of the gastrointestinal tract and digestive system.
D. List the solid organs of the abdomen.
E. List the hollow organs of the abdomen.

Abdominal Cavity

The two major body cavities are the thorax and the abdomen. The abdomen is inferior to (lies lower in the body than) the thorax.

The superior boundary of the abdomen is the diaphragm. The inferior boundary is at the level of an imaginary plane between the pubis and the sacrum (Fig. 25.1). Immediately beneath this plane lies the pelvic cavity, which can be regarded as the lowermost part of the abdomen.

The abdominal cavity contains the liver, gallbladder and bile ducts, spleen, stomach, and intestines. Immediately behind the lining membrane, between it and the major back muscles and spine, lie the kidneys with their drainage tubes (the ureters), the adrenal glands, and the pancreas (Fig. 25.2). In this same plane, between the peritoneum (the cavity lining) and the spine, lie two major blood vessels, the aorta and the inferior vena cava, supplying the whole lower half of the body with blood. Many nerves and lymph glands accompany these large vessels. The organs and vessels are supported against the body wall by the peritoneum.

The lowermost portion of the abdominal cavity is called the pelvic cavity. In it lie the rectum, the urinary bladder, and, in the female, the internal reproductive organs. Strictly speaking, the urinary bladder is outside the cavity, as it lies between the pubic bone in front and the pelvic peritoneum behind. It is however a pelvic organ and is frequently injured when the pelvis is fractured.

The entire cavity is lined by a smooth, glistening, thin, transparent layer of tissue called the peritoneum. Except where organs lie immediately underneath it, the peritoneum lies directly over the muscles of the body wall which serve to protect the organs within. Peritoneum is reflected from the body wall to cover the organs within the abdomen, so that everywhere when two surfaces are in contact, the surfaces are peri-

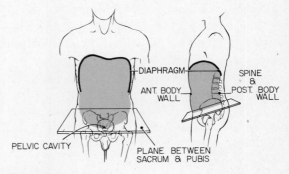

DIAPHRAGM

SPINE & POST. BODY WALL

ANT. BODY WALL

PELVIC CAVITY

PLANE BETWEEN SACRUM & PUBIS

Figure 25.1

The boundaries of the abdominal cavity are shown.

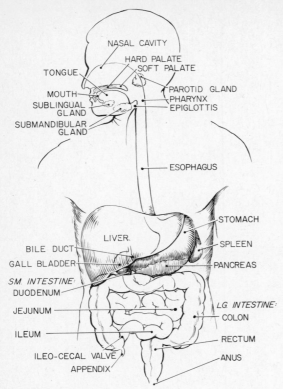

Figure 25.2

The digestive system is composed of several organs and extends through many divisions of the body, although it lies principally within the abdomen.

208

toneal. When peritoneum covers organs, it is called serosa.

Nearly all the organs within the abdomen are suspended there from the body walls by sheets of tissue called mesenteries. Mesentery is very delicate tissue formed by peritoneum. As peritoneum which lines the body cavity is reflected to cover the organs, it forms the mesentery. Mesentery carries blood vessels and nerves to all the organs. Mesenteric attachments allow some shifting in the positions of organs with regard to one another because they hang fairly freely. The continuous muscular activity of the bowel requires an easily movable organ, which is provided by a mesenteric attachment.

In the upper abdomen, the liver, spleen, and stomach are well protected by the ribs. In the lower abdomen, the pelvis gives much protection to organs.

In general, we can regard these organs, abdominal, retroperitoneal, and pelvic, as being

hollow or solid. Hollow organs are tubes through which materials pass. For example, the stomach and intestines conduct food through the body; the ureters and bladder conduct and store urine until it is expelled. Solid organs are solid masses of tissue where much of the chemical work of the body takes place. The liver, spleen, pancreas, kidneys, and adrenal glands are the solid organs of the abdomen. The stomach, duodenum, small intestine (jejunum and ileum), large intestine (colon), rectum, appendix, gallbladder, bile ducts, urinary bladder, and ureters are the hollow organs of the abdomen.

Injuries within the abdomen can involve either hollow or solid organs. In general, solid organs tend to bleed copiously when torn or injured. Hollow organs discharge their contents into the abdominal cavity when they are lacerated. These contents usually set up an intense inflammatory reaction, peritonitis, which is very painful. Bleeding from solid organs may be rapidly fatal and frequently causes shock.

Mesentery supporting hollow organs can be lacerated. In such instances, bleeding from the torn mesentery can be severe, and the organ torn away loses its blood supply. All such injuries require prompt care and usually operative treatment.

Digestive System

The digestive system is composed of the gastrointestinal tract (stomach and intestines), mouth, salivary glands, pharynx, esophagus, liver, gallbladder, pancreas, rectum, and anus. It transcends the boundaries of the abdomen and the thorax (Fig. 25.2). The function of this system is to prepare food which is eaten so that the individual cells of the body can be nourished. The process of digestion begins in the mouth.

Digestion of liquid and solid food, from the time it is taken into the mouth until essential compounds are extracted and delivered by the circulatory system to nourish all the cells of the body, is a complicated chemical process. In succession, different secretions are added by the salivary glands, the stomach, the liver, the pancreas, and the small intestine to convert food into basic sugars, fatty acids, and amino acids.

These products are then transferred to the liver in the blood from the intestine. In the liver these basic products of digestion are changed to materials that can nourish individual tissues and cells. The products are then pumped in the blood through the heart and arteries to the capillaries, where they pass through the capillary walls and the cell walls to feed all the cells of the body. Digestion within the small bowel produces many chemical compounds which are poisonous to the body. They cannot be passed safely into the general circulation until the liver has transformed them. The fact that all the blood leaving the intestine must pass first through the liver insures protection for the body as a whole.

Mouth. The mouth consists of the lips, cheeks, gums, teeth, and tongue. A mucous membrane lines the mouth. The roof of the mouth is formed by hard and soft palates (Fig. 25.2). The hard palate is a bony plate lying anterior, while the soft palate is a fold of mucous membrane and muscle that extends posteriorly into the throat. It is adapted to hold food that is being chewed and to initiate swallowing. Three pairs of glands discharge a constant flow of saliva into the mouth, which must normally be kept moist.

Salivary glands. The three paired salivary glands, located on each side of the lower jaw just under the tongue, on each side of the lower jaw just below the angle of the mandible, and on each cheek in the tissue just in front of the ears, produce nearly one and one half liters of saliva daily. Saliva is poured into the mouth through salivary ducts, and is approximately 98 percent water; the remaining 2 percent is mucus, salts, and organic compounds. Mucus serves as a binder for the chewed food being swallowed and as a lubricant within the mouth.

Digestive enzymes actually accomplish the chemical conversion of food within the gastrointestinal tract, breaking it down from starch, fat, and protein to simple sugars, fatty acids, and amino acids. There is only one digestive enzyme in saliva, ptyalin, which initiates the digestion of starches, converting them to simple sugars. Other enzymes exist in the secretions from the stomach, pancreas, and small bowel.

Pharynx. The pharynx, or throat, is a tubular structure, about five inches long, extending vertically from the back of the mouth to the esophagus and trachea. The trachea or windpipe through which we breathe lies just in front of the esophagus. It is connected with the pharynx by the larynx, or voice box. The larynx is covered by a leaf-shaped valve called the epiglottis. An automatic movement of the pharynx permits the epiglottis to close over the trachea when swallowing is initiated so that liquids and solids are moved into the esophagus and away from the windpipe.

Esophagus. The esophagus is a collapsible tube about ten inches long. It extends from the end of the pharynx to the stomach and lies just anterior to the spinal column in the chest. Contractions of the muscle in the esophagus propel food through it toward the stomach. Liquids pass with very little assistance. Semisolid foods seldom take more than ten seconds to pass through the esophagus to the stomach.

Stomach. The stomach, an abdominal hollow organ, is located in the upper left portion of the abdominal cavity; it has a J shape. Muscular movements and gastric juice which contains much mucus convert ingested food to a semisolid mass. Approximately one and one-half liters of gastric juice are produced each day and pass into the small intestine.

In one to three hours, the semisolid food mass is propelled by muscular contractions entirely into the small intestine. Poisoning or any reaction to trauma may paralyze muscular action and cause the retention of food in the stomach. In these instances, only vomiting or a stomach pump can empty this organ.

Only one digestive enzyme is produced in the stomach, pepsin. This agent initiates the digestion of proteins.

Pancreas. The pancreas, a flat, solid organ, lies below and behind the liver and stomach and behind the peritoneum on the spine and muscles of the back. It is oriented transversely in the upper abdomen. It contains two kinds of glands.

One kind secretes nearly two liters of pancreatic juice daily. This juice contains many enzymes acting in the digestion of fat, starch, and protein and it flows directly into the duodenum through the pancreatic ducts. This secretion is most important in the digestion of food.

The other kind of gland, called the "islets of Langerhans," does not connect to any duct but secretes its products into the bloodstream across the capillaries. These islets produce a hormone, insulin, which regulates the amount of sugar in blood. Several other hormones also are secreted in the islets of Langerhans. These hormones affect many other digestive processes.

The pancreas is firmly fixed in position and is not easily damaged. If it is injured, the loss of enzymes from a torn pancreatic duct into the abdominal cavity can cause a particularly severe peritonitis and hemorrhage.

Liver. The liver is a large solid organ which takes up most of the area immediately beneath the diaphragm, particularly on the right side. It is the largest solid organ in the abdomen and consequently the one most often injured. It is a vital organ with several functions. Poisonous substances produced by digestion are brought to it by the blood and rendered harmless. Factors necessary for blood clotting and for the production of normal plasma are formed here. Between one-half and one liter of bile is made by the liver daily to function in the normal digestion of fat. The liver is the principal organ for the storage of sugar for immediate use by the body. It also produces many of the factors which aid in the proper regulation of immune responses.

Essentially, it is a large mass of blood vessels and cells packed tightly together. For this reason the liver is very fragile and relatively easily injured. Blood flow in the liver is very high since all the blood that is pumped to the gastrointestinal tract passes through the liver before it returns to the heart. In addition, the liver receives a generous arterial blood supply of its own. Hemorrhage from a severe liver injury may be quickly fatal.

Biliary system. The liver is connected to the intestine by a ductal system consisting of the gallbladder and the bile ducts. These are properly considered hollow organs. The gallbladder is a reservoir for bile received from the liver, which it discharges into the duodenum through the common bile duct. The presence of fat in the duodenum triggers a contraction of the gallbladder so that it can empty. It usually contains two to three ounces of bile. The liver is connected directly to the duodenum by the bile ducts while the gallbladder is a pouch connected to the common bile duct. Stones can form in the gallbladder and can pass into the common bile duct to obstruct it. Obstruction of the duct so that bile does not pass into the duodenum rapidly produces jaundice (yellowing of eyes and skin) and must be corrected promptly by an operation. Injuries of these organs, gallbladder and bile ducts, are not common.

Small intestine. The small intestine, the major abdominal hollow organ, is so named because of its diameter in comparison with the large intestine and stomach. It includes the duodenum, jejunum, and ileum.

The duodenum, about twelve inches long, passes from the stomach to the jejunum. Most "stomach ulcers" are really ulcers of the duodenum. A part of this organ lies behind the peritoneum and closely curls around the head of the pancreas. The duodenum is thus well protected and injuries of it are rare, but they do occur, particularly from steering wheel impacts against the abdomen. Such injuries are very serious because they are difficult to treat and are usually associated with an injury of the pancreas. The duodenum is the part of the bowel into which secretions from the pancreas and liver empty to take part in digestion.

The jejunum and ileum together measure more than twenty feet on the average and, with the duodenum, make up the small bowel. The jejunum is the first half and the ileum the second half. The small intestine empties into the large intestine through the ileocecal valve between the ileum and cecum, the first part of the large bowel. This valve should allow passage of bowel content in only one direction, that is, into the colon. The junction of small and large bowel is normally in the lower right side of the abdominal cavity.

The small intestine lies entirely free within the abdomen, supported by its mesentery, which is attached to the back wall of the body. Arteries from the aorta to the intestine and veins carrying blood to the liver lie in this supporting tissue. These vessels may be damaged in instances of abdominal injury. Within the small intestine are the bile, pancreatic juice, and small bowel secretions. Some three liters of small bowel juice containing mucus and potent enzymes are secreted daily.

Bile, produced by the liver and stored in the gallbladder, is emptied as needed into the duodenum. It is greenish-black in color but, through changes during digestion, it gives feces a typical brown color. It is very important in the emulsifying and digesting of fatty food. Cholesterol is also secreted in the bile. Pancreatic and small bowel juices contain the powerful chemical enzymes which carry out the final processes of digestion of proteins, fats, and carbohydrates. Within the small bowel, food is digested (broken down to its basic chemical constituents). The products of digestion, water, and ingested vitamins and minerals are then absorbed for transportation to the liver.

Large intestine. The large intestine (the colon), another major hollow organ, is about five feet long. It encircles the outer border of the abdomen around the small bowel. It lies partly behind the peritoneum (both ascending and descending portions) and partly on a mesentery, hanging free like the small bowel. It is most susceptible to injury at those areas where it changes from a fairly fixed to a freely movable organ. The major function of the colon, which it shares with the very end of the small bowel, is absorption of water. Primarily, however, water absorption takes place in the terminal ileum. Stool is formed in the colon and passed out of the body through the rectum and anus.

Appendix. The appendix is a small tube closed at one end, three or four inches long, which opens into the cecum in the lower right side of the abdomen. It may easily become obstructed and as a result, inflamed. Appendicitis, which is the term for this inflammation, is one of the major causes of severe abdominal distress.

The appendix is a vestigial organ and has no major function in the human being. In early life, it may play a role in the development of the normal immune response. In later life it is simply present. It does not have any role in the usual processes of digestion.

Appendicitis is a severe and relatively common disease. It produces abdominal pain and tenderness in the right lower abdominal quadrant. Generally, when treated promptly it is a relatively innocuous problem. If, however, appendicitis is neglected so that the appendix ruptures, a much more serious situation exists. Whenever appendicitis is suspected, the best course is prompt transfer of the patient to the Emergency Department.

Rectum and anus. The lowermost end of the colon is the rectum. It is a large hollow organ adapted to store quantities of feces until they are expelled. It lies in the hollow of the sacrum within the pelvic cavity. At its terminal end is the anal canal, lined by normal skin and approximately two inches long. The rectum and anus are supplied with a complex series of circular muscles, called sphincter muscles, which can control the escape of liquids, gases, and solids from the digestive tract. In general, the most distal anal sphincter, voluntarily controlled, can prevent or permit the escape of gas and some liquid. True rectal control is given by a broad shelf of muscle called the levator ani, which forms the entire pelvic floor.

Sensation within the rectum and anus is very specialized. The rectum is adapted to expand and at a critical point to dispel its contents. Some rectal tumors fill up the organ and trigger this expelling reflex but cannot in turn be expelled. The resulting urge to defecate which cannot be satisfied is called tenesmus. Within the short terminal anal canal, sensation is that of the skin. Excoriations, irritations, and lacerations are every bit as painful as if they were on a finger or toe. In addition the anus is richly supplied with nerves. An irritation here may result in profound reflex changes.

Peristalsis. There are two layers of involuntary muscle throughout the wall of the entire intestinal tract from esophagus to rectum. Wavelike contractions, called peristalsis, of these muscle layers propel food and products of digestion through the tract. When peristaltic waves are especially strong or when they are interrupted by an obstruction so that the content cannot be propelled along, the contraction causes a painful cramp which is called colic. Colic has a very characteristic pattern. A cramp occurs and pain rapidly rises to a very severe level; it abruptly decreases and disappears as the bowel

211

relaxes. In the initial stages such cramps may occur every two to three minutes. As obstruction persists and the bowel proximal to the obstruction dilates, the waves of contraction diminish in number and strength.

Normal peristalsis is responsible for the bowel sounds which can be heard if one listens to the abdomen with a stethoscope. These represent the passage of gas and fluid through a narrow hollow organ.

Spleen. The spleen, a major solid organ, is smaller than the liver. It too is filled with large blood vessels and is even more fragile. The spleen is found in the upper left side of the abdomen just beneath the diaphragm. It is fixed in position by three major ligaments (bands of tissue).

These can easily tear out of the spleen in a severe accident. Bleeding from a ruptured spleen may be very severe and controllable only by removal of the organ. Injuries that produce fractures of the lower three or four ribs on the left side are likely to cause injury of the spleen also. The spleen is not required for life nor is it associated with the digestive tract. The major function of this organ is in the normal production and destruction of blood cells. Its function, if it is injured, can be assumed by the liver and bone marrow.

Genitourinary organs. The solid and hollow organs comprising this dual-purpose system in the abdomen are considered in Chapter 28, The Genitourinary System.

CHAPTER 26

Injuries of the Abdomen

GOAL I. Know the characteristics of severe abdominal injuries.

OBJECTIVES

A. Name the injuries that can be caused by improperly adjusted seat belts.
B. List the characteristics of severe abdominal injuries.
C. List the characteristics of hollow organ injuries.
D. List the characteristics of solid organ injuries.
E. List the characteristics of injury of the abdominal blood vessels.
F. Describe the difference between open and closed abdominal injuries.

GOAL II. Understand the procedures for treating severe abdominal injuries.

OBJECTIVES

A. Describe the methods used for evaluating a patient with an abdominal injury.
B. List the vital signs which should be recorded for a patient who has an abdominal injury.
C. Describe the procedures used in the treatment of a patient with a severe abdominal injury.
D. List the steps in the treatment of a patient who has sustained a severe abdominal injury and is vomiting.
E. List the steps in the treatment of a patient with an abdominal evisceration.
F. List the steps in the treatment of a patient with a foreign object protruding from the abdomen.

Abdominal injuries may be closed or open, and they may involve hollow or solid organs.

Closed injuries are those in which the abdomen is damaged by a severe blow, such as hitting a steering wheel or the dashboard of a car or being tackled in football, but in which the skin remains intact. Open injuries are those in which a foreign body has entered the abdomen, opening the peritoneum-lined cavity to the outside. Stab or gunshot wounds are open injuries.

Some penetrating injuries may be only a laceration of the abdominal wall itself; one may not be able to tell whether the penetration extends all the way into the abdominal cavity. In the case of a gunshot wound or a stab, the EMT must always assume that the bullet or knife has entered the abdominal cavity and should give emergency care as if that were the case. In treating penetrating abdominal wounds, the only certain way to determine if organs have been injured is to explore the abdomen at an operation and look at each organ. Often, the only way to be certain if penetration has occurred at all is to explore the abdomen. Thus, each penetrating wound must be treated as if it had entered the abdomen and injured one or several organs.

The abdomen contains both hollow and solid organs, any of which may be injured. The hollow organs usually contain a digesting stream of food. Rupture or laceration of these organs will allow their contents to spill into the peritoneal cavity where an intense inflammatory reaction will be caused by the food (digested or undigested) and the bowel contents, gastric fluid, and other digestive enzymes. This reaction produces a prompt and severe abdominal tenderness, muscular rigidity, and intense pain.

The solid organs have a rich blood supply; injuries of these organs usually cause severe hemorrhage. Blood within the peritoneal cavity is not very irritating; signs of these injuries may first be seen as changes in pulse and blood pressure.

Either closed or open abdominal injuries may involve the aorta, the inferior vena cava, or any of the other large blood vessels. In such instances hemorrhage is severe and may rapidly be fatal.

Signs of Abdominal Injury

The method of evaluating an abdominal injury is the same for blunt and penetrating injuries. The patient is permitted to lie supine as comfortably as possible, with knees slightly flexed, supported by pillows or splints when needed. Clothes should be removed or loosened. A rapid assessment of his condition can be made by simple inspection. Vital signs are recorded as an initial step.

At the first inspection, note how the patient is lying. A patient with severe abdominal disease or injury prefers to lie still without much movement, usually with the legs drawn up. Rather rapid, shallow breaths prevent much movement of the abdominal contents. A patient with acute pancreatitis or a ruptured appendix may lie on the right side with legs drawn up. Motion of the body or the abdominal organs irritates the inflamed peritoneum and causes much pain, which the patient instinctively tries to avoid.

Look for skin wounds through which bullets, knives, or missiles may have entered. Always check for corresponding exit holes in the patient's back or sides. Penetrating objects such as knives should be noted, stabilized, and left alone after supportive bandaging. Bruises or tire marks are important clues to the cause and severity of any blunt injury. Steering wheels, seat belts, and arm rests can cause such bruises and frequently leave marks in the pattern of the wheel, belt, or rest. The location of bruises or wounds is a clue to the organs that may be injured underneath. With severe lacerations of the abdominal wall, bowels may be protruding through the wound (evisceration).

The initial evaluation must include recording vital signs, especially the patient's pulse, blood pressure, and rate of respiration. Many abdominal emergencies, aside from those which cause severe bleeding, can cause a rapid pulse and low blood pressure. It is imperative that a record of these findings be made as early as possible and periodically thereafter to help the physician evaluate the progress and severity of the disease when he first sees the patient at the Emergency Department.

The patient may tell the EMT how and where the abdomen hurts. He may feel nauseated or may vomit. A patient who sustains abdominal injuries may have a stomach full of food or drink. If vomiting occurs, especially in a patient who is comatose or nearly so, it is imperative that the EMT keep the throat clear of vomitus so that it is not aspirated into the lungs. Turn the patient's head to one side and try to keep it lower than the chest. It is important to note what has been vomited: undigested food, blood, mucus, or bile.

The initial evaluation should allow one to determine the type of injury, its possible extent, and the presence of shock. Other measures can then be undertaken as outlined below. The patient should be transported to the hospital as rapidly as possible.

Blunt Abdominal Wounds

Blunt abdominal wounds may cause severe bruises of the abdominal wall. Within the abdomen, the liver and spleen may be lacerated. The intestine may be ruptured. Supporting

214

mesenteries may be torn, with injury of the vessels in their tissues. The kidneys may be ruptured or torn from their arteries and veins. The bladder may be ruptured, especially in a patient who has been drinking heavily and whose bladder may be full and distended. These patients may have severe intra-abdominal hemorrhage as well as peritoneal irritation and inflammation from the ruptured hollow organs.

Place the patient supine in a comfortable position with head turned to one side. Clear the mouth and throat of vomitus. Note signs of shock: pallor, cold sweat, a rapid, thready pulse, or low blood pressure. Control external bleeding by local pressure. Assist respiration by clearing the airway and using oxygen when needed. Rapid and gentle transportation to the Emergency Department must be provided as soon as possible.

Injuries from seat belts and shoulder belts. Some special considerations in diagnosis apply to injuries caused by the use of seat belts. Many thousands of injuries have been prevented and many lives have been saved by the use of seat belts. Patients who would have been thrown out of smashed cars literally owe their survival to seat belts that have immobilized them. However, the improper application of a belt occasionally causes a blunt injury of the abdominal organs.

Lap seat belts should be worn so that they are below the iliac crests of the pelvis (Fig. 26.1). They should restrain the bony pelvis at the hip joint. If the seat belt is too high and is fastened above the iliac crest, a sudden deceleration or an abrupt stop of the vehicle may cause an injury of the abdominal contents (hollow and solid organs and the great blood vessels) as the belt squeezes them against the spine. Injuries of the pelvis and lumbar spine can also occur as a result of the improper use of seat belts. These injuries include fractures of the pelvis, separation of the pubic symphysis, and compression fractures of the lumbar spine. The use of the belt in these cases has often converted what could have been a fatal injury to a manageable fracture.

Diagonal safety belts that run over the shoulder can cause injuries of the upper part of the trunk, such as a bruised chest, fractured ribs

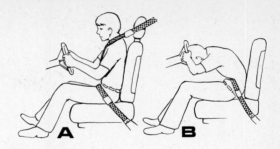

Figure 26.1 a–b

a, A seat belt and shoulder belt properly worn are shown. *b,* If the seat (lap) belt is worn too high, the belt itself may injure an abdominal organ. If no shoulder belt is worn, the upper part of the body can be thrown forward, often causing the head to strike against the steering wheel.

215

or sternum, or a lacerated liver. There are, however, far fewer head and neck injuries when this type of belt is used in conjunction with a lap seat belt and a head rest. Diagonal or shoulder belts have also helped much in reducing the number of abdominal injuries. The diagonal belt (shoulder belt) should never be used alone, as it has caused decapitations when the rest of the body was not restrained. Safety belts have saved many more people than they have injured; but their use must be governed by a proper understanding of what they can and cannot do.

Suspect a safety belt injury in all patients from automobile accidents. If there is any sign of an abdominal injury, handle the patient as described earlier in this chapter. When examining the abdomen, look for any contusions or belt marks which may be a clue to possible internal injuries.

Penetrating Abdominal Injuries

The penetrating abdominal wound presents a very special problem. One may have considerable difficulty in determining for certain without an operation if an instrument or missile has penetrated the abdomen, and if it has, what organs it injured. It is proper to assume that major damage has occurred even if no obvious signs are present immediately, since such signs often develop slowly. In these injuries, hollow organs are usually lacerated. The major result is the discharge of their contents into the abdomi-

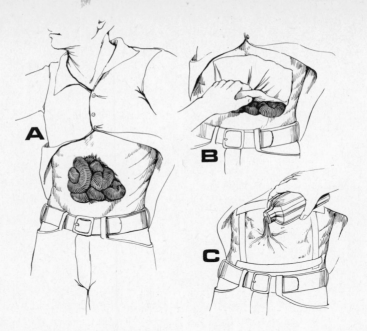

216

Figure 26.2 *a–c*

a, An Abdominal evisceration is a wound allowing the contents of the cavity to lie outside the peritoneum. *b,* Do not attempt to replace the eviscerated organs. Cover them with a clean, preferably sterile, dressing. *c,* Moisten the dressing with sterile solution.

nal cavity, with resulting inflammation. If major blood vessels are cut or if major solid organs are lacerated, hemorrhage may be rapid and severe.

Initial steps in the care of these patients are those already outlined. Note the areas of the abdomen where penetration has occurred. Note exit wounds. If a penetrating instrument is still in place, leave it. If it is impossible to transport the patient without removing it, cut it off carefully a few inches from the abdominal wall. If it is difficult to cut off, bandage it so that external bleeding is controlled and the penetrating instrument is stable. Do not withdraw it. Control obvious external bleeding with pressure. If the patient vomits, protect him from aspirating the vomitus. Finally, make him as comfortable as possible and transport rapidly and gently to the Emergency Department.

Eviscerations. When a severe abdominal lacerating wound has resulted in an evisceration, the abdominal organs lie outside the abdominal

cavity. Do not try to replace the organs within the abdomen. Cover them with a moist, clean, preferably sterile dressing. If sterile gauze compresses are available, they should be moistened with fluid from an IV bottle and used. Clean sheets or towels may be used. It is of utmost importance that one cover these organs to keep them moist and warm (Fig. 26.2). Do not cover the extruding viscera with material that clings or loses its structure when wet, like toilet tissue, paper towels, or absorbent cotton. Much time will be lost in removing the mess. The entire abdomen may be covered with clean aluminum foil secured in place with a clean sheet. The purposes of retaining moisture and heat are both served by this material.

Give necessary emergency treatment as already directed and transport the patient rapidly to the Emergency Department. Eviscerations are a first priority emergency and must be repaired by a physician at an operation as soon as possible.

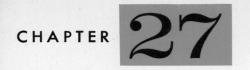

The Acute Abdomen

GOAL I. Know the characteristics of an acute abdomen.

OBJECTIVES

A. Describe the signs and symptoms of an acute abdomen.
B. List the common causes of an acute abdomen.
C. List the differences between localized and diffused abdominal pain.
D. Describe how diseases cause the signs of acute abdomen.

GOAL II. Understand the procedures for treating a patient with an acute abdomen.

OBJECTIVES

A. List the steps of an orderly examination for an acute abdomen.
B. List the vital signs which should be observed and recorded in examining a patient with an acute abdomen.
C. Describe why it is important to maintain an airway, administer oxygen, and prevent or treat shock in the patient with an acute abdomen.
D. Explain why patients with an acute abdomen should not be given anything to eat or drink.

The term *acute abdomen* is one sanctioned by time and used by members of the medical profession to indicate the presence in a patient of an abdominal disease causing irritation or inflammation of the peritoneum and consequent severe pain. All penetrating abdominal wounds and all blunt injuries severe enough to damage abdominal organs result in the development of the signs of an acute abdomen. These signs are abdominal tenderness and distention. The patient generally complains of abdominal pain. In this chapter, however, we are concerned with the development of this clinical picture without any preceding injury.

The term *abdominal catastrophe* is occasionally used to denote the most severe form of an acute abdomen. Neither term, acute abdomen or abdominal catastrophe, is exact; and neither term refers to a disease of any specific organ. Both mean the presence of severe abdominal disease, which is usually sudden in onset. Since many diseases in many different organs result in the same signs of pain and tenderness in the abdomen, it is possible to consider them all under these terms. It is frequently difficult for a skilled practitioner or surgeon to determine exactly what is causing an acute abdomen. The EMT must be able to recognize the existence of such an abdominal condition; he need not necessarily know the exact cause.

Conditions giving rise to acute abdominal signs are frequently sudden in onset and rapidly progressive. They may quickly result in death. The overriding principle of emergency care in these conditions is correction of life-threatening problems and transportation of the patient to a hospital without delay. Such conditions may require emergency operative procedures which must not be delayed.

The Signs of Acute Abdominal Distress

The signs of an acute abdomen arise from irritation or inflammation of the peritoneum. The condition, which is called peritonitis, always manifests itself as abdominal pain and tenderness when the abdomen is palpated or moved. The degree of pain and tenderness usually correlates with the severity of the inflammation within.

The sensory nervous supply of the peritoneum is rich and twofold. The parietal peritoneum (lining of the wall of the abdomen) receives its innervation from the somatic sensory portion of the lower intercostal and lumbar nerves. The peritoneum of the central portion of the diaphragm is supplied by the phrenic nerve. The lateral diaphragmatic peritoneum is supplied by the intercostal nerves. Sensations so served are similar to cutaneous sensations; and, though the peritoneum is insensitive to light touch, it is very sensitive to irritation, heavy touch, stretch, pressure, and temperature change. It can localize the irritating point well.

The visceral peritoneum (serosa, or covering of the organs) is supplied by the sympathetic chain and vagus nerves. Visceral sensory nerves are less able to localize pain. The type of pain perceived is limited to that arising from activation of stretch receptors, caused by distention in organs or forceful contraction of the organs. This type of activation is usually interpreted as colic.

The twofold nature of peritoneal innervation, somatic and visceral, gives rise to the phenomenon of referred pain. In this instance an irritated peritoneal surface over an organ may give rise to pain on the surface of the body which is served by the same area of the spinal cord as the irritated organ. Acute cholecystitis may cause pain in the shoulder, since the sympathetic nerves serving the gallbladder rise in the same area as the somatic nerves innervating the skin of the shoulder. There is no shoulder problem, but each set of nerves is activated.

Peritonitis always causes ileus (paralysis of normal intestinal motion). It is not uncommon to see abdominal distention in these patients from retained gas and feces. In the presence of such paralysis, nothing that is eaten will be passed out of the stomach or through the bowel. Vomiting is the only way in which the stomach can empty itself and it usually does so. Normally, muscular activity in the bowel is continuous as long as the patient is active. As soon as irritation causes a disturbance in the action of the bowel, distention proximal to the area of disturbance is seen.

Peritonitis also is always associated with a loss of body fluid into the abdomen. This loss results in a relative decrease in the volume of the circulating blood (hypovolemia) and may eventually result in shock. Depending on the stage of the development of peritonitis when the patient is seen, he may have normal vital signs or he may have a very rapid pulse and low blood pressure. If peritonitis is associated with hemorrhage, the signs of shock are much more acute.

The common signs and symptoms of acute abdominal disease are these:

1. Abdominal pain, local or diffuse
2. Abdominal tenderness, local or diffuse
3. A quiet patient who does not want to move because it hurts
4. A patient who is breathing rapidly and not deeply because a deep breath hurts
5. Rapid pulse (tachycardia)
6. Low blood pressure
7. A tense, often distended, abdomen

Varying degrees of each of the above conditions may exist. Pain may be sharply localized or diffused. When localized, it gives a clue to the cause. Tenderness may be minimal or it may be such that the patient will not allow his abdomen to be touched. He "guards" it with his muscles so that the abdominal wall is absolutely rigid. The position of the patient in bed is an important clue. In some diseases, patients can obtain comfort only by lying in one position. The patient with appendicitis may draw up the right knee.

218

The patient with pancreatitis may lie curled up on the right side. Each position tends to relax muscles adjacent to the inflamed organ and to lessen pain.

If breathing is painful, severe peritonitis may exist. Pulse and blood pressure may be greatly changed or not altered at all. They usually reflect the severity of the process and its duration. Distention can easily be gauged by looking at the patient's abdomen. Distention is apparent within a few hours after intestinal muscular activity has ceased.

Examination of the abdomen may be briefly accomplished in these steps:

1. Look at the patient to determine whether he is restless or quiet, whether motion causes pain, or whether any characteristic position, distention, or abnormality is present.
2. Feel the abdomen gently to see whether it is tense (guarded), or soft.
3. Determine whether the patient can relax his abdominal wall on command.
4. Determine whether the abdomen is tender when touched.

Such an examination can be done very quickly and will yield much information. Do not prolong this examination as the physician will do it in much more detail at the hospital. Carry out all abdominal palpations very gently. Occasionally an organ within the abdomen will be very much enlarged and very fragile. Palpation has been the cause of rupturing aneurysms of the aorta or lacerating the spleen.

Causes of Abdominal Disease

The abdominal cavity contains the solid and hollow organs making up the gastrointestinal and genitourinary systems. These organs are wholly covered with peritoneum, which lines the inside of the cavity and the outside of the organs. The entire cavity normally contains a very small amount of peritoneal fluid bathing the organs. Any condition which allows pus, blood, feces, urine, gastric juice, intestinal content, amniotic fluid, dead tissue, or severely inflamed tissue to lie within this cavity can give

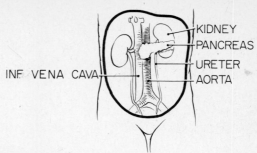

Figure 27.1

The major organs lying behind the peritoneum are shown. Diseases in these structures can cause peritoneal irritation.

219

rise to the signs of an acute abdomen.

Among the common diseases which produce these signs are acute appendicitis, perforated peptic ulcer, and cholecystitis (inflammation of the gallbladder). The list of diseases that can produce an acute abdomen is long and includes nearly every abdominal problem. Rarely, and most often in children, a primary infection of the peritoneum can occur. This infection similarly can give rise to the signs of acute abdominal inflammation.

The peritoneum is richly supplied with nerves which are sensitive to the presence of inflammation. Disease·or inflammation of organs which lie behind the peritoneum (Fig. 27.1). or beneath it in the pelvic cavity similarly can result in all the signs of peritonitis produced by actual inflammation within the cavity itself.

Pancreatitis can produce so severe an inflammation that it is hard to distinguish from a perforated ulcer. Kidney stones causing ureteral colic are frequently associated with paralysis of bowel action. One of the very common causes of an acute abdomen in the female is pelvic inflammatory disease, usually of the fallopian tubes and surrounding tissue. It is one of the major differential diagnoses in female patients with suspected appendicitis. Infections of the upper. and lower urinary tracts (respectively kidney and ureter, bladder and urethra) may also cause peritoneal irritation.

The aorta lies immediately behind the peritoneum on the spinal column. In older people it can often develop weak areas which swell, called aneurysms. The development of such a swelling at a weak spot is rarely associated with symptoms because it occurs slowly. If this weak area ruptures, however, massive hemorrhage may occur and some of the signs of an acute peritoneal irritation arise, along with severe back pain, because the peritoneum is rapidly stripped away from the body wall. In such instances, peritoneal signs are associated with profound shock.

The Care of the Patient with an Acute Abdomen

The signs indicative of an acute abdomen justify a working diagnosis of some serious abdominal surgical emergency. There should be no delay in transporting the patient to the Emergency Department.

Vomiting is not uncommon with these patients as the emergency frequently develops just after the patient has eaten a large meal or has done much heavy drinking. The patient's throat and airway must be cleared of vomited material and kept clear.

The administration of oxygen may be necessary. Usually there is no specific block in the exchange of air in the lung nor in obtaining air. Pain makes it physically difficult to breathe, and supplemental oxygen should be used to compensate for a small respiratory volume.

Under no circumstances should a patient with acute abdominal signs be given anything to eat or drink. Ingestion of food or fluid can only make worse many of his symptoms. If an emergency operation is required, the presence of food in the stomach will make it much more dangerous. In the presence of peritoneal irritation and intestinal paralysis, food will not pass out of the stomach and will only increase its distention and further aggravate vomiting.

No matter how distressed the patient is, the EMT should not give any medication for pain nor give any sedation. The examining physician must know exactly where and how much it hurts. Medication frequently masks these findings and may delay an ultimate diagnosis until it is too late to effect proper treatment.

Do not attempt to diagnose the causes of the patient's disease, but listen to the description of the location of pain and tenderness and the account of the severity of symptoms. The EMT must record the patient's description of how the process started and the vital signs as soon as possible so that the physician may know what these were when the patient was first seen. Shock is common with these patients. It must be recognized early, for its presence makes rapid transport to the hospital even more imperative.

Make the patient as comfortable as possible; conserve body heat with blankets; start an IV as directed by the doctor; and transport the patient gently and expeditiously to the hospital.

CHAPTER 28

The Genitourinary System

GOAL I. Know the structures and functions of the genitourinary systems in the male and female.

OBJECTIVES

A. Describe the structures and functions of the urinary system.
B. Describe the structures and functions of the genital system in the male.
C. Describe the structures and functions of the genital system in the female.

The urinary and genital systems are commonly discussed together because their various organs and passages develop embryologically from the same precursors and because they thus share many structures. Usually, the urinary and male genital systems are considered together. The female genital system is considered separately.

The urinary system controls the discharge of certain waste materials filtered from the blood. The genital system controls the reproductive processes from which life is created. The kidneys are retroperitoneal, solid urinary organs. The bladder and ureters are the hollow organs of this system (Fig. 28.1). The female genitalia—uterus, ovaries, and fallopian tubes—are contained almost entirely within the pelvis. The male genitalia lie outside the abdomen.

Urinary System

Kidneys. The body has two kidneys. They lie on the posterior muscle wall of the abdomen behind the peritoneum. The kidneys are vital organs. They rid the blood of toxic waste products and control its balance of water and salt. If the kidneys are destroyed or for any reason no longer function adequately, a condition known as uremia occurs. Waste accumulates within the bloodstream; the balance of salt and water is disturbed; and death may ensue.

Nearly 20 percent of the output of the heart each minute passes to the kidneys. Large vessels attach the kidneys directly to the aorta and inferior vena cava. Blood flow in the kidneys is high. Almost 1,500 liters of blood are circulated each day through the kidneys where waste products and water are filtered out constantly to form urine. The kidneys continuously concentrate this urine by reabsorbing the water as it is collected through a system of specialized tubes within the organ. These tubes finally unite to form the renal pelvis, a cone-shaped collecting

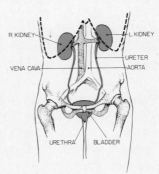

Figure 28.1

Kidney, ureters, bladder, and urethra constitute the urinary system, which is closely attached to the aorta and inferior vena cava.

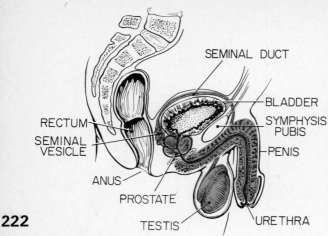

Figure 28.2

The male genital system, shown here in cross section, includes seminal vesicles and seminal ducts, prostate gland, testicles, urethra, and the penis.

222

area which connects the ureter and the kidney. Normally, each kidney drains its urine into one ureter, which passes to the bladder.

Injuries of the kidney, like those of other solid organs, can cause severe bleeding and disruption of function. In addition, renal (kidney) injuries can result in direct leak of urine into the surrounding tissues.

Ureters. Although each kidney is usually drained by one ureter, there may be multiple tubes. The ureter passes from the kidney along the surface of the posterior abdominal wall and drains into the urinary bladder within the pelvis. The ureters are small-diameter (0.5 cm.), hollow, muscular tubes. Peristalsis is present in these tubes to move the urine to the bladder. Injuries of ureters are rare because they are small and well protected. Such injuries result in a leak of urine into the surrounding soft tissue. These injuries must be promptly treated, as urine in tissue is extremely irritating. Diagnosis and treatment of these injuries require specialized hospital equipment and procedures.

Urinary bladder and urethra. The urinary bladder is situated immediately behind the pubic bone in the pelvis. It is covered by peritoneum and hence lies outside the abdominal cavity and in front of it. The ureters enter at its base and posterior. It in turn empties to the outside of the body through the urethra. In the male, the urethra passes from the anterior base

of the bladder into the penis (Fig. 28.2). In the female, the urethra opens at the front of the vagina (Fig. 28.3).

Urine, the product of blood filtration in the kidneys, passes through the ureters into the urinary bladder where it is stored. When the bladder becomes full, sensory cells send messages to the brain notifying it that the bladder is ready to empty. When it is time to void (urinate), the urinary bladder contracts, forcing urine through the urethra to the outside of the body. The normal adult forms one and one-half to two liters of concentrated urine every day. This waste is extracted from the blood circulated through the kidneys, which totals 1,500 liters daily.

Genital System

Genitalia. The genitalia include the male and and female reproductive organs and the male urethra. The male and female reproductive organs have certain similarities and, of course, basic differences. They allow the production of sperm and egg cells and appropriate hormones, the act of sexual intercourse, and, ultimately, reproduction.

Male reproductive system and organs. The male reproductive system includes the testicles, vasa deferentia or seminal ducts, seminal vesicles, prostate gland, urethra, and penis (Fig.

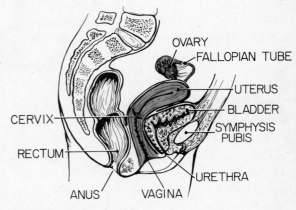

Figure 28.3

The female genital system, shown in cross section, is composed of ovaries, Fallopian tubes, the uterus, cervix, and vagina.

28.2). Each testicle contains specialized cells and ducts. Certain cells produce male hormones; others develop sperm. The hormones are absorbed directly into the blood from the testicles. Semen, or seminal fluid, contains sperm cells carried up each seminal duct (vas deferens) from a testis to be mixed with fluid from the seminal vesicles and prostate gland. The seminal ducts (vasa deferentia) travel from the testicles up beneath the skin of the abdominal wall for a short distance; then they pass through an opening into the abdominal cavity and down into the prostate gland to meet the urethra. The seminal vesicles constitute small storage sacs for sperm and seminal fluid. These vesicles also empty into the urethra at the prostate.

The prostate gland is a small gland that surrounds the urethra where it emerges from the urinary bladder. Fluids from the prostate gland and from the seminal vesicles come together during intercourse. During the act of intercourse, special mechanisms in the nervous system prevent the passage of urine into the urethra. Only seminal fluid, prostatic fluid, and sperm pass from the penis into the vagina during ejaculation.

The penis has a special type of tissue called erectile tissue. The special tissue is largely vascular and when filled with blood, causes the penis to distend into a state of erection. As the vessels fill under pressure from the circulatory system, the penis becomes a rigid organ which can enter the vagina. The urethra in the penis, which carries urine during urination, carries seminal fluid and sperm during ejaculation. Certain spinal injuries and some diseases cause a permanent and painful erection called priapism. It is easy to ascertain the presence of this condition, and it should not be overlooked.

Female reproductive system and organs. The female reproductive organs include the ovaries, fallopian tubes, uterus, and vagina (Fig. 28.3).

The ovaries, like the testicles, produce sex hormones and specialized cells for reproduction. The female sex hormones are absorbed directly into the blood. A specialized cell, called an ovum, is produced with regularity during the adult female's reproductive years. The ovaries release a mature egg, or ovum, approximately every twenty-eight days. This egg travels through the fallopian tubes to the uterus.

The fallopian tubes connect with the uterus and carry the ovum to the cavity of the uterus. The uterus is a pear-shaped body with muscular walls. It is a hollow organ. A narrow opening from the uterus to the vagina is called the cervix. This opening provides for the passage of sperm into the uterus, or for the passage of menstrual fluid into the vagina. When a baby is born, it passes from the uterus through the cervix to the vagina and then on to the outer world.

The vagina is a muscular, distensible tube connecting the uterus with the vulva (the external female genitalia). The vagina receives the male penis during intercourse, when semen and sperm are deposited in the vagina. The sperm may pass into the uterus and fertilize an egg, thereby resulting in pregnancy. Should the pregnancy come to completion, at the end of nine months the baby will pass through the vagina and be born.

The vagina also serves to channel the menstrual flow from the uterus out of the body.

Menstrual cycle. The menstrual period is the end of the monthly female reproductive cycle. During the adult female's active sexual life (from the start of her first menstrual period at about age twelve, until she passes through menopause at about age fifty) a woman has monthly periods of menstruation. Each month the endometrium (lining of the uterus) is stimulated by the female sex hormones to form a special bed. This bed is prepared so that if a sperm and an ovum unite, making a fertilized egg, the uterus will be ready to receive it and provide a place for it to grow. Approximately fifteen days after a menstrual period ceases, an egg is produced by one of the ovaries. This egg travels into the uterus through the fallopian tubes.

If a sperm is able to travel from the vagina through the cervix and to fertilize the egg, either in the uterus or in the fallopian tubes, the fertilized egg will settle in the uterus and begin to grow in the lining there, where a bed has been forming since the end of the previous menstrual period. Such an event is the start of a pregnancy which will go on for nine months. During this nine-month period, the uterus will become larger to accommodate the growing baby; and at the end of that time the baby will be expelled through the vagina, that is, be born.

If the egg is not fertilized, there will be a menstrual period. During the period, the uterus will shed its recently formed special lining, which is really a very thin layer of cells and blood. The lining, in the form of the menstrual flow, will pass out of the uterus into the vagina and out of the body. The flow will last about five days.

At the end of this time the flow will cease; the uterus will begin to prepare a new lining as a bed to receive a new egg; and the cycle will be repeated.

CHAPTER 29

Injuries of the Genitourinary System

GOAL I. Know the characteristics of injuries of the genitourinary system.

OBJECTIVES

A. Describe the characteristics of injuries of the urinary system.
B. Describe the characteristics of injuries of the genital system in the male.
C. Describe the characteristics of injuries of the genital system in the female.

GOAL II. Understand the procedures for treating injuries of the genitourinary tract.

OBJECTIVES

A. Describe the evaluation of a patient with a urinary tract injury.
B. Describe the procedures used by the EMT in treating injuries of the urinary tract.
C. Describe the procedures used by the EMT in treating injuries of the male genitalia.
D. Describe the procedures used by the EMT in treating injuries of the female genitalia.

Kidney

Injuries of the kidney are not common. They may result from blunt or penetrating trauma. The intensity of a blow required to damage the kidney is such that the injury is almost always associated with fractured ribs or other severely injured intra-abdominal organs. The kidneys lie in such a well-protected area of the body that a penetrating wound nearly always involves other organs as well as the kidney or its vessels.

A history, or physical evidence, of an abrasion, laceration, ecchymosis, or penetrating wound in the region of the lower rib cage, the flank, or the upper abdomen should make the EMT suspect accompanying kidney damage. The patient found to have fractures on either side of the lower rib cage or of the lower thoracic or upper lumbar vertebrae must also be considered a likely candidate for a kidney injury (Fig. 29.1). Force sufficient to fracture ribs or vertebrae is strong enough that associated soft-tissue damage is often inevitable.

Signs and treatment of renal injury. Except for the cutaneous signs of severe injury, bruises, and such, the evidences of damage of the kidney will not be manifest on external examination of the patient. Shock may be seen promptly when the injury is associated with significant blood loss. Since the function of the kidney is the formation of urine, an injury will usually be associated with blood in the urine (hematuria). Thus, any urine passed by the patient while under observation by the EMT should be measured and saved for a

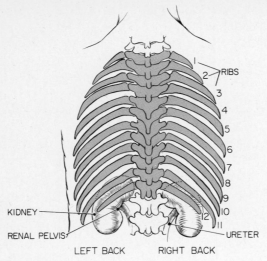

Figure 29.1

In a posterior view, the close relationship of the lower ribs with the kidneys on either side of the body is shown. Fractures of the ribs or vertebral bodies in this area are often associated with lacerations of the kidneys.

detailed microscopic examination at the hospital. A definitive diagnosis of the presence, the nature, and the severity of a kidney injury depends upon diagnostic studies available only in a hospital.

When one sees a patient who, because of the nature of his injury or because he has passed blood in the urine, is suspected of having sustained kidney damage, place him at total rest. Monitor vital signs carefully until arrival at the Emergency Department. The presence of shock or the severity of associated injuries may make transportation to the hospital a truly first priority emergency.

Urinary Bladder

Injury of the urinary bladder is usually a rupture caused by blunt trauma or penetrating laceration. In either event, urine is spilled out of the bladder into the surrounding tissue. Any urine that is passed through the urethra is likely to be bloody. Blunt injuries of the lower abdomen or pelvis frequently cause an explosive rupture of the urinary bladder, particularly when it is full and distended. Fractures of the pelvis are commonly associated with rupture or perforation of the urinary bladder, which is torn by the

sharp bony fragments (Fig. 29.2). Sudden deceleration, especially if the bladder is full, can literally shear the bladder off the urethra. Penetrating wounds of the lower mid-abdomen or perineum can all directly involve the bladder. A history of any of the above types of injury, or evidence on physical examination of trauma in the lower abdomen, pelvis, or perineum, or blood at the external urethral meatus all point to an injury of the urinary bladder. Final documentation of the presence and severity of an injury of the urinary bladder depends upon making X-ray studies.

Since the function of the urinary bladder is to be a reservoir for the storage of urine, any urine passed by a patient with suspected bladder injury should be noted; the specimen must be saved for presentation to the Emergency Department for a detailed analysis.

When possible injury of the urinary bladder exists, keep the patient at absolute rest and monitor vital signs. The presence of associated injuries or shock will dictate the urgency of his transport to the Emergency Department.

External Male Genitalia

Injuries of the external male genitalia include all the types of soft tissue injuries—avulsions, lacerations, abrasions, penetrations, and contusions.

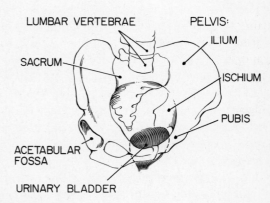

Figure 29.2

From an oblique anterior view, the close relationship of the urinary bladder and the bony pelvic ring is shown. A fracture of the pelvis is commonly a cause of a bladder laceration.

Rarely are these injuries life-threatening. They are uniformly extremely painful and generally a source of great concern to the patient.

Penis-urethra. Avulsion of the skin of the penis, particularly in the uncircumcised individual, can occur, especially in industrial accidents. When such a patient is seen, the denuded penis should be wrapped in a sterile dressing moistened with sterile saline solution before transportation to the Emergency Department. An effort should be made to salvage the skin and preserve it. It should be wrapped in a sterile gauze moistened with sterile saline.

Amputation, partial or complete, of the penile shaft demands immediate attention to blood loss, which can be effectively managed through the use of a tourniquet on the remaining stump. The injured penis should be dressed with a moist, sterile dressing for transport. If a complete amputation has occurred, an effort must be made to locate the amputated part so that it can be used in a possible reconstruction. The recovered part should be wrapped in a sterile, moist dressing. Very occasionally, the EMT will see a patient who has amputated his own penis. This is a violent gesture caused by mental disease. The rules noted above apply, together with those for managing a disturbed patient.

The acute angulation of the erect penis with respect to the anterior abdominal wall can result in a so-called fracture of the penis, a laceration of the supporting tissue of the organ. The injury may occur during particularly active sexual intercourse. It is always associated with intense pain, ecchymosis, and fear. Apply ice locally during transport to the Emergency Department. An operative procedure may be required to repair this injury.

Laceration of the frenulum of the penis (the ridge of skin below the head of the penis) is an accident which usually occurs when the penis is erect. It can be associated with profuse bleeding. Pressure on the bleeding area will usually be sufficient to stop the hemorrhage, but occasionally the placement of sutures will be required for complete control. Pressure, however, will control bleeding until suturing can be done.

The foreskin on occasion can be caught in the zipper of the trousers. This is a situation usually seen in children. If it is found that only one or two teeth of the zipper are involved, an attempt at unzipping should be made. With an agitated child or where a long segment of skin is trapped, simply cut the zipper out of the trousers to make the patient more comfortable for transport to the Emergency Department. Tears of the foreskin also are encountered rather often. The resultant bleeding is usually easily controlled with local pressure.

Urethral injuries in the male are uncommon, and there is little one can do for emergency care. No effort should be made to remove a foreign body lodged in the urethra unless it protrudes from the external urethral meatus and is known to be smooth surfaced. Lacerations of the urethra in the male can result from straddle injuries, pelvic trauma, or penetrating wounds of the perineum. They can be associated with brisk bleeding from the external urethral meatus. Pressure to occlude the urethra can control the blood loss. The final definition of the nature and extent of urethral injury depends upon detailed diagnostic studies to be done under sterile conditions in the hospital. Since the urethra is the conduit for urine, the passing of any urine and the presence or absence of blood in the urine are facts of utmost importance, which should be recorded. Any voided urine should be saved for a later examination at the hospital.

Scrotum-testis. Avulsion of the scrotal skin, with or without associated injury of the scrotal contents, can occur. When possible, recover and preserve the scrotal skin in a sterile, saline-moistened dressing for possible use in reconstruction. The denuded scrotal contents or the perineal area should be dressed with a sterile, saline-moistened dressing for the movement of the patient to an Emergency Department. Bleeding can be controlled with pressure over the dressing.

Direct blows on the scrotum and its contents can result in rupture of the testes or a significant accumulation of blood about them. The application of a generous ice pack to the scrotal-perineal area is desirable while transporting the patient.

The treatment of injuries involving the male external genitalia requires a few general rules applicable to a number of specific instances.

1. These injuries are extremely painful. Make the patient as comfortable as possible.
2. Use sterile moist compresses to control bleeding and cover denuded areas.
3. Never move or manipulate impaled instruments or urethral foreign bodies.
4. If possible, always identify and bring detached parts (foreskin, penis, testicles) with the patient.
5. Remember that these are rarely life-threatening injuries. The presence and severity of other wounds dictate priorities of care.

228

Internal Female Genitalia

The uterus, ovaries, and fallopian tubes are subject to the same kinds of injuries as any other internal organ. However, they are rarely damaged because they are small and well protected by the pelvis. Unlike the bladder, they do not lie adjacent to the bony pelvis and are not injured when it is fractured.

The pregnant female may suffer a rupture of the uterus from a blunt injury or laceration by a penetrating wound simply because the organ is so large it is easily injured. These are very serious injuries and usually result in loss of the life of the fetus in the uterus. They can also cause severe hemorrhage and peritonitis. The leaking of amniotic fluid (a special fluid surrounding the fetus) into lacerated veins can cause sudden and severe derangements in clotting within the blood vessels. Any major blunt or penetrating injury in the pregnant female becomes a much more severe problem because of the enlarged uterus.

External Female Genitalia

The external female genitalia include the vulva, the clitoris, and major and minor labia (lips) at the entrance of the vagina. The female urethra enters the anterior vagina.

Injuries of the external female genitalia can include all the types of soft-tissue injuries. These genital parts have a rich nerve supply, and injuries of them are very painful. Lacerations, abrasions, and avulsions should be treated with moist compresses, local pressure to control bleeding, and a diaper-type dressing to hold

bandages in place. Major bleeding will require control in the operating room. Under no circumstances should dressings or packs be placed in the vagina.

Foreign bodies should be left alone after stabilization and these patients transported promptly to the Emergency Department. Contusions and other blunt injuries may require careful in-hospital evaluation.

In general, although these injuries are painful, they probably are not life-threatening. Bleeding may be a copious but it can usually be controlled by local compression. Priorities of need for transportation to the Emergency Department are dictated by associated injuries, amount of hemorrhage, and the presence of shock.

Sexual assault and rape. Instances of sexual assault and rape are all too common. Often the EMT can do little beyond soothing and calming the patient and providing quick transportation to the Emergency Department. Genitalia should **not** be examined by the EMT unless obvious bleeding or laceration requires the application of a dressing. The patient should be advised not to wash, douche, urinate, or defecate until after the physician has had an opportunity to make an examination at the Emergency Department. Other injuries, such as fractures, lacerations, or unconsciousness should be treated according to all the appropriate routine procedures.

The EMT should obtain as clear a history of the incident as possible. Questioning and any necessary treatment should be handled quietly, as speedily as possible, and away from onlookers. A calm, professional manner is called for, with no display of personal curiosity.

The EMT must be aware that a patient has the right to refuse assistance and to refuse to be taken to the Emergency Department. Such refusal can occur in cases of rape or sexual assault because of the wish to avoid publicity. It can also happen that although assistance may have originally been requested, it is refused after arrival of the EMT at the scene. This too is the patient's prerogative, if the patient is rational. Assistance from a rape counseling center, many of which have recently been established, can often be helpful.

VII
Medical Emergencies

CHAPTER 30

Heart Attack

GOAL I. Understand the mechanisms and therapy of acute myocardial infarction.

231

OBJECTIVES

A. Explain the function of the blood supply to the heart.
B. Describe the process of atherosclerosis.
C. Describe the varied presentations of actue myocardial infarction (AMI).
D. Describe the physical findings of AMI.
E. Describe the therapy of AMI.

GOAL II. Understand the differences between angina pectoris and acute myocardial infarction.

OBJECTIVES

A. Describe the usual presentation of angina.
B. Describe the differences between angina and acute myocardial infarction.

GOAL III. Understand the mechanisms and therapy of heart failure.

OBJECTIVES

A. Describe the changes in the heart with heart failure.
B. Describe the clinical picture of congestive heart failure.
C. Describe the therapy of congestive heart failure.

Heart disease is the leading cause of death in the United States, accounting for nearly half a million deaths per year. Most of these are associated with atherosclerosis, or coronary artery disease. The immediate cause of death is usually acute myocardial infarction (heart attack).

Cardiac Function

In order for the myocardium (heart muscle) to carry out its pumping function, it must have a continuous supply of oxygen. Blood vessels called the coronary arteries carry oxygen to the myocardium. When the heart must increase its work, as during periods of physical exertion or mental stress, the myocardium requires more oxygen and therefore more blood flow. In the normal heart the increased amount of blood is easily supplied by dilation of the coronary arteries, which increases blood flow. Disease within these arteries interferes with their ability to dilate and to carry blood, and can reduce the amount of oxygen available to the myocardium. Myocardial infarction (MI—death of heart muscle) or angina pectoris (chest pain, generally considered to mean only the pain of too little oxygen in the heart) both are conditions arising from a reduced oxygen supply.

The coronary arteries originate at the base of the aorta just above the aortic valve. The right coronary artery supplies the right ventricle and, in most people, the underside of the left ventricle. The left coronary artery has two branches, both supplying the left ventricle.

The disease process which can damage the coronary arteries, as well as other arteries of the body, is called atherosclerosis. Atherosclerosis begins with the deposit of fat laid down just beneath the endothelium (inner cell layer) of the artery. Deposits may be apparent as early as age eighteen. As the person grows older, more fat is deposited, until the lumen (the inside diameter) of the artery is narrowed. Deposits are usually present by age twenty-five. As these deposits grow, they finally disrupt the endothelial covering and cause scarring or fibrosis of the artery. Calcium deposited within the scar still further narrows the lumen of the artery (Fig. 30.1 *a*).

Finally, by age forty-five to fifty-five, occlusion of the artery may be so extensive as to limit any increase in blood flow to the heart at times of peak activity such as running or taking exercise. Therefore, during these periods the oxygen supply of the heart can no longer equal its requirements for oxygen.

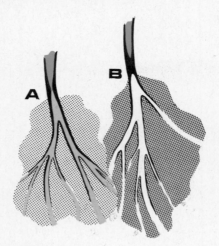

Figure 30.1 *a–b*

a, A severely narrowed coronary artery is shown. The heart muscle supplied by this vessel is ischemic (lacking in oxygen) but not dead. *b*, Complete occlusion of the coronary vessel has occurred with thrombosis. The muscle supplied by this vessel is now dead. A myocardial infarction has occurred.

Angina Pectoris

If the heart has too little oxygen for its needs for more than several seconds, severe pain will occur. This pain is called angina pectoris. Since the occurrence of angina pectoris indicates coronary artery disease, it is important to understand the pain and to recognize it.

Angina pectoris occurs when the need of the heart for oxygen exceeds its supply; therefore it generally occurs at times when the heart is working hard—periods of physical or emotional stress. The key characteristic of angina pectoris is a pain which comes on with exertion and is relieved by rest. The pain is felt substernally; it radiates to the jaw or arms, especially the left arm; it is described as a pressure sensation or a squeezing sensation "like someone standing on my chest." It lasts usually three to eight minutes and rarely longer than ten minutes. It may be associated with shortness of breath, nausea, and sweating. The pain should be relieved promptly when the oxygen supply of the heart equals or exceeds the demand, as would occur when the physical or emotional stress diminishes or ceases.

Angina pectoris is treated with a medicine called nitroglycerine. It is provided as a small white tablet (one-half the size of aspirin) which is placed under the tongue. Nitroglycerine works in seconds to diminish the work of the myocardium and to reduce the oxygen need, thereby relieving the pain of angina pectoris. Although angina pectoris is painful, it does not mean the death of the myocardium and does not lead to the death of the patient or to permanent damage of the heart.

Myocardial Infarction

If the narrowing of the coronary artery by atherosclerosis is severe enough or if a blood clot forms at the point of the narrowing (Fig. 30.1 *b*), then the oxygen supply in the area of the heart served by that artery can be so diminished that the heart muscle dies. This condition is a myocardial infarction.

Myocardial infarction occurs predominantly in the left ventricle. The left ventricle is a thick-

232

walled chamber that produces the high systemic blood pressure; therefore it requires much more oxygen than does the lower pressure, right ventricle. The left ventricle suffers most from a lack of oxygen. A myocardial infarction has serious consequences. These are:

1. Sudden death from arrhythmias (unorganized beating of the heart)
2. Congestive heart failure
3. Shock

Sudden death. It is estimated that between 30 to 50 percent of all patients who suffer a myocardial infarction die before they can reach the hospital. These deaths occur because of extensive abnormalities of the heart rhythm (arrhythmias) which prevent any effective pumping action of the heart. The chance of an arrhythmia occurring after a myocardial infarction is greatest within the first hour after the infarct and diminishes to only a small risk after three to five days.

Congestive heart failure. Failure of the heart occurs when the muscle is so damaged by the infarction that it can no longer pump enough blood for the needs of the body. This event occurs anytime after an infarction but it usually is manifest between the third and seventh day after the heart attack. These patients may have pulmonary edema (fluid in the lungs) with frothy pink sputum; they may have difficulty breathing; there may be evidence of generalized edema in the body.

Shock. Cardiogenic shock is an early complication of an infarction which occurs within twenty-four hours of the event and means that the heart has been so damaged that it is unable to sustain a normal systemic blood pressure. This condition is discussed in Chapter 9, Shock.

Clinical Presentation of Acute Myocardial Infarction

An acute myocardial infarction may have the following signs:

1. Sudden onset of weakness, nausea, and sweating without a clear cause
2. Chest pain
3. Sudden arrhythmia with syncope (fainting)

4. Pulmonary edema
5. Sudden death

Unfortunately, the first presentation of coronary heart disease may be sudden death, and 30 to 50 percent of all patients with myocardial infarction may never reach the hospital. Fifty percent of these people will have had no previous knowledge of any heart disease, while the other 50 percent will have had the diagnosis of coronary artery disease made prior to their sudden death. The sudden death of myocardial infarction, caused by an arrhythmia, usually is a result of ventricular fibrillation. The chance to save such a patient exists only if someone begins CPR promptly. Ventricular asystole, the lack of any heartbeat, may also be a cause of sudden death, but the incidence of this particular event is hard to determine since many dangerous ventricular arrhythmias rapidly end in asystole if no treatment is given.

The chance of sudden death is extremely high at the instant of the infarction; therefore, this moment is the most dangerous time for the patient. Rapid institution of basic life support has been and can be successful in resuscitation of many patients with this disease.

The vast majority of patients with acute myocardial infarction who do not die with the onset of the infarct develop chest pain. Classically, this pain is

1. Substernal in location
2. Squeezing in quality or character
3. Longer lasting than thirty minutes
4. Not related to exertion and not relieved by rest or nitroglycerine
5. Perceived as radiating to the jaw, to the left arm, or to both arms

The pain of a myocardial infarction differs from angina pectoris in two ways.

1. The pain of an acute myocardial infarction lasts longer than that of angina pectoris. Whereas anginal pain usually lasts no longer than three to ten minutes, the pain of an acute myocardial infarction lasts thirty minutes to hours.
2. The pain of myocardial infarction, unlike that of angina pectoris, is not related to

233

exertion or mental or emotional stress. It is not relieved by rest or by nitroglycerine. The pain of a myocardial infarction may come on at any time, waking one from sleep or occurring when the individual is sitting quietly reading.

About 90 percent of those with an acute myocardial infarction develop some sort of cardiac arrhythmia—usually extra beats arising in the damaged ventricle. These extra beats, called ventricular premature contractions, may group together and produce a serious disturbance called ventricular tachycardia. If ventricular tachycardia persists it deteriorates into ventricular fibrillation, which is a cause of sudden death. Some patients with myocardial infarction may not feel pain but may notice the irregularity of the heartbeat. The episodes of ventricular arrhythmia may cause syncope (fainting). Therefore, patients who develop a sudden syncope must be treated as suspect for acute myocardial infarction, especially if they noted any chest pain or discomfort prior to or after the faint.

The sudden onset of left ventricular failure, causing pulmonary edema, may be the first sign of an acute myocardial infarction and should be treated as such. If the amount of damage caused by the infarction is great enough, the heart can no longer pump blood effectively. Since myocardial infarction occurs in the left ventricle and not ordinarily in the right ventricle, the left ventricle will have reduced pumping capability and cannot pump out the blood coming from the lungs, but the right ventricle will continue to function well and will keep pumping blood into the lungs. Pressures within the lung capillaries will rise and fluid will pour out from the blood vessels into the pulmonary alveoli (air sacs). The lungs literally fill with fluid and the patient feels as if he were drowning. He cannot breathe enough to get oxygen from the air and develops a marked feeling of shortness of breath; at times the fluid in the alveoli may actually come out his mouth and nose as pink foam. If such a patient has no past history of shortness of breath or heart failure and if the pulmonary edema is sudden in onset, he should be reated as if the episode were an acute myocardial infarction.

Treatment for the pulmonary edema should be instituted at the same time.

Because the left ventricular muscle is damaged by the myocardial infarction, the amount of blood pumped per minute falls. An occasional patient who does not note pain or does not experience an arrhythmia may develop a feeling of sudden extreme weakness. He may tell someone he is suddenly too weak to stand or walk. This extreme weakness is probably a result of the fall in cardiac output. Such an individual should be assumed to be having an acute myocardial infarction and be so treated.

Physical Findings of Acute Myocardial Infarction

The physical findings of an acute myocardial infarction are variable.

Pulse. Generally the pulse rate is increased as a normal response to stress, fear, or the actual injury of the myocardium. Since arrhythmias are the rule rather than the exception, an irregularity of the pulse may be noted. In some cases of acute infarction, bradycardia (an abnormal slowing of the pulse) develops rather than tachycardia (an abnormally rapid pulse).

Blood pressure. Blood pressure falls as a result of diminished cardiac output and diminished capability of the left ventricle to pump.

Respirations. Respirations are normal unless pulmonary edema occurs. In this case there are rapid, shallow respirations.

General appearance. The patient appears quite frightened. A cold sweat is frequently present. The patient may feel nauseated and may vomit. The skin is often pale gray.

Patient's mental status. One of the unexplained aspects of an acute myocardial infarction is the fact that many patients have an almost overwhelming feeling of impending doom. They are convinced—almost resigned—that they are about to die.

Approach to the Patient

In the conscious patient in whom heart disease or an infarct is suspected, the following steps are appropriate.

234

Reassurance. Act professionally, be calm, speak to the patient calmly in a moderate voice. Inform him that there are trained people present to care for him and that he will shortly be taken to the hospital. Remember, all patients are frightened; some may act carefree; some may be demanding; but all are frightened. The professional attitude of the EMT will be the single most important factor in gaining the patient's cooperation.

History. Take a brief history from the patient himself or those about him. Simultaneous with one EMT's taking a history, the other should obtain and record vital signs, noting the time they are obtained. Pulse, blood pressure, and respiratory rate are vital pieces of information.

Position. If a myocardial infarction is suspected, place the patient in a semi-reclining position, loosen shirt or blouse, remove jacket or any restricting or cumbersome garment.

Oxygen. Administer oxygen by facemask.

ECG. If electrocardiographic leads are available and the EMT is trained to place them, do so to obtain and monitor the patient's heart rhythm and rate.

IV. If the EMT is trained to give an intravenous infusion, he may start an IV with dextrose solution. It should be run very slowly.

Hospital advice. If telemetry is available, call the Emergency Department and request that a physician monitor the patient's status. Report the patient's vital signs, history, medications being taken, and treatment instituted. Take care not to frighten the patient. Further treatment should be undertaken only under supervision of the emergency physician. Once the physician agrees that the situation is stable, transport the patient to the hospital, continuing telemetry en route.

Records. If no telemetry is available, call the nearest hospital and alert the Emergency Department as to the status of the patient and your estimated time of arrival. Leave a copy of the ambulance record with the patient at the hospital receiving area. If possible, give an additional oral report at the Emergency Department.

Congestive Heart Failure

Physiology. Regardless of whether the heart has been damaged by valvular disease, sustained hypertension, or coronary heart disease, the pumping function of the left ventricle may be impaired. When the muscle can no longer contract well, several adaptations take place in the heart in its attempt to maintain an adequate cardiac output. When these adaptations fail, congestive heart failure may develop on a chronic basis.

The common adaptations are these:

1. The heart rate increases.
2. The size of the left ventricular chamber enlarges in an attempt to increase the amount of blood pumped per minute.

235

Unfortunately, the left ventricle can increase in size only in response to an increase in the pressure required to fill it. The increased pressure can only be a result of a pressure rise in the capillaries and veins of the lungs. If the pressure in the pulmonary capillaries exceeds 25 to 30 mm Hg (normal is below 12 mm Hg), fluid passes through the capillary walls and into the alveoli. Pulmonary edema develops. It may occur suddenly, as in a myocardial infarction, or slowly over months, as in chronic congestive heart failure.

Presentation. Once fluid passes from the capillaries to the alveoli, the patient has a marked sensation of shortness of breath. The fluid tends to make the lung stiffer; therefore, the patient breathes rapidly but with shallow respirations. Regardless of the speed with which fluid accumulates in the lung, the patient experiences greater difficulty breathing while lying than standing or sitting. When lying flat, the increased return of blood to the right ventricle is delivered to the lungs and further congests the pulmonary circulation.

The patient with chronic congestive heart failure generally has marked shortness of breath, mild or pronounced agitation, and insists on sitting upright. Chest pain may be present, but it is not generally a part of congestive heart failure. Vital signs will reveal a normal or somewhat high blood pressure, a rapid heart rate, and rapid, shallow respirations. If one listens to the patient's chest with a stethoscope, the sound of air bubbling through the fluid in the alveoli and bronchi may be heard. This sound is called "rales." It is a sound much like sand falling on an empty tin can. Wheezing may also be heard. In severe congestive heart failure, these sounds are heard from the apex to the base of the lungs. They are best heard by listening at the back of the patient's chest.

Treatment. The EMT must treat the patient as if he were having an acute myocardial infarc-tion in addition to heart failure. Vital signs and monitoring of heart action must be obtained. Oxygen therapy should be given. The patient should be allowed to remain in an upright posi-tion with his legs down. It is important to reas-sure the patient and attempt to calm him. Prompt transportation to the Emergency De-partment is essential.

236

CHAPTER 31

Stroke

GOAL I. Understand the causes of stroke and its effects on the person.

OBJECTIVES

A. Define stroke.

B. List the causes of stroke.

C. Describe the presenting symptoms of stroke.

D. List the effects of stroke on the body.

GOAL II. Understand the procedure for the immediate care of the stroke patient.

OBJECTIVES

A. Describe the initial evaluation of the stroke patient.

B. Describe the immediate care of the patient with stroke.

C. List precautions to be taken which are unique to the stroke patient.

Normal function of the brain requires a continuous supply of oxygen and glucose and, therefore, a continuous blood flow. Interruption of a flow in a cerebral artery for more than six minutes usually causes irreversible damage in the area of the brain supplied by that artery. Since specific areas of the brain correspond with specific functions (for example, interruption of blood flow on the left side of the brain will cause speech problems in righthanded individuals), the results of damage in the brain depend on the area of the brain destroyed. A lack of blood flow in the entire right side of the brain will cause paralysis of the entire left side of the body.

Causes of Stroke

A stroke (cerebro-vascular accident, or CVA) may be caused by any interruption of blood flow which lasts long enough to damage the brain. The clinical features of the stroke will depend on the amount and site of the brain damage. Although the damage may be extensive enough to cause death, this event is uncommon. The natural history of a stroke is gradual improvement of the patient and partial or complete return of function.

Interruption of cerebral blood flow may be a result of one of a number of events.

1. Occlusion of a cerebral artery can result from clot formation (thrombus) at the site of damage within the artery. Such damage is usually from atherosclerotic vascular disease.

2. Rupture of an artery can cause bleeding into the brain (Fig. 31.1). The bleeding may cause spasm of the leaking artery and further interruption of blood flow within the vessel. Brain damage may result directly from the hemorrhage into tissue or from the impaired circulation.

3. A blood clot formed elsewhere, usually

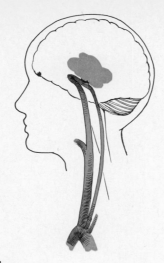

Figure 31.1

In this schematic illustration, the two internal carotid arteries are shown supplying blood to the brain. A rupture of a branch of one of them has resulted in a hemorrhage within the brain (intracerebral hematoma).

within the heart, may travel to a cerebral vessel as an embolus and occlude it.

The most common cause of a stroke is clotting of a cerebral vessel at an area of atherosclerotic disease. This event generally occurs in the elderly individual with high blood pressure (hypertension). Males and females are equally affected.

Bleeding from a cerebral artery may occur in the young or the old. It too is associated with hypertension, and in young people it is generally caused by an aneurysm in the vessel. The aneurysm is a weakened, bulging area of the blood vessel.

An embolism in a cerebral vessel occurs most often in individuals with heart disease. Frequently valvular heart disease or any heart disease that causes an abnormal rhythm, usually atrial fibrillation, is the cause of the clot which passes to the brain.

Manifestations of Stroke

These three different events that can interrupt blood flow to the brain cause three distinct clinical pictures. Clotting of a cerebral artery causes a lessening of body function, generally without pain or seizures. An arterial rupture is frequently accompanied by a severe headache with rapid loss of consciousness. A cerebral embolism may also occur suddenly with a convulsion or paralysis or the abrupt loss of consciousness.

Regardless of the different onsets of a stroke, the final manifestation is made up of variable signs and symptoms, depending on the area of the brain damaged.

Strokes may produce the following effects:

1. Paralysis of extremities, unilateral or bilateral
2. Diminished consciousness, varying from coma to confusion or dizziness
3. Difficulty with speech or vision
4. Convulsions (although many individuals have epilepsy or experience convulsions from other causes without any damage to the brain whatsoever)
5. Headache alone

Care of Patient with a Stroke

The initial care of the patient with a stroke should include the careful observation of vital signs.

Is respiration regular or irregular? Certain characteristic hesitancies in the breathing pattern occur in some patients with stroke. Others may have very rapid, but not labored, respirations. Is the frequency of breathing sufficient or will supportive respiratory assistance be required?

Taking a pulse both at the wrist and the throat can be important. It is helpful to observe early in the course of a stroke whether both carotid pulses (one on each side of the throat) are present or absent. When palpating the pulse, its regularity or lack of regularity should be noted. An irregularity of the pulse may indicate underlying heart disease and therefore suggest a cause for the stroke.

The blood pressure should be taken. A very high blood pressure associated with a slow pulse is often a sign of marked swelling of the brain. Immediate care by a physician is necessary for this patient.

Additional problems specifically relating to the patient with a stroke, and to his family, are also extremely important in the overall care. Anything that will increase the anxiety of the patient must be avoided; overly energetic handling on the part of the EMT or the family may aggravate the stroke. The single most important aspect of emergency treatment for this patient is thoughtful, tender, loving care. In this time of crisis, both the patient and the family need calm reassurance.

Even though the patient may be unable to speak and may appear to be unconscious, he may be able to hear and comprehend what is taking place around him. Look for signs which indicate he understands his situation.

Oxygen should be administered only if there is breathing difficulty or cyanosis. When lifting and transporting the patient, always protect paralyzed arms or legs.

Nothing should be given by mouth, as the throat may be paralyzed. If the patient is unconscious or comatose and choking on his own saliva, transportation should be on the side, preferably with the paralyzed side down. Clear the airway by suction, and give oxygen. Transportation to the Emergency Department must be as gentle as possible.

239

CHAPTER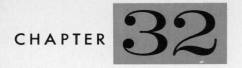

Diabetes Mellitus

GOAL I. Understand the causes and complications of diabetes mellitus.

OBJECTIVES

A. Explain the mechanism of sugar digestion.
B. Describe the symptoms of diabetes mellitus.
C. List the symptoms of diabetic coma.
D. List the symptoms of insulin shock.

GOAL II. Know the treatment for the complications of diabetes.

OBJECTIVES

A. Describe the therapy for the conscious diabetes patient.
B. Describe the therapy for the unconscious diabetes patient.

A certain amount of sugar is always present in a normal person's blood, for all cells require sugar as an energy source to function properly. Diabetes mellitus (commonly called sugar diabetes) is an inherited disease in which the body is unable to utilize sugar normally as an energy source because of a deficiency of insulin, a hormone produced by the pancreas.

Insulin is a substance necessary to enable sugar in the blood to enter the cells of the body. Diabetes mellitus occurs when inadequate amounts of insulin are secreted by the pancreas.

Diabetes mellitus is treatable. Some diabetic patients are able to control their disease by proper diet alone; others do well with pills; many require an injection of insulin once or twice a day. Insulin introduced into the body has an action similar to that produced by the pancreas. The amount of insulin taken must be balanced against the food intake of the diabetic patient, since some sugar is present in all foods.

If there is not enough insulin in the blood, the glucose (sugar) in the blood cannot be utilized by the cells of the body because it is not released to them. The glucose retained in the blood will rise to an extremely high level, which will indeed force some sugar into the cells, but the high concentration is not enough to keep them from being starved. The high level of sugar in the blood has an extremely harmful effect, however, as it leads to an excessive loss of both sugar and fluid in the urine. The loss of sugar and fluid in the urine causes the classic symptoms of uncontrolled diabetes mellitus: polyuria (frequent urination) and polydipsia (frequent drinking of liquids to satisfy thirst).

Diabetic Coma and Insulin Shock

The patient with diabetes may become an emergency case because of one of two conditions: diabetic coma or insulin shock.

Diabetic coma. The body will attempt to overcome the lack of sugar in its cells by using other foods for energy, and will draw upon the fat it has stored. Unfortunately, the use of such sources is not only inefficient but the waste products from the use of fat for normal energy requirements markedly increase the acidity of the blood. If the loss of fluid and the increase of acidity are severe enough, diabetic coma will occur. In this condition, the sugar level in the blood is very high, but the sugar level does not directly cause the coma. The presence of acidic waste products in the blood and the loss of fluid cause the coma. Both these conditions are brought about by the imbalance between the sugar in the blood and in the body cells.

242

Development of coma commonly occurs when a diabetic patient who is untreated or who fails to take prescribed insulin undergoes some sort of stress, such as an infection. The patient may then be found comatose with the following physical signs:

1. Air hunger, manifested by rapid and deep sighing respirations (Kussmaul respiration)
2. Dehydration (dry, warm skin and sunken eyes)
3. A sweet or fruity (acetone) odor on the breath, caused by the acid in the blood
4. A rapid, weak pulse
5. A normal or slightly low blood pressure
6. Varying degrees of unresponsiveness

Insulin shock (hypoglycemia). Insulin shock may result when too much insulin has been given, or when the patient has not eaten enough food, or has exercised excessively. Sugar is rapidly driven out of the blood and into the cells, and not enough sugar remains available in the blood for the use of the brain. Since the brain requires as constant a supply of glucose as it does of oxygen, unconsciousness and permanent brain damage can quickly occur if blood sugar remains low.

Insufficient sugar in the blood (hypoglycemia) is associated with the following signs and symptoms:

1. Normal respiration
2. Pale, moist skin
3. Dizziness; headache
4. Full, rapid pulse
5. Normal blood pressure
6. Fainting; seizures; coma

Diagnosis and Treatment

If a diabetic patient becomes an emergency case, it may be difficult for an inexperienced person, even knowing the patient has diabetes, to tell the difference between the signs of diabetic coma and insulin shock.

In cases of sugar imbalance from either cause, if the patient has not yet reached the coma stage, he may feel sick or be only semiconscious. But he can frequently inform the EMT about the exact cause of his illness. In taking care of an ill diabetic patient, ask him or his family these two questions:

1. Have you eaten today?
2. Have you taken your insulin today?

If the patient has eaten but has not taken insulin, the problem is probably diabetic coma. If the patient has taken insulin but has not eaten, the problem is probably insulin shock. A diabetic patient will usually know what is the matter; so listen carefully.

If the patient is unconscious, the EMT may be able to decide on the basis of the signs and symptoms discussed above whether the problem is diabetic coma or insulin shock. The primary visible difference will be the patient's breathing —deep sighing respirations in diabetic coma and normal respirations in insulin shock. A diabetic patient who is unconscious and having seizures is more likely to be in insulin shock. All noticeable differences are compared in Table 32.1.

Care for these conditions includes these steps:

1. The patient in diabetic coma (too much blood sugar) needs insulin and perhaps other medication. Transport this patient to the hospital immediately for proper medical care.
2. The patient in insulin shock (low blood sugar) needs sugar in his system. The administration of any sugar solution may promptly reverse insulin shock.
3. The EMT should check the patient for an A.M.A. Emergency Medical Identification Symbol (Fig. 4.5), which may be found as a wallet card, necklace, or bracelet. It will advise if the patient has a known

TABLE 32.1
DIAGNOSTIC SIGNS IN DIABETIC EMERGENCIES

	DIABETIC COMA	INSULIN SHOCK
HISTORY		
Food	Excessive	Insufficient
Insulin	Insufficient	Excessive
Onset	Gradual—days	Sudden—minutes
Appearance of patient	Extremely ill	Very weak
Skin	Red and dry	Pale and moist
Infection	May be present	Absent
GASTROINTESTINAL SYSTEM		
Mouth	Dry	Drooling
Thirst	Intense	Absent
Hunger	Absent	Intense
Vomiting	Common	Uncommon
Abdominal pain	Frequent	Absent
RESPIRATORY SYSTEM		
Breathing	Exaggerated air hunger	Normal or shallow
Odor of Breath	Acetone odor usual (sweet, fruity)	Acetone odor may be present
CARDIOVASCULAR SYSTEM		
Blood pressure	Low	Normal
Pulse	Rapid	Normal, may be rapid
VISION	Dim	Diplopia (double vision)
NERVOUS SYSTEM		
Headache	Present	Absent
Mental State	Restlessness merging into unconsciousness	Apathy, irritability merging into unconsciousness
Tremors	Absent	Present
Convulsions	None	In late stages
URINE		
Sugar	Present	Absent
Acetone	Present	May be present
IMPROVEMENT	Gradual, within 6 to 12 hours following administration of insulin	Immediate improvement following oral administration of carbohydrates (glucose, candy, orange juice, ginger ale, sugar.)

243

medical problem and can possibly save the EMT from having to grope for a diagnosis.

When undecided, give sugar. Because it is often difficult to determine the precise nature of the diabetic condition, **sugar should be given to any unconscious or semiconscious diabetic patient, even though the final diagnosis may be diabetic coma (too much sugar in the blood).** The reason for giving sugar is that untreated insulin shock (too little sugar in the blood) resulting in unconsciousness can quickly cause brain damage or death. As a matter of priority, the patient in insulin shock is far more critical and far more likely to have brain damage than the patient in diabetic coma. If the EMT gives sugar to a patient in insulin shock, he may save the patient's life or avoid brain damage. The patient in insulin shock should respond promptly to the giving of sugar and awaken within one to two minutes. A person having such a reaction must be transported to a hospital as soon as possible. By the time he reaches the hospital, he may have responded to the sugar. Whether he requires hospitalization is then a decision for his physician to make.

On the other hand, if the EMT gives sugar to a patient in a diabetic coma, there is little risk of seriously worsening his condition. Brain damage or death will occur, if at all, only after a longer period, during which a physician's assistance can be obtained. Diabetic coma requires hours of insulin and fluid therapy, which should be done only under a physician's care. Prompt transportation to the Emergency Department with all usual precautions is indicated.

In the conscious patient, sugar cubes, granulated sugar, candy, or any fruit juice (sweetened with additional sugar if available) will reverse an insulin reaction. If the patient is unconscious, and therefore not able to swallow, intravenous glucose should be given. The proper dose is 50 ml (one ampule) of a 50-percent solution of Dextrose in water, administered steadily over three to four minutes intravenously.

Do not attempt to put liquid into the mouth of an unconscious individual as it may be aspirated into the lungs. If it is not possible to give an intravenous solution, a cube of sugar or concentrated glucose may be placed under the tongue of an unconscious person, as some sugar is absorbed through the lining of the mouth. The patient should be observed closely by the EMT until the sugar cube or glucose tablet has dissolved, because it could become displaced from under the tongue and lodge in the patient's esophagus or trachea.

CHAPTER 33

Dyspnea

GOAL I. Understand the causes and mechanisms of shortness of breath.

OBJECTIVES

A. Define dyspnea.

B. List the medical causes of shortness of breath.

C. Describe the means by which the blood acquires oxygen and loses carbon dioxide.

D. Describe how the level of carbon dioxide in the blood affects respiration.

E. Describe the effects of excess carbon dioxide in the body.

F. Describe how the level of oxygen in the blood affects respiration.

GOAL II. Understand problems of the lungs and other problems that cause shortness of breath and know the appropriate treatments for these problems.

OBJECTIVES

A. List the causes of chronic lung disease.

B. Describe the clinical presentation of lung disease.

C. Describe the clinical findings of lung disease.

D. Describe the emergency treatment of lung disease and special precautions for such treatment.

E. Define asthma.

F. Describe the emergency therapy for asthma.

G. Describe hyperventilation and the therapy for it.

Dyspnea is defined as the "sensation" of shortness of breath. It is a symptom the patient complains of, and it may be accompanied by signs of labored or difficult breathing. Difficult breathing or the sensation of dyspnea may result from a variety of medical or traumatic causes. The traumatic causes of breathing difficulty are discussed elsewhere (Chapter 6, Injuries of the Chest); the discussion in this chapter is limited to dyspnea from nontraumatic causes.

Causes of Dyspnea

Medical problems where dyspnea, or evidence of breathing difficulty, is present include:

1. Acute pulmonary edema
2. Obstruction of the airway by aspiration of vomitus or foreign objects
3. Chronic obstructive lung disease (emphysema or chronic bronchitis)
4. Asthma or allergic reactions

5. Dyspnea without lung abnormalities (hyperventilation)

Obstruction of the airway may occur in semiconscious and unconscious individuals as a result of the position of the head, obstruction by the tongue, or aspiration of vomitus. Proper opening of the airway by neck extension may solve the problem, but hyperextension may be done only after a head or neck injury has been ruled out. If simple opening of the airway does not correct the breathing problem, a search for upper-airway obstruction should be undertaken. Upper-airway obstruction should be considered first in any dyspneic patient who has been eating just before the onset of breathing trouble, in crawling babies, and in young children.

Pulmonary Physiology

The major function of the lung is to provide oxygen to the blood and to take carbon dioxide from the blood and expel it from the body in the expired air.

In order to carry out the exchange of oxygen and carbon dioxide properly, there must be no impairment of the flow of inspired and expired air to and from the areas of pulmonary blood flow. The problem in most disorders of the lung is that pulmonary blood flow is so located that damage of the airway or of the lung itself can prevent the exchange of gases. Also, abnormalities of the pulmonary blood vessels themselves may interfere with blood flow and thus with the proper delivery of oxygen.

Any type of lung disease that causes too little oxygen to enter the blood is detrimental to the body. An excessive level of carbon dioxide may also have an adverse effect. The stimulus that causes an individual to breathe is the level of carbon dioxide in the arterial blood. If the carbon dioxide in the blood drops below its normal level, one automatically breathes at a lower rate per minute and less deeply. This response, which causes less carbon dioxide to be expired, allows the amount in the blood to rise and the level to return to normal. On the other hand, should carbon dioxide build up in the arterial blood, one breathes at a more rapid rate and more deeply, "blowing off" carbon dioxide and thereby lowering its amount in the arterial blood. The arterial level of carbon dioxide is controlled breath by breath and is so regulated that very little variation in its level occurs in the normal healthy person.

Carbon dioxide and oxygen levels in arterial blood. If, because of any kind of lung disease, the vessels or airways are deranged so that the blow-off of carbon dioxide is impaired, its level in the blood begins to rise. If the carbon dioxide rises rapidly, or even slowly, to high levels, the respiratory center (the area in the brain that senses the level of carbon dioxide and controls respiration) is narcotized (depressed). This carbon dioxide narcosis may be so severe and the respiratory center so depressed that the patient fails to have a stimulus to breathe at all, as far as carbon dioxide is concerned. Respiration will then cease unless a secondary drive for respiration takes over. Fortunately, a second stimulus does exist. A low level of oxygen in the blood will also impel one to breathe, although this oxygen stimulus is not as strong as the carbon dioxide drive.

Chronic Obstructive Lung Disease

Chronic obstructive lung disease is a slow process of disruption of the normal airways, the alveoli, and the pulmonary blood vessels. The process may be a result of lung damage by repeated infections or by inhalation of toxic industrial agents. Most commonly, the combination of damage from cigarette smoking and frequent lung infections is the cause. In one form, the patient's arterial oxygen level falls and the arterial carbon dioxide level rises. If infection of the lung is added to this chronic condition, the carbon dioxide level may quickly rise to the point of suppressing the breathing drive. Patients with chronic lung disease cannot handle pulmonary infections well because the existing airway damage causes them to be unable to cough up the mucus or sputum produced.

In another form of chronic lung disease, there is no retention of carbon dioxide but low oxygen levels are present.

Clinical presentation. The patient with chronic obstructive lung disease (emphysema or chronic bronchitis) is generally elderly. The chest has a barrel-like appearance because air is continuously trapped within the lung. Generally, the patient may have lost weight slowly and will be thin. He may be only semiconscious or unconscious from carbon dioxide narcosis. He will appear in respiratory distress, using accessory muscles to breathe, including the muscles in the neck and shoulders to expand the chest. He will purse his lips to puff air out.

The history, if obtainable, will reveal a sudden increase in shortness of breath on top of a long history of dyspnea, although there rarely is any history of chest pain. The patient will probably have had a recent "chest cold" and may have noted fever as well as inability to cough up sputum. If he can cough up sputum, it will be thick and green or yellow in color. He will be a smoker.

Blood pressure will be normal and the pulse rapid, occasionally irregular. Particular attention must be paid to the respiratory rate. It may be rapid or it may be very slow (carbon dioxide narcosis). Listening to the chest will reveal rales, wheezes, and rhonchi (a whistling, snoring sound), but sounds of breathing may be very hard to hear and often may be heard only high up on the posterior chest.

Approach to the patient. As always, the patient's status (vital signs) should be noted, with particular attention to the respiratory rate. Reassurance should be given and a kind, professional approach assumed. Oxygen treatment should be given. However, great care must be taken to observe the respiratory rate and to judge the effectiveness of the respirations. Repeated evaluations, at least every five minutes, are necessary until the Emergency Department is reached. This care is important as the rise of arterial oxygen may diminish the respiratory drive while the carbon dioxide level remains high. It takes a long time to correct a high arterial carbon dioxide level, but the oxygen content may rise at once when enriched air (air with oxygen) is given. If the respirations fall below twelve per minute, breathing assistance with a bag and mask should be given. Oxygen should

be continued. The patient should be urged to breathe as deeply as he can.

Asthma

Bronchial asthma may occur at any age. The disease is caused by abnormal spasm of the airway passages, which produces a characteristic wheezing as the patient attempts to breathe out. Usually no abnormality in the level of blood gases, oxygen, and carbon dioxide occurs, and between attacks many patients have normal lung function. An allergic response to a bee sting or to substances injected, ingested, or inhaled may produce an acute asthmatic attack.

Clinical presentation. The patient may be young or old. There is obvious respiratory distress, and the wheezing on expiration may be heard without the stethoscope. While the individual can draw air in without much difficulty, the expiration or the outflow of air is greatly restricted. The restriction causes the person to labor to push each breath out. The effort to exhale is tiring and frightening to the subject.

The history is one of episodic attacks of shortness of breath, with the patient completely normal between the episodes. Since the public generally tends to call all lung trouble asthma, it is important to find out whether the patient has recurrent attacks of this nature but can breathe normally at other times. Always ask the patient to describe what he means by asthma.

Chest pain is rarely present. The pulse rate will be normal and the blood pressure may be slightly elevated as a consequence of the tension and anxiety the person feels or the medication that likely has been taken to alleviate the attack. The respiratory rate will also be increased.

Approach to the patient. Patient status (vital signs) should be assessed and a history obtained. Reassurance and oxygen therapy should be given. The person should be allowed to sit up, as breathing will be much easier in this position. If the respiratory distress is severe, an IV should be started. Many persons with asthma have medications to take when an attack occurs. These medications should be sought and administered with the assistance of the EMT. Transportation to the Emergency Department should be rapid and gentle.

247

Dyspnea without Lung Abnormalities (Hyperventilation)

Clinical presentation. Hyperventilation is described as over-breathing to the extent that arterial carbon dioxide is abnormally lowered. When over-breathing blows off too much carbon dioxide, the blood pH will be raised above normal. The body will experience alkalosis, which is the cause of many of the symptoms associated with over-breathing. It is a common response to psychological stress—almost as common a reaction as headache or stomach upset. One can produce some of the symptoms in one's self by breathing as deeply and as rapidly as possible for three to five minutes. However, an individual often will not realize he has been hyperventilating.

The patient is generally terrified of death. He may feel that it is not possible to get enough air into his chest, despite the fact that a larger quantity than usual is being exchanged. Dizziness and a faint feeling are common. Often the person experiences a sensation of numbness or tingling of the hands and feet, which may also be described as being cold. Fainting may occur. Sticking, stabbing chest pains that increase with respiration may occur. Vital signs reveal rapid breathing and a high-pulse rate (tachycardia) with normal blood pressure.

Differential diagnoses. Other illnesses may cause a reaction that looks like simple over-breathing. The principal means of the body for the defense of pH (keeping a normal level of acidity of blood) is to vary the respiratory rate. If the blood pH falls (becomes acid) from diabetic ketoacidosis, from acidosis due to poor tissue perfusion (following cardiac arrest), or from the ingestion of acid, the body attempts to return the pH to normal by blowing off carbon dioxide.

Blood clots that have migrated to the lung and formed a pulmonary embolism can also bring on hyperventilation.

Approach to the patient. The patient's status should be assessed and a history obtained. The key to treatment is kindness and reassurance.

A maneuver to build up the blood carbon dioxide is to ask the patient to breathe into a paper bag. This will cause him to rebreathe his own exhaled breath and raise the arterial carbon dioxide. Do not worry about oxygen; the patient will receive sufficient oxygen, as exhaled breath is not exclusively carbon dioxide.

The patient should be transported rapidly to the Emergency Department. It is easy for the EMT to make an incorrect diagnosis and all these patients should be seen by a physician for a definitive diagnosis.

248

CHAPTER # 34

Unconscious States

GOAL I. Know the causes and types of loss of consciousness.

249

OBJECTIVES

A. List the common causes of unconsciousness.
B. Describe the differences in the causes of loss of consciousness.
C. Explain what brings on unconsciousness in the common faint.
D. Name the types of convulsions in epilepsy.
E. Understand how a convulsion is brought on.

GOAL II. Know the appropriate emergency therapy for an unconscious person.

OBJECTIVES

A. Describe the general care of an unconscious patient.
B. Describe the care of a person who has fainted.
C. Describe the treatment of and special considerations for the person who has a convulsion.
D. Describe the treatment of the patient who has taken a drug overdose.

In caring for the unconscious patient, the EMT's approach should be directed initially toward treatment for the unconsciousness and then toward determination of the specific cause. Some of the illnesses accompanied by unconsciousness have been discussed in other chapters of this book. In this chapter, a discussion of the common faint, epilepsy, and reaction to drug overdose will be presented.

Emergency Care

In every unconscious patient care must be taken to assure an open airway and to provide respiratory support when necessary. A supine unconscious patient may be in danger of aspiration of vomitus or other oral contents and suffocation from an obstructed airway. If injury of the neck has been ruled out and the airway opened, the patient should be placed on one side, face down, with care being taken to keep the airway open. He must be transported in this position with continued monitoring of respiration.

A history should be sought regarding previous unconsciousness, epilepsy, or any known medical illness, including details of drug usage and the possibility of a drug overdose. A check should be made for a medical identification symbol for a possible clue to the cause of the unconscious state. Emergency Department personnel will be aided by a knowledge of the patient's history.

Verify vital signs and the presence of any injuries. Note whether the pupils of the eyes are constricted or widely dilated. Transport the patient promptly to the Emergency Department.

The Common Faint

The exact mechanism of the common faint is unclear, but apparently a marked slowing of the pulse occurs without an increase in blood flow per heartbeat, resulting in diminished cerebral function. Near faints can usually be avoided by having the patient lie down quickly and by elevating the legs. An increased return of blood to the heart counteracts the effect of the slow pulse and cerebral blood flow then becomes adequate to sustain consciousness. The common faint is not dangerous unless the patient is somehow maintained in an upright position. No specific therapy is necessary other than treatment of any injuries sustained because of falling during the faint.

Epilepsy

Epilepsy is a common condition usually easily controlled by medication. Uncontrolled, it is manifested by convulsions (in epilepsy often called seizures), generally followed by unconconsciousness. Epilepsy may occur as a result of an old brain injury with a scar, acute head trauma, a brain tumor, or a cerebral embolus (a blockage of blood flow inside the brain).

There are two types of convulsions: grand mal (major seizures) and petit mal (seizures which do not cause unconsciousness and which in fact may not be detectable except by trained personnel). A grand mal seizure is manifested by a burst of brain cell activity leading to uncontrollable contractions of the muscles of the body. Contractions of the jaw muscles lead to biting tongue or lips. Loss of bladder or bowel control is common and urination or defecation may take place.

Management. Basically, keep the patient from hurting himself during the attack and assure an open airway and proper respiration during the unconscious state. A "bite stick" (padded tongue blade) may be placed between the patient's teeth to keep him from biting his tongue if it can be inserted easily. Do not ever place fingers between the teeth. The patient's head, arms, and legs should be protected but not rigidly restrained. Contractions of all chest muscles may cause the patient to appear to have an airway obstruction and to turn blue. Normal respiration almost always follows the seizure activity, and the lack of respiration during the attack rarely presents a problem unless several convulsions follow each other in quick succession (status epilepticus). In the latter case, attempts at artificial respiration must be made but are extremely difficult to carry out because of the convulsive movements of the patient.

Following the seizure, an epileptic patient should be transported to the Emergency Department. Since most epileptic patients take some type of medication, a search for it should be made and it should be taken to the hospital.

Drug Overdose

General considerations. In general, the emergency treatment for all drug overdoses is to support the patient until the drug may be cleared or metabolized by the body. In some cases, such as insulin or heroin overdose, treatment may include the use of a specific antagonist. For an insulin overdose, sugar (preferably given in intravenous solution) will reverse the unconscious state. In both instances, definitive therapy must be given rapidly or brain damage may occur.

Therapy. In most overdose states, the primary depression after loss of consciousness will be of the respiratory center. Great care must be taken to insure that the airway is open and that artificial respiration is given if necessary.

If there is a fall in blood pressure, the patient's legs should be elevated slightly. The response of the pupils of the eyes to light should be noted. Widely dilated pupils are characteristic of overdoses of such drugs as barbiturates, whereas constricted pupils occur with the use of narcotics such as demerol or heroin.

Since cardiovascular collapse with resultant shock is an occasional occurrence with overdose, preparation for intravenous infusion should be made prior to transportation.

250

CHAPTER 35

Communicable Disease

251

GOAL I. Understand what constitutes a communicable disease.

OBJECTIVES

A. Define a communicable disease.
B. List modes of transmission of a communicable disease.
C. Define terms used when referring to a communicable disease.

GOAL II. Understand the role of the EMT in dealing with a communicable disease.

OBJECTIVES

A. Define the EMT's role in the control of a communicable disease.
B. List measures to be taken by the EMT to minimize his personal exposure to a communicable disease.
C. List measures the EMT must take in the maintenance of his vehicle when it is exposed to a communicable disease.
D. List measures the EMT must take in handling a patient with a communicable disease.

GOAL III. Know the characteristics and basic epidemiology of the more common communicable diseases.

OBJECTIVES

A. List the sources of common communicable diseases.
B. List the incubation periods of common communicable diseases.
C. List the mode of transmission of common communicable diseases.
D. List communicable diseases for which immunizations are available.
E. State the difference between period of incubation and period of communicability.

A communicable disease is a contagious disease, one which can be transmitted from one person to another. Communicable diseases can be transmitted directly by contact with an infected person, by ingestion of infected food, or by infection of an open skin wound. They can be transmitted indirectly by contact with contaminated objects, such as soiled dressings or clothing from an infected person. Indirect contact implies that the person being infected was not directly in contact with the host or carrier but touched some object that had been contaminated.

Inhaling the droplets spread from an infected person when he coughs or sneezes or inhaling dust contaminated with infecting agents is a third common mode of contracting disease. Depending on the disease, simple precautions can be taken by the EMT to protect himself, other personnel, and the vehicle from contamination. Risks do exist in handling these patients, but with care they can be minimized.

Infection refers to the state produced in a host by the invasion of an infecting or pathogenic organism (virus, bacterium, or parasite). Contamination is the presence of an infectious agent on body surfaces, in water or food, or on objects such as dressings. A host is the organism or person in whom an infectious agent resides. A host is infected. A carrier is a person who may transmit an infective disease but himself have no evidence of it. A carrier may occasionally be immune to the disease but still be able to transmit it.

A reservoir is the place where the infecting organisms live and multiply. The source of infection is the thing, person, or substance from which an infectious agent passes to a host. Sometimes the reservoir is also the source of the infection. The communicable period is the time during which an infectious agent may be transferred from one host to another. The incubation period is the time between infection of an individual and the first appearance of the signs of the disease in that individual.

The Role of the Emergency Medical Technician

In the control of communicable disease, the role of the EMT is to protect himself, other personnel and patients, and the emergency vehicle from contamination. The EMT should have regular physical examinations and yearly chest X rays. The EMT should wash his hands regularly both before and after working with a patient, and should air and clean the emergency vehicle between each transportation of patients. Routine cleaning of the floors, walls, and emergency equipment with soap and water is most important in eliminating sources and reservoirs of infection. Disposable equipment should be used whenever possible.

An EMT who knows in advance that he will be transporting a patient with a communicable disease should carry a disposable gown and mask and should remove all unnecessary equipment from the vehicle. Once the patient has been

removed from the vehicle, all contaminated linen, dressings, and disposable equipment should be placed in a disposable bag. The ambulance should be aired for one to two hours. It should then be thoroughly scrubbed with soap and water. All surfaces should then be scrubbed again for five minutes with a disinfecting agent such as 80 or 90 percent isopropyl alcohol, or a formaldehyde-alcohol preparation, or a phenolic germicide solution. Respiratory equipment in particular is a potential reservoir and source of infection, primarily by the droplet spread of bacteria. Disposable oxygen masks and suction tubing and tips should be used whenever possible.

It is wise for the dispatcher to keep the medical record of the EMT at hand. If a patient with chicken pox requires transportation, it should be done by technicians who have had the disease. In their absence, precautions listed in Table 35.1 can be observed. The medical record should also show an up-to-date notation of the EMT's own immunizing shots.

If it is not known until after an ambulance run has been made that the patient had a contagious disease, the following steps should be taken:

1. Ambulance personnel must be notified and offered appropriate immunization promptly.
2. The ambulance should be thoroughly cleaned as described above.
3. All linen and other articles used that day should be regarded as contaminated.
4. If anyone else has been carried in the ambulance before knowledge of the contagious disease was obtained, the physicians attending that patient must be notified.

Generally, following these procedures will allow adequate protection of the EMTs themselves, other personnel, the vehicle, and the patients.

Communicable Diseases

Some communicable diseases with which the EMT should be familiar are described in Table 35.1.

TABLE 35.1
COMMUNICABLE DISEASES

Disease	Characteristics	Source	Mode of Transmission	Incubation Period	Period of Communicability	Care of Ambulance	Care of Personnel
Chicken pox	Acute febrile viral disease; itchy red rash which leaves scabs; more common in children	Respiratory tract secretions (scabs do not carry infection)	Direct contact; droplet contact	2 to 3 weeks	1 day before skin lesions appear to 6 days after skin lesions appear	Air; scrub; dispose of or boil linens	Wash hands; shower; change clothing
Diphtheria	Acute bacterial infection of throat, tonsils, nose, and sometimes skin with local pain and swelling	Discharge from nose and throat	Direct or indirect contact	2 to 5 days	2 to 4 weeks	Air; scrub; disinfect equipment; launder linen	Immunization; wear mask if not immune
German measles	Feverish viral illness with rash; more common in children; danger of birth defects if contracted during first 3 months of pregnancy	Discharge from nose and throat	Direct contact; indirect contact; droplet contact	14 to 21 days	1 week before rash appears to 4 days after rash appears	Air; scrub; launder linen	None
Gonorrhea	Bacterial venereal disease characterized by thick yellow urethral discharge in males; more difficult to detect in females and may lead to chronic infection	Exudate from mucous membrane	Sexual intercourse	3 to 4 days	Months or years unless treated	Air; launder linen	None

253

TABLE 35.1 (*Continued*)

Disease	Characteristics	Source	Mode of Transmission	Incubation Period	Period of Communicability	Care of Ambulance	Care of Personnel
Infectious hepatitis	Acute viral infection with fever; loss of appetite; jaundice; fatigue	Feces, urine, blood from infected person; dishes, clothing, or bed linen used by infected person; injuries from IV needles used for infected person	Fecal-oral contamination through handling clothes and linen; contaminated water, food, syringes; transfusion from infected person	15 to 30 days	Unknown	Air; scrub; launder linen	Wash hands, use precautions when disposing of IV material, needles, or instruments used for these patients
Malaria	Parasitic tropical disease with cyclic fever; chills, fatigue	Infective mosquito	Mosquito bite	12 to 30 days	Mosquito infection 1 to 3 years	Air; scrub; rid ambulance of insects	None
Measles	Acute viral disease; fever; bronchitis; red blotchy rash; common in childhood	Nose and throat secretions	Direct contact; indirect contact; droplet contact	10 days	4 days before rash appears to 5 days after	Air; scrub; launder linen	None
Meningitis	Acute bacterial disease with fever; severe headache; nausea; vomiting; coma	Nose and throat secretions	Direct contact; droplet contact	2 to 10 days	Varies	Air; scrub; launder linen	If close contact has occurred, see physician
Mononucleosis	Acute viral disease with fever; sore throat; lymph node swelling	Respiratory tract secretions	Unknown; possibly person-to-person oral route	2 to 6 weeks	Unknown	Air; scrub; disinfect articles soiled with nose and throat discharges	None

Disease	Characteristics	Source	Mode of Transmission	Incubation Period	Period of Communicability	Care of Ambulance	Care of Personnel
Mumps	Acute viral disease with fever; swelling and tenderness of the salivary glands	Saliva of infected person	Direct contact; indirect contact; droplet contact	12 to 26 days	7 days before swelling appears to 9 days after	Air; scrub; launder linen	None
Pneumonia	Acute viral or bacterial disease; fever; chills; cough; chest pain	Respiratory tract secretions	Direct contact; indirect contact; droplet contact	Varies	Varies	Air; scrub; launder linen	None
Poliomyelitis	Acute viral disease with fever; headache; gastrointestinal symptoms; stiff neck; paralysis	Nose and throat secretions; feces	Direct contact	7 to 12 days	6 weeks	Air; scrub; disinfect; launder linen; wash hands	None
Rocky Mountain spotted fever	Acute bacterial disease with fever; headache; rash over the body including palms and soles	Infected tick; reservoirs are rodents and dogs	Tick bite	3 to 10 days	Tick's life span	Destroy all ticks	Remove ticks without crushing, protecting hands with gloves if possible
Smallpox	Acute viral disease with fever; headache; abdominal pain; rash with scabbing eruptions	Respiratory discharge; scabs	Direct contact; indirect contact; droplet contact	7 to 16 days	From first symptoms to disappearance	Sterilize by vigorous cleaning using soap, water, and germicides burn linen and clothing	Revaccination
Scarlet fever	Acute bacterial disease with headache; fever, nausea; vomiting; sore throat	Respiratory discharge	Direct contact; indirect contact; droplet contact; carriers exist	2 to 5 days	Unknown	Air; scrub with germicide; boil linen	Wear mask; change; shower; boil clothes

TABLE 35.1 (*Continued*)

Disease	Characteristics	Source	Mode of Transmission	Incubation Period	Period of Communicability	Care of Ambulance	Care of Personnel
Syphillis	Acute bacterial venereal disease; primary lesion seen at 3 weeks as a hard sore which erodes; secondary skin eruptions appear during next 4–6 weeks; late disabling complications of heart and brain occur	Saliva; semen; blood; vaginal discharge during the infectious period	Direct contact through mucosal surface or open wounds; sexual intercourse	10 days to 10 weeks	Variable	Air and launder linens	If scratched or bitten, contact physician
Tuberculosis	Chronic bacterial disease; cough; fatigue; weight loss; chest pain; coughing up of blood	Respiratory secretions; occasionally milk	Direct contact; indirect contact; droplet contact	4 to 6 weeks	As long as live tubercle bacilli are excreted; carriers exist	Air; scrub; disinfect; burn disposable respiratory equipment; boil linens	Wear mask; chest X-ray yearly; skin test periodically
Typhoid Fever	Fever; loss of appetite; diarrhea	Feces and urine	Direct contact; indirect contact; raw fruits; vegetables; milk; carriers exist	2 weeks	As long as typhoid bacilli are excreted	Air; scrub; disinfect; burn linen contaminated with urine or feces	Wash hands
Whooping cough	Acute bacterial disease with violent attacks of coughing; a high-pitched whooping; common among children	Respiratory discharge	Direct contact; indirect contact; droplet contact	7 days to 3 weeks	7 days to 3 weeks	Air; scrub; boil linen	Change; shower; boil clothes

VIII
Childbirth and Special Pediatric Problems

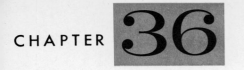

Childbirth

GOAL I. Know the procedures for treatment of pregnant women experiencing emergency problems.

259

OBJECTIVES

A. List four things to do for a pregnant woman with convulsions.
B. List four things to do for a pregnant woman who is hemorrhaging.
C. Describe four signs which indicate that delivery is imminent.
D. Identify three circumstances in which it will probably be necessary for the mother to deliver at the site.

GOAL II. Know the procedure for the delivery of a baby.

OBJECTIVES

A. Describe the preparation of the surface upon which the mother should lie for delivery.
B. Describe the position the mother should assume for delivery.
C. Describe the location of each of the EMTs during delivery.
D. List the steps to be taken in helping to deliver the baby.
E. Identify the characteristics of complicated deliveries.
F. Describe the procedures to follow in various complicated deliveries.

GOAL III. Know the procedures for caring for the baby after it is born.

OBJECTIVES

A. List the things to do for the baby after delivery.
B. Describe the procedure for separating baby and umbilical cord.
C. Describe the signs of a baby requiring resuscitation and the steps in providing resuscitation.
D. Describe characteristics of the premature baby and the procedures for its care.

GOAL IV. Know the procedures for care of the mother after childbirth.

OBJECTIVES

A. Describe procedures to assist the mother after a normal delivery.
B. Describe the procedures for treating a mother who has severe bleeding or other problems following delivery.

The delivery of a baby is an exciting event. The EMT may be called upon to help a mother deliver her baby when there is no time to take her to the hospital, when hospital facilities are not available, or when the hospital cannot be reached, as could be the case in a storm. This chapter contains information necessary to assist a mother in a safe and adequate manner. Always remember that in the great majority of cases the mother delivers her baby and the EMT only assists. The mother pushes the baby out. It is not pulled out.

260

Definitions

The anatomy of a nonpregnant woman and that of a woman eight months pregnant are shown in Figure 36.1. Some of the terms defined below are illustrated there.

Abortion—Delivery of the fetus before it is mature enough to survive out of the uterus.

Most states define this period as less than twenty weeks of pregnancy.

Amniotic sac (bag of waters)—A thin, membranous sack that surrounds the baby inside the uterus. During pregnancy, the fetus floats in about one-half to one liter of amniotic fluid inside the amniotic sac. During labor the sac breaks and the fluid gushes out of the vagina. This happening is normal and should be expected.

Birth canal—The vagina and the lower part of the uterus.

"Bloody show"—The mucus and blood that are discharged from the vagina when labor begins, usually one-half to one ounce. It is often very stringy.

Cervix—The lowermost part of the uterus. The cervix is a tube-like, muscular structure forming the lower part of the uterus. It opens into the vagina. The cervix dilates during labor to allow the baby to enter the vagina.

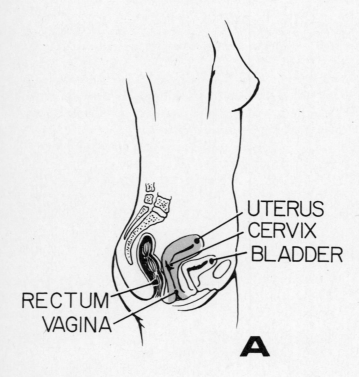

UTERUS
CERVIX
BLADDER
RECTUM
VAGINA
A

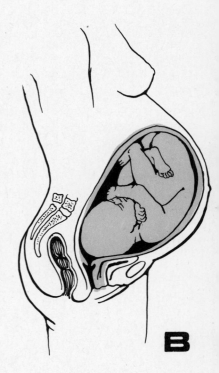

B

Figure 36.1 *a–b*

   The most important anatomic relationships in, *a*, a non-pregnant woman and, *b*, a woman at eight months of pregnancy are shown.

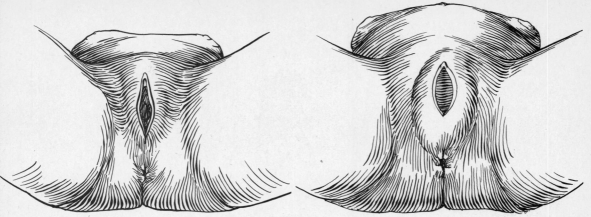

Figure 36.2

Two views of the entrance to the vagina are shown. The first is normal; the second shows crowning just prior to delivery.

Crowning (*bulging*)—The bulging-out of the vaginal opening that occurs when the presenting part of the baby presses on it. The presenting part, often the top of the baby's head, may or may not be visible at this time (Fig. 36.2).

Fetal death certificate—The certificate required when the baby is born dead (stillbirth). In most states stillbirths of less than twenty weeks pregnancy are regarded as abortions. Registration may or may not be required.

Fetus—The developing baby before it is born.

Labor—The process by which the muscles of the uterus open the birth canal and push the baby down and through it to birth. During the most active stage of labor, muscle contractions occur at two- to three-minute intervals and usually last thirty to forty-five seconds. Labor is divided into three stages: *First stage*, from the time the contractions begin (often as much as half an hour or an hour apart) until the cervix is fully opened. *Second stage*, from the time the cervix is fully opened until the baby is born. *Third stage*, from the time of the birth of the baby until one hour after the delivery of the placenta.

Live birth certificate—A certificate that a live birth has occurred, regardless of the length of the pregnancy. This registration is required by all states. The certificate may usually be signed by the person attending the birth, not necessarily by a trained medical person.

Perineum—The skin between the opening of the vagina and the anus.

Placenta (*afterbirth*)—A special organ of pregnancy attached to the wall of the uterus through which the baby receives its nourishment and gets rid of its waste products during the pregnancy. After the birth of the baby the placenta is expelled through the birth canal. The placenta is usually one-fifth the size and weight of the baby.

Presenting part—The part of the baby that emerges from the mother first. Usually the head comes out first (Fig. 36.3). A head-first delivery is called a cephalic delivery. When the buttocks or feet come first, it is called a breech delivery.

Umbilical cord—The rope-like attachment

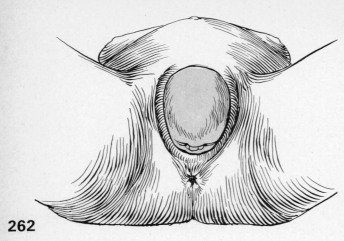

262

Figure 36.3

A view of the top of the baby's head as it presents is shown. This presentation is normal.

between the placenta and the infant's navel, usually about twenty inches in length. Through it, the infant receives nourishment from the placenta and passes waste back to the placenta before birth.

Uterus (womb)—The muscular organ that holds and nourishes the fetus. The uterus opens into the vagina through the cervix.

Vagina—The lower part of the birth canal opening to the outside (Fig. 36.2).

Equipment and Supplies

Each emergency vehicle should carry at all times a sterile delivery pack containing the items listed below:

1 pair of surgical scissors
3 hemostats or cord clamps
Umbilical tape or sterilized cord
Ear syringe, rubber-bulb type, for aspiration of the baby's mouth and airway
5 towels
1 dozen 4 × 4-inch gauze sponges
3 or 4 pairs of rubber gloves
1 baby blanket
Sanitary napkins (may be kept separate in an open box if they are sterile and individually wrapped)
2 large plastic bags

Predelivery Emergencies

In convulsions caused by epilepsy or by toxemia of pregnancy (eclampsia), place a padded tongue-depressor or a fold of a towel in the mother's mouth to prevent biting the tongue and to prevent the tongue from falling back and blocking the airway. Place the mother on one side and, when she regains consciousness and there is no danger of aspiration of vomitus or mucus, elevate the shoulders and head 30 to 40 degrees above the horizontal. Transporation to a medical facility should be as gentle as possible with the shoulders and head elevated.

Patients with convulsions, heart complications, lung complications, and other disturbances should be given oxygen. It will not harm the unborn baby.

Patients who are pregnant or thought to be pregnant may hemorrhage through the vagina. Patients who are losing blood in excess of a bloody show should **not** be examined vaginally. They should be treated as are other patients who are losing blood, that is, an intravenous infusion started, oxygen administered, and body temperature maintained. As a rule, a pregnant patient who is lying down should be encouraged to lie on one side or the other instead of the back.

If a woman in labor has sustained injuries, as in an automobile accident, the general principles of emergency care should be followed. Keeping the mother's respiratory and circulatory systems operative are of prime importance.

Evaluating the Mother

Upon arrival where a woman is in labor, the first decision to make is whether to transport her to a medical facility. As a general rule, it is preferable to do so. If the birth should occur during the trip and in a properly equipped vehicle, mother and baby can be cared for about as easily as in a home. In some circumstances, however, it is necessary to deliver the patient where the EMT finds her. These circumstances would include:

1. When the delivery can be expected within the next few minutes

2. When the medical facility can no longer be reached, as in a disaster or castastrophe
3. When there is no transportation available

To help determine whether the delivery can be expected within the next few minutes, the following questions must be answered. The mother may be asked the first two. The third must be answered by examination.

1. Has the mother ever had a baby before? A mother having a first baby usually has a slower labor, and it can be expected that she can be transported more readily.
2. Does she feel that she has to strain or move her bowels? If she is experiencing this sensation, it usually means that the presenting part is just inside the vaginal entrance and delivery will occur soon.
3. Is the vagina bulging or is the presenting part visible through the entrance (crowning)? Most of these patients will have the sensation of having to move their bowels. The EMT should look at the vaginal entrance (underwear should be completely removed) to see if it is bulging or if the presenting part is beginning to appear through it. The examination should be visual. Look but do not touch.

In general, a patient who is straining as if to have a bowel movement, whose vagina is bulging, or whose baby is beginning to crown through the vaginal entrance should not be transported. **Do not let this patient go to the bathroom.** Do not hold or tie the mother's legs together or have the mother cross her legs to restrain or delay delivery. Under these circumstances, it is best to prepare for the arrival of the baby.

Normal Delivery

Once it is decided there is no time to transport the mother to a hospital, have someone try to summon a physician to the house. If a physician cannot be obtained, try to find a woman who has had some experience in childbirth to help. The father or another person should be sent to seek this help, while the EMT makes preparations for the delivery of the baby.

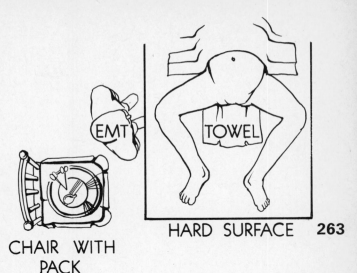

CHAIR WITH PACK

HARD SURFACE   263

Figure 36.4

In this view from above, the EMT is near the patient's right knee in a position to observe the entrance of the birth canal. The instruments are on a chair close at hand. Note the projection of the surface beyond the mother's vagina so that the baby may be delivered onto a shelf.

Remember that the mother delivers the baby, but the EMT can do certain things to help. Remember that you are helping the mother and protecting the baby. You do not pull the baby out. You guide it and support it as it passes through the vagina.

It is best for the mother to deliver on a hard surface which has been elevated to a height that makes it easy for the attendant to assist her. The hard surface may be softened somewhat by blankets, newspapers, folded sheets, or towels. Ordinarily, it will be necessary to have the patient in a bed. If there is enough assistance, the bed can be elevated by chairs. Table leaves, ironing boards, pieces of plywood, or something similar can be placed between the springs and the mattress to make the bed firmer and to prevent pooling of the amniotic fluid and blood that come with the baby. Large quantities of newspapers laid under the sheet may protect the mattress.

The patient should lie on her back with the knees up and the feet flat on the surface (Fig. 36.4). If possible, first put a stretcher on the bed or table and place the mother on it, as this will facilitate transportation later and permit a minimum of handling after delivery. Put a clean, folded sheet, blanket, or newspapers under the patient's buttocks to lift them about two inches off the surface. Have her bend the knees and spread the thighs apart. In an automobile, the mother may be placed flat on the seat with one leg bent and resting on the seat and the other bent with her foot resting on the floorboard.

Someone, the husband or another EMT, should sit at the mother's head to reassure her and encourage her in a quiet, comforting way. Frequently the mother will want to grip someone's hand. The person talking with the mother should be ready to assist if she vomits by turning her face to one side and cleaning out her mouth when necessary.

The EMT should stand on the right side of the patient if he is righthanded or on the left if lefthanded. If a table is used, there should be at least two feet of table beyond the mother's buttocks so that the slippery baby may be delivered onto a shelf (Fig. 36.4).

Opening the Delivery Pack and Draping the Mother

The emergency delivery pack should be placed on a table or chair beside the patient, on the same side where the EMT is working. Very often there is quite a gush of amniotic fluid, and the delivery pack should be placed so that it will not be contaminated. At the same time, it must be placed close enough that the EMT can reach the equipment easily. The EMT should wash his hands and put on a pair of sterile gloves.

Taking the first sterile towel, fold it and place it under the mother's buttocks in such a way that the hands do not touch the other linen or the patient. The next towel should be placed on the bed or table between the patient's legs just below the opening of the vagina, and the third towel should be placed across her abdomen. The remaining towels will be available for other use.

The Delivery

The EMT should stand in such a way that he can observe the vaginal opening constantly. Encourage the mother to relax and rest between contractions. She should not strain unless abso-

lutely necessary. Encourage her to breathe through her mouth as deeply as she can without discomfort.

She may protest that she has to move her bowels. Explain that this feeling is caused by the pressure of the baby's head on her rectum and that it is a normal sensation. Quietly reassure her that this is one sign that the baby will soon be delivered.

When the baby's head begins to push out of the vagina with each contraction, place the gloved hand (right hand for righthanded persons, left hand for lefthanded persons) on its head and exert very gentle pressure. Do not touch the mother's skin. The pressure you exert should be sufficient to allow the head to come out slowly, but it should not be enough to keep the head from being born. Do not let the head suddenly pop out of the vagina. Very often it may take two, three, or more contractions for the birth to occur. The hand should be removed from the head when the pushing-out force ceases, and be reapplied when it begins again.

When the baby's head is born, look and feel to see if the umbilical cord is wrapped around the neck. If it is, try to slip the cord gently over the baby's upper shoulder. If the cord is tightly wrapped around the neck, clamp it with two clamps placed 2 inches apart and then cut it between the clamps and unwrap the end from the baby's neck. Be careful not to tear the cord or to clamp or cut the baby's skin with the instruments.

When the baby's head is born, its face is usually turned down toward the rectum of the mother (Fig. 36.5). Commonly, the face then will turn toward one thigh or the other (Fig. 36.6). At this point the EMT should place his right hand (left hand for lefthanded persons) under the baby's head and support it as the mother pushes the rest of the baby out.

As soon as the chin is born and the face turns (or if the face doesn't turn and stays looking downward), the EMT should pick up the bulb syringe, compress it completely, and insert the tip gently into the mouth of the baby for a distance of about one or one and one-half inches and slowly release the compression. This procedure should suck out some mucus and water

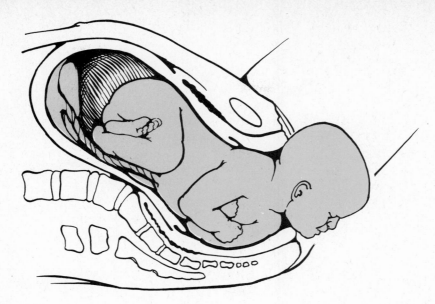

Figure 36.5

   A side view as the baby's head leaves the vagina shows the face pointed in the direction of the rectum.

from the baby's mouth. Next, expel the contents of the syringe on the towel lying across the abdomen, compress the syringe again, and re-insert it. Repeat the suction two or three times in the baby's mouth and once in each side of its nose.

After the baby's head is turned, the upper shoulder will usually become visible in the vaginal entrance (Fig. 36.7). As the baby's ab-domen and hips are born, the EMT should put his other hand under that part of the baby so that from that point on two hands are holding

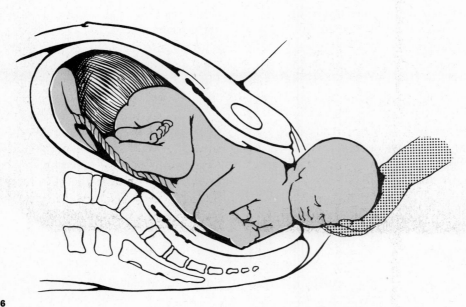

Figure 36.6

   A side view of the baby's head as it starts to rotate before the shoulders are delivered shows the face turning toward one thigh. The head must be supported by the EMT at this stage of the delivery.

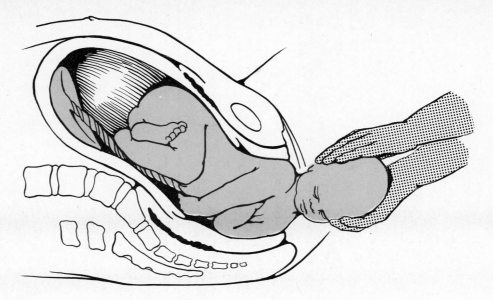

Figure 36.7

A side view shows the upper shoulder being delivered. Support of baby's head must be continued. Do not pull on the baby.

266

the baby. When the feet have been born, grasp them as shown in Figure 36.8. The EMT must be careful to hold the baby's head in such a fashion that the neck is not compressed. Do not hold the baby with its head straight down.

Remember that the baby will be very slippery and should be carefully placed on the table or bed as soon as this can be done. It is best that the baby be placed on its side with the head slightly lower than its body. Take a sterile gauze and wipe the blood and mucus from the baby's nose and mouth. Then suck out the nose and mouth again with the bulb syringe (Fig. 36.9). At all times the baby should be on its side with the head only slightly lower than the trunk. The baby should generally be at the same level as the mother's birth canal or below. Do not place the baby on the mother's abdomen.

By this time the baby is usually breathing on its own and its color will generally be pink. It is common, however, for the feet and hands to retain a blue color for a long period of time. It is usually necessary to suck out the baby's mouth and nose several times between the time of its birth and when it is taken to the hospital. The baby should be kept warm by a blanket or towel so arranged that only the baby's face is

exposed. The towel or blanket should be warmed to about 90° F temperature if possible.

Care of the Umbilical Cord

After the baby's nose and throat are clear and it is breathing, and after it is wrapped carefully, clamp the cord with two clamps 3 inches apart about 6 inches from the navel (Fig. 36.10). There is no hurry to carry out this procedure while the baby remains at the level of the birth canal. Then, use the sterile scissors to cut the cord between the clamps.

Working with the part of the cord still attached to the baby and using the umbilical tape from the pack, tie the cord off closer to the baby's naval about one inch from the clamp. Umbilical tape is used because the cord would be cut through by ordinary string or thread. Compress the cord slowly with the tape so that it does not cut through. Use a square knot and leave both clamp and tie on the cord. The portion of the cord running from the tie to the baby should not be pulled or stretched while the tape is being tied as it might tear off from the baby's abdomen.

Finish wrapping the baby in a sterile blanket or towel and carefully hand it to an assistant.

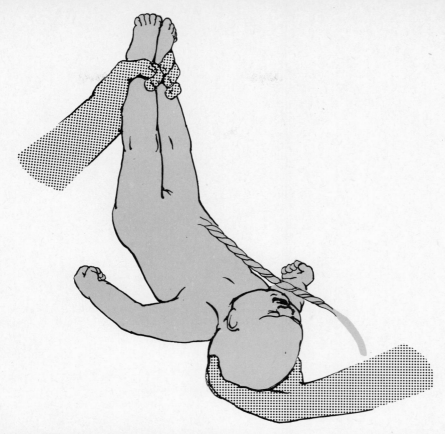

Figure 36.8

When the baby is fully delivered, remember that it will be very slippery and must be held firmly and carefully.

Management of the Placenta

With the delivery of the baby, the second stage of labor ends and the third stage begins. The placenta (afterbirth) usually separates from the uterus and is delivered a few minutes after the baby is born, but this process may sometimes take as long as fifteen to thirty minutes. If the placenta does not come out within twenty minutes, transport the mother and the baby without delay to the hospital so a physician can remove it. If the placenta does not deliver and there is

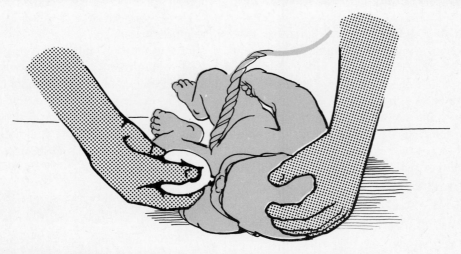

Figure 36.9

Using the bulb syringe, gently suck out the baby's mouth and nose until the airway is clear.

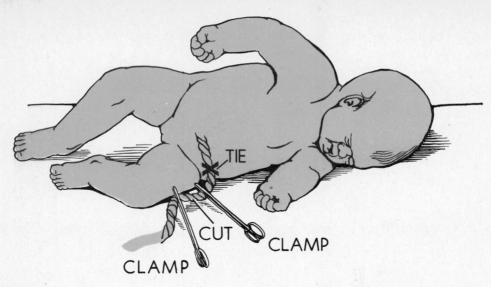

Figure 36.10

The umbilical cord should be clamped with two clamps 3 inches apart and 6 inches from the navel. The cord is then cut between the clamps. As an extra safeguard against bleeding, it is tied again, closer to the navel, with umbilical tape.

heavy bleeding, do not wait at all but transport the mother and baby immediately in an ambulance.

If the mother is hemorrhaging, do the following things during transport:

1. Place her in shock position with the legs elevated, and keep her warm.
2. Give oxygen.
3. Place a sterile pad (sanitary napkin) over the vaginal opening. Do not put anything into the vagina.
4. Gently massage the mother's lower abdomen to cause the uterus to contract and expel the placenta. You will feel a grapefruit-sized object, which is the uterus. Do not push the uterus toward the vagina, but rub it with a light circular motion. You will be able to feel it contract and become firm.
5. If the baby is in good condition, place the baby at the mother's breast and encourage it to nurse. The stimulation of the nipple may cause the uterus to contract and thereby reduce bleeding.

Normally, after the placenta comes out, there is a loss of about one-half pint of blood. Wrap the placenta in a towel or put it in a plastic bag. Always take the placenta to the hospital for a doctor to examine so he can be sure none of it is left in the uterus. Even a very small part of it retained in the uterus can cause continued bleeding and infection.

After the placenta is delivered, put a sterile pad over the vaginal opening. Lower the mother's legs and support them together. Normally, nothing more will be passed from the vagina. The mother, baby, and placenta are ready to go to the hospital. Record the time of delivery.

If the Bag of Waters Does Not Break

There is one unusual condition the EMT must be able to recognize. The amniotic sac (bag of waters) usually breaks open during the labor and fluid gushes from the vagina. If the sac does not break during labor, the baby may be born still enclosed in the sac. If this happens, use a clamp to puncture the bag at once and push the sac away from the baby's nose and mouth so it can breathe. Be sure to suck out the nose and mouth with the bulb syringe.

Resuscitation of the Newborn

When a newborn baby does not begin to breathe within about thirty seconds, and especially if the baby is limp at delivery, begin artificial ventilation. Do not use resuscitation equipment. Follow the resuscitation procedure described below.

1. Suction the airway as previously described.
2. Place the baby on one side with the head slightly lower than the body
3. Stimulate the baby by slapping an index finger against the bottom of the feet. The baby may breathe when this is done a few times. If he does not respond, begin the next step.
4. Using mouth-to-mouth resuscitation, breathe gently into the baby's nose and mouth with the force normally used to blow out a puff of cigarette smoke. Ventilate rapidly several times. If the baby breathes, give oxygen until the skin is pink and he is breathing well. If the infant does not breathe after several puffs, continue mouth-to-mouth resuscitation.
5. If you cannot feel a pulse after two minutes, begin cardiac compression. For a baby, use only an index finger to depress the infant sternum (see Chapter 10, Basic Life Support).
6. Continue cardiopulmonary resuscitation until the baby breathes or until it is pronounced dead by a physician. Transport the baby to the hospital as quickly as possible. Resuscitation continued for fifteen to twenty minutes has saved babies, without brain damage.
7. Keep the infant slightly warm at all times, but not hot. Warmth aids in his ultimate survival.
8. Some babies are born dead. If the death occurred several hours or longer before the birth, the baby may smell bad and the skin may show large blisters. The head may also be very soft. Under these circumstances, do not attempt to resuscitate the infant.

In the event of an apparent stillborn infant or the possibility of imminent death following birth, an EMT of any religion may baptize the newborn of Christian parents. The ceremony is done by putting a drop or two of water on the bare skin of the baby, preferably the head, while saying: "I baptize you in the name of the Father, and of the Son, and of the Holy Spirit." This exact form should be used. Efforts at resuscitation should be continued during and following baptism. Many parents will feel that baptism is not necessary, but others are greatly comforted by it.

Abnormal Deliveries and Serious Complications

Most deliveries are normal. However, the EMT must be able to recognize when there is a problem. When a problem is suspected, the mother should be transported to the hospital immediately. Here is a list of complications that can make a delivery difficult and hazardous for the mother and baby:

1. Breech presentation
2. Prolapsed umbilical cord
3. Excessive bleeding
4. Limb presentation (foot or arm protruding from the vagina)
5. Baby not delivered after twenty minutes of watching a mother who is having frequent contractions (one every two to three minutes)

Proper emergency care in these situations may save a life. The EMT must know what to do.

Breech delivery. Breech delivery is the most common "abnormal" delivery. The presenting part will be the buttocks or the feet of the baby instead of the head. Sometimes it is necessary to go ahead and help the mother deliver a breech baby. If the baby "won't wait" until the mother gets to the hospital, do the following things:

1. Position and drape the mother as usual.
2. Allow the buttocks and trunk of the baby to deliver spontaneously.
3. Support the baby's legs and trunk as they are delivered, letting the legs dangle astride your arm, with your palm under the trunk (Fig. 36.11).
4. The head then usually comes out on its own. Sometimes, however, the head does not deliver within three minutes after delivery of the waist and trunk. Do **not** attempt to pull the baby out. Transport the

269

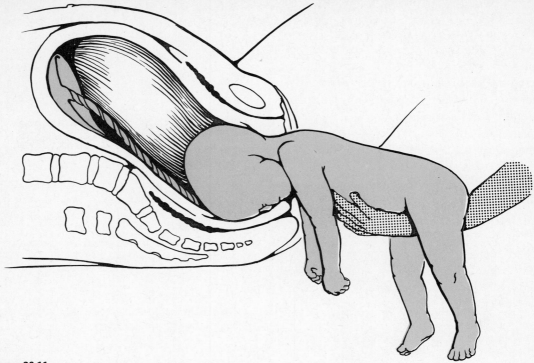

Figure 36.11

A breech delivery is shown. The attendant's hand supports the chest and abdomen of the baby as it is delivered. Do not pull on the baby.

mother and baby to the Emergency Department or get a physician's help at the home as quickly as possible. Meanwhile, attempt to keep the baby's airway open with a finger in its mouth so it can breathe.

5. After the head is delivered, give the same care previously described for the umbilical cord, placenta, baby, and mother.

Prolapsed umbilical cord. Prolapsed cord means that the umbilical cord comes out of the vagina before the baby. This complication usually occurs at the time the bag of waters breaks. The baby is in danger because the cord will be compressed against the pelvic wall by the baby. If the umbilical cord is visible outside the birth canal, put the mother in very severe shock position with the buttocks and legs much higher than the shoulders and have her lie on one side or the other. Wrap a sterile towel around the visible portion of the cord and protect it from being pressed by the mother's legs. If sterile saline solution is available, the sterile towel should be

moistened with the solution. Give the mother oxygen, keep her warm, and transport her to the hospital at once. Do not try to replace the cord in the vagina.

Excessive bleeding. If the mother bleeds more than usual (anything more than a bloody show before delivery or more than five soaked pads in the first thirty minutes after delivery) or if she goes into shock, do the following things:

1. Treat for shock and start an IV.
2. Place a sanitary napkin at the opening of the vagina, and when it needs to be changed, save the blood-filled pads for a future estimation of blood loss by the physician.
3. Do **not** put your hand into the vagina or pack anything into the vagina.
4. Do **not** hold the mother's legs together.
5. Keep any tissue passed and give it with the pads to the physician at the hospital.

Limb presentation. The presentation of a single arm or a single leg in the birth canal constitutes one of the most complex problems of delivery. This mother must be transported as quickly as possible to a hospital, for such a delivery will require trained obstetrical help.

Prolonged delivery. If the baby has not been delivered after twenty minutes of observing the mother with contractions every two to three minutes, the EMT may conclude that there will be a prolonged delivery. The mother should be transported to the hospital immediately.

Emergencies in Early Pregnancy

Delivery of the fetus and placenta prior to twenty weeks is called an abortion. The lay term is miscarriage.

Abortions frequently cause severe bleeding. Bleeding may be internal, that is, into the abdominal cavity. The EMT should **not** pull on the fetus or cord and should **not** put his hand into the mother's vagina, as fatal hemorrhage might be produced. The following things may be done:

1. Treat for shock.
2. Transport to the hospital.
3. Save any tissue the mother passes.

Twins

If the delivery is normal, the birth of twins should not be considered a complication. They are delivered one after the other, in the same manner as single babies. If the mother is not aware of the possibility of a multiple birth, the EMT should suspect twins if he sees that her abdomen is still large after one baby has been delivered. Labor contractions will begin again about ten minutes after the first baby is born; the second baby is usually born within forty-five minutes of the first. If the mother is to be transported after the birth of the first baby but before the second, she should be given oxygen during the transportation. She will feel more comfortable if she lies on one side.

When the first baby is born, clamp and cut the cord as instructed above to prevent possible hemorrhaging from the second baby through the umbilical cord. The second baby will probably be born prior to the delivery of the placenta of the first. Continue with the same procedure as in a single birth, and remember the importance of keeping the infants warm until they reach a hospital. Since twins are frequently born before they are full term, they might be small enough to be considered premature. It is even more important to keep premature babies warm.

Delivery without Sterile Supplies

At times it is necessary to assist a patient in delivering a baby when proper equipment and supplies are not available. The technique described below should be useful under those circumstances.

Clean sheets and towels which have not been used since their previous laundering are safe and may be used for preparing the patient. The EMT's hands should be washed as thoroughly as possible. Conduct the delivery of the baby as if gloves were available. As soon as the baby is born, use a clean finger to wipe out the baby's mouth, taking care not to initiate vomiting.

Do not attempt to tie or clamp the cord with string, thread, shoelaces, or the like, and do not cut the cord. Rather, keep the baby at the side of the mother's buttocks at the same level or below the entrance of her vagina but out of the pool of amniotic fluid and blood. As soon as the placenta is delivered, wrap it in newspaper or a towel, leaving it attached to the baby, and place it with the baby, who can now be moved. The placenta always should be slightly above the baby (Fig. 36.12). The baby and the placenta can now be transported safely.

The baby must be kept warm. If necessary, wrap it in an article of clothing, such as a shirt worn by the EMT. In case of hemorrhage by the mother, the baby can be placed at the mother's breast and the uterus gently massaged as previously described.

Premature Infants

Any baby weighing less than five and one-half pounds, or one born before eight months of pregnancy, should be considered premature. Facilities for weighing the baby will probably not be available; judgment must be made from the

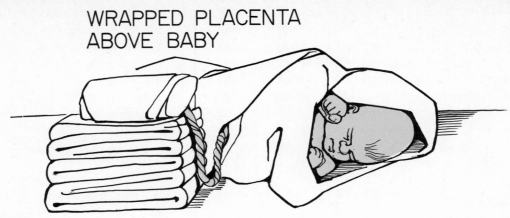

WRAPPED PLACENTA
ABOVE BABY

272   **Figure 36.12**

When sterile supplies are not available, the placenta, still attached by the umbilical cord, may be wrapped in a towel and kept with the baby. It should be placed slightly higher than the baby.

history the mother gives and by the baby's appearance. A premature baby will be much thinner, smaller, and redder than a full-term baby, and the head will be relatively larger.

Premature babies need special care if they are to survive. The smaller the baby, the more important is this care. With proper handling, infants weighing as little as two pounds or even less have a chance of living. There are five important things to remember in the handling of a premature infant.

1. Keep the baby warm. The maintenance of body temperature is extremely important. It should be wrapped in a warm blanket as soon as it breathes well, and kept in a place where the temperature is about 90° F. A serviceable makeshift incubator can be provided by wrapping the infant in aluminum foil. The head should be covered, but the face should be left uncovered.

2. Keep the mouth and throat clear of fluid and mucus. Wipe the blood and mucus from the nose and mouth with sterile gauze sponges. With the rubber bulb aspirator, gently suction out the mouth and each nostril. Be sure to squeeze the bulb and hold it squeezed before putting it in the baby's mouth or nose. Put the tip gently into the mouth or nose and release the bulb slowly.

3. Check to see if the cord is bleeding. Examine the end of the umbilical cord carefully, and if there is the slightest sign of bleeding, apply an additional clamp or tie. **Even the smallest amount of bleeding may be serious for premature infants.**

4. Give oxygen. It allows the baby to breathe more easily and is frequently a lifesaving procedure. It should be administered very gently and very carefully. Make a tent over the baby's head and let the oxygen enter it. Aim it at the top of the tent. If the baby is in a special carrier (see below), it will not be necessary to make the tent. Do not blow the oxygen in a stream directly over the baby's face. Oxygen may have certain special dangers for the premature infant, but given gently and for a comparatively short time (fifteen to thirty minutes), it should not be dangerous. (See Chapter 10, Basic Life Support, for a more detailed discussion on oxygen for the newborn.)

Turn the key on the oxygen cylinder very slowly until the oxygen bubbles freely through the water in the bottle attached to the cylinder. Ideally, about 70 to 100 bubbles a minute are recommended. If the color of the infant is not good, do not hesitate to increase the amount of oxygen and change the position of the infant slightly.

5. Don't infect the infant. The premature infant is very susceptible to infection and proper precautions to prevent it may mean

the difference between life and death. Be careful not to talk, sneeze, or breathe directly into the baby's face, and keep everyone else as far away as possible. This protection should be given any newborn baby, but it is even more important for the premature.

6. Radio the hospital so the staff will be expecting the mother and baby. Proceed carefully at a wise speed to the hospital.

Before transporting a premature infant, make definite arrangements with the hospital so admission will be as soon as you arrive. Whenever possible, have some member of the family accompany the infant in the ambulance. The physician at the hospital will want to talk with a member of the family.

Transport of the premature infant to the hospital. New transport techniques which have been developed for premature infants are related to the equipment to be used. The following discussion is general and assumes that only ordinary equipment will be available. Specific guidelines should be worked out by each Emergency Medical Service with hospitals in its locality.

Special use of infant carriers. In some areas of the country, and in most metropolitan areas, a special carrier for transporting the premature infant will be available. This unit will make proper infant care much easier. The EMT should be aware of these facilities and know in advance where to obtain special infant carriers.

Equipment in infant carriers. The premature infant carrier should contain the following articles:

Crib
3 hot water bottles with covers
1 quilted pad
1 baby blanket
1 diaper
1 room thermometer
1 rubber suction tube with glass trap (sterilized)
1 Kelly clamp (sterilized)
1 rubber suction bulb
1 rubber funnel with tube
1 oxygen cylinder (40 gals) with attachments
1 bottle of 70-percent alcohol

273

Before leaving on a call known to be a premature delivery, put very hot water in all three hot water bottles in the carrier. **Be careful to keep the bottles well covered to avoid any contact with the very tender skin of the infant, which burns easily.** Place one hot water bottle, in its cover, on the floor of the carrier under the crib and one in its cover on each side of the crib, tying the covers to the side bars to keep the bottles from falling.

Prepare the infant for transportation by removing the folded blanket and diaper from the crib, trying not to keep the carrier open any longer than necessary, in order to conserve heat. Place the infant in the blanket on the diaper as soon as possible, without removing its clothing, if any; keep the blanket away from the face so it can breathe freely. Then put it in the carrier as gently as possible. The temperature inside the carrier should be between 90° and 100°F. as registered on the thermometer. Be sure that the carrier is secure and will not move around.

CHAPTER 37

Pediatric Emergencies and Special Problems

GOAL I. Understand the special problems encountered in the ill or injured child.

OBJECTIVES

A. Describe the treatment for a child with an obstructed airway or a child requiring assisted ventilation or cardiac compression.

B. List the systolic blood pressure levels indicating shock in children in various age groups.

C. Describe how to estimate the volume of intravenous fluids that can be administered to a child safely.

D. List traumatic and nontraumatic causes of abdominal pain in children.

E. Describe how to treat a child with a high fever.

F. List some common causes of convulsions in children.

G. List the steps in treating a child who has ingested a poison.

GOAL II. Recognize the existence of Sudden Infant Death syndrome, and of abuse and sexual molestation of children, and know how to meet these situations.

OBJECTIVES

A. Define Sudden Infant Death syndrome.

B. List the identifying features of child abuse.

C. Describe the treatment of a sexually molested child.

Trauma is the leading cause of death in childhood. Prompt, effective action is especially important when treating injured children. A child's life saved offers the promise of years of productive activity. while an injury compounded by a mistake can result in crippling disability for life. Helping children is demanding, but it has rewards no other activity can match.

Some EMTs are completely comfortable when treating children; most, however, are not. A crying child in the midst of distraught parents and onlookers can challenge the confidence of the most seasoned professional. A knot in the stomach or a lump in the throat is not an uncommon reaction for anyone confronted with a seriously ill or injured child. Such a situation however requires calmness, deliberateness, and confidence. The EMT is trained to meet most of the specific situations that will arise, and he can do much better by maintaining his own self-control. When necessary, a good plan is to designate someone—a relative, friend, or onlooker—to help comfort parents.

Basic Life Support

The principles for the use of basic life support measures are the same for children as for adults. Possibly the child can tolerate cerebral hypoxia a minute or two longer than the adult whose brain may be supplied by aging arteries, but instituting support is urgent in both instances. Shock, cardiac arrest, respiratory arrest or insufficiency cannot be tolerated by the small human being for more than a very few minutes before some permanent damage occurs within a vital organ or system. The EMT should review Chapter 10, Basic Life Support, thoroughly.

Airway obstruction. As with the adult, airway obstruction is usually relieved by proper positioning of the head. In the older child, hyperextension of the neck and head will usually open the airway in the same manner as it does for an adult. The infant or the small child (under six years) breathes much more easily if the head is elevated and supported and the neck is not extended so far. The reasons for this difference are the extreme flexibility of the neck in the infant and small child and the fact that hyperextension may itself cause obstruction of the airway.

The presence of vomitus should be ascertained by sweeping a finger across the back of the pharynx. If the child has vomited, material in the upper airway must be removed, by suction if possible, before instituting ventilation.

With a child, removal of a partially obstructing foreign body in the airway should probably be carried out in the hospital. If the child can move air in and out past the obstruction, he should be introduced gently to the oxygen mask or given mouth-to-mouth ventilation while being transported promptly to the Emergency Department. Only when a foreign body has caused a complete airway obstruction should the EMT attempt to dislodge it. Procedures for dislodging a foreign body from the airway are described in Chapter 10. Briefly, the child may be turned over your forearm with his head lower than his waist and a series of sharp blows delivered between the shoulder blades. Alternatively, place a fist below the breastbone between the xiphoid process and the navel and deliver a rapid, upward thrust. Either of these methods will often be effective in dislodging a foreign body.

Oxygen. Oxygen should be given to all cyanotic or unconscious children and to all children in shock. If the child is conscious, the best test of a need for oxygen is whether or not he accepts it. If he is more comfortable with it than without it, the administration of oxygen is appropriate. The child should be introduced to the mask slowly and gently and, when possible, should be allowed to hold it. Some children are initially fearful of anything that covers the face.

Assisted ventilation. The indications for and the principles underlying the use of assisted ventilation in children are the same as for adults. Some specific considerations may be mentioned. Do not try to administer more than twenty breaths a minute. Assisted ventilation is effective if the chest rises and is allowed to fall between administered breaths. Do not blow harder through the child's nose and mouth than is necessary to make the chest rise. The smaller the child, the more likely one is to force air into the stomach. Should this distention occur, the air can be expelled by administering gentle pressure under the left ribs. The EMT must be prepared, as with adults, to clear vomited stomach contents from the pharynx promptly by suction or by lowering the patient's head and turning it to one side.

A plastic artificial airway, in an appropriate size, which can be slipped between the tongue and palate is often helpful in the resuscitation of an unconscious child. If the airway does not make ventilation easier, do not force the child to retain it. Assisted ventilation in children is best carried out by the simplest possible method. If mouth-to-mouth breathing is effective, do not hurry to substitute a mechanical respirator.

Cardiac arrest. As with the adult, no purpose is served by circulating unoxygenated blood. For this reason, give first attention to securing and maintaining an airway and restoring ventilation. Once the child is breathing spontaneously or when artificial ventilation has been instituted,

276

check for the heartbeat. If a pulse in the neck or groin cannot be felt, the EMT should stop for a moment, put an ear to the child's chest and listen. When a heartbeat cannot be detected, initiate external cardiac compression immediately.

Cardiac compression. To administer cardiac compression to an older child, place the heel of the hand over the lower half of the sternum. For the younger child and the infant, place only the tips of the index and middle fingers over the middle of the sternum, relatively higher than for the older child or adult. Alternatively, to give heart compression to the infant, one may place both thumbs side by side on the sternum with the hands encircling the chest, and compress the heart with the thumbs. When performing cardiac resuscitation alone on an infant, the EMT can position himself at the infant's head and encircle the chest with his hands, supporting the child's head with his wrists. He then places his thumbs on the sternum, his fingers behind the chest, and gives cardiac compression with his thumbs. The EMT should not attempt to exceed eighty to one hundred compressions per minute. This rate will still allow the heart to relax and refill between compressions.

The means of detecting the success of cardiopulmonary resuscitation are the same in children as in adults. Check the carotid or femoral pulses periodically. As with the adult, the carotid pulse may be easier to check than any other pulse in the body. Observe dilated pupils to see if they regain reactivity or constrict. Watch for consciousness to return, spontaneous breathing to be resumed, or a spontaneous heartbeat to be reestablished.

Bleeding and shock. Control of bleeding in children is best accomplished by direct pressure on the wound. All of the principles described in Chapter 8, Bleeding and Control of Bleeding, apply equally well in the pediatric patient. A tourniquet is used as a last resort, and the safest tourniquet is a blood pressure cuff applied above the wound and near either the groin or the shoulder. In children, inflation of the cuff to 150 mm Hg and in infants to 120 mm Hg will usually secure adequate control. A tourniquet inflated too tightly (over 200 mm Hg) may damage the vascular and nerve structures of a tiny

extremity. A loose tourniquet may actually increase blood loss. All the routine precautions for the use of a tourniquet must be observed.

Shock in injured children is almost invariably the result of loss of blood. If shock is suspected or confirmed, look for any blood loss which can be controlled. The most important indicator of shock is a low systolic blood pressure (two-thirds of the individual's normal). In children, shock is assumed to be present if the systolic blood pressure is below 50 in the preschool child, below 60 in the child under twelve, and below 70 in the teenage or young adult. Accurate determination of blood pressure in a child may require a special pediatric-size cuff. At least three sizes of cuffs should be carried on the ambulance as routine equipment.

In infants and children who have not been bleeding, shock is usually related to loss of tissue fluids, that is, dehydration. Diarrhea or vomiting can bring about dehydration in small bodies much more quickly than in larger ones. A dehydrated child must be regarded as desperately sick and should be transported to the Emergency Department as soon as possible.

All the supportive measures which have been described in Chapter 8, Bleeding and Control of Bleeding, and Chapter 9, Shock, are appropriate in the care of the child in shock or bleeding. A supine position with the legs slightly elevated, extremely gentle handling of the patient, some protection against the loss of body heat, control of obvious external bleeding, splinting of fractures to minimize further tissue damage and to help control bleeding are all vitally important factors.

In older children, fourteen years and above, the EMT will normally be qualified to institute intravenous infusions, which, however, should be undertaken only at the direction and usually at the specific order of a physician, with whom the EMT should be in contact. In pressing emergency situations, when the EMT must act independently, some general rules apply for the administration of intravenous fluids. An amount of intravenous fluid equivalent to 10 milliliters per estimated pound of body weight can be given to the pediatric patient in the form of normal saline solution, Ringer's lactate solution, or

Plasma-Lyte. The administration of this amount of fluid should result in an elevation of blood pressure above the level of shock or in a return to normal. If this amount of fluid does not change the blood pressure, the same amount may be given again as a repeat dose. The administration of fluid up to that level can be carried out as an emergency measure when the EMT does not have immediate direction or help at hand. No more than 20 ml per estimated pound of body weight should be given without the specific direction of a physician. It is extremely important that accurate records of the fluid given the patient be kept, since what he has received will largely determine what additional fluids will be given at the Emergency Department in the hospital.

While shock is a treatable state, the tissues of the body suffering inadequate perfusion will undergo permanent damage after a given period of time; so it is necessary to reverse a state of shock as soon as possible. If the state persists in patients for more than one or two hours, irreversible shock may develop. In this particular situation, no matter what treatment is administered (intravenous fluids, blood, correction of external bleeding, splinting of fractures, and the like), permanent damage of vital systems has occurred and the patient is likely to die. The EMT must realize that limits of time exist within which he can treat shock successfully and that he must employ all the means at his command to combat the state. He should also be aware that, although shock may not be present upon first examination of an injured person, it can develop after the passage of some time. Prompt transport of the patient to the Emergency Department is essential.

Specific Injuries and Problems

Head, neck, and spine injuries. Head injuries are common in children. They require the same careful treatment that they do in adults. The unconscious child should not be moved until an airway is secure and breathing and circulation are restored. In the unconscious child, as in the unconscious adult, the possibility of a broken neck should be assumed until it is ruled out, and

the patient should be treated accordingly. The natural tendency to pick up a child in one's arms must be resisted. If the neck or back has been broken, spinal flexion is the most dangerous possible movement. The use of a spineboard to move the patient is as important for children as for adults. Fortunately, the light weight of a child generally makes the use of a spineboard considerably easier.

In the absence of an identifiable spinal injury but in the presence of a head injury, the child should be transported on the left side with head slightly elevated on a blanket or a pillow. Considerable attention must be given to securing and maintaining an airway.

Fractures, soft-tissue injuries, chest injuries. The principles outlining the treatment of these injuries are identical in children and in adults. Review Chapters 6, 14, 16, 17, 18, 19, and 20 for the appropriate treatment of these problems.

Abdominal injuries. Penetrating abdominal injuries and eviscerations are less common in children than they are in adults. Blunt abdominal wounds resulting in rupture of the spleen, liver, or intestine occur somewhat more often in children, usually as a result of falls or automobile accidents. These internal injuries are frequently difficult to diagnose. Often, abdominal pain is the only clue. Even when abdominal pain seems to be improving, a child who has sustained an injury from such an accident should be checked by a physician, as shock can develop later. Gentle handling, rapid transport to the Emergency Department, and a careful and continued monitoring of vital signs are the essentials in emergency treatment for these patients.

Abdominal pain. The most common serious cause of abdominal pain in children is appendicitis. The age range is broad. The disease can be seen in newborn infants, preschool children, schoolchildren, and adults of all ages. In infants and preschool children, the diagnosis is extremely difficult; the only signs may be that the child is fussy and has no appetite. Vomiting may or may not occur. Fever is usually present. Abdominal pain is the most important sign. A child who fits this picture must be taken to the Emergency Department for the doctor to decide whether he has a mild case of gastroenteritis or appendicitis requiring an operation. Even the doctor may need to observe the child over some hours before he makes any decision.

In very young children, usually under the age of five, intussusception is another relatively common cause of severe abdominal pain. Intussusception is the name given to a condition in which a portion of the gastrointestinal tract becomes telescoped within the next portion and continues telescoping on down the bowel. Most commonly the ileum becomes telescoped into and entrapped within the colon. The characteristic picture is severe intermittent abdominal cramping. The infant or child may seem completely normal between the cramps. The child may also pass a dark, black-red liquid stool with this condition.

Intussusception is a severe abnormality and may require an operation to treat. Certainly, the pain associated with intussusception is so severe that the EMT must be at once alerted to the presence of a serious disease. These children must always be transported to the Emergency Department as soon as possible for the attention of a physician.

In general, the problem of abdominal pain in children requires prompt diagnosis by a physician. The EMT should not try to define the cause of the problem, but only its presence, and should proceed to transport the child with little loss of time.

Special Problems Seen in the Pediatric Patient

Fever. Children with fever are sick. Children commonly respond to illness with the development of some degree of fever. Although a minor elevation of temperature is usually not serious, it should not be ignored. Often the presence of the fever indicates some condition which requires prompt attention. Occasionally a child may respond to relatively minor illness or injury with the development of a disproportionately high fever. Regardless of what causes it, a fever in the range of 103° to 104° F and above can be dangerous itself because of the effect of the hyperthermia (high heat) on the body. In some children a high fever is usually accompanied by a convulsion.

The child with a particularly high temperature should be cooled before and during transportation to the Emergency Department. Frequently, simply controlling the fever may contribute significantly to the overall well-being of the patient. Remove the clothing and cover the child with a towel saturated with tepid water. Do not use ice water as it may produce such a violent shivering reaction in the patient that his temperature actually rises because of the muscular activity of the body. Do not use rubbing alcohol for the same reason. Do not submerge the child in a tub or basin of water.

Convulsions. Convulsions are common in very young and preschool children, and, as stated, are frequently associated with a high fever. They are very frightening to those who have never seen or treated them.

The convulsing child must be protected from injuring himself until the seizure passes. The classical practice of placing a mouthpiece between the teeth to prevent the patient from biting the tongue and to help keep the airway open is acceptable if it can be carried out easily. In some instances, forcing the jaws apart to place a mouthpiece over the tongue has resulted in more injury than would have been caused by the seizure. For this reason, many authorities no longer recommend this practice. To help protect the child from injuries of other parts of the body during the seizure, the EMT may use blankets or other padding.

It will be helpful to the physician who attends the patient if the EMT can report which parts of the body were twitching. Often parents are too upset to give this information.

Ordinarily, the seizure will be over before the EMT arrives. Observations concerning the onset of the seizure, the extremities involved, and the child's movements should, however, still be clear in the minds of those who witnessed the convulsion, and the EMT may be able to obtain information from them. He should do so, particularly if they are bystanders who will not be going to the hospital.

The child will be in a post-seizure state and may be dazed or even unaware that a seizure has

279

occurred. In this situation the EMT should make the child comfortable and transport him as gently as possible to the Emergency Department. The only effective treatment for a convulsion at the time it occurs is the immediate intravenous injection of an anticonvulsant medication. This medication can only be given at the direction of a physician. Its use requires a specific order identifying the medicine to give and specifying the quantity. If the child is still experiencing a seizure or undergoes a convulsion while under the care of the EMT, a physician may be contacted for advice, but the EMT can give the anticonvulsant injection **only if the physician specifically prescribes it.** If the convulsing child has fever, his temperature should be controlled as described, both before and during transportation to the hospital.

Regardless of the apparent cause, any child developing a convulsion for the first time must be checked by a physician. Most seizures in childhood are harmless. However, the development of a convulsion can signify a serious problem such as meningitis, a brain tumor, or a severe injury. If the child has had previous seizures, the parents should bring his medications to the hospital for the receiving physician in the Emergency Department to examine.

Poisonings. Children are curious and like to examine by feeling, tasting, or sniffing. Frequently they are exposed to substances which are harmful, and all too frequently a considerable dose may have been swallowed before anyone is aware of the child's activity.

If the substance has been spilled by the child, promptly remove it from any part of the body by flooding with tap water. Contaminated clothing must also be removed. Special attention must be given to the eyes. Wash them out gently but thoroughly and as promptly as possible. Save all substances that may be needed later for analysis. Take the bottle or tube or a sample of the substance itself to the Emergency Department. This sample may be a piece of contaminated clothing or washings from the skin or even a small bottle of vomitus if the container of the original substance is not available. Identification of the substance is essential for selection of the best antidote or treatment.

Generally, if the child has swallowed a toxic substance, vomiting should be induced to reduce the amount of substance in the stomach. Give a dose of syrup of ipecac, followed by one or two cups of water.

In some very specific instances vomiting should **not** be induced to treat poisoning because it will damage tissues further or allow the spread of a dangerous substance to other areas.

Do **not** induce vomiting:
1. When the poison is a strong acid
2. When the poison is a strong alkali (lye or Drano, for example)
3. When the poison is a petroleum product (kerosene, furniture polish)
4. When the poison is an anti-emetic (anti-vomiting) drug
5. When the poison is strychnine
6. When the poisoned child is unconscious, semiconscious, convulsing, or in shock

If there is any suspicion that the child has swallowed a caustic material such as lye or a strong acid, he should be very quickly taken to the Emergency Department. Often the only way to determine whether the esophagus has been severely burned is for a physician to inspect it under anesthesia. Treatment for this condition will require hospitalization.

Contagious diseases. Occasionally, children with measles, mumps, chicken pox, or other contagious diseases must be transported by the EMT. Ordinarily symptoms of these diseases are obvious. Measles and chicken pox, when fully developed, cause rashes; mumps causes a swelling and tenderness of the tissues directly in front of and below the ear. Even when there are no symptoms, it is wise for the EMT to check for a history of exposure to any one of these three frequently occurring diseases when a child is feverish. Emergency Department personnel should know that the child may have a contagious disease so they can avoid placing it in contact with other patients.

Provided moderate care is exercised and the child is not excessively handled or allowed to cough on the transporting EMTs, and provided further that the EMTs practice careful hand-

280

washing technique, the danger to the personnel transporting an infected child is minimal. The ambulance and its contents must be carefully cleaned to protect the next passenger.

Many other communicable diseases can occur in children. A thorough discussion of the proper means of handling patients with communicable diseases in an emergency situation is contained in Chapter 35, Communicable Disease.

The transportation of infants. Some general principles govern the transportation of sick or injured infants. Infants exposed to the air generally lose body heat, unless the environmental temperature is close to 98° F. Sick or severely injured infants are at great risk from bacterial contamination. Thus, provision should be made for protecting the infant from cold and from direct bacterial contamination from the hands, noses, and mouths of the attendants.

An infant carrier should provide access to the child so that his airway may be cleared and artificial ventilation maintained where it is necessary. Obviously, the carrier should allow the baby to be completely in view. It should also provide a means of keeping the baby warm. An infant in a carrier with supplemental oxygen and attended by the EMT does not normally require high-speed transportation to the hospital.

Newborn babies should be transported in clean incubators which allow oxygen enrichment of the air and control of both humidity and temperature. The infant's head should be accessible, and appropriate sizes of tracheal intubation equipment and ventilatory equipment should be at hand. Space in an ambulance is at a premium and the transportation of an infant does not occur frequently. For these reasons, the special equipment for transporting infants or young children should be maintained at the ambulance base and placed in the ambulance only when needed.

Baptism. Occasionally the EMT will be faced with the problem of a dying child. If the child has not been baptized, it is possible that the EMT can provide comfort to the family by baptism. The rite is extremely simple and involves saying, "I baptize you in the name of the Father, and of the Son, and of the Holy Spirit." Drops of water placed on the forehead are appropriate but not essential for baptism. A witness to the ceremony is desirable but also is not essential. If the infant or child has already been baptized, doing so again in an emergency situation is not harmful.

Sudden Infant Death Syndrome (SIDS). The sudden, unexpected death of an infant in its crib is an emergency with which the EMT may be confronted, for some ten thousand babies die in this way in the United States each year. Sudden Infant Death Syndrome (SIDS) is the leading cause of death in infants after the first few weeks of life. At the present time the cause of this particularly tragic event is unknown. The occurrence cannot be predicted; similarly, it cannot be prevented. Death usually occurs during sleep in an apparently healthy infant and may not be discovered until sometime during the night or the following morning.

In this particular situation the EMT must expect to encounter anguished parents. Efforts to assist the baby will help them as much as anything that can be said to them. The administration of CPR before and during transportation to the Emergency Department should be undertaken. Transportation should be carried out as quickly as possible. It is a wise procedure to notify the receiving department of the hospital, in advance, of the nature of the case being transported.

Child abuse. The intentional injury and abuse of children is a far more common occurrence today than many people realize. An important fact in child abuse is that the episodes are often repeated with progressive severity. They frequently result in permanent disability or the death of the child.

It is necessary that the EMT know some of the identifying features pointing to child abuse. Among these are an adult's story which does not ring true or which does not account for all of the injuries that are observed. Many injuries on a child's body in different stages of healing are also characteristic of child abuse. A history of previous injuries with suspicious stories and conflicting descriptions of the "accident" from different observers can frequently be obtained.

The EMT does not make the diagnosis of child abuse. The EMT observes and records his find-

281

ings and the history as it is given to him. These findings are transmitted to the physician at the Emergency Department. If a suspicion has been raised, it is appropriate and important that the EMT voice it to the medically concerned personnel, as well as reporting to the other authorities discussed later in this section.

Parents and babysitters are by far the most frequent child abusers. The child so abused needs medical care and protection; the abuser himself needs counseling and may require psychiatric care. An obvious case of serious child abuse may arouse strong emotions in the EMT and severely challenge his ability to conduct himself in a professional manner. It is necessary, however, that the EMT treat this situation as he should all others, calmly and as efficiently as possible.

When abuse is suspected, the child should be taken to the Emergency Department no matter how trivial the injury appears to be. State laws require the reporting of any suspicion of abuse to police and to the child protection services of the community. These specific agencies are responsible for determining whether the suspicion of child abuse is valid, and, if so, what corrective measures are necessary. Agencies are, however, powerless to protect the child from any further injury unless the suspicion of the abuse is reported to them. Every EMT should know his responsibility as defined by the laws of his state regarding suspected cases of child abuse. Failure to report a suspicion of abuse ultimately may

cause more serious injury or cost the child's life.

The sexually molested child. Sexual assault of children of both sexes is not uncommon. Most victims of rape range from ten to nineteen years of age. Younger children are more frequently the victims of other types of sexual assault, commonly called fondling or sexual molestation.

The procedures outlined in Chapter 29 for dealing with adults in such cases apply also to dealing with children and their parents. The EMT should review the section on sexual assault in that chapter. Important points are restated briefly below.

No examination of genitalia should be made unless obvious bleeding requires application of a dressing. Both child and parents should be cautioned that the patient should not wash, urinate, or defecate before examination by a physician. Other conditions, such as fractures, lacerations, or unconsciousness, should be appropriately treated.

Quiet, professional conduct is mandatory for the EMT. In situations where curious onlookers are apt to gather, an important consideration should be shielding the patient and removal from the scene as quickly as possible. Obtaining a history from adults is particularly important when the patient is a child.

If it is known at the time of dispatch that a female child is involved, a female EMT, nurse, or other attendant should accompany the ambulance when possible.

IX

Mental Health Problems

CHAPTER 38

The Disturbed and Unruly Patient

GOAL I. Know the behavioral manifestations reflecting psychological and psychiatric reactions in patients who experience injuries, sickness, or disaster.

OBJECTIVES

A. Describe the psychological and psychiatric reactions of patients with injuries or illness.
B. Describe the psychiatric problems of the dying patient.

GOAL II. Know the many organic states causing disordered behavior.

OBJECTIVES

A. List specific organic diseases or conditions associated with disturbed behavior.
B. Describe the range of psychiatric or behavioral disturbance seen in response to injury, illness, or disease.
C. Describe the specific means by which the EMT may treat unruly or disturbed behavior in given instances.

GOAL III. Know the behavioral manifestations reflecting primary emotional or psychiatric disease or are associated with organic brain dysfunction and know the emergency treatment of these manifestations.

OBJECTIVES

A. Describe the emergency treatment for the suicidal patient.
B. Describe the behavior patterns of the emotionally disturbed patient.
C. Describe the behavior of the aged senile patient with organic brain disease.
D. Establish appropriate priorities of psychiatric and medical care for suicidal or disturbed patients.
E. Describe the situations in which additional aid is required.
F. Describe the appropriate areas of help available to the EMT in treating the emotionally disturbed patient.
G. Describe the legal limitations imposed on the EMT in treating the emotionally disturbed patient.

In almost any crisis requiring the services of an EMT, changes occur in the emotional states of the people involved, members of their families, and bystanders. Reactions can range from controlled expressions of fear and anxiety to acute disturbances of thinking, feeling, and behavior, depending upon the nature of the crisis and the way in which it is handled, as well as upon the emotional stability of those associated with the event.

The EMT, arriving early at the scene because physical injuries have occurred, is also usually the first professional person to deal with emotional behavior. By proper treatment of acute reactions, major problems can often be prevented from developing. Fires, floods, tornadoes, and other natural disasters produce a pronounced effect on the emotional well-being of those affected. The EMT can be of invaluable assistance in this period of shock and may help prevent delayed or more serious reactions.

The EMT also often encounters primary psychiatric emergency problems, ranging from disorders related to drug or alcohol abuse to mild or serious forms of behavioral disorganization. These disorders must be distinguished from disturbed behavior as a result of a crisis.

Many manifestations of disturbed behavior are associated with or result from physical conditions, such as a head injury, a severe infection, a toxic reaction, or diabetes. Others do not appear to have an observable physical basis.

The Psychological Aspects of Injuries and Sickness

General reactions. When the EMT responds to an emergency, one of his most important responsibilities is to assess accurately the patient's mental condition and emotional reaction. To what degree is the patient frightened, anxious, or grief-stricken? How are these feelings manifested? How does a sense of helplessness affect the patient? Frightened patients, if they talk at all, are frequently irrational and incoherent. If the EMT observes this reaction, he can ask the patient about fear and relieve much of it just by listening to the answer. The question and an attentive response will reassure the patient that his feelings are important; it is comforting and calming to be treated as an individual and to realize that someone cares or is concerned about one's situation.

Many patients are very anxious when injured or ill. They may exhibit irrational behavior,

misrepresent the nature of their injuries, breathe so rapidly that they hyperventilate and sometimes lose consciousness, cry, laugh, seem very angry or aggressive, run in circles, or otherwise show completely inappropriate reactions. The EMT, in command of his own feelings and behavior, can best help these people by working in a calm, efficient manner, by showing kind concern, and by letting the patient know that he is regarded as a whole person rather than just a collection of injured parts. Such an attitude encourages trust, provides emotional comfort, and relieves anxiety. If the patient is unable to think or act in an orderly or controlled fashion, the EMT must "take over," at least temporarily, and give directions on what to do and how to do it, step by step.

If family or friends are with the patient after an accident or in other crises, the EMT should deal with them as well as with the patient. The most comforting support one can provide is to demonstrate emotional stability under stress, to perform competently and kindly, and to provide reassurance through proper actions that all that can be done is being done in the best interests of the patient. It is also important that the EMT do everything possible to protect the patient and family from undue stress and embarassment arising from what they may say in their confusion or from their fear of how they may appear.

Natural disasters usually involve more than one individual, and therefore some knowledge of group and crowd control is useful for the EMT. Generally, when normality is upset, people immediately try to create order, either by reestablishing old rules or developing new ones. They seek leadership in these efforts, and the EMT can prevent much confusion and wasted effort by assuming the leadership role at once and selecting assistants to be responsible for immediate tasks. These tasks may range from searching for additional victims to setting up shelters. The mobilization of all available resources may be one of the most important tasks the EMT can perform.

Alcohol. One of the most frequent causes of abnormal or unruly behavior the EMT may encounter will probably be that caused by acute

286

alcoholic intoxication. However, it should never be assumed that abnormal behavior in a person who has been drinking is always the result solely of the use of alcohol; diabetes and head injuries are only two of the many conditions that often produce a picture similar to alcoholic intoxication. Intoxicated patients should be examined closely for associated injuries before or during transportation.

Many patients who are acutely intoxicated will exhibit the appearance and demeanor of being in full possession of their faculties. However, incoherence, loss of memory, aggressive behavior, and unconsciousness are more common in acute alcoholic intoxication. A firm but gentle verbal approach is usually most effective. Discussions should be avoided because they often lead to arguments and physical demonstrations.

The person who has suddenly ceased drinking after a prolonged period of alcohol consumption may develop alcoholic hallucinations or outright delirium tremens (DTs). In these conditions, he may be agitated, afraid of what he sees, incoherent, occasionally "high" to the point of mania, or convulsing. A patient with the DTs is a desperately sick patient who may readily succumb to cardiovascular collapse.

In general, there are different local rules in communities in the United States for handling the patient in whom an alcoholic or drug reaction is strongly suspected. These patients may be disruptive in the Emergency Department. In several areas, detoxification centers exist. Each EMT must be familiar with local policy regarding patients suffering from uncomplicated episodes of alcohol or drug abuse.

Drugs. The EMT will probably encounter many persons under the influence of various kinds of drugs. The problems that are created by drugs are considered in Chapter 39, Alcohol and Drug Abuse. Overdoses of narcotics, analgesics, or hypnotics ordinarily result in a patient who requires cardiac and pulmonary support, since these agents severely depress the central nervous system.

The EMT may encounter patients under the influence of hallucinogens, such as LSD, mescaline, or psilocybin. An overdose causing un-consciousness is unlikely; however, occasionally one sees a "bad trip" or panic state caused by the altered state of consciousness these drugs induce. "Talking the patient down" is the correct approach. The EMT should be quiet, relaxed, sympathetic, and supportive. The patient must be reassured that the state is transient and will pass as the drug is cleared from the body. Restraints should not be used as they may only make an unruly patient worse. **Do not leave this patient alone.**

Occasionally a patient will be seen with acute central nervous system stimulation from the use of stimulants ("uppers") such as the amphetamines. Again, gentle treatment and talking down the restlessness, excitability, talkativeness, and irritability constitute the proper approach.

In all the foregoing instances, where drug intoxication is suspected, prompt transportation to the Emergency Department should be undertaken.

The Emotionally Disturbed Person

People who are emotionally upset manifest their problems in a variety of ways. The disorder may be temporary and mild, or brief but acute. It may be very serious and long lasting. Contrary to popular opinion, most emotionally disturbed people are not unruly nor do they demonstrate bizarre behavior. A wide range of behavior is seen in patients who are disturbed.

Occasionally, the EMT may be summoned to treat an individual who is disturbed or unable to take care of himself. A depressed person who feels hopeless and abandoned may have made a suicide attempt. An aggressive individual may threaten harm to others; he may recognize what he is doing but be unable to control the anger or panic. Some disturbed individuals are unable to interpret their surroundings correctly or to recognize the nature of their actions, thus endangering themselves or others. Elderly people may be found wandering in the street. Living alone, they may become confused and unable to take physical care of themselves. The EMT may encounter an individual who has sustained a physical injury or illness but who is also showing signs of mental disturbance.

When responding to a psychiatric emergency, the EMT should assess the need for help as quickly as possible. If the patient has a dangerous weapon such as a gun or a knife, or is at a dangerous height threatening to jump, the police should be summoned before any other action is taken. They can be asked to stay nearby or out of sight, if possible, until the need for their help is evident. Their support may be required in a similar manner with the aggressive, belligerent person who does not appear willing or able to cooperate. The presence of a psychiatrist or a clergyman may also be required at the scene.

In establishing the priorities of care, a psychiatric emergency must sometimes take precedence over a medical emergency. In a case where a homicidal or suicidal act is possible, medical care may necessarily have to be delayed. On the other hand, if serious physical disability or death seems imminent, medical care should assume first priority and the EMT should make an effort to assist a patient if he can.

Approach to the patient. The EMT should attempt to obtain from the patient, his family, friends, or bystanders any information that may shed light on the present behavior or that will reveal whether the patient has acted in a disturbed manner before. He should find out if possible under what circumstances this or previous disturbed behavior occurred, whether the patient has ever been treated for mental disorders and whether he has been under medical care. Other information to be sought should include opinions on what seems to have brought on the present emergency, whether the patient has been taking drugs or medicines of any kind, and whether he has been exposed to toxic chemicals.

Following an evaluation of the situation, and when support is nearby, the EMT should approach the patient in a quiet, unhurried manner. Many disturbed patients are frightened and panicky. Anything the EMT can do to reduce their fright and panic will be helpful. The EMT should not touch the patient unless there is an immediate and obvious need for medical treatment or physical restraint to prevent the patient from harming himself or others. Instead, the EMT should identify himself and talk to the patient in a reassuring way, trying to find out what

is the trouble. The EMT must take time. It may be necessary to listen to the patient for a while. Most disturbed persons will become calmer when dealt with in a straightforward, direct manner.

If the patient is potentially aggressive or hostile, it would be wise to have at least two people in the room. The EMT should try to involve the patient in making the decision to go to a hospital if this course appears indicated, and should try to avoid the use of strong-arm tactics or restraining devices. Rather than be taken on a stretcher, the patient will probably prefer to sit in the ambulance. This courtesy should be allowed, although the patient should never sit in the seat with the driver. At least two people should accompany the patient in the vehicle in close proximity in case control or restraint should become necessary.

When the EMT is unable to approach an extremely disturbed patient alone or with a companion, four or five persons may be required; their presence alone may induce the patient's cooperation.

The suicidal crisis. The suicidal crisis encompasses a wide range of behavior from the actual act of taking one's life to the mere expression of the thought about doing so. The crisis period is usually limited and, with appropriate help, an individual may pass through this critical time and again be able to function.

While there are no hard and fast rules for the successful treatment of the suicidal person, several general principles should be known.

1. Suicidal behavior is frequently a disguised attempt to communicate a need.
2. Whether the communication is a direct or a disguised cry for help, recognition of the need can aid the EMT in understanding the nature of the problem. All such attempts or gestures must be taken seriously. When talking with a suicidal person, it is important for the EMT to establish a trusting relationship. A harsh or a critical attitude toward the patient's wishes or attitude or toward behavior which seems strange should be avoided. An understanding attitude is required to develop a trusting relationship with the patient.

3. A calm, decisive, reassuring, and common-sense approach to the suicidal individual can greatly aid the present treatment and future outcome.

4. During the initial crisis, to keep the patient alive, the EMT may need to act in ways he normally would not to satisfy the patient's childlike whims. A broadminded and sympathetic response is imperative.

5. During the process of intervention, the EMT may experience personal feelings which are difficult for him to handle. It is crucial that he recognize his own feelings and their potential influence upon the suicidal person. He must expect an emotional reaction in himself and not allow it to appear in his dealings with the patient.

Both physical and emotional or psychological first aid may be necessary in the treatment of the suicidal person. If the patient has already harmed himself, physical needs—for example, treatment for a slashed wrist or a drug overdose—should be immediately attended. Sometimes, especially in the case of medications or foreign objects that have been swallowed, the need for physical emergency treatment will not be obvious. The EMT must obtain as much information and data as possible and transmit them to the Emergency Department personnel, no matter how absurd the reports may seem.

During all stages of intervention, precautionary measures against a repeated or sudden additional suicide attempt should be taken. Firearms, medications, and other objects that are potentially lethal should be removed from the patient's grasp. **He should not be left alone at any point, or for any moment, whether at home or in the ambulance.**

The Dying Patient

Most of the time the EMT's contact with the dying patient will be limited to someone who is slipping in and out of consciousness, but there may be occasions when a dying patient is clearly in touch with what is happening. The EMT must be reassuring and unusually sensitive to this patient's apprehensions. Stress that everything possible is being done to transport the patient to the hospital as quickly as possible and that expert help will be available there.

Although attention to physical needs will be paramount, the EMT must be attentive to the patient's emotional needs and possible desire to send instructions or messages to others. An offer of the EMT to make himself available to survivors will make the thought of death less frightening for the patient. Last messages or directions of dying patients must be noted. Frequently, they will have legal importance. Should the EMT be attending both a dying patient and a potential survivor who is aware of the situation, the EMT should reassure the survivor that personnel in the Emergency Department will be able to assess the severity of the patient's condition and will do all they can to save him.

At all times, the EMT must be aware of and master his own feelings. Dealing with death causes anxiety for all persons in the health professions. If the EMT is aware that this perfectly normal reaction affects everyone, there will be a significantly smaller chance that his own feelings about death will interfere with his proper treatment of the dying patient.

Physical Causes that Can Be Misinterpreted

Diabetes. Not infrequently a diabetic patient will take an overdose of insulin, or will not eat sufficient food to cover the insulin he regularly takes. He will then exhibit the unsteadiness, slurred speech, tremors, weakness, and abnormal behavior which are easily mistaken for alcoholic intoxication. This misdiagnosis has led to the death of diabetic patients in "drunk tanks" of jails. A direct question to the patient about diabetes or a search for an identifying tag, locket, or card may be rewarding, both to the patient and the EMT.

Head injury. A person may be rendered confused or speechless by an injury of the head which may not be apparent without a careful examination. The assumption that the patient is drunk or incapacitated because of drug use should not be made màde without examination and questioning.

Other conditions. Severe infections with generalized sepsis and high fever may render a patient delirious or incoherent. Toxic reaction to many substances other than alcohol and drugs can similarly produce bizarre behavior. In the former instance, an infected lesion will usually be seen and a fever or other sign of infection will be present. The diagnosis of a toxic reaction may be difficult.

Conclusion

Each state has its own laws relating to the management of the emotionally disturbed person. The EMT should be familiar with the laws in his area relating to involuntary transportation, entering homes, and applying restraints. It is important to remember that people engaged in emergency care, other than members of law enforcement agencies, are **not empowered to restrain or transport a patient forcibly against his will.** The EMT may not act in such a manner even if requested to do so by members of the patient's family. He may intervene only to the extent that any private citizen would to prevent the patient from doing bodily harm to himself or to others. Most important, it is essential for the EMT to remember to take time in dealing with disturbed persons, to control his own fear, to speak in a calm, reassuring manner, and to try to convince the patient that he is only seeking to provide help.

In dealing with all emergencies causing disturbed or unruly behavior, the EMT should recall that, just as the symptoms of a medical disease or injury are the indicators both of the condition of the patient and bodily attempts to deal with it, so the symptoms of an emotional disturbance are indicators both of the disorder and the means by which the patient is attempting to cope with a problem.

290

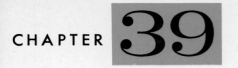

Alcohol and Drug Abuse

GOAL I. Understand the role of alcohol and other compounds in situations which may confront the EMT.

291

OBJECTIVES

A. List the commonly used drugs by type of reactions produced.
B. List the various drugs and materials subject to abuse.
C. List the various substances which may be accidentally ingested and which may produce adverse reactions.
D. List the most common types of drugs abused.
E. List major clinical effects produced by drugs that are commonly abused.
F. List the disease processes that alcohol or drug abuse can mimic.

GOAL II. Know the principles of immediate care of patients who have abused alcohol or drugs.

OBJECTIVES

A. Describe the immediate care of patients who have abused alcohol or drugs.
B. Describe the immediate care of a patient with an allergic drug reaction.
C. Describe how the EMT can be of assistance in identifying specific offending substances.
D. Describe local rules pertaining to the care of patients who have abused alcohol or drugs.

Introduction

A drug is any substance which can produce an effect on the mind or the body. Undesirable reactions occur with the use of almost every drug. These reactions often require emergency medical treatment. Adverse reactions result when individuals accidentally or intentionally misuse any of the compounds listed below:

1. Alcohol
2. Prescription drugs
3. Non-prescription or over-the-counter medicines
4. "Street" drugs (drugs obtained by illegal means)
5. Household or industrial chemicals

In addition, many drugs may elicit severe allergic responses in patients who have become sensitive to them. These responses are not necessarily the result of intentional or accidental misuse of the drug; however, they may require emergency medical care.

Relatively few of the deaths from drug abuse are related to narcotic addiction. The classic example of a misused drug in society today is alcohol. However, only 5 percent of all alcoholics are typical "skidrow drunks."

In the following discussion, drugs will be categorized according to their principal effects on the body rather than by their scientific or chemical classifications. Most drugs which are knowingly misused are taken either for their stimulating, depressing, or hallucinatory effects on the mind.

Though drug use results in various reactions, only five major effects from drugs need to be noted in a guide for emergency care. A classification of drug effects into the five groups is given in Table 39.1. The physical effects, which are often extremely unpleasant and even life-threatening, as well as the mental and emotional effects mentioned earlier, are also noted.

Because of the prevalence of problems related to the use of alcohol, it is considered in a separate section.

292

TABLE 39.1
CLASSIFICATION OF DRUG EFFECTS

Agents	Familiar Names	Undesirable/Dangerous Effects
Drugs Which Stimulate—The Uppers		
Amphetamines	Bennies, speed	Nervous system stimulation (the jitters, headache, sleeplessness, incessant speech, convulsions)
Caffeine	Coffee, colas	
Anti-asthmatics	Adrenalin, aminophylline, isoproterenol	Increased heart rate, blood pressure, and breathing rate
Vasoconstrictors	Decongestants	
Cocaine	Snow, coke	Extreme depression when stopped
Drugs Which Depress—The Downers		
Alcohol		Nervous system depression (lethargy, sleepiness, coma, decreased response to pain, respiratory depression, death)
Barbiturates	Phenobarbital, seconal, reds	
Marijuana*	Grass	
Narcotics	Morphine, codeine, heroin	Impaired coordination, judgment, and reflexes
Tranquilizers	Thorazine, Valium	Constipation
Anticonvulsants	Dilantin	Tremors, especially with withdrawal
		Low blood pressure
		Withdrawal symptoms may be painful, even life-threatening
Drugs Which Cause Hallucinations		
LSD	Acid	Hallucinations
Peyote		Dangerous psychiatric behavior, including suicide attempts
Mescaline		Panic reactions
		Impaired judgment
Drugs Which Elicit Allergic Reactions		
Antibiotics	Penicillin, Sulfas	Anaphylactic shock—acute, life-threatening, asthmatic-like attack
Iodines	Expectorants	
Virtually any other drug		Rashes, hives
		Swelling, bruising
		Fever
Miscellaneous, Undesirable Drug Reactions		
Virtually any drug taken in improper amounts	Digitalis	Alterations in heart function
	Potassium	Confusion, incoordination
	Reserpine	Vomiting
	Steroids	Bizarre, unilateral muscle spasms are associated with major tranquilizers like thorazine
	Tranquilizers	

* Also has minor hallucinogenic properties

Drug Abuse

Individuals who use drugs may present many situations and problems of concern to the EMT. The narcotic analgesic medications, which are central nervous system depressants, include heroin, morphine, opium, methadone, and meperidine (Demerol). When an overdose of any of these compounds is taken, the patient may become comatose and his respirations slow and shallow. Adequacy of respiration must be ascertained immediately, since it is usually the life-threatening factor for this patient. If needed, an airway must be secured and respiratory support provided.

Overdoses of hypnotics, sedatives, alcohol, and tranquilizers, often known as "downers," are frequently encountered. These agents also tend to depress respiration. The principles of emergency care for these patients involve securing and maintaining an adequate airway and providing appropriate respiratory support during transportation to the Emergency Department.

The EMT may encounter patients under the influence of hallucinogens. Drugs in this group of compounds include LSD, mescaline, psilocybin, and peyote. Overdose with these agents to the point of unconsciousness and coma is unlikely, but the EMT must occasionally treat a patient on a "bad trip" or in a panic state because of altered perceptions induced by these drugs.

Occasionally, but not as often, this same type of reaction will be seen following the use of marijuana. To a certain degree, marijuana is an hallucinogenic as well as a depressant drug. Insofar as it alters the state of consciousness to produce hallucinations, it may cause the occurrence of panic as a result of its use.

In general, the emergency care for these patients involves emotional support and, wherever possible, avoiding the use of restraints. It should go without saying that these patients must not be left alone during their care or transportation to the Emergency Department.

Central nervous system stimulants, "uppers," include amphetamines, caffeine, cocaine, antiasthmatic drugs such as adrenaline and aminophylline, and vasoconstrictor drugs used as decongestants. The use of these drugs induces in the patient a characteristic set of symptoms, including excitement, restlessness, irritability, and talkativeness. Uncommonly, their use may result in unconsciousness. If coma is seen, the patient must be checked immediately for signs of cardiorespiratory failure and, when it exists, an appropriate form of treatment should be instituted. Respiratory failure is not uncommon with the use of cocaine because of its direct depressant effect on the respiratory center of the brain.

The EMT may have occasion to see patients suffering from an acute drug-withdrawal syndrome. The use of some drugs, especially over a long period of time, may result in physiologic dependence on the drug. Sudden withdrawal from the drug may cause a varied set of symptoms. For example, withdrawal from barbiturates can cause anxiety, tremors, nausea, fever, delirium, convulsions, and ultimate fatality. Withdrawal from heroin or methadone, although probably seen much more frequently, is usually less dangerous. The symptoms of heroin and methadone withdrawal are multiple, however, and may be of significant discomfort to the patient.

In instances of drug ingestion or injection, it is important that the medical personnel in the Emergency Department be told as much about the number and type of drugs taken as possible. All readily available material around the patient—in his residence, if the EMT finds the patient there, or on his person—which might help to identify the drugs should be transported along with him to the hospital. However, a person who is believed to have had a drug overdose should be transported to the Emergency Department as quickly as possible without waiting to search.

One must also keep in mind that any patient may have taken any one of a large number of drugs and often may have taken several in various combinations. The combination of specific drugs with a large quantity of alcohol is a particularly common incident which can be very dangerous. The patient suffering from multiple drug ingestion must be treated as a priority one emergency, since each drug may increase the effect of the others and their combined effect may be much more rapid and powerful than that of any one alone.

Alcohol Abuse

Alcohol, a central nervous system depressant, is misused more than any other drug in society today. Alcohol-related problems comprise a large portion of Emergency Department work. It has been estimated that nine million Americans are alcoholics and that for each individual so afflicted, four additional persons are adversely affected. Statistics show that 50 percent of traffic fatalities, homicides, suicides, general accidents, and violent attacks are associated with the use of alcohol.

The major signs of acute alcohol intoxication and the additional associated problems that can arise from chronic alcohol use are listed in Table 39.2. Problems associated with acute alcohol intoxication or with the chronic use of alcohol have not been differentiated from one another since they all may require emergency care and are associated with the same cause.

It must be emphasized that the use of alcohol can produce physical signs that mimic other disease processes and can occasionally produce states indistinguishable from them. Uncontrolled diabetes, head injuries, cerebral palsy, life-threatening infections with delirium, and toxic reactions often resemble drunkenness. Diabetic patients have been left unaided in jail drunk tanks and even in Emergency Departments because the personnel have interpreted the symptoms as those of acute alcohol intoxication or withdrawal. In many instances these patients have died. It is necessary, then, to recognize alcoholism as the disease it is and to be able to differentiate the signs of acute or chronic alcohol use from the signs and symptoms of severe organic illness.

Ordinarily, the EMT will be concerned with the patient who has consumed a large quantity of alcohol and is drunk. The intoxicated patient may exhibit aggressive, inappropriate behavior and be uncooperative in other respects. He often has difficulty with coordination and balance. These patients may fall easily and injure themselves. Adequate precautions must be taken for their protection.

Occasionally a patient may have consumed enough alcohol to develop the signs of severe

294

TABLE 39.2

SIGNS OF ALCOHOL USE THAT REQUIRE IMMEDIATE ACTION

1. Depression of nervous system (lethargy, sleepiness, coma, decreased response to pain, respiratory depression)
2. Impaired coordination, judgment, reflexes
3. Tremors, especially with withdrawal
4. Excessively low blood pressure
5. Painful withdrawal symptoms (withdrawal can be life-threatening)
6. Aggressive, inappropriate behavior
7. Gastritis with vomiting, bleeding, dehydration
8. Depression of respiration to level of respiratory arrest
9. Grand mal seizures (can precede delirium tremens)
10. Delirium tremens (terrifying mental confusion, constant tremor, fumbling movements of the hands, fever, dehydration, rapid pulse rate)
11. Wernicke's encephalopathy (characterized by muscular incoordination, ocular disorders and mental confusion)
12. Korsakoff's psychosis (including memory loss and disinterested behavior)
13. Musculoskeletal trauma of unexplained origin and in various stages of healing

central nervous system depression with respiratory difficulty. In this instance he may require cardiopulmonary support en route to the hospital.

A specific problem associated with the use of alcohol is a result of withdrawal from it. In the course of a prolonged drinking episode, the patient may stop consuming alcohol because he can no longer procure any, because he is sick, or because he makes a resolution to stop drinking. Two situations (alcoholic hallucinations and delirium tremens) may arise from an abrupt withdrawal from alcohol after its prolonged use. These situations are each part of the same process but differ in degrees of severity. Alcoholic hallucinations are the perception of figures, usually animals, in various attitudes about the patient. Ordinarily, this is a temporary but frightening state, which can be treated relatively well by reassurance. Delirium tremens (DTs or the rum fits) is a much more severe complication caused by sudden withdrawal from alcohol.

DTs usually occur from one to seven days after withdrawal. They are characterized by restlessness, fever, sweating, confusion, disorientation, delusions, hallucinations, agitation, and even mania with wild behavior. It is extremely important that the EMT recognize this patient's actions as those of a confused and very sick person and administer the appropriate help in this situation. Delirium tremens itself has a relatively high mortality rate, and it too must be distinguished from any other disease or injury which its appearance might be masking. Three specific dangers exist with the occurrence of delirium tremens.

1. While restless, the patient may injure himself or others. The EMT must protect the patient, but not necessarily with restraints, since the use of restraints usually only increases agitation.
2. Convulsions can be seen with acute alcohol withdrawal, and the EMT should be prepared to treat seizures should they occur.
3. Because of agitation, fever, and sweating, the patient loses a considerable amount of water and may become dehydrated. The risk of hypovolemic circulatory collapse

or shock is significant in this patient. Accordingly, during transportation to the Emergency Department, careful monitoring of blood pressure must be maintained. If the blood pressure falls, intravenous infusion should be started to counteract hypovolemic shock.

Emotional support through which the patient is comforted and helped to understand what is taking place can often reduce agitation and consequently diminish the incidence of further injury or shock.

Apart from these specific considerations, the treatment of the patient who is acutely intoxicated with alcohol follows the treatment of other patients intoxicated with central nervous system depressants and may require all the available support techniques up through formal cardiopulmonary resuscitation.

The Emergency Care of a Patient Who Misuses Alcohol or Drugs

As with all emergency patients, the EMT must decide the priorities of care for the problems presented by the patient who misuses alcohol or drugs. Where they are required, basic life support measures (Chapter 10) must be instituted immediately and should override other considerations in treating these patients until some stability of the cardiorespiratory system has been achieved. Otherwise, the major elements of care for these patients include the following steps.

1. **Induce vomiting.** If the patient has taken the overdosed drug within the past thirty minutes, vomiting should be induced by the administration of syrup of ipecac, followed by warm water. Specific contraindications exist, however, for the use of vomiting. Patients who have swallowed lye, strong acids, petroleum compounds, or antiemetic drugs, or those who are semiconscious or comatose should not be made to vomit. When vomiting is induced, the EMT must be prepared to suction the vomited material from the patient's mouth and throat to clear the airway.

Often the overdosed drug will cause a marked

295

irritation of the gastrointestinal mucosa or lining and will in this manner cause the patient to vomit. Since the patient may be semiconscious or comatose as a result of the action of the drug, the aspiration of vomited material into the lungs can cause serious pulmonary damage. He must be positioned on one side with the head down to avoid aspiration. The EMT must be prepared to remove all vomited material from the pharynx promptly.

2. Prevent self-injury. The EMT should be prepared for a generalized convulsion in the patient who has taken an overdose of hallucinogenic or stimulatory agents and is having a severe excitatory reaction. Protect this patient from falls, from injuries as he strikes fixed objects, from hitting himself, or from biting his tongue.

3. Maintain the level of consciousness. If the patient is showing the signs or symptoms of central nervous system depression—that is, lethargy, sleepiness, decreased response to pain, or respiratory depression—he should be stimulated constantly by gentle shaking, pinching, and conversation to determine the initial level of consciousness and to keep him awake. Frequently, keeping the patient sitting up, moving, or walking is very helpful. These maneuvers may be sufficient to produce adequate spontaneous respiration while en route to the Emergency Department. If the patient is allowed to pass into semiconsciousness or coma, respiratory depression follows and he may not be able to continue breathing in that state. If respiratory depression is so profound that breathing has ceased, artificial ventilation is required with all means at the disposal of the EMT.

4. Instill confidence. When hallucinogenic agents, stimulants, and occasionally alcohol are used, panic reactions, hallucinations, and abnormal psychological states may be observed. These reactions may also be associated with the abrupt discontinuation of the use of the drug. In a patient exhibiting such agitated behavior, the appropriate treatment is to "talk him down." The EMT should approach the patient in a quiet, relaxed, and sympathetic manner and talk. The patient must be assured that his mental condition is the result of the use of the drug and that it will return to normal when the drug is eliminated from the body. The EMT who exhibits calm self-control and provides guidance in this situation can frequently calm this patient with conversation alone. The use of physical restraints is to be avoided unless absolutely indicated, because the patient may harm himself or violently attack others. Generally, the use of restraints for such a patient results in increasing unruly and disturbed behavior considerably.

5. Evaluate further injuries. If fractures, lacerations, or internal injuries are suspected or observed, follow standard procedures to control obvious bleeding and immobilize injured areas. A person in a generally depressed state because of the use of alcohol or drugs can sustain serious bodily injuries but not exhibit the normal sensations of pain. These injuries must not be overlooked in the initial evaluation of the patient's condition. Diagnostic wisdom is required to differentiate a depressed level of consciousness as a result of alcoholic intoxication from the effects of an actual head injury. Since over 50 percent of all traumatic injuries are associated with the apparent ingestion of alcohol, being able to distinguish the effects of an injury from the effects of alcohol becomes particularly important.

Two additional problems are pertinent when one is evaluating the condition of the patient with alcohol or drug overdose. The first of these is that addicts are prone to develop serious infections and hepatitis from contaminated injections and contaminated drugs. Although superficial infections of the extremities are easily recognized, deep-seated infections within the body are not. For example, infections of the spine, pelvis, brain, liver, or heart valves may be present. Symptoms associated with these processes may be mistaken by the patient and medical personnel for withdrawal symptoms and proper treatment for the problem be withheld because of the mistake.

A second problem is that patients under the influence of narcotic or other depressant drugs have been observed to fall into stupor or coma in contorted positions. In consequence, circulation of blood in a limb may be reduced so much

296

that muscle is destroyed or nerves damaged. The physical findings will be a cold, swollen, paralyzed, cyanotic, anesthetic limb.

Associated with the destruction of muscle in the particular compartment of the limb (compartment syndrome), a brown urine is produced as the body tries to clear material from the damaged muscle through the urinary tract. The passage of this material, called myoglobin, damages kidneys and may result in complete kidney failure.

The finding of a damaged limb under these circumstances indicates an acute physical emergency. An immediate operation for decompression of the limb may be required, even if the patient is still under the influence of the drug. Emergency measures the EMT may employ include repositioning the limb to facilitate blood flow, elevating it, cooling it (without placing ice directly on the skin), and immobilizing it. The patient should be taken to the hospital immediately.

6. Observe for allergic reactions. An allergic reaction, although not associated with drug abuse, can be mistaken for a drug reaction, particularly if the allergy is severe. The primary danger in allergic reaction is the development of anaphylactic shock. In this situation, the history the patient can give is of great value and he can usually identify the offending agent.

Respiratory support measures are essential in treating anaphylactic shock. Spasm of the bronchial passages and production of large amounts of mucus in the airway may lead to asphyxiation. Cardiovascular collapse may complicate this emergency.

Definitive treatment for anaphylactic shock is the administration of epinephrine intravenously. The use of this drug may be ordered only by qualified medical personnel. If the reaction from the allergic response only involves a gastrointestinal disorder, a skin rash, or itching, the patient should be transported to the Emergency Department and observed for possible progression of the symptoms and for evaluation by a physician.

7. Observe for shock. As previously stated in the discussion on delirium tremens, and in occasional other instances, the patient may de-velop symptoms of shock. The EMT should be aware of this possibility, observe carefully for signs of it, and be prepared to give appropriate treatment.

Conclusion

In addition to providing the immediate medical care described above, the EMT must gather material and information that will assist the hospital staff in diagnosing and treating the suspected drug problem. To aid in identifying the offending substance, look for medication containers and pills near the patient. Try to obtain samples of vomitus, urine, and fecal material, and question other individuals in the area concerning the habits of the patient. Be alert to the fact that several substances may be used concurrently or that drugs may be mislabeled, which can lead to confusing symptoms. Mislabeling is especially common with street drugs. As much information as can be gathered should accompany the patient to the hospital.

Finally, transport the patient to the Emergency Department as quickly as possible. Be alert for all of the possible complications noted. Never make a judgment that the patient is in satisfactory condition and can be discharged. Never leave the patient alone until he has been transferred to the care of appropriate medical personnel at the Emergency Department for final evaluation.

The EMT must also be aware of all local rules pertaining to the care of alcohol or drug abuse patients. In many large communities, specific detoxification centers exist for the reception of these patients when there is no question of associated illness or injury. Local arrangements differ from area to area in the United States, and the EMT is responsible for a clear knowledge of rules in his community.

Do not overlook the following facts:

Drug abuse and psychiatric disease are often related.

Street drugs are frequently contaminated or diluted with dangerous as well as unsterile substances. They are the source of infection as well as cross-reaction to the substances used in diluting them.

Alcoholism may be complicated by a variety of other problems. Also several bona fide diseases, such as diabetes, epilepsy, head injury, or outright psychosis, can be mistaken for drunkenness.

Treatment of the alcoholic patient or the drug abuser does not end with detoxification for a specific episode. Ongoing treatment may last the extent of the patient's life. His chances, however, for surviving to enter a course of such treatment may at one time depend entirely on timely intervention by the EMT.

X

Environmental Injuries

CHAPTER 40

Heat Exposure

GOAL I. Understand the types of heat exposure and their effects on the body.

OBJECTIVES

A. List the causes of heat exposure.
B. Point out the common factor in all causes of heat exposure.
C. Point out the differences in the various causes of heat exposure.
D. Describe the importance of the skin as an organ of the body.
E. Point out other areas or organs which are endangered as a result of heat exposure.

GOAL II. Understand the rationale and methods of emergency burn treatment.

OBJECTIVES

A. Explain the importance and methods of rating burns.
B. List the common factors in treatment of all burns.
C. Describe differences in treatment of specific burns.
D. Describe systemic complications of burns.

GOAL III. Know the procedures for evaluation and treatment of patients with heat exposure.

OBJECTIVES

A. Describe the signs and treatment of heat exhaustion.
B. Describe the signs and treatment of heat stroke.

Under the term heat exposure we include several environmental injuries: thermal burns, burns from electrical current, chemical burns, burns resulting from radiant energy, and systemic reactions to heat. These injuries have only one factor common to all of them, which is that the human organism has received, either locally or over its entire surface, a concentrated or diffuse dose of excess energy for which its normal protective mechanisms are insufficient.

Burn injuries are generally rated in terms of damage of the integument. Specifically, they are classified in percentage of surface damaged and depth of damage through the various layers of skin. The anatomy of the skin is considered in some detail in Chapter 12. To review, the skin is basically a two-layered structure consisting of an outer epidermis and an inner dermis. The epidermis is made up of tough, keratinized (horny) cells which constantly are being sloughed away from the body.

Between the dermis and the epidermis lies a

productive layer which continuously gives rise to new cells to form the epidermis as the old cells are sloughed away. Within the inner layer, the dermis, are contained various organs of the skin: the hair follicles, the sweat glands, the sebaceous glands producing oil which lubricates hair and skin, the nerve endings, and blood vessels. Beneath the dermis is the subcutaneous fatty tissue and beneath this tissue are the muscles of the body, enclosed in fascial layers and surrounding the skeleton.

The functions of the skin are many. It serves to isolate the body in its environment, to protect the body from bacterial invasion, to control the temperature of the body, to retain the fluids of the body, and to furnish a myriad of details about the external environment to the brain through its nerve endings. Any damage of this surface covering allows a break in these mechanisms. Through such a damaged area an overwhelming bacterial infection may invade the body. If the damage is great enough, the regulatory function of the skin in terms of maintaining normal body temperature and normal fluid balance is lost. If enough skin is damaged, its ability to inform the patient of environmental changes is similarly lost.

People do not commonly regard the skin as an organ of the body. It is, however, the single largest organ of the body and because of the multitude of its functions, it is one of the most important. Damage of this organ is of grave concern.

Thermal Burns

The most common type of burn is the thermal, or heat, burn. The seriousness of the burn can be measured. It depends upon the degree of the burn (depth of the skin injured) and the amount of the body surface involved. Burns can be classified in degrees from one through six. A first degree burn is limited to the most superficial layer of the epidermis and results only in erythema (reddening) of the skin (Fig. 40.1 *a*). A second degree burn causes damage into but not through the dermis and characteristically results in the appearance of vesicles (blisters) in the skin (Fig. 40.1 *b*). A third degree burn is one in which the full thickness of the skin is destroyed down to the subcutaneous fat (Fig. 40.1 *c*). In this burn the skin may appear pale, dry, and white; it may even be brown or charred. Clotted blood vessels may be seen through the skin as though one were looking at them through parchment. A fourth degree burn involves destruction of the skin and the subcutaneous fat. A fifth degree burn involves destruction of the skin, the fat, and the underlying muscle. A sixth degree burn involves destruction through all the structures, including the supporting bone.

With burns more serious than second degree, there is destruction of the sensory nerve endings of the skin. The burned area is consequently insensitive. However, the area surrounding the burn will not have all nerve endings destroyed and may frequently be extremely painful.

The amount of body surface that is burned is very important in determining the seriousness of the burn. A very rough but reasonably accurate estimate of the amount of body surface burned is determined by the rule of nines. This rule, which applies specifically in adults and older children, divides the body into sections, each of which constitutes approximately 9 percent of the total area. The diagrams in Figure

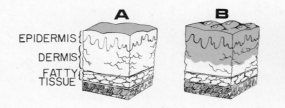

EPIDERMIS
DERMIS
FATTY TISSUE

Figure 40.1 *a–c*

The three common degrees of thermal burn injury are shown. *a*, A first degree burn causes epidermal injury and is manifested by cutaneous erythema and pain. *b*, A second degree burn causes a partial destruction of the dermis and is characterized by blisters (vesicles). It too is painful. *c*, A third degree burn causes complete epidermal and dermal destruction. It is not painful.

302

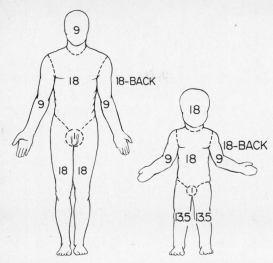

Figure 40.2

In the adult, most areas of the body can be divided roughly into portions of 9 percent, or multiples of 9. This division, called the rule of nines, is useful in estimating the percentage of body surface damage an individual has sustained in a burn. In the small child, relatively more area is taken up by the head and less by the lower extremities. Accordingly, the rule of nines is modified. In each case, the rule gives a useful approximation of body surface.

40.2 indicate the application of this rule. In infants and younger children a considerably greater proportion of the body is taken up by the head and a smaller proportion by the lower extremities. Accordingly, the rule is modified for these patients. Strictly, the rule of nines allows only an approximation of the burned surface area of the body, but it is useful in early estimates, which are the only instances in which the EMT is involved. The physician can obtain a more accurate representation of the percentage of body surface burned.

By knowing the degree of the burn, the approximate percentage of the body that has been burned, the location of the burn, accompanying complications, and the age of the patient, one can classify the severity of thermal burn injury as critical, moderate, or minor. Such a classification is essential in a disaster where many injured patients are involved and where triage separates the patients into emergency cases and cases for whom treatment may be delayed. A summary of the three classifications follows.

Critical (severe) burns—This category includes:

1. All burns of whatever degree and extent if they are complicated by respiratory tract injury and other major injuries or fractures
2. Third degree burns involving critical areas such as the face, hands, or feet
3. Third degree burns which involve more than 10 percent of the body surface
4. Second degree burns which involve more than 30 percent of the body surface

Moderate burns—This category includes:

1. Third degree burns of 2 to 10 percent of the body surface which do not involve the face, hands, or feet
2. Second degree burns which involve 15 to 30 percent of the body surface
3. First degree burns involving 50 to 75 percent of the body surface

Minor burns—This category includes:

1. Third degree burns of less than 2 percent of body surface if no critical areas involved
2. Second degree burns involving less than 15 percent of the body surface
3. First degree burns of less than 20 percent of the body surface

In evaluating a patient who has sustained a burn, age and general condition must also be considered. A moderate burn in an aged patient who is chronically ill should be classified as critical in terms of the immediate treatment required because of the patient's general condition apart from the burn.

The care of thermal burns. The care of thermal burns depends on the percentage of burned body surface involved. In no instance should grease (butter, lard, vaseline, mineral oil, or other ointments) be applied to a burn. For first or second degree burns, such as a person might receive from leaning against a hot stove, the EMT should:

1. Immerse the burned part in cold water for two to five minutes.
2. Cover the burn with a sterile dressing or clean sheet.
3. Use cool wet applications for relief of pain.
4. Transport the patient to the Emergency

303

Department, continuing cool applications en route.

For extensive first or second degree burns and for all third degree burns the procedure set forth below should be followed.

1. Examine for and relieve any respiratory distress. Always anticipate respiratory difficulty when there are burns around the face and neck or when the patient has been exposed to hot gases or smoke.
2. Cover the burned area with a sterile dressing or a clean sheet. Use cool wet applications for relief of pain.
3. Treat the patient for shock if it is apparent.
4. Transport the patient to the Emergency Department, continuing the cool applications en route.

Severe pain, which may accompany first or second degree burns or may exist at the edges of a third degree burn, is best relieved by injected analgesic medications. These drugs must be given by a qualified person on a doctor's order. Such an injection should **not** be given by the EMT. The patient should first be examined by a doctor who will prescribe an injection if needed; it will be given at the hospital.

Local treatment with cool compresses remains the best emergency treatment for burn pain. Third degree burns, which destroy nerve endings, are often not painful enough to require such treatment before the patient reaches the hospital. In burns of this degree and increasing severity, initial efforts are best directed at general support and resuscitation of the patient.

Chemical Burns

Chemical burns are common, especially in industry. Chemicals that cause severe burns are classified as acids or alkalis. Strong acids or strong alkalis can burn any area of the body they contact; but they most often contact and affect the skin, mouth, and eyes. Generally speaking, alkali burns are the more serious because these compounds penetrate deeper and burn longer. When such burns occur in a factory, laboratory, or shop, common emergency measures may have been carried out by trained per-

sonnel before the arrival of the EMT. Whoever gives initial treatment should follow certain guidelines, which are given below.

Strong chemicals burn rapidly; there is no time to waste. The area of contact should be flushed at once with water, without delaying even for removal of clothing (Fig. 40.3). Continue to flood the area with water while clothing is being removed and afterward. The most effective flooding is achieved under a large shower head. It may be effectively done with a hose attached to a faucet; but the force of the stream of water should be taken into consideration if a hose is used. A hard blast of water against already damaged tissue will cause additional injury. While the EMT should keep the flow as full as possible, it should be gentle, not powerful.

Alkali burns. When alkali burns caused by sodium hydroxide or potassium hydroxide have occurred, the affected area should be flooded with water. Dry lime should be brushed off and water should be used only if available in very large amounts for rapid flushing because water will convert the dry lime to a dissolved, active, burning alkali. All the patient's clothing should be removed so that any residual amounts of chemical retained in creases of the clothing

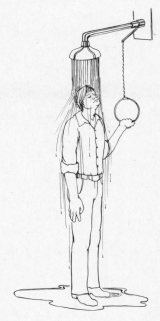

Figure 40.3

For a chemical burn, immediate flushing with water is imperative.

304

may not later come in contact with the skin. Shoes and stockings should be removed.

For alkali burns specifically, a solution of a mild acid may be used to neutralize the alkali. One or two teaspoons of vinegar (acetic acid) to one pint of water may be flushed over the burned area, but only after it has been thoroughly washed with water.

Acid burns. With strong organic or mineral acids, flush the burned area with water and remove all clothing, as prescribed for major alkali burns. After flushing thoroughly with water, one may flood the affected area with a solution made of one teaspoon of baking soda to a pint of water. The soda will tend to neutralize any remaining acid.

It is impossible to state exactly how long a part burned with chemicals should be irrigated with water. In general, the water should be allowed to run over the burned area for a period of time long enough that the EMT is certain all the chemical is flushed from the skin. Frequently the patient will be able to tell him that irritation has ceased or pain has diminished as the chemical is removed.

Because phenol is soluble in alcohol, it has sometimes been stated that a burn resulting from the application of phenol on the skin should be flushed first with alcohol. However, alcohol in large quantities is often not available. Not uncommonly, also, such flushing spreads the phenol over a considerably larger area of skin than would normally be affected had alcohol not been used. The best treatment for burns from this and other organic chemicals still remains prolonged rinsing with water, as described.

Special care of the eyes. The eyes must be given special care. Chemical burns of the eyes are pressing emergencies and much permanent damage can result from a very short exposure of these tissues to a chemical. The eye should be flooded with water as prescribed for the other areas of the body, using either a bulb syringe or a gentle flow from a faucet. Flushing should be continued for at least five minutes for acid and as long as fifteen or twenty minutes for alkali burns. The EMT may be obliged to support the patient's head under a faucet and hold the eyelids open while effecting this treatment because

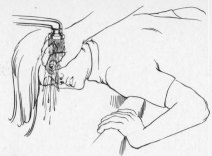

Figure 40.4

It is imperative that eyes injured by a chemical be flushed with copious amounts of gently flowing water for a long period of time.

305

it will usually be impossible for the patient to cooperate (Fig. 40.4). He will probably be in much pain and agitated.

Under no circumstances should any chemical antidotes, such as vinegar, soda, alcohol, or other compounds, be used in treating chemical burns of the eyes. Only water may be used.

The aftercare for both acid and alkali burns is similar. Cover the burn with a sterile dressing and immediately transport the patient to the Emergency Department. The aftercare for burns of the eyes should be to close the eye gently with the eyelid, dress it with a very soft pad, and transport this patient at once to the Emergency Department.

Swallowed Chemicals

Chemicals which have been swallowed are discussed in the general chapter on poisons (Chapter 45).

Electrical Burns

Electrical burns may be more serious than they seem at initial observation. In general the entrance wound is small, but the electric current characteristically destroys a considerable volume of tissue underneath what is an apparently innocuous skin wound (Fig. 40.5). Emergency care for electrical burns consists of covering the site with a dry sterile dressing and transporting the patient to the Emergency Department. There are commonly two burns on the body, one at the point where the current has

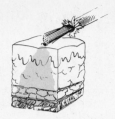

Figure 40.5

While the cutaneous wound of an electrical burn may be very small, the volume of destroyed tissue beneath it is very large.

306

entered the body and one at the point where it has left. The EMT should be sure to look for a second burned area and treat it as he did the first.

In general such burns are associated with broken or downed electrical lines. Because of the risk of injury for the EMT and additional injury to the patient from electrical contact, these patients must not be touched or removed from automobiles across which electric lines are draped or approached in a danger area unless personnel specifically trained in electrical hazards are present to direct and assist. Treatment must be delayed until it is safe for assistance to be given. The EMT should read and reread Chapter 43, Electrical Hazards, and never fail to take all proper precautions.

A major complication of electrical burns is cardiac arrest, either as cardiac standstill or, more commonly, as ventricular fibrillation. Fibrillation is an uncontrolled and ineffective beating of the heart, which can be induced by the sudden passage of a current of electricity through it. The local injury in these burns is rarely of immediate concern, but respiratory and cardiac arrest are. Usually respiratory arrest occurs first and if not promptly treated is rapidly followed by cardiac arrest. Attention for the patient with an electrical burn must be directed at cardiopulmonary resuscitation first rather than to local care of the burn. The extent of tissue damage, cutaneous and muscular, from electrical burns may not be entirely apparent until some days after the burn has occurred. Characteristically, these wounds grow larger and larger in their initial stages as the damaged tissue dies.

All the precautions for treating the patient surrounded by electrical hazards must still be observed by the EMT even when the patient's problems are serious or critical. An EMT who has been injured, perhaps fatally, will be of no assistance to the patient.

Radiation Burns

Nuclear radiation and solar radiation (from the sun) can both cause severe generalized burns.

Nuclear burns. Injury from nuclear radiation is discussed in Chapter 42, Radiation Exposure. The exposure of the whole body to a certain level of nuclear radiation may be lethal. An important point to remember is that when radiation injury occurs simultaneously with a burn, implying that the patient has been close enough to the fireball to sustain thermal as well as radiation injury, each injury tends to make the other worse. A 20 percent, second degree thermal burn, which usually is considered a moderate burn, is rendered critical if it is accompanied by significant radiation exposure.

Solar burns. Solar burn (ordinary sunburn) can require emergency care. First and second degree burns are easily incurred when proper precautions against overexposure to the sun are neglected. When a person has received sufficient radiation from the sun to cause many large blisters, or in some cases one large overall blister, he has sustained a second degree burn of the surface of the body involved. He must be treated as he would be for any other thermal burn of this extent and degree.

Ordinarily, first degree burns are minor burns that rarely involve more than a limited area of skin. These are by far the commonest burns sustained from solar radiation. They are extremely uncomfortable. The best immediate emergency treatment is the gentle application of tepid or cool water or wet, cool cloths.

The occasional person who has large expanses of skin exposed to the sun for even a short period of time without proper conditioning can sustain a first degree burn of nearly the whole body. The results of this exposure are extreme discomfort and perhaps some systemic signs, which generally should pass in a matter of twenty-four or forty-eight hours; but for that period of time the patient may require treatment, hospitalization, and sedation for discomfort.

Heat Exposure

Athletes and workers engaged in outdoor activities are susceptible to illnesses from exposure to heat, especially in the warmer areas of the world, and in all areas in the warmer periods of the year. Illnesses from exposure to heat are often seen in industries where furnaces or ovens are involved in routine processes. Over-exposure to heat occurs most commonly in the early part of a warm period of the year before people have adjusted to higher temperatures. Most often affected are those who are not in good physical condition and those who have not taken the care to condition themselves gradually to increased heat.

When one exercises or labors hard, heat is created in the body. The body automatically reacts to dissipate the excess heat by sweating. When a person perspires, salt and water pass through the sweat glands to the surface of the skin. The water evaporates from the surface, and the process of evaporation cools the body. The salt is left on the surface and is usually washed off the next time the patient bathes.

Some specific syndromes are the result of exposure to heat. These are:

1. Heat cramps
2. Heat exhaustion
3. Heat stroke

Heat cramps. Painful muscle spasms of the arms and legs following strenuous exercise are occasionally seen in persons who otherwise seem to be in very good condition. Very hot weather or prolonged exposure to the sun is not always necessary for heat cramps to occur. Industrial workers more often experience this type of cramp than do athletes.

Normal contraction and relaxation of muscles requires a rather strict balance within the muscle of water and salt. All the tissues in the body are bathed in intracellular and extracellular fluids which have specific concentrations of salt in water. When a person perspires excessively, both water and salt are lost and reserves of each

within the body become depleted. The individual normally interprets this depletion as thirst. If he satisfies his thirst by drinking large quantities of water without taking any additional salt, he depletes his body of salt. A result of this abnormality of salt and water concentration within the tissue is an involuntary, uncontrolled muscular spasm which causes the characteristic cramp.

Generally, people with heat cramps need more salt. Frequently heat cramps can be avoided if a person swallows a salt tablet along with the water that he drinks during a very hot day or when he is working or exercising vigorously in the sun. If cramps have developed, however, they usually will stop when the patient is given a glass of salt water, made by mixing one teaspoon of table salt to a quart of water. Drinking this solution can rapidly reverse the cramping. If there is any indication of a more serious condition, the patient should be transported immediately to the Emergency Department where it will be the responsibility of the attending physician to complete the diagnosis.

Heat exhaustion. Heat exhaustion (heat prostration or heat collapse) is a common illness caused by heat. It is manifested principally by the signs of peripheral vascular collapse, which are weakness or faintness, dizziness, headache, loss of appetite, and nausea. The patient may appear ashen gray and his skin may be cold and clammy. Vital signs usually, however, are normal. The body temperature may even be below normal.

Commonly, heat exhaustion occurs in an otherwise fit person who is involved in extreme physical exertion in a hot environment. Under these conditions the muscular mass of the body and the brain require an increased blood flow. Similarly, an increased blood flow is required by the skin so that heat may be radiated from the skin and sweat may be made. Heat exhaustion is a manifestation of the fact that the vascular system is inadequate at that particular time to meet the demands placed upon it by skin, muscle, and viscera. The patient is, in essence, in a state of mild shock.

He should be treated as though he were in shock. He should be placed in a cool room, supine, and made comfortable. He may require an intravenous infusion of fluid, if a physician directs it. He should rest to allow his vascular system an opportunity to meet the demands placed upon it.

This state is one of the most common of the illnesses induced by heat. It is ordinarily very promptly reversed and non-fatal. It is significantly aggravated by preexisting conditions such as cardiovascular disease, vomiting, or diarrhea. In any instance where a prompt recovery is not seen after rest in a relatively cool area, the patient should be transferred immediately to the Emergency Department for more vigorous fluid and electrolyte therapy.

Heat stroke (sunstroke). A sunstroke is more accurately called heat stroke, since both terms indicate a similar complex of symptoms; but it is not necessary for the patient to be exposed to the sun for this state to develop. Of all the systemic diseases resulting from heat exposure, heat stroke is by far the least common but by far the most serious. Normally a person who is exposed to a particularly warm environment or who actively exercises or works in such an environment automatically activates the body mechanisms for losing heat. Heat is radiated from the skin through an increased cutaneous circulation and the evaporation of sweat. Some heat is radiated in the exhaled breath. The control of heat within the body is a complex mechanism deep within the most primitive part of the central nervous system. It is a regulatory mechanism that is found at almost all levels in the development of warm blooded animals. Heat stroke represents a failure of the heat regulatory mechanism of the body.

Persons who experience heat stroke are usually those who have worked in a very warm, humid environment for a prolonged period of time. Experimentally, as individuals have worked for longer periods of time in hot environments, they have been found to sweat less. The person who develops heat stroke is one in whom sweating has ceased. Thus the major

mechanism for heat loss by the body no longer functions. As heat builds up within the body, generated by metabolic activity, the body temperature rises. In the face of rising body temperature, metabolism itself becomes greater, and the cells, particularly those in the central nervous system, are damaged.

The signs of heat stroke are quite obvious. The patient will have a warm dry skin with a temperature of 105 degrees or even higher. There will ordinarily be a history of prolonged exposure to heat, usually within a humid environment where it is particularly difficult for sweat to evaporate. Coma or near coma or diminished cerebral function exist. Early in the course of the disease the pulse is rapid and full. As the changes of heat stroke become established and tissue is damaged by body heat, vasomotor collapse occurs, blood pressure falls, and the pulse becomes rapid and weak.

Heat stroke is a true emergency. All untreated victims of heat stroke will die. They may die even when treated. The first portions of the body affected in heat stroke are cells within the central nervous system. In a person who sustains a heat stroke but does not die, permanent central nervous system damage may be the result if the condition is allowed to persist for any significant period of time. Recovery from heat stroke is entirely related to the rapidity with which treatment is instituted and the vigor with which it is pursued.

The emergency care for the patient with heat stroke is designed to rid the body of excessive heat as rapidly as possible. Temperature must be reduced to below 100 degrees if at all possible. This can be accomplished by immersing the patient in the bathtub in water cooled with ice, or by using wet sheets or wet compresses and fans while transporting the patient to the hospital. Treatment for shock by intravenous infusion may also be required. Cooling must be continued during transportation, and the patient must be taken to the hospital as a priority one emergency.

CHAPTER 41

Cold Exposure

GOAL I. Understand the types and effects of cold exposure on the body.

309

OBJECTIVES

A. Describe the importance of the wind-chill factor.
B. Explain the methods of heat loss from the body.
C. List the clinical injuries of cold exposure.
D. Explain the factors aggravating cold exposure.

GOAL II. Know the procedures for treating persons suffering from cold exposure.

OBJECTIVES

A. Describe the keystones of treatment of cold injuries.
B. Identify the methods of heat conservation.
C. Recognize the stages through which tissues pass as they are warmed.

The human body may be injured by exposure to temperatures at or below freezing for a long period of time or by exposure to extreme cold for only a very short period. Exposure can injure the surface of the body, causing defined local tissue damage; or it can result in profound generalized body cooling, ultimately causing death. Two factors have an important influence upon the development of cold injury:

1. The temperature of the environment
2. The velocity of the wind

Thermal Conductivity of the Environment

That the environment can conduct heat away from or to the body is an important factor in the development of cold injury. If a hand or any part of the body, particularly if it is wet or even slightly damp, comes into contact with very cold metal, the skin instantly adheres to the metal. Both metal and moisture are excellent thermal conductors. The hand becomes literally frozen to the metal because the moisture on and within its surface promptly freezes. Cloth fabrics are poor heat conductors; and thin, dry, silk or cotton gloves may prevent such an injury, even though they provide no appreciable insulation from the cold.

Still air is a very poor heat conductor, and a person in dry clothes standing still in a windless area can tolerate very low temperature for quite some time. The combination of cold and wind is much more dangerous in the development of freezing injuries. The chilling effect of a temperature of 20° F combined with a wind of thirty-five miles per hour is equal to the chilling effect of 20° below zero with no wind. From these measurements, a term called the wind-chill factor has been developed. The factor allows technicians and medical personnel to relate cold injuries to what the temperature would have to be if there were no wind at the time of exposure. For instance, a person exposed

THE WIND-CHILL FACTOR

Wind Speed	Degrees Fahrenheit (Dry-Bulb Temperature)													
	35	30	25	20	15	10	5	0	−5	−10	−15	−20	−25	−30
	Equivalent Degrees at Indicated Wind Speed													
Calm	35	30	25	20	15	10	5	0	−5	−10	−15	−20	−25	−30
5 mph	33	27	21	16	12	7	1	−6	−11	−15	−20	−26	−31	−35
10 mph	21	16	9	2	−2	−9	−15	−22	−27	−31	−38	−45	−52	−58
15 mph	16	11	1	−6	−11	−18	−25	−33	−40	−45	−51	−60	−65	−70
20 mph	12	3	−4	−9	−17	−24	−32	−40	−46	−52	−60	−68	−76	−81
25 mph	7	0	−7	−15	−22	−29	−37	−45	−52	−58	−67	−75	−83	−89
30 mph	5	−2	−11	−18	−26	−33	−41	−49	−56	−63	−70	−78	−87	−94
35 mph	3	−4	−13	−20	−27	−35	−43	−52	−60	−67	−72	−83	−90	−98
40 mph	1	−4	−15	−22	−29	−36	−45	−54	−62	−69	−76	−87	−94	−101

Labels within table: COLD, VERY COLD, BITTER COLD, EXTREME COLD

Figure 41.1

Using the wind-chill factor, the equivalent cooling power of various wind conditions is shown. For example, under calm conditions a temperature of 15° F has a cooling power of 15°, but when accompanied by a ten-mile-an-hour wind the cooling power is equal to a temperature of −2° F.

310

to −30° F in a storm with a forty-mile-per-hour wind, would suffer the same exposure as if he were at −101° F on a still day with no wind at all. The velocity of the wind markedly increases the chill of the air and aggravates the resulting injury. Figure 41.1 is a representation of the results of the wind-chill factor for various degrees Fahrenheit at various velocities of wind. Table 41.1 lists a variety of ways of estimating wind velocity from easily observed signs.

Heat Regulation

The temperature of the human body must be maintained within a very narrow range (75° to 112° F) simply for survival. For proper bodily function the range is considerably narrower, within one or two degrees of 98.6° F. The human body is a heat-generating mechanism in which metabolism results in the production of warmth. The body also gains heat from external sources such as the sun, fire, or the ingestion of warm food. It maintains its proper functional temperature by balancing the heat internally generated or externally gained by that appropriately lost. There are five major ways in which the body may lose heat.

1. *Conduction*—The direct transfer of heat by contact of the body with a cooler object allows conduction of heat to the cooler object.
2. *Convection*—When cool air moves across the body surface, heat is transferred to the cooler air, warming it and cooling the body.
3. *Evaporation*—When water on the surface of the body is transformed from a liquid to a vapor, heat is required by the process of evaporation and is lost from the body.
4. *Respiration*—When inspired air is raised to the body temperature in the lungs and then exhaled, heat is lost through respiration.
5. *Radiation*—Heat can be radiated by the body to the environment.

For the purpose of heat regulation, the body consists of a core (the brain, heart, lungs, and major abdominal organs) and a shell (the skin, muscles, and extremities). When exposed to

TABLE 41.1

VISUAL ESTIMATION OF WIND VELOCITY*

Observed Phenomena	Descriptive Terms	Wind Speed (mph)
1. Smoke rises vertically; flag lies limp.	Calm	0–1
2. Smoke drift shows direction of wind; leaves on trees move slightly; flag barely moves.	Light air	1–3
3. Wind is felt on face; leaves rustle; flag occasionally moves out a little from staff.	Light breeze	4–7
4. Leaves and small twigs are in constant motion; flag stands out from staff at 30–45° angle.	Gentle breeze	8–12
5. Dust is raised; loose paper blows about; small branches move.	Moderate breeze	13–18
6. Small trees begin to sway; flag stands out at 90° angle.	Fresh breeze	19–24
7. Large branches are in motion; whistling is heard in telephone wires; flag stands out straight from staff and flutters vigorously.	Strong breeze	25–31
8. Whole trees are in motion; it is inconvenient to walk against the wind; light loose objects are lifted from the ground; flag whips about wildly.	Moderate gale	32–38
9. Twigs are broken off trees; automobile in motion trembles; telephone lines whine loudly.	Fresh gale	39–46
10. Trees bend sharply; slight structural damage may occur; both vehicles and pedestrians are seriously impeded.	Strong gale	47–54
11. Trees may be uprooted; structural damage is considerable.	Whole gale	55–63
12. Severe damage occurs.	Storm	64–72
13. Walking against wind is nearly impossible; destruction is widespread.	Hurricane	72 plus

* Reprinted by permission from George L. Cantzlaar, *Your Guide to the Weather*, Barnes & Noble, Inc., New York, 1964, p. 135.

cold, the body attempts to increase internal heat production by muscular activity (shivering) and by increasing the basal metabolic rate at which food stored within the body is burned. Heat loss is decreased by reducing the circulation of blood in the shell. When these compensatory mechanisms fail, injury from cold can occur in two ways.

1. The core temperature is maintained but the shell temperature falls. A spectrum of lesions occurs:

    Frost nip
    Superficial frostbite
    Deep frostbite
    Chilblains
    Trench foot (Immersion foot)

2. When both core and shell temperature are lost, systemic hypothermia occurs; all body processes slow, and the patient will die if not treated.

When functioning in a cold environment, the EMT must be able to protect both himself and the patient against serious heat loss from all causes.

Conduction and convection losses may be prevented by imposing insulating material of relatively low thermal conductivity between the body and the outside air. Such materials are wool, Dacron, foam, or down. The use of the layer principle of clothing is effective in preventing either overheating or excess chilling since one or more layers may be added or subtracted as necessary. Air is caught between layers of clothing and is warmed by the body. If the air remains dry and trapped, a warm layer surrounds the body and maintains an appropriate body temperature. Eskimos have used this principle of clothing for many years.

Water conducts heat 240 times faster than air; perspiration-soaked clothing allows considerable chilling. An injured person should be protected with appropriate dry insulating material both over and underneath him. Neither patient nor EMT should touch cold metal with bare unprotected skin, nor should they sit or be placed directly in the snow or on the cold ground. Direct-conduction heat losses can be serious in each instance.

Heat loss from convection alone is prevented

by wearing windproof garments and by seeking shelter during periods of cold and high wind. A typical occurrence of cold injury today from convection alone is the development of frostbite in a skier, who often sits on a lift exposed to a relatively high wind. Any areas of skin not properly protected are extremely vulnerable under these conditions.

Radiated heat loss generally occurs with an uncovered head.

Evaporative loss of heat occurs, for example, when one is exposed in clothing wet by rain or perspiration and the clothing gradually dries. If one is accidently splashed with supercooled gasoline, or any other volatile liquid hydrocarbon, prompt evaporation of the compound may cause local freezing and damage of the skin because of the combined loss of heat from evaporation of the liquid and conduction of body heat through it.

Those areas of the body where the surface area is large compared to the volume, such as the head, the ears, the hands, must be adequately covered to minimize loss of heat from conduction, convection, and radiation. The use of a protective, oil-based ointment on the nose, the lips, and the cheeks markedly lessens the effects of convection. Avoiding tight clothing, especially gloves and shoes, will help maintain normal circulation and minimize the effects of cold on the extremities. One should be able to curl one's toes comfortably within boots used for skiing or in snowy areas. Alcohol and tobacco both interfere with the proper regulation of the circulation in the small vessels in the skin and the extremities. They cause vasodilation and uncontrolled heat loss. Their use should be strictly avoided during exposure to very low temperatures. The internal production of heat can be enhanced by the ingestion of frequent snacks, especially of warm food or drink.

Cold Injuries

Injuries from cold are usually sharply localized. Systemic hypothermia or severe cooling of the entire body is a rare phenomenon but a very serious one. It occurs mainly in three groups of people:

1. Hunters, hikers, skiers, or climbers exposed to unusually severe weather
2. Inadequately clothed persons exposed to ordinary cold
3. Alcoholic or other very ill persons whose normal defenses to cold are insufficient and who become exposed for long periods of time to ordinary cold.

Freezing temperatures affect the cells in the body in a predictable fashion. Much of the content of a cell is water; when it is subjected to excessive cooling, the cell freezes and is no longer able to function. The resulting ice crystals may destroy the cell. Local cold injuries are manifestations of injuries of the capillary blood vessels and other tissue components in the skin and the deeper tissues.

The cell injuries are all essentially the same, varying only in degree and in the depth to which the tissue exposed has been injured. The duration of the exposure, the temperature to which the skin has been exposed, and the wind velocity are the three most important factors in determining the severity of a cold injury.

Local injuries. Local injuries from cold fall under the overall term of *frostbite*. Several degrees of injury can exist however. Freezing of a part of the body occurs when not enough heat is available to counteract external cold. Predisposing factors include:

1. Inadequate insulation from cold and wind
2. Restricted circulation because of arterial disease or tight clothing, especially footwear
3. Fatigue
4. Poor nutrition
5. The use of alcohol
6. The normal responses of the body in maintaining its core temperature by shunting blood flow away from the shell

The most commonly affected parts of the body are the hands, feet, ears, and exposed parts of the face. All of these areas are located far from the heart and subjected to a normally rapid heat loss because of a large surface area to volume ratio.

Frost nip or incipient frostbite. Frost nip usually involves the tips of the ears, the nose, the cheeks over the zygomatic processes, the chin, the tips of the fingers, or the tips of the toes. It occurs in conditions of high wind or extreme cold or when both co-exist. It is manifested as a sudden blanching or whiteness of the skin. A person is often not aware that he has a frost nip until someone tells him his skin appears to be pale or glassy. Frost nip comes on slowly, is painless while developing, and often goes unnoticed by the person. If this injury is identified early there is usually no tissue damage and it can be treated quite effectively by the firm, steady pressure of a warm hand, by blowing hot breath on the spot, or by holding nipped fingers motionless in the armpit. The area should not be rubbed and most especially should not be rubbed with snow. As warmth and color return there will be tingling about the injured region. After thawing has taken place, the skin may turn red and may superfically shed by flaking over the next several days.

Superficial frostbite. A superficial frostbite usually involves the skin and the superficial tissue just beneath it. In this condition the skin has a white, waxy appearance and is firm to the touch; but the tissue beneath it is soft and resilient. This finding is presumptive evidence that only the skin and the subcutaneous tissue are involved. This patient should be taken indoors, protected from the cold, and subjected to the same steady, careful, local rewarming as described above. Rubbing of the area is not done as it will only further injure already damaged tissue. As the injured area thaws, it is at first numb, then mottled blue or purple. It will probably swell because the capillaries are injured and plasma can leak into the tissue. It may begin to sting and burn because of the injured nerves. If the frostbite is severe and involves tissue beneath the outer layer of the skin, there may be enough vessel damage and plasma leak to cause the development of blisters. Throbbing, aching, and burning of the injured area may last for some weeks. It may remain permanently red and tender and become extremely sensitive when again exposed to cold. Subsequently, the body area should always be protected with a dry warm covering.

Deep frostbite. Deep frostbite is an extremely serious injury usually involving the hands and the feet. The tissues are cold, pale, and solid. This patient should be taken as quickly as possible to the Emergency Department. Meanwhile he should be kept dry, provided external warming, and given cardiopulmonary resuscitation if necessary. Tissues deep to the skin and subcutaneous layers are usually injured and may be completely destroyed.

In these cases, the injured area turns purplish blue and becomes extremely painful after thawing. Large blisters or gangrene may develop in the first day or two. The amount of permanent tissue damage depends on the degree of the temperature and the duration of the freezing. The injury is worse if the person is wet or if the tissue has been exposed to cold metal and then torn or avulsed when separated.

Frequently the injured extremity has been partially or completely thawed by the time the EMT sees the patient. If such is not the case, the part should be thawed by a rapid rewarming in a warm water bath. This is the treatment that will be instituted at the medical facility. If a long delay is anticipated in reaching the Emergency Department, the EMT must know how to conduct proper rewarming, when warm water and containers are available. The temperature of the water should be kept between 100° and 105° F. A thermometer should be used to make certain that the temperature does not exceed 105° F. This temperature was designated at the International Medical Conference on Frostbite held at Fairbanks, Alaska in February 1964. It is within the range of temperatures attained by the body and is just 6–7° F warmer than normal body temperature. The warmth of the water must be maintained by continuously adding fresh warm water. Heat is lost promptly from the bath as the cold extremity is immersed in it. A clean container large enough to allow the extremity to be immersed entirely within it without touching the sides or bottom is required. Water should be heated in a separate container and added slowly with stirring, while the extremity is temporarily removed. Heat must be evenly distributed throughout the water bath, and the temperature kept constant at 100–105° F. Rewarming is continued until the frozen area is deep red or bluish in color. The procedure may require half an hour or more. Concurrently, the patient's body temperature must be maintained by the use of warm drinks, warm clothing, warm blankets, and protection in a warm room.

Since severe pain usually accompanies thawing, the need for analgesic medication should be anticipated. Infection is always a danger in these wounds and will markedly aggravate any tissue damage. Bandage the thawed parts very gently with sterile, lightly applied dressings; leave blisters unopened; separate the toes and fingers with sterile, soft gauze pads. If the time required to transport the patient to the Emergency Department will be particularly long, gently wash the thawed area with germicidal soap; dry it thoroughly with sterile pads; and bandage it with a sterile dressing prior to transportation. Transportation should be as soon as possible, with the patient lying down, and the extremity elevated. Refreezing must be avoided at all costs.

Chilblains. Chilblains result from repeated exposures of the bare skin to temperatures in the low sixties or below for prolonged periods. The injury results in a red, swollen, hot, tender, itching area usually on the fingers or toes. Chilblains recur in the same area during cold weather. In between periods of recurrence, the area is usually red and rough. This lesion is commonly seen on the bare extremities of women and children. It represents a chronic injury of the skin and the peripheral capillary circulation. There is no treatment for it once the skin injury has been established except to prevent recurrence and protect the injured area when exposure to cold is necessary.

Trench or immersion foot. Trench foot, or immersion foot, results from the wet cooling of an extremity over hours or days at temperatures which are slightly above freezing. It is commonly seen in seamen who have been shipwrecked and in soldiers forced to remain in trenches or to sit or stand for prolonged periods of time with their feet in water or mud. If one is unable to remove wet shoes and stockings for long periods of time, trench foot or immersion foot results. The lesion represents primary dam-

age of the capillary circulation of the skin, which may progress to cause necrosis or gangrene of skin, muscle, and nerves. Malnutrition and stress aggravate the degree of the injury.

Initially the extremity is cold, swollen, waxy, mottled, and possibly numb. After it is warmed, it becomes red, swollen, and hot; blisters may develop. Gangrene may eventually occur; and disability may last for months or years. A variation of the injury, warm water immersion foot, has been seen in troops fighting in the tropics. The basic lesions are similar.

Emergency treatment consists of removing wet footgear, gently warming the cold extremity, preventing infection with local cleaning and sterile dressings, and the administration of general supportive measures such as intravenous fluids to maintain the circulation as much as possible. Blisters should not be opened. The patient should be transferred directly to the Emergency Department as soon as possible.

General treatment for local injuries. Some general statements can be made concerning the emergency treatment of local cold injuries.

Only the most superficial frostbite can be treated in the field with direct application of body heat. The patient with a deep frostbite should be taken immediately to the Emergency Department.

Putting clothing over the frostbite will help prevent further injury. The part should never be rubbed, chafed, or manipulated.

Even if the patient must walk on a frostbitten foot or leg, he must be taken as rapidly as possible to an Emergency Department for definitive medical care. Experiences in recent years in Korea and Alaska indicate that walking even long distances on a frostbitten limb will not lessen the chance of successful treatment **if the limb has not been thawed.** It must be emphasized, however, that **once a frozen limb has been thawed, the patient becomes a stretcher case.** Attempts to walk on a thawed limb, with the resulting exposure to refreezing, are extremely painful and dangerous. This patient must be transported supine with the limb protected.

The appearance of blisters in a frostbite is generally a good prognostic sign, indicating that damage of only a partial thickness of the skin

314

exists and that the patient may recover. Blisters should not be opened. They should be protected with a dry sterile dressing.

The following *Don'ts* should be observed.

Don't make matters worse. Treat injured parts extremely gently to prevent further damage of the tissue.

Don't apply pressure or constriction on the injured area; the tissue should be bandaged lightly to protect it from contamination.

Don't under any circumstances rub or abrade the tissue. Frozen cells contain ice crystals which can cut or destroy the tissue.

Don't apply snow or thaw the part in cold water. This is no more sensible than treating a burn by putting it in a fire.

Systemic hypothermia. General severe body cooling is known as systemic hypothermia. It can occur at temperatures well above freezing. It is usually caused by exposure to low or rapidly dropping temperatures, cold moisture, snow, or ice. Contributing factors are hunger, fatigue, and exertion. It is commonly seen in alcoholic patients who have collapsed in snowbanks, and in hikers who have been exposed to temperatures close to 32° F when the weather is both windy and wet. If environmental temperatures are significantly below freezing, hypothermia may be accompanied by varying degrees of frostbite. Accurate recognition of systemic hypothermia requires the use of a clinical thermometer which can reach a low temperature.

Generalized body cooling makes itself manifest in five stages:

1. Shivering, which is an attempt by the body to generate heat
2. Apathy, sleepiness, listlessness, and indifference, which may accompany rapid cooling of the body
3. Unconsciousness with a glassy stare, a very slow pulse rate, and slow respiratory rate
4. Freezing of the extremities
5. Death

Stage 3 generally follows stage 2 very rapidly. When the body core temperature falls below 95° F (rectal), sustained shivering begins. As cooling proceeds, clumsiness, fumbling, stumbling, falling, slow reactions, mental confusion, and difficulty in speaking follow. Death may occur within two hours of the onset of the first symptoms. When working under dangerous meteorological conditions, one must always be alert for the development of systemic hypothermia in one's self or one's companions.

Systemic hypothermia is an acute priority one medical emergency and requires the rapid transfer of the patient to the Emergency Department. The basic principles of emergency care are these:

1. Prevent further heat loss.
2. Rewarm the patient as rapidly and safely as possible.
3. Be on the alert for complications.

For the patient with mild to moderate hypothermia (rectal temperature of 81° to 95° F, with the patient conscious), further heat loss is prevented by moving the patient out of the wind, replacing wet clothing with dry, and adding appropriate insulating material. External heat should be provided the patient in any way possible—hot water bottles, electric blankets, campfires, body heat from rescuers, or any other means. Because the patient is unable to generate adequate body heat of his own, merely placing him in a blanket or sleeping bag is not sufficient. He can be put into a prewarmed sleeping bag if external heat is used to maintain the warmth. Internal heat, if the patient is conscious, may be given as hot liquids, and calories may be added as sugar or glucose tablets or in hot sweet drinks. If it is available, the single most effective way of warming the patient with systemic hypothermia is to immerse him in a tub of warm water kept between 105° and 110° F.

If the patient is in a state of severe hypothermia (rectal temperature below 81° F, or unconscious), significant dangers exist from cardiac arrhythmias and rewarming shock. Cardiac arrhythmias, most particularly ventricular fibrillation, occur when the heart reaches low temperatures. Arrhythmias are the common cause of death in these patients. Rewarming shock occurs as the circulatory system of the body warms and dilates before the heart becomes able

315

to support the expanded circulation within a dilated system.

Very little time should be spent trying to warm these patients in the field. They should be evacuated as rapidly as possible to an Emergency Department where equipment for rapid rewarming and provision for cardiac intensive care is available. During transportation to a medical center, the patient's head should be kept lower than the feet, sudden jolts should be avoided, and further heat loss prevented. An intravenous infusion of 5 percent dextrose and water or balanced electrolytes should be started. Cardiorespiratory function must be monitored very closely. Cardiopulmonary resuscitation may be necessary. Initial rewarming should be underway during transport; oxygen certainly should be given.

Do not assume that these patients are dead, though they may look ghastly. In the hospital some may be rewarmed rapidly under close observation. Rewarming may even be done much more safely and more effectively than with more conventional methods by using warm peritoneal dialysis fluid within the abdominal cavity or a pump oxygenator to support the circulation and warm the blood directly.

In general the injured or ill person is more susceptible to frostbite and systemic hypothermia than a normal person. Chilling predisposes one to the development of shock, and shock aggravates the effects of further chilling. These patients must be transported as rapidly as possible to the Emergency Department while measures are instituted for local or general treatment immediately.

Any ambulance service located in an area where cold weather search and rescue may be needed should provide its crews with specific survival training for these conditions. A knowledge of existing weather conditions and the likelihood of weather change is always required. Thorough familiarity with the area is needed. Proper clothing must be provided. Even short rescue missions should not be undertaken without proper provisions in the vehicle for extra clothing and food. On prolonged missions, not shaving and not washing the face will give considerable extra protection against cold. As with many other hazards, one of the first considerations of the EMT must be his own protection so that he may remain capable of helping others.

316

CHAPTER 42

Radiation Exposure

GOAL I. Know the principles of safe handling of patients exposed to ionizing radiation.

OBJECTIVES

A. Name the different kinds of ionizing radiation.
B. Name the physical and chemical forms in which ionizing radiation may be present.
C. Describe the methods by which ionizing radiation may enter the body to cause damage even though the radiation itself may not be able to penetrate the skin
D. Describe a sign which would indicate the possible presence of radioactivity in an accident.
E. Name the three safety principles which are important in avoiding dangerous exposure to radiation.
F. State the principles of radiation decontamination.
G. State where one can obtain expert advice concerning possible patient exposure to ionizing radiation.

Man has always been exposed to minute amounts of radiation through cosmic rays and naturally occurring radioactive minerals. However, radiation at a high level is a relatively new danger. With the development of atomic energy for peaceful uses, many persons now come into contact with radioactive materials through their work. In addition, the nuclear power industry, which processes, fabricates, and transports fuel materials, is an increasing source of accidental contamination or exposure. Many more persons are exposed to radiation through X-ray examinations but this exposure is at a controlled level that should do little or no harm. Everyone should know some basic facts concerning radiation hazards.

Radiation is a form of energy transmission. Anything that blocks the radiation absorbs the energy of the beam. The absorption of energy by living tissue can cause damage. Many forms of radiation exist, among them light, sound, and radioactivity. All can be harmful at high levels.

Light is a form of radiation which includes visible and invisible portions of a spectrum. Invisible light, infrared or ultraviolet, contains much thermal energy (heat) and can cause burns. Visible light is normally not dangerous but at intense levels it can injure the retina of the eye.

Sound waves are another form of the transmission of energy. They offer no known threat unless the acoustic decibel limit exceeds established standards of safety or unless exposure to very loud sounds is constant over a prolonged period of time.

The most hazardous form of energy radiation cannot be perceived by hearing, seeing, or feeling. It is ionizing radiation, which has the unique property of being able to disrupt atoms and so

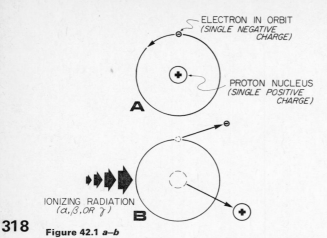

ELECTRON IN ORBIT
(SINGLE NEGATIVE CHARGE)

PROTON NUCLEUS
(SINGLE POSITIVE CHARGE)

A

IONIZING RADIATION
(α, β, OR γ)

B

318

Figure 42.1 a–b

a, Hydrogen is the smallest atom. It is comprised of a proton (with a positive charge of 1) in its nucleus and an electron (with a negative charge of 1) in orbit about the nucleus. *b*, The sketch shows ionizing radiation striking the hydrogen atom, causing it to split apart. The proton and electron fly into space as a positive ion and a negative ion.

damage cells and tissues of the body. The atom, once thought to be the basic particle of all matter, is composed of several smaller particles, some bearing no electrical charge, some bearing either a positive or negative charge, and all having different masses. The atom itself is electrically neutral and physically stable. There are the same number of electrons (negatively charged particles) orbiting it as there are protons (positively charged particles) in its nucleus. Atoms are stable building blocks of matter until their atomic structures are altered. Ionizing radiation has this effect of altering the atomic structure (Fig. 42.1).

When radiation strikes an atom it can disrupt the atom's electrical balance and therefore its stability, causing it to split apart. The smaller parts into which it separates are either positive protons or negative electrons. Each of these electrically charged subatomic particles is called an ion. The energy which has converted the electrically stable, or neutral, atom to charged ions is thus called ionizing radiation. Three significant types of ionizing radiation exist: alpha particles, beta particles, and gamma rays.

Alpha particles are the positively charged protons from the nucleus. They do little damage because they are weak enough to be absorbed by a sheet of paper or by clothing.

Beta particles, the negatively charged electrons, are capable of producing somewhat more injury but are absorbed by heavier clothing. Alpha and beta particles are dangerous only if inhaled or swallowed so that they damage body tissues internally. Inhaling smoke with these particles in it, eating or drinking food or liquids with particles in them, or rubbing particles into a wound or onto the skin are the usual sources of radiation contamination.

Gamma rays are emitted spontaneously by a radioactive substance. They are extremely penetrating and thus more dangerous. They are virtually the same as X rays, but X rays for medical diagnosis are given with short exposures that cause minimal damage unless used too often. Gamma rays, which easily pass into and through the body, contain large amounts of energy and can do much cellular damage (Fig. 42.2).

Gamma radiation and X rays are measured in roentgens (r). One roentgen equals the amount of radiation that will produce one unit of ionization in one cubic centimeter of dry air under standard temperature and pressure conditions. Most radiation meters may be read in milliroentgens (one thousandth of a roentgen) as well as roentgens. Roentgens are measured specifically as the amount of ionizing radiation delivered at a given surface.

The radiation absorbed by tissue is somewhat less than that delivered. Absorbed radiation is measured in rads (radiation absorbed dose). This measurement takes account of the delivered radiation as well as the type of tissue into which it passes. The difference between rads and roentgens for gamma and X rays is so small as to have no practical significance.

How Radiation Affects the Body

Because life is dependent upon billions of individual body cells, the destruction of a large number of them by destroying their individual atoms results in radiation sickness and sometimes in death. This loss of cells occurs with exposure to a large dose of radiation.

The degree of radiation sickness depends upon the total dose, the type of radiation delivered, and whether part or all of the body is ex-

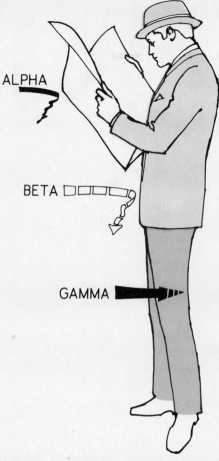

posed. For example, large doses of radiation to an arm may cause loss of the arm but have only a limited effect on the rest of the body. Most important is the amount of radiation received by the whole body or by its important organs (Fig. 42.3).

It should be emphasized that all radiation has some effect on cells of the body. Controlled doses for limited periods of time are tolerated well, but the EMT must not forget that radiation always causes some cellular changes. We have found out what limits are tolerated, but this does not mean that repeated exposure to these limits should be undertaken. Care in dealing with sources of ionizing radiation is mandatory at all times.

319

Figure 42.2

The three basic types of ionizing radiation are alpha, beta, and gamma. The sketch shows what the radiation from each type will penetrate. Alpha radiation will penetrate only thin materials; it can be absorbed by a newspaper. Beta radiation will penetrate somewhat thicker materials; it can be absorbed by layers of clothing. Gamma radiation will penetrate all but the densest materials; its rays can be absorbed only by a lead shield, a stone or earth wall several feet thick, or the equivalent of these.

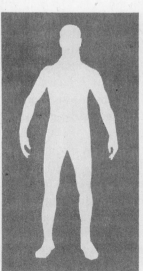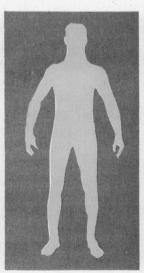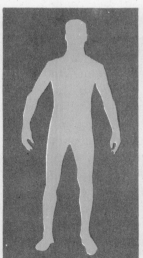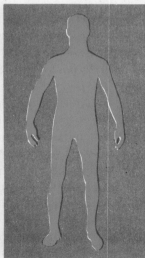

Figure 42.3

The degree of damage the body would suffer from exposure to various degrees of radiation (the entire body exposed) is demonstrated above. A person exposed at a rate of 100 roentgens per hour (100 r/hr) over a short period of time would be able to tolerate the dose. Exposure at a rate of 200 r/hr over an equal period of time would make him sick, and a rate of 300 r/hr over an equal period of time would make him very sick. Prolonged exposure to 300 r would inevitably lead to his death. Exposure at a rate of 400 r/hr for the same period of time would cause death rapidly.

Protection from Radiation

The amount of radiation damage that a person receives depends upon the following factors:

1. Strength of the radiation source
2. Type of radiation—alpha, beta, or gamma
3. Duration of exposure to the radiation
4. Area of the body that receives the radiation
5. Distance from the source of radiation
6. Shielding from the source of radiation

In rescue work, brief exposure is of great importance. Shielding is too cumbersome, and distance hampers effective rescue work. By dividing the work among as many rescuers as possible and working rapidly, exposure of any one person can be kept to a minimum and the absorbed dose may be negligible. By limiting exposure of a person to sixty seconds in the presence of a 100 r/hr source, only a 1-2/3 r total dose would be received. This quantity of radiation is insignificant as a one-time exposure.

Shielding, if placed over the source of radiation rather than over the rescuer, is a second wise approach. The best protection against most gamma rays is a lead shield one to two inches thick; however, any material of great mass such as concrete, brick, or earth can be a relatively effective shield.

Radiation can be transmitted directly through the air or indirectly on particles of dust or smoke. Deposits of radioactive material that enter the body by being inhaled or swallowed can be extremely dangerous because they will continue to expose cellular structures to radiation until the particles are passed out of the body or until they undergo radioactive decay. For this reason, the EMT should wear a filtration mask if a radiation hazard is suspected. Smoking or eating near radiation sources must be avoided, as these are the most common ways in which radiation-contaminated materials are inhaled or swallowed.

Accidents Involving Radiation Hazards

The vast majority of accidents involving radioactive materials occurs in facilities which

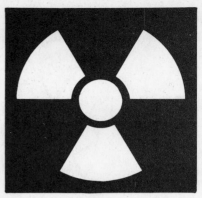

Figure 42.4

This sign is the universal radiation symbol, a purple propeller on a yellow background. It is used to indicate radioactive sources, containers of radioactive material, and areas where radioactive material is stored or used. Exercise caution wherever you encounter it.

use these materials daily. The EMT should seek and follow the professional advice that is readily available to him in these centers.

Transportation of radioactive materials is now a common occurrence. Accidents occasionally happen in circumstances where professional guidance is unavailable. In these cases the EMT should know how to evaluate the dangers involved in a rescue operation. All radioactive substances are kept in labeled and shielded containers when not in use. Radioactive material shipped by interstate commerce must comply with the regulations of the Interstate Commerce Commission (ICC), which prescribes rules for the packaging and labeling of materials and sometimes for the marking of vehicles. Shipments must be identified with a bright purple propeller on a yellow background (Fig. 42.4). Certain radiation materials must be accompanied by professional personnel at all times during transit.

Probably the only real hazard of injury from radiation in a transportation accident would occur if a relatively large, powerful radiation source, such as a material that produced gamma radiation, became unshielded and persons unaware of the danger remained in the radiation field. The most likely ways this kind of accident could happen would be as a result of a fire, where a container might rupture or be destroyed, or in a violent collision resulting in a spill of the radioactive material.

Wherever accidents involve powerful gamma radiation sources, lead shielding or other material of great mass (concrete or metal walls, ditches, earth banks, even vehicles or heavy equipment) should provide sufficient protection for those in the vicinity.

In an explosion or fire, radioactive material may be carried on dust or smoke particles; every precaution must be taken to avoid the problem of contamination in this way. The best protection against radiation contamination from dust is protective clothing. Several layers of clothing, including hat, gloves, and a filtering mask, will protect one from most radioactive dust. The more tightly woven the clothing, the greater the protection against the radioactive particles. Masking tape should be placed at cuffs and across button openings to close these passages to dust and other particles.

If it is suspected that radioactive material is on the clothes or shoes of the EMT or the patient, they should stop at the edge of the exposed area and remove as much contaminated clothing as possible. The EMT should wash both himself and the patient if they are badly contaminated. By carrying out this simple procedure, he will greatly reduce the hazard to all personnel involved. Radiation will be significantly reduced and, with a little care, contamination will not be carried elsewhere. Water used for washing becomes contaminated itself and should be kept in a covered container for proper disposal.

If clothing and other material removed from patients or the EMT is suspected of carrying radiation particles, it should be put into covered metal containers with tight lids—galvanized garbage cans, for example. Disposal of the clothing into this container should be done as it is removed so that the number of people handling it is minimized. The can should be sealed and labeled. Appropriate ultimate disposal should be arranged through the Nuclear Regulatory Commission (NRC) or the state health department.

Do not permit spectators to enter an area suspected of having radioactive material present. Above all, permit nothing to be picked up and handled or removed from the accident scene. Do not gather up clothing and materials lying on the ground. Do not burn materials, as burning will only put contaminated particles into the air in the form of radioactive smoke and ashes. Do not bury materials, as you may be in the wrong location and cause others to be unknowingly exposed at a later date. Only certain areas are designated for radioactive disposal. These areas are under federal or state control.

Rules of Safe Rescue

The only method of detecting radiation hazards is by use of a Geiger counter, ionization chamber, or other instrument designed to detect radiation signals. These instruments are most useful in detecting gamma radiation, which is stronger than alpha or beta particles. A Geiger counter measures the rate of radiation and usually expresses it as roentgens or milliroentgens per hour. Most emergency vehicles do not carry a Geiger counter, but the EMT should know where to procure one immediately and how to use it. Special training is necessary to operate the device, but anyone who can read and interpret a car speedometer can learn to use the counter.

In the future, as the use of radiation materials throughout the country increases, Geiger counters and similar devices may become standard emergency equipment. When readings are expressed in roentgens or milliroentgens per hour, the EMT should be able to convert this reading into a practical statement of radiation dose. For example, if you are working while exposed to ionizing radiation at a constant reading of 100 milliroentgens per hour, in two hours you will receive 200 milliroentgens, or 0.2 roentgens. If you work for ten hours, you will receive ten times the 100 milliroentgens per hour—that is, 1,000 milliroentgens, or 1 roentgen. Neither 0.2 or 1 roentgen is hazardous when received over such extended periods.

One must test a Geiger counter frequently to be certain of its accuracy. It is a rather delicate instrument which should not be dropped or handled roughly. On the other hand, when maintained properly, it will give an accurate reading.

The EMT should not hesitate to provide

emergency care for a patient exposed to radiation. The rule is, "Get in and get out of the exposure area quickly." The EMT should remove both patient and self from hazard as soon as possible, even if it means violating some of the other rules of emergency care. Situations that require immediate extrication of patients regardless of consideration of radiation safety would be impending explosions, fire, threat of collapse of a building, hazard of poisonous gas, or a downed power line in the close vicinity.

A rescuer who takes a calculated risk in entering an area of radioactivity should remain as briefly as possible and should not reenter the field without appropriate clearance.

Exposure of the whole body to 100 roentgens (100 r) in one hour (which would be the same as 50 r per hour for two hours or 200 r per hour for thirty minutes) has little or no life-threatening effect. If a reading of 500 r per hour showed on the meter, a rescuer could go into the area for twelve minutes and receive exposure equivalent only to 100 r. If the risk is small, or if it must be taken to carry out a rescue operation, the EMT should proceed, keeping in mind the three most important factors that determine how much radiation will be received:

1. Length of time exposed
2. Distance from the source of radiation
3. Amount of shielding from the source of radiation

Information gained from witnesses or experts in the area and the use of a Geiger counter will be helpful in determining what the risk will be during an emergency procedure.

Once the patient has been extricated, notify the hospital that a radiation patient is being brought in and start lifesaving procedures immediately. A patient exposed to radiation who has had clothing removed and has been thoroughly washed presents little danger to those

transporting him. A person is not made radioactive by receiving alpha, beta, or gamma radiation. This fact is obvious when one considers that a chest X ray does not cause radioactivity in the exposed individual. However, if the source of the radiation remains on the patient's clothes or skin, danger of exposure is still present. The precautions discussed in this chapter are to avoid such a situation.

Decontamination

Decontamination of the patient and the EMT includes removing all clothing and then taking a shower, with particular attention to the hair and parts of the body that have apposing surfaces, that is, rub together. These areas are buttocks, upper thighs, upper arms and chest, and between the fingers and the toes. A tub bath is not as effective as a shower because it does not remove the particles as efficiently. All ambulance equipment, linens, cots, and fittings may be contaminated. Before equipment can be reused, it must be checked by local radiation authorities. Before the ambulance is used again, it must be decontaminated by washing inside and out to remove any radioactive dust. **Washing must be carried out under the direction of local authority.**

Emergency Medical Service personnel in any given area should inform themselves regarding the local regulating body for radioactive material. Initially, the regulation of all ionizing materials was under the direction of the Atomic Energy Commission. This board has been replaced by the Energy Resources Development Administration. Two functions are served by this administration: research and development of nuclear energy and regulation of the use of nuclear materials. This second function is carried out by the Nuclear Regulatory Commission (NRC). In approximately one-half of the states in the United States, the functions of the NRC are delegated to the state health department.

CHAPTER 43

Electrical Hazards

GOAL I. Know the hazards which may be present in electric wires and common electrical equipment and recognize the precautions needed in dealing with such hazards.

OBJECTIVES

A. Name materials that conduct electric current.
B. Name materials that do not conduct electric current and are therefore good insulators.
C. Describe the conditions necessary for the flow of electric current.
D. List the most commonly encountered electrical hazards.
E. Describe how to recognize high voltage in a downed electric wire.

GOAL II. Understand the injuries which may result from electric shock and know the treatment of patients with such injuries.

OBJECTIVES

A. List the type of injury which is the most common result of electric shock.
B. Describe the method of immediate treatment for electrical burns.
C. Describe how electric shock may affect the heart and respiration.
D. List the causes of death from electric shock.
E. List the precautions necessary in dealing with electrical hazards.

The EMT must understand the basic principles of handling electricity and be able to recognize electrical hazards. **When problems arise he must always seek help from qualified individuals, such as electricians or electric utility company personnel.** The EMT must take every precaution to prevent himself or others from being injured in efforts to administer aid to persons involved in electrical accidents.

Electricity is an energy flow that can pass along specific conductors. Materials that do not allow the passage of electrical current are said to be non-conductors and are used to insulate electrical wires. Water, most metals, wet ground, and human beings are good conductors of electricity. Dry air is not a good conductor.

The flow of electric current (electricity) along a conductor will take place only when there is a source of current and the circuit is complete, or when there is a path to the ground. Completion of a circuit from the source of the energy to the ground or to another cable will allow a continuous passage of electricity through the wires. Wires must be intact and all connections must be complete for an electric current to flow. If the circuit is broken, current will not flow until the circuit is restored again through some conductor. In the example of a broken electrical cable, the circuit is completed again as soon as the cut end of the cable hits the ground or anything else through which current can pass to the ground. When a person touches a "hot" wire, he, in effect, becomes the electrical conducting device and the current will pass through him to the ground, causing considerable damage and possibly death.

Since electricity readily flows through water, wet ground is a good conductor and can create an extremely hazardous situation where electricity is concerned. Many persons have been electrocuted working with electrical equipment while standing in water or on wet ground.

It is important to know that low voltage electrical sources, even common house voltage, can send enough current through the body to cause serious injury or death. A massive electrical charge in contact with the human body causes burns through all tissues and can result in sudden death from damage of the cells of the nervous system or the heart.

Electricity and the Heart

The rhythmic contractions of the heart which cause blood to circulate through the body are the result of periodic stimulation of the heart muscle by a special network of nerves. Electric shock affects these nerves and causes a change in the pattern of the heartbeat, which can then become totally disorganized. Such noncoordinated beating is called fibrillation. It is completely ineffective in circulating the blood. The patient is in actual cardiac arrest exactly as if his heart had ceased to beat altogether.

Electrical Hazards

Electrical equipment. Emergency situations arise most frequently from the use of defective electrical equipment or appliances or the misuse of such equipment. Generally, power tools and power equipment and home appliances such as toasters, washing machines, and dryers are the sources of problems. Persons injured in an electrical accident in the home may still be in contact with the electrical source when the EMT arrives at the scene of the accident. Care of the injured

person cannot be undertaken until the electrical source has been de-energized, either by turning off the master switch or by pulling the cord of the appliance free from its electrical connection.

Contact with overhead or underground wires. Other serious electrical hazards are overhead or buried lines, which may be accidentally contacted. Overhead contact can occur when cranes, derricks, or ladders are used near power lines or when persons are installing television or radio antennas. Contact with buried lines may occur when persons plant trees, or shrubbery, or install fence posts.

At accident locations, when cranes or other equipment have come into contact with overhead wires, the injured person will frequently fall clear of the equipment. If the equipment is still in contact with the wires, the EMT must be sure that no one touches the equipment in attempting to aid the injured person. Further, no one should touch an injured person who is still in contact with the equipment. If electrical utility personnel are not available, but if proper tools and protective equipment such as lineman's gloves, boots, and hot sticks are available, and if the EMT has been **thoroughly trained** in the use of this equipment, he may attempt to pull the injured person away from contact with the energized source. In all instances where overhead lines have been contacted by cranes, derricks, or antennas, the electric utility company must be notified and necessary help obtained from them to cut off the power source.

Fallen wires. Fallen wires as the cause of an accident are another frequent hazard. The electric utility company must **always** be called to the scene for assistance. The EMT should stay clear of the downed wires and keep bystanders and others out of the area (Figs. 43.1 & 43.2). High voltage conductors may arc or burn or the ends of the cable may whip or roll around, endangering persons at the scene. Where conductors have fallen across a fence, a car, or any other metal object, these items too will become energized.

Fallen wires may trap persons inside automobiles or other vehicles. No attempt should be made to approach the vehicle until the wires are clear or de-energized. Injured persons trapped in these vehicles should be advised of what-

324

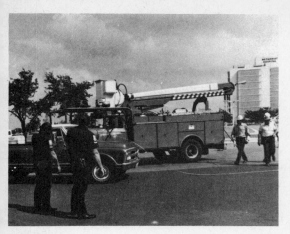

Figure 43.1

A pick-up truck has a "hot" wire draped across its hood. The EMTs have advised the injured patient to remain quietly in the cab and wait for the wire to be removed by an electrical company crew. The EMTs themselves stand well back from the wire and await the trained personnel, who are approaching.

ever medical care they can provide for themselves or others in the vehicle. Occasionally, a situation demands immediate resolution. Only if proper tools and protective equipment are available, and then only if the EMT is thoroughly trained in their use, may he attempt to clear the vehicle of wires and proceed with the rescue. Trapped persons should usually be instructed not to attempt to leave the vehicle until it is de-energized. Any contact between the person in the vehicle and the ground, such as a hand on the car and a foot on the ground, will immediately make him the electrical conductor to the ground, since most cars are insulated by their tires. The result can be a severe burn or an electrocution.

In only one circumstance is it vital that the trapped person attempt to leave the vehicle. If the vehicle is on fire as a result of the accident, attempts should be made to put out the fire with the proper fire extinguishing equipment. If it is not possible to put out the fire, it may be necessary to give the trapped person instructions to jump clear of the vehicle, emphasizing the absolute need that there must be no body contact between the vehicle and the ground at the same time. Ordinarily, one does **not** instruct the patient to jump clear of a vehicle entangled in downed electrical wires.

Electrical Injuries

Electrical injuries are generally of three types.

1. Electrical burns. Characteristically, electrical burns are seen at two points on the body, where the current entered and where it left. Again characteristically, there may be very small areas of visible burn on the skin but very extensive damage in deeper tissues. All degrees of burn are seen. The burn is the result of the heat generated by the current as it enters and leaves the body. In nearly every patient where sufficient current has been received to cause a burn, one will be able to see two burns. When the point of exit has been the patient's feet, there may be no damage of the shoes, but the feet should be checked carefully. Proper initial treatment for these burns is a sterile dressing.

2. Cardiac and respiratory arrests. Although there may be no visible burns, the passage of an electric current through the body may result in cardiac or respiratory arrest because of the direct effect of the current on the nervous system or on the mechanism controlling the heartbeat. The effect of electricity on the body causes fibrillation of the heart and respiratory arrest, which are the mechanisms of death by electrocution. These conditions obviously must be treated immediately with CPR as described in Chapter 10, Basic Life Support.

325

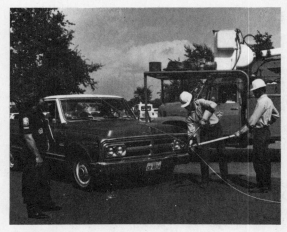

Figure 43.2

Electrical company personnel, wearing specially treated protective gloves, cut the wire with special equipment, thereby breaking the electrical circuit and rendering the wire harmless. The EMTs are still standing back.

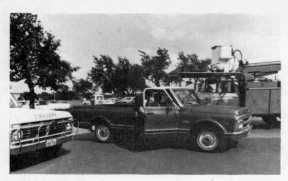

Figure 43.3

With the electrical hazard removed, the EMTs are able to enter the truck and treat the patient inside.

326

3. **Fractures.** Fractures may frequently occur as secondary injuries after or during electric shock. They usually are the result of falls. Sometimes the patient may have been hurled against an unyielding surface as a result of the electric shock. The shock itself may cause muscle spasm strong enough to cause a fracture. After proper resuscitation has been carried out, these fractures are treated as routinely as any other fractures according to the procedures outlined in Chapters 16 through 20 (Figs. 43.3 & 43.4). Fractures should be suspected in these patients and must be sought by the EMT.

Electrical Equipment

It is not the intent of this text to provide in-

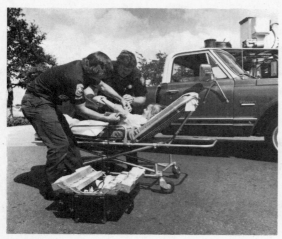

Figure 43.4

The patient has been removed from the truck and placed in a litter preparatory to being transported to the hospital in the ambulance. A splint is being applied to her arm.

formation for the EMT in the proper handling of uncontrolled electrical hazards. It is, however, necessary that the EMT know the types of electrical equipment available for handling wires, how this equipment should be used, and what its limitations are. Once again the point is emphasized that unless he has been thoroughly trained by experts in handling electrical wires and equipment, the EMT should not attempt a rescue without proper aid.

Very occasionally, however, a situation will arise where appropriate aid from utility company personnel cannot be obtained. If the EMT is located in areas where this is likely to happen, he should seek instruction in the proper management of downed wires before an emergency situation arises where only he is available to provide help.

Polydacron rope. Normally a hundred feet of half-inch, non-conductive rope is used to pull wires off vehicles. This rope is specially prepared from polydacron material and is completely non-conductive if it is absolutely dry. To pull a wire from a person, one end of the rope is thrown under the wire and one over the wire. The rescuer then takes the ends of the rope and quickly pulls the wire away. Rapid removal of the wire minimizes the chance of additional electrical arcing and burns. Attention must be given to the fact that **the rope must be dry.** Since water is a good conductor, even non-conductive rope covered with water will allow electricity to pass along it to the rescuer via the water.

"Hot sticks," lineman's gloves, and rubber boots. Hot sticks are specially designed tools used by electrical linemen to manipulate energized wires. They are specially treated by the manufacturer to prevent moisture from penetrating the wood. Wood is non-conductive if it is absolutely dry. Hot sticks should be used only in conjunction with tested lineman's rubber gloves, which have leather protectors and cotton inserts, and preferably with rubber boots too (Fig. 43.5).

The hot sticks may be used to push or pull the person from the wire or the wire from the person. In moving either the patient or the wire, caution must be taken that the live wire does not whip around like an unattended fire hose. Pulling with the hot stick rather than pushing will

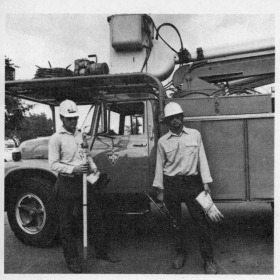

Figure 43.5

    The electrical company trained personnel are holding "hot sticks," hot stick cutting tools, and protective gloves. Special boots are also available for wear when needed.

allow the greater degree of control. Again it must be emphasized that hot sticks are non-conductive only so long as they are absolutely dry. Lineman's gloves and boots must be periodically tested to see that there are no holes through which electricity could pass into contact with the body of the person wearing them.

    Precaution: Never cut an electrical wire. If one attempts to cut the wire he will be much too close to the electrical charge and may receive severe burns from the flash, from the ends of the wire as they whip free, or through the wire cutters as they pass through the energized wire.

    Recall that protective or safety electrical equipment must be tested periodically to be certain that it remains non-conductive. It should be graded for work on high voltage or low voltage lines. A knowledge of the voltage being carried by a line may help considerably in selecting the type of equipment used to make a rescue.

327

CHAPTER 44

Water Hazards

GOAL I. Know the different types of water-related medical problems.

OBJECTIVES

A. Define drowning.
B. List the characteristics of hypothermia.
C. Define breath-holding blackout.
D. List injuries which can result from diving into shallow water.
E. List the most frequently encountered problems in scuba diving.
F. Define decompression sickness.
G. Define nitrogen narcosis.

GOAL II. Understand the treatment of water-related medical problems.

OBJECTIVES

A. Describe the methods of rescue and resuscitation.
B. Describe rescue and resuscitation methods for a patient who has a suspected neck injury.
C. List the steps in treating the patient with hypothermia.
D. Describe the treatment of a scuba diver who suffers descent problems.
E. Describe how to correct nitrogen narcosis.
F. Describe the treatment of air embolism.
G. Describe the prevention and treatment of decompression sickness.

Accidents related to aquatic activities may demand immediate emergency care to prevent death or permanent injury. Each year about seven thousand people in the United States die as a result of accidents in the water. Many of these lives could be saved with proper attention to basic principles of rescue and life support. In some instances, the emergency measures are as simple as removing the patient from the water and clearing the airway. At the other extreme, aquatic problems may require treatment in recompression chambers and attention by personnel with special training in diving medicine.

The most frequent problems associated with aquatic accidents are the least serious. Ear disorders account for nearly 90 percent of all the medical problems encountered and are certainly not life-threatening, many times not particularly serious. Drowning and other life-threatening situations account for 5 percent of water accidents. The final 5 percent of such accidents are generally traumatic and involve specific injuries sustained in water from too-shallow dives, deep dives, dives with diving equipment, or exposure to sharks and venomous marine organisms. In general, these injuries are not life-threatening.

Some, however, may be severe or fatal.

Drowning

The term most commonly used to define aquatic accidents is *drowning*. The term is a non-specific diagnostic term and frequently is used to denote any water death or near-death; but the great majority of water accidents, even those resulting in severe disability or death, do not involve any consideration at all of drowning.

Drowning is specifically defined as suffocation in or under water. A distinction is made between those persons drowning in fresh water, as in the backyard swimming pool, and those drowning in salt water, as in the ocean. This distinction is significant only when a considerable volume of water has entered the air passages.

In most drownings or near-drownings, little water reaches the lungs because the larynx is extremely sensitive to any foreign material introduced into it. An individual's first reaction when water enters the mouth and nose is to cough and swallow while trying to take a deep breath. If the head is under water, he may involuntarily inhale large amounts of water as well as swallow a considerable quantity. If water enters the trachea or larynx, an immediate irritative response resulting in laryngeal spasm occurs; this spasm effectively seals the airway from the passages of the mouth and nose. A very small amount of water, perhaps as little as a teaspoonful, will have entered the lungs at this stage. Rescue at this point requires immediate effective clearing of the airway. The patient will usually promptly respond to artificial ventilation.

In many instances the drowning person remains in laryngeal spasm until he has ceased attempting to breathe. Again, in these instances water will not have passed into the lung; the person suffers primarily from hypoxia because air cannot pass through the larynx when it is in spasm. Resulting tissue damage from insufficient oxygen may be severe.

Artificial ventilation must be used in an attempt to minimize the effects of hypoxia and to support the patient until spontaneous breathing returns. Usually, as unconsciousness deepens, laryngeal spasm will relax and the patient can be ventilated. Oxygen must be used in the resuscitation of these patients, as in any other patient whose major problem is hypoxia. If unconsciousness and laryngeal relaxation occur while the person is still underwater, little water enters the lung because he is no longer inhaling or swallowing.

In persons in whom large quantities of water have entered the lungs, the water is relatively quickly absorbed through the surface inside the lung. Fresh water tends to be absorbed promptly from the lung into the bloodstream and to dilute the normal body salts profoundly. Dilution directly damages blood cells and the cells of the pulmonary membranes and may cause their rupture. Sea water on the other hand is approximately two to three times more concentrated in salt than are the normal fluids within the body. It tends to pull water out of the body tissues and into the lung, causing the development of pulmonary edema. This condition causes difficulty in transporting oxygen across the pulmonary membranes into the blood. Any contaminants in the water—chemicals, bacteria, and algae—all cause direct irritation of the very delicate pulmonary membranes; all result in problems that must be treated at the hospital.

Emergency care for all these conditions is cardiopulmonary resuscitation. Provision for clear airways and prompt ventilation must be made. Usually, the major injuries suffered by the patient result from hypoxia. Therefore, the use of oxygen in resuscitation must always be considered.

Diagnosis and Initial Treatment

Two immediate observations are valuable in assessing a water accident. The first is to determine whether it was a surface or underwater accident and, if underwater, whether skin diving or scuba equipment was being used. The second important observation is to determine when the accident occurred.

By far the great majority of water sports accidents fall into the surface category with no specific equipment being used. Accidents associated with deeper dives in which breathing equipment is used can be divided into several categories. Each category has specific physical injuries that pertain to it, as well as specific treatments.

The fate of a person threatened with drowning, whether it is a surface accident or one deep under the water, is determined by five considerations:

1. The speed of the rescue
2. The immediate clearing of the person's airway
3. The immediate institution of artificial ventilation or cardiopulmonary resuscitation with supplemental oxygen
4. The innate ability of the person to recover
5. The kind of water in which he was submerged

In all cases, a drowning person must be brought to the surface promptly if he is to have a chance to survive without injury. Artificial ventilation or cardiopulmonary resuscitation should be started immediately and continued until the patient has either revived or has been pronounced dead by a physician. If there is no physician at the accident scene, resuscitation efforts should continue until the patient has been transported to the Emergency Department. Definite decisions for continuing treatment can be made there.

Frequently, problems associated with drowning or near-drowning do not become apparent until the effect of the absorption of large quantities of fresh water or the development of pulmonary edema is well established. The EMT is not involved with this situation. Simply, he must provide cardiopulmonary support until the patient arrives at the hospital.

Rescue

Normally, the first person to see someone in trouble in the water should perform the rescue, if he has the skills. If the first person is unable to make a rescue, he should note the exact location of the one in trouble and seek help urgently. The safety of the rescuer must always be considered. Many double drownings occur when untrained persons attempt swimming rescues. The role of the EMT is to provide expertise in extrication of injured persons from the water, resuscitation, and emergency transport.

The rescuer need not be a swimmer to assist a person in trouble on the surface of the water. One can often hold out a pole or throw such things as a rope (being sure to hold onto one end of it), an empty gasoline can, a picnic jug, or plastic bottle—anything that will float. If the swimmer is too far away to be reached by a thrown object, often a boat or log, a paddle board, an inflated inner tube, or other large floating object can be pushed out to him. An inflated spare tire mounted on its rim is available in the trunks of most cars; it can easily support two or more persons if it is put into the water, rim and all.

To be efficient in water rescue, the EMT should develop a prearranged plan for the steps to pursue. A good knowledge of the measures necessary to insure water safety is needed. When a rescue from the shore as described above cannot be made, a boat rescue may be used. Under these circumstances, the EMT must wear a life jacket for his own safety. Personnel working where currents are swift must be secured to shore or boat by a lifeline. Excessive clothing and boots should be removed when weather permits.

Only trained water safety personnel should ever attempt a swimming rescue. It is tragic enough to lose one person to drowning without losing the would-be rescuer also. The rule of "Throw, tow, row, and only then go" should be remembered in making water rescues (Fig. 44.1).

331

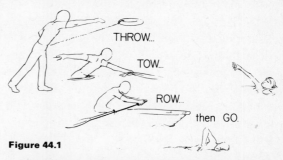

THROW...

TOW...

ROW...

then GO.

Figure 44.1

Swimming rescues must not be attempted by untrained personnel who cannot handle panic-stricken persons in the water. Always follow the sequence outlined above. Throw a floatable object to the swimmer, or tow him in by pole or rope. If these approaches are not successful, try to reach him in a boat. Only when these courses have been exhausted, and only if the EMT is capable of doing it, should a swimming rescue be attempted.

The EMT who works in an area where water sports are common should know the resources available for assistance in water rescue, emergency transportation, and recompression. Many fire departments have water rescue squads. The Coast Guard can provide emergency evacuation from almost any coastal area. Arrangements can be made with military commands for mercy flights to recompression chambers.* Diving clubs and explorer posts frequently have water rescue units.

If the swimmer cannot be seen but the area of the accident is identified, organized recovery methods should be started by expert swimmers, using wading, swimming, and surface-diving methods. Paddle boards may be helpful in reaching a person some distance from the shore, and they make good recovery floats. The use of a skin diver's snorkel and facemask or water goggles may improve a rescuer's chance of finding someone on the bottom. If the location of the drowning is known and the victim cannot be seen, or skilled lifesavers are not available, a very last resource is the use of a T-bar grappling iron with 3-gang (cod) hooks or any kind of strong hook. The use of this drag may cause a serious wound in the rescued person, but it may allow recovering him from the water soon enough for resuscitative measures to be instituted. It may also muddy the water so much that other divers may have difficulty seeing the victim underwater if the drag is unsuccessful.

Removal of someone from the water with a suspected injury of the spine as a result of a diving, skiing, or boating accident involves the same principles used anywhere in the handling of a patient with a suspected spinal injury. If the patient is unconscious, and particularly if there are marks about the head and face indicating contact with some object, he must be treated as if he definitely has an injury of the spine. If the patient is conscious, ask if there is loss of feeling or diminished sensation in the extremities, paralysis or weakness in the arms or legs, and paraesthesia (tingling).

It is not uncommon to find these persons in a face-down position on the surface. The extremely important steps of turning the swimmer to a face-up position while he is still in the water, administering mouth-to-mouth ventilation, and stabilizing the body and neck on a floating board are illustrated in Figure 44.2. When possible, the patient should be secured to a spineboard before being taken from the water and should be lifted out head first. Some improvising may be necessary. For example, childrens' water skiing belts make good cervical supports and will float, allowing control of both head and neck.

Resuscitation

When artificial ventilation is indicated, it should be initiated as soon as it can be done effectively, even before the person has been removed from the water (Fig. 44.2). Artificial ventilation can be given in shallow water or while the rescuer supports the patient by hanging onto a boat or any other sturdy floating object, or to the side of a pool or dock. Most recreational swimming accidents occur within fifty feet of the shore or a swim float. Getting air into the lungs without delay is vital; it may be lifesaving.

If cardiopulmonary resuscitation is required, it should be started as soon as the patient is supine on a support with the neck stabilized.

Specific Aquatic Problems

Surface-related problems. Virtually all the problems that the EMT will encounter arising from water hazards will be related to activities on the surface of the water. These include routine swimming accidents, swimming pool accidents, water skiing accidents, and injuries related to standard diving and water activities. They are discussed below in order of their frequency.

Swimmer's ear. Swimmer's ear is a nonemergency condition which results from inflammation in the external ear canal. Warmth and moisture within the canal can contribute to the

---

* Two diving and recompression centers in the United States are manned twenty-four hours a day. One is at Brooks Air Force Base, San Antonio, Texas (telephone [512] 536-3278). The other is at the Navy Experimental Diving Unit, Panama City, Florida (telephone [904] 234-4355). Immediate information about a diving problem or the location of the nearest recompression facility may be obtained from either of these centers.

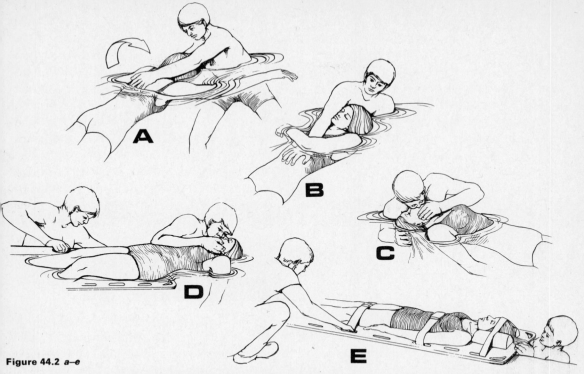

Figure 44.2 *a–e*

a, A swimmer with a spinal injury is often found face down in the water. *b*, Turn the patient in the water while supporting the head and neck as one unit. *c*, Institute artificial respiration at once without waiting to remove the patient from the water. *d*, Continue ventilation while a spineboard is floated under the patient, maintaining support of the head and neck until the board is in place. *e*, The secured patient is ready for transportation. Should spontaneous breathing not have been restored, artificial respiration should be continued during extrication from the water and during transportation to the Emergency Department.

growth of infecting organisms picked up during swimming or diving. It is unlikely that an EMT will be consulted for this problem, but it is by far the most common problem associated with aquatic activities. Ordinarily, the ear itches. The ear canal should not be probed; definitive treatment should be sought from a physician. Progression of the condition may lead to serious external or middle-ear infections.

Panic. When submerged for even very short periods of time, many persons panic and struggle to reach the surface. Struggling frequently continues to the point of exhaustion or causes the person to sink farther into the water. Investigations have shown that panic is the major contributing cause of death in the majority of drownings associated with scuba diving as well as with ordinary activities on the surface of the water. Panic is an integral part of water hazards. It can begin a cycle that can lead to the death of the patient (Fig. 44.3).

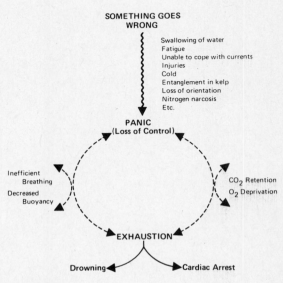

Figure 44.3

A schematic drawing shows the effect of panic in water accidents, where it can often contribute to the death of the person who loses control of himself.

Hypothermia. Water is a considerably more effective conductor of heat than is still air. Most deaths from water accidents in the very cold climates of the United States, from planes which have fallen in water or from ships that have sunk, are attributed to progressive hypothermia and cooling of the patient's core temperature. Emergency medical treatment for this type of problem must include attention to the patient's body temperature. When the already-cooled patient is removed from the water and exposed to air, a further heating loss occurs from evaporation and the body temperature may continue to drop.

334

The drop in body temperature in a person submerged for a prolonged period of time contributes to a comparable decline in body functions, making it progressively more difficult for the person to save himself by getting out of the water or swimming to safety. On the other hand, the progressive decline in body temperature in the person who has apparently drowned has some protective effect on the tissues of the body. Metabolism is reduced and the effects of hypoxia are minimized, making it possible for some persons who have been submerged for a considerable period of time to be resuscitated, with ultimate return of completely normal function.

Breath-holding blackout. A common occurrence in swimmers who are trying to prolong their capacity to stay under the water is breath-holding blackout. In order to improve the ability to hold their breath, divers will sometimes hyperventilate (breathe deeply several times in quick succession) before entering the water. In this manner a significant decrease in the blood level of carbon dioxide is achieved, and the individual, who normally depends on the presence of carbon dioxide in the blood to provide the stimulus to breathe, can remain much longer without breathing. He is then at risk from a diminishing level of oxygen in the blood, which can cause loss of consciousness and subsequent drowning.

Associated injuries. Serious injuries can be associated with aquatic accidents. These include hyperextension or hyperflexion injuries of the neck from diving accidents, encounters with marine animals, collisions with boats and propellers, and a variety of other occurrences. The presence of these injuries complicates the rescue and treatment of someone who seems to be drowning. Particular attention must be given to extrication from the water and resuscitation of the patient with a possible spinal injury in order not to compound it (Fig. 44.2).

The effects of injuries from marine animals are varied. Bites from sharks are a major source of soft-tissue injuries which may be extensive. In addition to CPR, attention must be given to treating the bite itself or stopping bleeding. The effects of injuries from venomous marine animals are considered in Chapter 45, Poisons, Stings, and Bites.

Problems Related to Open-Circuit Scuba Diving

Problems related to diving are becoming much more frequent in the United States. Sports divers, who number nearly three million people, are subject to a number of problems, which can be divided into three categories:

1. Descent problems
2. Bottom problems
3. Ascent problems

Descent problems. Injuries related to descent are compression problems, commonly called squeeze problems or squeeze injuries. Specifically, an area in the body, normally hollow and containing air at atmospheric pressure, is subjected to a squeeze as the diver descends if the passage connecting the area to the throat or mouth is blocked. Pressure within the cavity then cannot equalize readily with the increased external pressure. Such areas are the middle ear, the sinus cavities, the lung, and the facial area which includes and surrounds the eyes and nose, commonly called the mask area. Ear and sinus problems can also arise when a diver descends rapidly. Pressure inside the cavities is not equalized with external pressure, as would be the case if the diver paused at intervals during descent. Ordinarily, pain prevents further descent and in effect limits the damage.

Uncomplicated squeezes of these areas are not emergency conditions and do not require medical follow-up. Sinus squeeze and mask squeeze may be treated by cold packs. Ear compression (ear squeeze) can be complicated by rupture of the eardrum. This injury requires immediate treatment to minimize the chances of middle-ear infection, hearing loss, and disturbance of balance. When a ruptured eardrum is suspected, the EMT should transport the patient to the Emergency Department promptly.

If cold water enters the middle ear the diver may lose his sense of balance. In this circumstance a scuba diver may panic and rapidly sprint to the surface with a lung full of air under excess pressure, thereby developing one of the major problems of ascent, air embolism. A section is devoted to this problem later in the chapter.

An exceedingly rare descent condition is severe lung compression (thoracic squeeze) which occurs only when the diver descends deeply and rapidly while holding his breath. In this situation, external compression of the lung can result. Emergency treatment here is resuscitation and life support during transporation of the patient to a medical facility.

Bottom problems. Bottom problems are related to the duration and the depth of a given dive. They are common in divers using rebreathing or deep-sea diving equipment, but, except for nitrogen narcosis, they are rarely observed in sports divers. Five specific conditions exist. Each one can lead to unconsciousness underwater and drowning. Treatment for all of them includes prompt rescue and basic life support. These major problems are discussed in the following paragraphs.

1. Nitrogen narcosis—If a diver descends too deeply, the increasing pressure of nitrogen in his body has an effect on the brain similar to that of alcoholic intoxication. This condition has been called "rapture of the deep." It is immediately corrected by rising to shallower water. Failure to ascend may allow the diver to become so narcotized that he disregards his own safety; he may even discard his breathing equipment while underwater.

2. Oxygen toxicity—Virtually nonexistent in scuba diving, oxygen toxicity occurs when pure or enriched oxygen mixtures are used instead of air. The first symptom may be a convulsion. Other signs include dizziness, numbness, and muscle twitching. Immediate correction usually follows ascent and a switch to breathing plain air instead of a mixture enriched with oxygen. Since the condition is unpredictable and occurs without warning, usually only at greater depths, the EMT will not normally be involved with primary care in such a case.

3. Carbon dioxide toxicity—Again, virtually nonexistent in scuba diving, carbon dioxide toxicity occurs with the use of special rebreathing types of equipment. When carbon dioxide is not reabsorbed adequately by the equipment, it accumulates in the diver himself and causes shortness of breath, headache, and panic. Ascent and exposure to uncontaminated surface air readily correct the situation.

4. Hypoxia—A diminished oxygen level in the blood (hypoxia), occurring from exhaustion of oxygen in the air supply, from faulty breathing equipment, or from other causes, produces unconsciousness. Drowning will result unless prompt rescue and resuscitation are instituted.

5. Carbon monoxide poisoning—If a compressor used to fill an air tank for pressurized diving equipment has faulty connections, the tank may be filled with air contaminated with carbon monoxide. (The preparations are frequently made by the diver himself.) The symptoms of carbon monoxide poisoning underwater are the same as those on the surface and include headache, shortness of breath, and ultimately unconsciousness. Drowning will result unless rescue and resuscitation are promptly instituted.

Ascent problems. There are two major problems associated with ascent from diving. Both are caused by breathing gas under pressure while submerged. In its most serious form each requires recompression of the patient for definitive treatment. These problems are:

1. Air embolism
2. Decompression sickness

1. Air embolism—The most dangerous and most common, yet least recognized, hazard in scuba diving is air embolism. It can occur in dives as shallow as six feet if the diver holds his

335

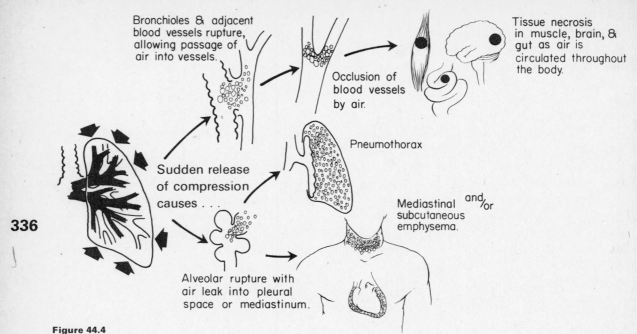

Bronchioles & adjacent
blood vessels rupture,
allowing passage of
air into vessels.

Occlusion of
blood vessels
by air.

Tissue necrosis
in muscle, brain, &
gut as air is
circulated throughout
the body.

Sudden release
of compression
causes . . .

Pneumothorax

Mediastinal ^{and}/_{or}
subcutaneous
emphysema.

Alveolar rupture with
air leak into pleural
space or mediastinum.

336

Figure 44.4

Air in the lung rapidly expands when compression on the outer chest is suddenly released. The resulting rapid pressure outward can rupture alveoli and bronchioles and create the conditions shown above.

breath in a rapid ascent. Air embolism occurs when water pressure on the chest is rapidly reduced and air within the lung expands as a consequence. Too rapid an expansion can rupture alveoli within the lung and damage the adjacent blood vessels. Additionally, air can be forced from the lung into the pleural space or into the mediastinum to create a pneumothorax or a pneumomediastinum (Fig. 44.4). Air can then be forced from the lung into the blood vessels to travel as emboli in the vascular system to any part of the body. Air bubbles in vessels act as plugs, preventing body tissue from receiving its normal supply of blood and oxygen. Brain damage is obviously the most serious result of air embolization (Fig. 44.4).

Signs and symptoms of an air embolus are:

1. Mottling (blotching) or itching of the skin
2. Froth, often bloody, at the nose and mouth
3. Pain in muscle, joints, tendons, or the abdomen
4. Difficult breathing, with chest pain
5. Dizziness and vomiting
6. Difficulty in speaking and in seeing properly
7. Possible paralysis and coma

Immediate treatment is rescuing the patient from the water, keeping him calm and quiet, and giving basic life support during transportation to the Emergency Department. Oxygen inhalation and artificial ventilation are used when necessary. The patient should be kept on the left side with the head and chest lower than the feet, as this position may reduce the chance of air embolization to the brain. The airway should be kept clear.

The patient may require immediate recompression in a pressure chamber. The EMT should keep himself informed on the location of the nearest recompression chamber and maintain advance arrangements that will permit prompt access to this chamber when necessary. Failure to recompress the patient immediately can result in permanent brain damage.

2. Decompression sickness. The "bends," caisson disease, or decompression sickness are all names for the same condition, which is primarily caused by bubbles of nitrogen gas plugging small vessels within the body. In contradistinction to air embolism, decompression sickness is related to the depth and duration of a dive. Ordinarily, sports scuba divers exhaust their air supply before sufficient nitrogen has been absorbed into the body tissues to make them subject to this condition when they ascend.

In any situation where a person breathes air under pressure, as in diving, he absorbs much more than the usual amount of air into his tissues. Inspired air is primarily nitrogen, oxygen, and carbon dioxide. Oxygen and carbon dioxide rapidly diffuse throughout the body and present no problems in blood or tissues; nitrogen, however, which is absorbed into fat, is released slowly and carried as small bubbles in the blood. As long as the high pressure of the dive is maintained, nitrogen is released very slowly and the bubbles remain very small. When pressure is released quickly, as it is if a diver ascends rapidly without pause, nitrogen is released rapidly and the bubbles become much larger, actually obstructing the vessels in which they lie. The result is decompression sickness, or the bends. The term bends has been given to this disease because patients generally assume a bent-over posture from joint pains when these areas are involved. Symptoms are directly referable to the obstructed arteries, which may be muscular, cerebral, skin, or visceral.

If one ascends from a dive at a rate not exceeding 25 feet per minute and pauses for ten minutes at specific levels, depending upon the depth and duration of the dive, he allows his body to be depleted of nitrogen gradually and avoids the bends. Specific dive tables are available which give the rate of ascent and the number and length of pauses that must be made for a dive of given duration at a given depth. If these tables are followed, the bends ordinarily will not occur.

Decompression sickness can also occur if one flies too high with a very rapid ascent in an unpressurized airplane. Here, the person is breathing air at pressures considerably less than normal. The nitrogen previously absorbed into the blood and tissues at normal atmospheric pressures is rapidly released, as described above.

The proper treatment for decompression sickness is recompression. The patient is placed in a pressure chamber and subjected to high pressure once again. Nitrogen which has been released into the blood is forced back into the tissues, bubbles are reduced in size, and the symptoms subside. The patient may then be gradually decompressed to allow him to exhale all the excess nitrogen slowly and steadily. If a recompression chamber is not immediately available, recompression may be attempted by having the diver descend to specific depths in the water and reascend over a period of time, pausing for periods at various levels. This treatment is to be used only if no other is available.

Administration of intravenous fluids before recompression may help improve circulation and minimize permanent injury.

Damage from the bends is usually transient. However, if a block has occurred in a major cerebral or spinal vessel, enough tissue may have been injured to produce a permanent effect. Prompt treatment with special equipment is the best preventive.

Oxygen should be administered while en route to a recompression chamber to attempt to minimize brain damage. Additionally, the EMT should get as much information from the patient as possible concerning the depth and duration of the dive, and should note the patient's physical appearance, strength, and mental clarity. These data will facilitate the selection of treatment tables which will be used by chamber personnel.

Decompression sickness may present a wide range of symptoms, from minor skin rashes and joint pains to very serious central nervous system complaints. Symptoms of decompression disease may not occur until some hours after a dive is concluded while those of air embolism may be immediate. Decompression symptoms and air embolism symptoms and their treatments are very similar. The most dangerous error in dealing with these conditions is to fail to recognize that the patient has either an air embolism or decompression sickness. In either case, recompression is the primary treatment and must be speedily provided.

337

CHAPTER 45

Poisons, Stings, and Bites

GOAL I. Be aware of the general scope of the common forms and problems of poisoning.

OBJECTIVES

A. Define a poison.

B. List the common categories of poisons in the household.

C. List the systems of the body which may be affected by poisons.

D. List the steps that should be taken in attending a patient who has ingested a poison.

E. Name the circumstances under which vomiting should *not* be induced for an ingested poison.

F. Describe the method used to induce vomiting.

G. Describe the emergency treatment of a patient who has had contact with a surface poison.

GOAL II. Be familiar with the problems associated with poisonings by plants.

OBJECTIVES

A. List the various body systems that can be affected by poisonous plants.

B. Describe the emergency treatment for a patient who has ingested a poisonous plant.

GOAL III. Be familiar with the problems associated with insect bites and stings.

OBJECTIVES

A. List the common classes of insects which can cause painful or harmful bites.

B. Describe the two types of responses the body makes in reaction to an insect bite or sting.

C. Describe the emergency treatment of a patient who has an allergic reaction to an insect sting.

D. Describe the signs, symptoms, and emergency treatment of a patient who has been bitten by a black widow spider.

E. Describe the signs, symptoms, and emergency treatment of a patient who has been bitten by a brown recluse spider.

GOAL IV. Know the problems related to the bites of poisonous snakes.

OBJECTIVES

A. List the poisonous snakes of the United States.
B. Describe the physical characteristics of pit vipers.
C. List the signs, physical findings, and emergency treatment of a patient who has been envenomated by a pit viper.
D. Describe the physical characteristics of coral snakes.
E. List the physical signs and symptoms and emergency treatment of a patient who has been envenomated by a coral snake.

340

GOAL V. Know the problems related to the injuries which persons can receive from marine animals.

OBJECTIVES

A. Describe the types of injuries which marine animals can produce in human beings.
B. Describe the emergency treatment for a patient who has received a stinging injury from the tentacles of a jellyfish.
C. Describe the signs and symptoms and emergency treatment of a patient who has received a puncture wound from the spine of a sea urchin.

A discussion of the most serious poisons, stings, and bites with which the EMT will come into contact forms the material of this chapter. It is separated into the following sections: General Poisons, Plants that Poison, Insect Bites and Stings, Spider Bites, Snakebites, and Injuries from Marine Animals.*

Each year in the United States an estimated one million children and thousands of adults accidentally swallow potentially poisonous substances (Fig. 45.1). When the large number of intentional poisonings is also considered, the magnitude of the poisoning problem becomes apparent.

There are 580 Poison Control Centers throughout the United States where information may be obtained on the emergency treatment of patients with suspected poisoning. In

* Grateful acknowledgment is made of valuable information contained in *Dangerous Plants, Snakes, Arthropods and Marine Life of Texas,* edited by Michael D. Ellis.

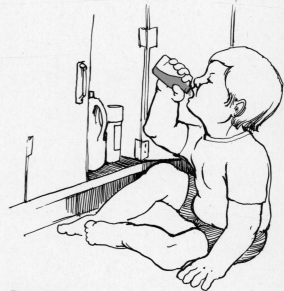

Figure 45.1

A curious child will try to taste or swallow almost any substance. A common victim of accidental ingestion of dangerous compounds is the unwatched toddler.

addition, Poison Control Centers may help in determining the components of commercial products and in identifying symptoms that may result from contact with them. Most of the centers operate twenty-four hours a day. Each community Emergency Medical Service should be prepared to contact the nearest Poison Control Center for information when it is needed.

General Poisons

A poison can be defined as any substance that produces a harmful effect on the body processes. It may act by modifying the normal metabolic functions of cells or by directly destroying them. Poisoning may result from ingestion, inhalation, injection, surface contact, or absorption through skin and mucous membranes of substances in toxic amounts.

The first consideration in treatment of poisoning is to determine whether a poisoning actually has occurred. The person who has merely swallowed some substance is not necessarily poisoned. Some substances are harmless and require no treatment. Others require nothing more than drinking a glass of milk or water to minimize the chances of an upset stomach. However, one should suspect poisoning in any patient with an unexplained severe or acute illness.

Some of the more common symptoms of poisoning include nausea, vomiting, abdominal pain, diarrhea, pupillary dilation or constriction, excessive salivation or sweating, abnormal respiration, unconsciousness, and convulsions. If respiration is inadequate, cyanosis (bluish color of lips and skin) will occur. Chemical burns or inflammation will result from skin contact with corrosive substances.

An important aid in assessing and confirming the existence of poisoning is to search the area where the patient was found or where he has recently been. Objects at the scene, such as bottles or containers (especially medicine bottles) or remains of food or drink, may prove to be important. Gases and some other substances in the area may sometimes be detected by smell.

If the patient vomits, all or part of the vomitus should be collected and taken to the hospital Emergency Department as it may aid in identifying the poison. The importance of taking along a labeled container of the suspected poison, if possible, cannot be overemphasized. Accurate and rapid identification may be facilitated by having the precise spelling of a brand name or reading the components of the product on the label. If other sources of information fail, the label will provide the name of the manufacturer, who can possibly be contacted. Further, the amount left in the container can provide an estimate of the maximum amount of a product that could have been ingested. By bringing the container with the patient, proper treatment may be expedited and a life perhaps saved.

Ingested Poisons

Poisonous substances most likely to be ingested can include foods, drinks, drugs, household products, and plants. Poisonous plants are discussed in a later section of this chapter.

Children are usually involved in accidental poisonings, while adults are more frequently involved in suicide or murder attempts or overconsumption of alcohol or drugs. For a detailed discussion of this last topic, see Chapter 39, Alcohol and Drug Abuse.

Treatment. When it has been determined or is strongly suspected that a poisoning has occurred, appropriate first-aid measures should be instituted at once. Many persons think there is an antidote (a substance that neutralizes the poisonous effects of other substances) for most or all poisonous agents, but unfortunately this is not true. There are very few actual antidotes, and these few generally require a physician's direction for use. Good emergency treatment and supportive care are the best resources of an EMT in treating a patient who has been poisoned.

Dilution. In general, the most important treatment for ingested poisons is to dilute the poison in the stomach and then to induce its removal by vomiting. Both these treatments require that the patient be conscious. To dilute the poison, have the patient drink one or two glasses of milk or water.

Vomiting. Observe the patient carefully, especially his state of consciousness, before deciding to induce vomiting. Vomiting can sometimes be

341

more harmful than helpful. If in doubt about inducing vomiting, seek advice from a physician or from the Poison Control Center.

Do not induce vomiting under the following circumstances:

1. If the patient is unconscious or convulsing (as vomitus could be aspirated into the lungs)
2. If the swallowed poison is a strong corrosive such as acid, lye, or drain cleaner, or if it has caused burns of the lips and throat (since bringing it back up will only cause additional burns)
3. If the poison contains kerosene, gasoline, lighter fluid, clear or free-flowing furniture polish or other petroleum distillates (as it could cause chemical pneumonia if aspirated into the lungs)

If vomiting is to be induced, however, the most effective way for patients one year of age or older is to administer one tablespoonful of syrup of ipecac, followed by a glass of water. Most patients will vomit within fifteen to twenty minutes. If no vomiting has occurred after twenty minutes, the dose may be repeated **once only.** If vomiting is induced, the patient must be observed at all times to avoid aspiration of the vomitus into the lungs. Placing him on one side with the head and trunk sloping slightly downward will facilitate vomiting and help prevent aspiration as well.

Absorbents. Activated charcoal is an effective absorbent of many toxic substances. The EMT should check with a physician or the Poison Control Center to see whether its use is indicated in any particular instance.

Activated charcoal inhibits the vomiting action of ipecac. Thus, if ipecac has been administered, activated charcoal should be given only after the patient has vomited. Activated charcoal is administered by mouth. Mix one or two tablespoonfuls in eight ounces (a glassful) of water immediately before giving it to the patient. It should not be mixed and allowed to stand before it is drunk, for the charcoal will settle to the bottom of the glass.

Soothing agents. Also useful in cases involving ingestion of substances that are irritating to the

gastrointestinal tract are demulcents such as aluminum hydroxide gel, milk of magnesia, or milk. These agents are soothing and help to decrease gastrointestinal irritation.

Inhaled Poisons

For poisons that are inhaled, such as natural gas or carbon monoxide, the first rule in aiding the patient, and perhaps in protecting one's self, is to move the patient into fresh air immediately. Supplementary oxygen may also be given if needed. If the patient is not breathing, start artificial respiration promptly and continue it until breathing returns. Cardiopulmonary resuscitation may be required.

Injected Poisons

Drug overdosage by injection is almost always a result of drug abuse. For a discussion of this problem, see Chapter 39, Alcohol and Drug Abuse. Poisonous bites and stings (which are also injected poisonings) are discussed in more detail separately in this chapter.

Symptoms produced by injected poisons are:

1. A delirious state
2. Pain
3. Tenderness at the site of injection
4. Swelling at the site of injection
5. Unconsciousness
6. Diminished function or failure of respiratory and circulatory systems.

If swelling is apparent in any extremity, immediately remove all rings, watches, and bracelets. Constricting bands may be applied above and below the site of bite or injection. Such a band is not a tourniquet and, properly applied, should not produce the effect that a tourniquet does. The band should be applied tight enough to stop the flow of blood in the superficial veins but not in the arteries. The patient's pulse below the constricting band should remain evident. Apply the bands above and below the site of the bite or injection, just at the borders of the swelling. Be prepared to move the bands as the swelling progresses.

342

Surface (Contact Poisons)

Some substances may cause tissue irritation or destruction by contact with the skin, mucous membranes, or eyes. These substances include corrosives, like acids, alkalies, and phenols, as well as other less destructive compounds. Contact with these agents will cause inflammation or chemical burns in the affected areas.

The irritating or corrosive poison should be removed from the patient as soon as possible. For skin contact, washing the affected area thoroughly with soap and water is indicated. If the patient's clothing is contaminated, direct a stream of water under the clothes even while they are being removed to aid in removing the corrosive rapidly. Chemical irritants in the eye should be treated by copious washing of the eye (Chapter 24, Injuries of the Eye, Face, and Throat). Do not waste time attempting to neutralize acids or alkalies, as it has been shown that rapid, thorough flushing with water is more valuable in preventing further injury.

Plants that Poison

Several thousand cases of poisoning from plants occur each year, many of them resulting in severe reactions in the patients. Poisonous plants are growing in yards, gardens, houses, and offices. The high incidence of such poisonings indicates that most children and many adults are unaware of the dangers that may arise from eating or even nibbling the most innocent-looking plant. A poisonous plant can affect the circulatory, gastrointestinal, or central nervous systems, or it can irritate the skin. Manifestations of the poisoning frequently overlap; however, certain plants have a predominant effect on one primary system.

Circulatory Disturbances

The patient, within thirty to fifty minutes following ingestion of a poisonous plant, may present the classical signs of circulatory collapse: rapid heart rate, falling blood pressure, sweating, cyanosis, and weakness.

Plants that can produce circulatory collapse are:

Autumn crocus	Lantana	Poison hemlock
Baneberry	Lily-of-the-valley	Potato (sprout)
False hellebore	Mistletoe	Rhododendron
Foxglove	Monkshood	Rosary pea
Green hellebore	Mountain laurel	Snakeberry
Indian poke	Oleander	Yew

Treatment. There is no antidote for most plant poisonings and therefore the treatment of the circulatory collapse should be the same as for any other cause of shock. Place the patient in a supine position with the legs elevated, keep him warm, give intravenous infusions, and transport him to the Emergency Department. Administer cardiopulmonary resuscitation as needed. If the patient is alert and conscious, vomiting should be induced with syrup of ipecac. Remember to collect the vomitus and also to take a sample of the ingested plant to the hospital if at all possible.

Gastrointestinal Disturbances

Small amounts of some plants can produce severe gastrointestinal disturbances whereas large amounts of others are required to produce symptoms. Vomiting and diarrhea may develop within twenty to thirty minutes following ingestion.

Plants that can produce gastrointestinal disturbances are:

Baneberry	Inkberry	Oleander
Bloodroot	Iris	Pigeonberry
Caladium	Jack-in-the-pulpit	Poinsettia
Castor bean	Larkspur	Pokeweed
Daffodil	Mayapple	Precatory bean
Fly mushroom	Mistletoe	Rosary pea
Four o'clock	Morning glory	Snakeberry
Foxglove	Narcissus	Wisteria
Hyacinth	Oak	Yew

Treatment. As there is no specific antidote for most plant poisonings, this patient should be given all the support measures needed and transported to the hospital for care by a physician. It is very important to take a sample of the ingested plant to the hospital so that it can be identified. The vomitus should be collected, as it may also help the physician identify the poisonous plant.

343

Central Nervous System Disturbances

Poisonous plants may produce various symptoms of nervous system disturbance, including depression, hyperactivity, hyperexcitement, stupor, mental confusion, or coma.

Plants that can produce nervous system disturbances are:

Apple (seed)	Fly mushroom	Poison hemlock
Apricot (pit)	Green hellebore	Potato (sprout)
Autumn crocus	Hemp	Precatory bean
Baneberry	Indian poke	Rhododendron
Bleeding heart	Jimson weed	Rhubarb (blade)
Carolina jessamine	Larkspur	Rosary pea
(same as yellow	Lima bean	Snakeberry
jessamine)	(some varieties)	Sweet pea
Cherry (pit), both	Marijuana	Thornapple
cultivated and	Monkshood	Water hemlock
wild	Morning glory	Yellow jessamine
Daffodil	Mountain laurel	(same as
Dutchman's	Narcissus	Carolina
breeches	Oleander	jessamine)
False hellebore	Peach (pit)	

Treatment. Treatment should be primarily directed toward basic life support. Vomiting should not be induced if the patient is stuporous or unconscious. The patient should be taken to the hospital at once.

Skin Irritants

Through skin contact, some plants can produce severe itching and burning and cause blister formation. Rarely do these types of plants produce systemic reactions of a severe nature.

Plants that may produce skin irritations are:

Buttercup	Iris	Poison ivy
Christmas rose	Mayapple	Poison oak
Dumbcane	Oleander	Poison sumac
(dieffenbachia)	Poinsettia	Yew
Four o'clock		

Treatment. Emergency treatment of skin irritation should consist only of a thorough cleansing of the skin with soap and water.

A specific risk exists with dieffenbachia, one of the most frequently seen plants in homes and offices these days. A piece of this plant put into the mouth can cause sufficient irritation and swelling of the mucous membranes to produce difficulty in swallowing, breathing, and speaking (thus the common name—dumbcane). If the swelling is severe enough, the airway can become completely closed and the patient will be in danger of suffocation. Emergency treatment consists of opening the airway, using an artificial airway if necessary, giving oxygen, and transporting the patient to the Emergency Department at once.

Insect Bites and Stings

Several classes of insects can give painful and harmful bites or stings. These classes include bees, wasps, ants, scorpions, caterpillars, and spiders. Spider bites are discussed separately.

Bees, Wasps, and Ants

Stings from bees and wasps are among the most common insect bites—more common than all other insect bites combined. The stinging organ of the bee, wasp, or ant projects from the posterior portion of the insect's abdomen to inject venom into the individual's skin. A wasp or ant may use its stinger repeatedly, but the honey bee leaves its stinger and venom sac attached to the skin. It is the only species of insect which does so. Identification of the offender may be difficult as bees and wasps usually quickly fly away after stinging their victims.

Symptoms associated with bee, wasp, and ant stings may be a local response, a systemic or allergic response, or both.

Local response. Most individuals stung by insects suffer from local reactions only. These reactions consist of pain, redness, itching, and swelling in the form of a white, firm, elevated skin wheal. Although the swelling may be excessive and produce apprehension and fear in the patient, the symptoms are usually of short duration and will gradually resolve themselves without medication. Moderate application of ice will help control the pain.

A suspected honey bee sting should first be treated by carefully scraping the stinger and its attached venom sac from the skin. Forceps should **not** be used, as squeezing the sac will only inject more venom into the patient.

Systemic allergic response. It is estimated about 5 percent of Americans are hypersensitive

344

or allergic to the venoms of the bee, wasp, or ant. Approximately half of the four hundred deaths reported each year caused by venomous insects and animals are caused by the stings of bees and wasps, especially of the honey bee.

The symptoms of a hypersensitive reaction begin with generalized itching, skin wheals, weakness, headache, difficulty in breathing, anxiety, and abdominal cramps. The patient may then develop the classic symptoms of shock which frequently precede death. All these symptoms can develop quickly. Death has been reported to occur within sixty minutes from the time of the sting. Urgent treatment is requisite once allergic manifestations become evident.

Treatment. Basic life support as needed must be promptly instituted, with the maintenance of an airway, ventilation, and heartbeat. The patient should be given oxygen as required. In addition, the following supportive measures should be taken.

1. If the bite or sting is on an extremity, place a tourniquet immediately above the injury to try to prevent dispersal of the venom throughout the system.
2. If the stinger with its venom sac is present, carefully scrape it from the skin.
3. Place an ice bag over the area of the bite, to decrease absorption of the poison.

Transport the patient to the Emergency Department without delay. His life may depend upon prompt treatment beyond emergency basic life support.

Scorpions

Scorpions will not sting unless greatly provoked; children receive most scorpion stings. The toxin is injected by a stinger located at the tip of the scorpion's tail. Except for a particular variety in the Southwest, most scorpions in the United States produce innocuous stings. An ordinary scorpion sting produces a swelling which varies from slight to pronounced and results in pain and, at times, skin discoloration.

The sting of a scorpion located in Arizona can cause a severe systemic reaction, including skeletal muscle contractions, respiratory arrest, excessive salivation, gastric distention, a rise in blood pressure, pulmonary edema, convulsions, and congestive heart failure.

Treatment. Treatment for ordinary stings consists of local pain relief only, usually accomplished by applying an ice bag to the site of the bite. Application of ammonia solution on the area is also often helpful in relieving pain.

Emergency treatment for the sting of the dangerous Southwest scorpion is directed to basic life support. Antivenin, which may be administered by a physician, is available in areas where this scorpion exists. Therefore, a physician should be contacted and the patient transported to the Emergency Department at once, as in other instances of severe envenomation.

Puss Caterpillar (Tree Asp)

A variety of caterpillar or asp (an insect, not the snake) with a painful sting is frequently found eating the leaves of trees and bushes in the fall months, but it may also be present in the spring. Clusters of venomous spines are intermingled with fine hairs on its back so that the slightest brush against it can produce a sting from several spines without contacting either head or tail. Classically, there is an immediate severe burning and painful sensation at the site of the sting with redness and swelling, followed within ten minutes by the radiation of pain into the axillary (armpit) or inguinal (groin) areas.

Treatment. Treatment is primarily directed to relieving the rather severe pain. Application of an ice or an artificial coolant bag to the affected areas is helpful. The swelling and pain can persist for more than twenty-four hours.

Spider Bites

The black widow spider and the brown recluse spider produce poisonous bites; both are relatively common in some areas of the United States. Envenomations from these spiders are very painful and occasionally life-threatening. It is very important to identify the spider which delivers the bite as numerous kinds of spiders are capable of producing an irritating but non-poisonous bite.

345

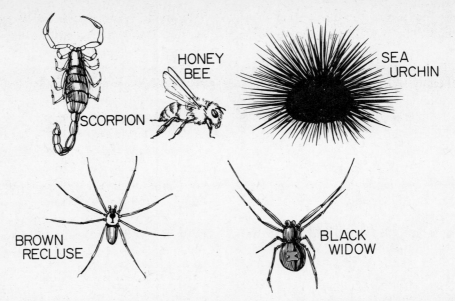

SCORPION

HONEY BEE

SEA URCHIN

BROWN RECLUSE

BLACK WIDOW

Figure 45.2

Many common animals that injure by biting or stinging are illustrated. Characteristic markings identify the black widow spider and the brown recluse spider. The stings of the scorpion and the honey bee are in the tails. The sting of the sea urchin is at the tips of the spines.

Black Widow Spider (Hourglass Spider)

The female black widow spider is also called the hourglass spider because of its marking (Fig. 45.2). It is glossy black with a distinct red or yellowish-orange marking in the shape of an hourglass on the belly. No marking shows on the spider's back. Both large and small specimens are seen; the largest is about $1\frac{1}{2}$ inches long with its legs extended.

The patient may not even have felt the bite when it was delivered, and there may be no sign at the place bitten. Occasionally, two tiny red dots may be seen. Initially there may be pain at the site of the bite for an hour or two. Later, muscular cramps may develop in the involved extremity and spread to the muscles of the patient's back. The pain then characteristically spreads to the abdomen, where muscles may assume a boardlike rigidity. Tightness in the chest, difficulty in breathing, nausea, vomiting, and sweating are frequently present.

Death has been only rarely reported.

Treatment. Other than basic life support and the application of a cold pack to the bite, there is no specific emergency treatment to be rendered by the EMT. However, antivenin for the black

widow spider bite and other drugs are available for administration by the physician. It is, therefore, of utmost importance that the offending spider be identified if at all possible. When a diagnosis of black widow spider bite is made or suspected, the patient should be transported to the Emergency Department and placed under the care of a physician.

Brown Recluse Spider (Brown Spider, or Fiddleback Spider)

The brown recluse spider is usually smaller than the black widow spider and will measure about one inch long with its legs extended. It can be identified by the violin-shaped or fiddle-shaped marking on its back (Fig. 45.2). A bite usually occurs while an individual is in a little-used storage area, an attic, a cellar, an old unused building—hence the name *recluse spider*.

The bite may or may not be felt; however, the bitten area becomes red, swollen, and tender, often within ten hours. A small blister is generally present. Several days later a black eschar (scab) develops, which sloughs (drops off) in a day or two, leaving a draining ulcer. Formation of another scab, sloughing off, and enlargement of the ulcer are repeated, sometimes for weeks. In some cases chills, fever, nausea, and vomiting occur.

Death has only rarely been reported.

Treatment. As with the black widow spider bite, basic life support should be carried out. Identification of the spider is very important as it greatly aids a physician in treatment.

Snakebites

Each year in the United States, forty-five thousand snakebites are reported, of which seven thousand are inflicted by venomous snakes. During the past five years, the number of deaths from poisonous snakebites in this country has not exceeded twelve each year. Approximately 30 percent of all bites by venomous snakes show no evidence of envenomation; that is, the reptile does not inject poison in every bite.

In the United States, there are approximately 120 species of snakes, about 20 of which are poisonous. The venomous species include all the rattlesnakes, among which are the Western diamondback, the Eastern diamondback, the prairie, timber, red, Pacific, Mojave, black-tailed, and sidewinder rattlesnakes. Other snakes which are venomous are the water moccasin, sometimes called the cottonmouth, the copperhead, and the coral snake. Because there are so many different kinds of snakes in the United States, identification of the one which has bitten the patient becomes extremely important. One should use a proper source book to check for distinguishing characteristics instead of relying only on a general knowledge of color and markings for identification. Any snake with a rattle on its tail is venomous regardless of its color.

Pit Vipers

The rattlesnake, cottonmouth snake, and copperhead are called pit vipers because they bear a characteristic deep pit located between the eye and the nostril (Fig. 45.3). This pit is a heat-sensing organ which allows the pit viper to make a direct hit on a warm-blooded animal even when he cannot see it. Another characteris-

tic of the pit viper is a set of elongated hollow fangs in the upper jaw, which fold against the roof of the mouth. When striking, the snake extends these fangs and injects poison from its venom sac. The pit viper also has vertical, elliptically shaped pupils and a somewhat flat, triangular head.

The cardinal signs of envenomation by a pit viper are severe burning pain and immediate swelling about the fang marks. The swelling and pain usually develop within five to ten minutes and spread slowly over the next eight to thirty-six hours. If these local signs do not occur within an hour or so, one can be almost certain that envenomation has not occurred. Bleeding under the skin and discoloration of the surrounding area may develop within several hours of envenomation. This reaction will be followed by hemorrhagic blisters, and, as time passes, some degree of local anesthesia (numbness) will be noted.

The systemic signs, which may or may not occur after the local signs, are weakness, sweating, faintness, nausea, vomiting, tachycardia (an abnormally rapid pulse), and hypotension (low blood pressure). The EMT should remember that, as with any other type of trauma, there

347

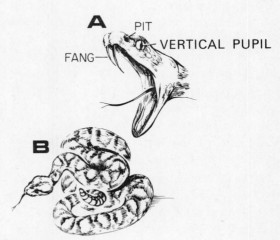

Figure 45.3

The pit viper is the most common poisonous snake in the United States. Several species of rattlesnake, as well as the cottonmouth moccasin and the copperhead are all pit vipers. *a,* Some characteristics of pit vipers are shown: a hinged, long pair of fangs, a vertical slit for the pupil, and the pit (the heat-sensing organ) between the eye and the nose. *b,* A rattlesnake coiled and ready to strike shows the typical flat, triangular head.

are degrees of injury and that either a minimal or a large amount of poison may have been injected. Emergency treatment by the EMT in most instances will be mainly supportive. The steps of emergency care are as follows:

1. Calm and reassure the patient, who will often be excited or hysterical. The patient should lie down, be quiet, and be kept warm. He should **not** be given alcohol.
2. Clean the bite with soap and water or an antiseptic solution.
3. Locate the fang marks and wrap *soft* rubber tubing ($\frac{1}{2}''$ Penrose drain) about the extremity both above and below the fang marks. The tubing should be very lightly applied to occlude only the lymphatic tissues and superficial venous blood flow. It should not occlude arterial or deep venous flow.
4. Immobilize the extremity with a splint.
5. Check the patient's vital signs, blood pressure, pulse, and respiration.
6. Minimize the development of shock by the use of blankets and elevation of the feet. If the patient develops shock, start IV solutions and give oxygen.
7. Apply an ice bag or chemical coolant bag if a physician so directs. Under **no** circumstances should the extremity be **packed** in ice.
8. Transport the patient to the Emergency Department, giving advance notice of the type of case being brought in. Antivenin, which may be given by a physician, must often be procured elsewhere. The hospital can begin the search as soon as it learns of the need.

If the EMT reaches the patient within twenty to thirty minutes of the time he was bitten, and **If** the patient already shows definite signs of envenomation, and **If** a physician concurs, a sterile surgical knife blade may be used to make an incision about one-half inch long by one-fourth inch deep over each fang mark. Suction cups or local massage of the tissue will then help remove some of the injected venom. Suction by mouth is not recommended—not because of the possibility that the poison will enter a cut in the mouth

of the EMT but because the human mouth harbors so many different toxic bacteria that the bite could become secondarily infected. Incision with suction later than thirty minutes from the time of envenomation is not recommended. The Emergency Department should be kept constantly informed of the patient's vital signs and general condition during treatment and transportation, as further definitive measures may be directed by the physician.

The EMT will seldom be involved in the use of antivenin, but he should know that the larger zoos in the United States usually stock supplies of snake antivenin and have emergency programs for dispensing them, as well as a list of the names and addresses of consulting physicians in the area. In addition, there is a national antivenin index which is maintained by the Oklahoma City Zoo. During the day the phone number is (405)424-3344. During the night or on weekends it is (405)271-5454.

Coral Snake

The coral snake is a small, shy, and docile snake. It averages less than two feet in length and has a body diameter of about three-eights of an inch. It is very colorful, with bright red, yellow, and black rings encircling its body in regular order. The arrangement of the colored rings helps to distinguish the coral snake from nonpoisonous snakes that also have red, yellow, and black rings. In the coral snake, the red ring always touches the yellow ring. The distinction is made easy to remember by the well-known verse:

> Red on yellow
> Will kill a fellow.
> Red on black,
> Venom will lack.

The coral snake belongs to the same group of snakes as the cobra, mamba, and krait. Its poison is the most toxic of any of the poisonous snakes in the United States. Fortunately, it is responsible for only 1 to 2 percent of snakebites in this country. Its fangs are unlike those of the pit viper in that there are several pairs of short, rigid, grooved fangs at the end of the upper jaw. Therefore, the coral snake must use a chewing motion to inject its poison. Because of its small mouth and teeth and limited jaw expansion, the coral snake usually bites its victim on a small part of the body—a hand, a foot, especially a finger. Following the bite of a coral snake, one can find one or more tiny punctures or scratchlike wounds in the area of the bite.

The signs and symptoms of the coral snake bite are completely different from those of the pit viper's bite. Following envenomation by a coral snake, there are only minimal local signs of pain and swelling. Ecchymosis (blackening) and tissue necrosis (decay of flesh) usually do not occur, and other signs and symptoms develop only after one to seven hours. The venom of the coral snake is neurotoxic; that is, it has its effect on the central nervous system. Patients may complain of depression or apprehension or euphoria. The neurotoxicity of the poison affects the cranial nerves, resulting in paralysis of respiratory movements and of the eyelids and eyeball movements.

Treatment. The EMT, if at all possible, should identify the snake. Antivenin is available, but most hospitals or doctors will have to order it from a central supply area, often in another city. Therefore, the need for it should be made known as soon as possible.

The steps of emergency care are these:

1. Immediately quieten and reassure the patient. Do not give alcohol.
2. Flush off the area of the bite with one to two quarts of water to wash away any poison left on the surface of the skin.
3. Lightly apply a soft-rubber tubing about the extremity above the bite.
4. Splint the extremity to minimize the spread of the venom to the central nervous system.
5. Check the patient's vital signs and continue to monitor them.
6. Keep the patient warm, elevate the lower extremities, and give IV solutions to help prevent shock.
7. Give artificial ventilation with oxygen if needed.
8. Apply an ice bag or coolant bag to the bite area if the physician so recommends. Under **no** circumstances should the extremity ever be **packed** in ice.
9. Transport promptly to the Emergency Department, giving advance notice that the patient has been bitten by a coral snake.

Incision and suction are not recommended in the case of a coral snake bite, as there is little local effect from this bite. The danger is to the central nervous system.

Injuries from Marine Animals

Although over one thousand species of marine animals are poisonous to eat or are capable of inflicting injury upon humans, there are only six major types of injury mechanisms. These are outlined in Table 45.1.

Each type of injury has its own emergency medical treatment, also outlined in Table 45.1. Except in the case of fish poisonings, the emergency treatment usually results in a definitive cure. However, complications do arise, and for this reason, anyone receiving an injury from a marine animal should have follow-up care by a physician.

In terms of frequency, injuries from marine animals are uncommon. These animals are not aggressive. Most injuries are self-inflicted; for example, the patient has swum into the tentacles of a jellyfish, stepped on a stingray, or fallen onto a sea urchin. These three injuries are the ones which most frequently occur with marine animals.

In localities where marine animal injuries are likely to occur, additional emergency supplies as indicated in Table 45.1 should be kept on hand. Note particularly those items which are out of the ordinary (bottle of meat tenderizer, drying powders such as talcum or flour, a spatula or knifeblade, and water heating arrangements, such as a pan and a can of Sterno). Further treatment may be required, especially for a patient who has eaten a poisonous fish.

The EMT should familiarize himself with unusual marine animals in his locality and with specific treatments and antivenins for injuries inflicted by them.

349

TABLE 45.1

GUIDE TO DIAGNOSIS AND EMERGENCY TREATMENT OF MARINE ANIMAL INJURIES

Type of Injury	Marine Animal Involved	Emergency Treatment	Possible Complications
Trauma (bites and lacerations)	Major wounds by: Shark Barracuda Alligator gar	Control bleeding Prevent shock Give basic life support Splint the injury Secure prompt medical care	Shock Infections
	Minor wounds by: Moray eel Turtle Corals	Cleanse wound Splint the injury	
Sting (by tentacles)	Jellyfish Portuguese man-of-war Anemones Corals Hydras	Inactivate the area with alcohol and sprinkle with meat tenderizer Coalesce with powder and scrape the area[1]	Allergic reactions Respiratory arrest
Puncture (by spines)	Urchins Cone shells Stingrays Spiny fish (catfish, toad, or oyster fish)	Inactivate with hot water[2]	Allergic reactions Collapse Infections Tetanus Granuloma formation
Poisonous bite (by fangs)	Sea snake Octopus[3]	Give basic life support	Paralysis Myoglobinuria Respiratory arrest
Poisoning (by ingestion)[4]	Puffer fish Scromboids (tuna species) Ciguatera (large colored fish) Paralytic shell fish	Give basic life support; prevent self-injury from convulsions	Allergic reactions Asthmatic reactions Paresthesia, numbness Temperature reversal phenomena Respiratory arrest and circulatory collapse
Miscellaneous: Shocks Skin rashes	Electric fish Marine parasites	No treatment required; injuries usually self-limiting	Electric fish or electric eel may precipitate a panic reaction

[1] The intense burning pain resulting from the sting of the jellyfish is produced by nematocysts (stinging cells) on the tentacles. Even when the sea creature is washed up on shore, the stinging cells remain potent for several days. In treating the sting, 95-percent alcohol "fixes" the nematocysts on the skin and prevents further stinging, and the meat tenderizer neutralizes the protein toxin of the nematocyst. Powder dries the area and causes the stings to stick together so they can be more readily removed by scraping.

[2] A toxin is introduced with some of the puncture wounds from this group. In any case, the wounds are excruciatingly painful. It appears that the foreign material or poison introduced into the wound is heat-sensitive. Dramatic treatment results occur with soaking in quite hot water for thirty to sixty minutes. Be careful, however, not to scald the patient with water that is too hot, as the pain of the wound will mask his normal reaction to heat.

[3] Only one species of octopus, the blue ringed octopus of Australia, is known to have inflicted fatal bites to persons.

[4] Should ingestion of a poisonous fish be suspected, reference to Halstead's *Poisonous and Venomous Marine Animals of the World* or seeking immediate assistance from poison control centers is suggested.

XI

Emergency Vehicles and Equipment; Patient Handling and Extrication

46

Emergency Vehicles, Equipment, and Maintenance

GOAL I.   Be familiar with the medical requirements and the design criteria of emergency medical care vehicles.

OBJECTIVES

A. Define an ambulance.
B. Identify the basic medical requirements for an ambulance.
C. Identify the design criteria for an ambulance.
D. Compare helicopters and surface vehicles for advantages and disadvantages as ambulances.

GOAL II.   Know the equipment necessary for an ambulance to meet national standards.

OBJECTIVES

A. List the categories of equipment to be carried on an ambulance.
B. Identify the essential equipment in each category.

GOAL III.   Understand the importance of and the procedures for emergency vehicle maintenance.

OBJECTIVES

A. Describe the daily inspection of an ambulance.
B. Describe the cleaning and decontamination processes necessary for an ambulance.
C. Describe the 1,000-mile servicing procedure for an ambulance.

For many decades following introduction of the first motor-driven ambulance in 1906, the vehicle most frequently used as an ambulance was the hearse, because it could provide transportation of an individual in a recumbent position on a portable litter (stretcher). Very few supplies were carried and there was limited space for an attendant. Now, however, hearses are being rapidly withdrawn from this dual service as better equipped and more ample vehicles are being utilized.

In recent years manufacturers have enlarged and improved the ambulance so that it no longer resembles the hearse. They have responded to the EMTs' need for more working room and have provided space for oxygen devices, for at least the essential equipment recommended by the American College of Surgeons, and for an additional litter. These additions have resulted in greater length, width, and height of the patient compartment. In a highly competitive and limited-output industry, these improvements are costly. Manufacturers welcomed the consolidated recommendations of ambulance operators, physicians, and automotive design engineers who, through the National Academy of Sciences/National Research Council and the Department of Transportation, established national standards. These standards have resulted in greater uniformity of design and equipment and provided not only for the scientific needs of today but also for adaptation to future advances without the necessity of radical changes in design.

The most pressing needs which the modern ambulance must meet are: increased space for performing cardiopulmonary resuscitation in transit, a ceiling height sufficient for adequate gravity flow of intravenous fluids, installed suction and oxygen devices, two-way radio communication, storage room for equipment, facilities for safeguarding personnel and patients, and equipment for light-rescue operations.

Basis for Increased Ambulance Capability

Regardless of whether ambulances are used in urban or rural areas, they should be standardized to carry the minimum recommended equipment. The need for equipment for safety and rescue work and for road clearance, for example, can be as necessary in a city as in a rural area, should a disaster or public disorder impede the response of rescue vehicles or make roadways impassable.

Continued research and development of larger vehicles as mobile life-support units may be necessary, but the recommended standard ambulance can at present provide all the supplies and space necessary for lifesaving care at an accident scene and during transport. One type of larger vehicle, now in use sparingly, which has proven its worth and should be given

further study is an intensive-care transfer vehicle. There are problem patients who will succumb if left in the original hospital to which they were admitted or if they are transferred by surface or air vehicles in use today. Many of these patients can survive if a special transfer unit with more sophisticated diagnostic and treatment equipment is available.

NAS-NRC Definition of an Ambulance

An ambulance is defined as a vehicle for emergency care, especially designed to provide a driver compartment and, preferably separate, a patient compartment which can accommodate two EMTs and two litter patients so positioned that at least one of the patients can be given intensive lifesaving care during transit (Fig. 46.1).

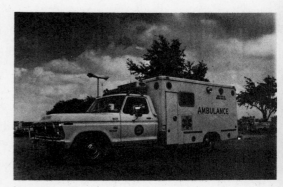

Figure 46.1

A modular ambulance which meets standards established by the National Academy of Sciences/National Research Council is shown.

Such a vehicle must carry equipment and supplies to provide emergency care at the scene of an accident and during transport, to safeguard personnel and patients under hazardous conditions, and to carry out light-rescue procedures. It must have two-way radio communication capability between the ambulance and the Emergency Services dispatcher, the authorities, and the hospital, and walkie-talkie communication between the EMTs. It must be designed and constructed to afford maximum safety and comfort so that moving the patient does not aggravate an injury or create complications.

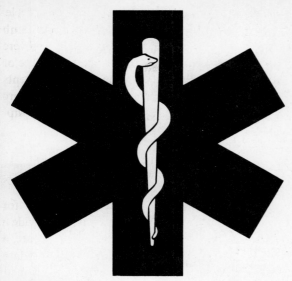

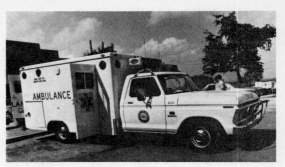

Figure 46.3

An ambulance is shown with side door open. The Star of Life emblem is seen on the door.

355

Figure 46.2

The Star of Life emblem is displayed on the sides, rear, and roof of vehicles that meet federal specifications as licensed ambulances.

Restrictions on Designation as an Ambulance

To qualify as an ambulance, a vehicle must meet all requirements stated in the above definition. Unless it is fully equipped and manned to serve as an ambulance, no vehicle employed for transport of non-emergency patients (litter, wheelchair, or seated cases) or especially designed as a mobile coronary unit or a mobile operating room unit should be licensed as an ambulance. Neither should it be permitted to use ambulance identifying colors or insignia, flashing lights, or warning signal devices.

Federal specifications for the ambulance have been determined (*Federal Specifications—Ambulance—Emergency Care Vehicles*), and no ambulance may be purchased with federal matching funds unless they are followed. Pertinent portions of these specifications are discussed below.

Uniformity of External Identification

So that the ambulance will be universally differentiated from all other vehicles, the recommended exterior color is basically white in combination with orange (strip), with blue lettering and emblems. The material used for the emblems and markings shall be reflectorized blue and white. The Star of Life emblem (Fig. 46.2) shall be on the sides (Fig. 46.3), rear, and roof. Unless otherwise required by state or local regulations, the rotating, roof-mounted beacon, the upper-body corner lights, and warning lights mounted on the radiator grill shall be flashing blue and white. The audible warning signal shall be intermittent so that drivers of other vehicles can recognize the sound. The word AMBULANCE shall be in mirror image on the front of the vehicle for ready identification by a driver ahead when seen in the rear-view mirror (Fig. 46.4).

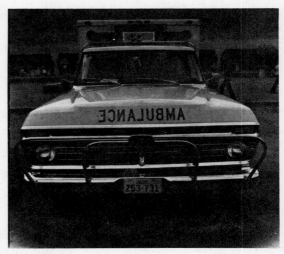

Figure 46.4

On the front of the vehicle, the word *Ambulance* is spelled backward so that it will read correctly when viewed in a rear view mirror.

Chassis

The chassis shall provide optimal smooth-riding qualities, have a road clearance of at least six inches when loaded, give protection in fording water up to twelve inches in depth and have a heavy braking system. A fuel range of at least 150 miles is required. Higher road clearance or a four-wheel-drive capability may be necessary where geographic location and off-highway operations dictate these needs. The ambulance body may be mounted on a passenger or truck chassis. General federal motor vehicle safety standards for ambulances shall be those applicable to the chassis employed.

The overall length of the ambulance may vary according to whether the patient and driver compartments are constructed as a single unit or the driver's cab is mounted separately. In either case the minimal interior length of the patient compartment shall be 116 inches, the maximum length of the entire vehicle over bumpers shall not exceed 22 feet, and the height at curbside shall not exceed 110 inches, including roof-mounted equipment but excluding two-way radio antennas.

Ambulance Body

The body must be crashworthy, free of interior protruding objects that can be dangerous to patients and technicians, air-conditioned, easily cleaned, insulated, and large enough to accommodate two litter patients, two EMTs, and all installed and portable equipment and supplies necessary for optimal patient care. Windows are not recommended except in the front, rear, and curbside door of the patient compartment. Direct access between the driver and patient compartments is desirable. If there is a passageway, a door shall be provided that can be secured on the driver's side. In either case, there shall be a window and a means of voice communication between the driver and patient compartments. The driver shall be shielded from light in the rear compartment at night.

Dimensions of the patient compartment. There must be a clear space of 25 inches at the head and 15 inches at the foot of a 76-inch litter in the patient compartment. The minimal inside width shall provide for two 23-inch–wide litters with sufficient space between them to permit a technician in kneeling position at the side of a patient to perform external cardiac compression. Thus a free 25-inch working area is required, part of which might be unobstructed space for the lower legs and feet of the EMT beneath the second litter or beneath a squad bench. The minimal accepted inside ceiling height is 60 inches.

All equipment necessary for patient care in transit must be installed, secured, or stored in cabinets or drawers inside the patient compartment. By eliminating side windows, greater space for storage is available.

Speed and Acceleration

The fully loaded ambulance must be provided with a power train of such speed and acceleration that it is capable of rapid dispatch to the scene of an emergency, of maintaining its position in traffic on modern highways, of avoiding hazardous situations in moving traffic, and of moving faster than traffic when necessary. The criteria of speed and acceleration are designed to insure safety of the ambulance in traffic on interstate highways. Training, judgment, and primary concern for the safety of the patient will determine the manner in which the driver uses these high-performance capabilities, which must never be employed unsafely or irresponsibly.

Emergency-Care Equipment and Supplies

Basic requirements. For purposes of estimating space requirements for installed, portable, and stored equipment and supplies, and locating them for optimal accessibility, designers must be familiar with the size, weight, shape, and power requirements for each item.

Design must not be limited to accommodation of contemporary equipment and supplies. Allowance should be made for inevitable scientific advances in emergency care and for new and refined equipment that can be expected to appear. Video facilities have joined radio transmission between ambulance and Emergency Department, and telemetry of diagnostic signs, proven effective from thousands of miles in space, has also proven useful on earth. However, as EMTs become more highly trained, physicians in Emergency Departments will become more and more willing to depend upon the EMT's interpretation of diagnostic signs, and will utilize more voice communication in consultation and treatment.

The location of equipment and supplies should be dictated by the relative importance of accessibility, with priority given to items necessary to cope with life-threatening conditions. The equipment and supplies necessary for airway care, artificial ventilation, suction, and oxygenation must be within reach of the EMT at the head of the litter. Those for cardiac resuscitation, control of external bleeding, administration of intravenous agents, and monitoring blood pressure shall be available at the side of the litter.

To the greatest extent possible, equipment and supplies must be so standardized and durable as to make possible any necessary interchange between ambulances or between ambulances and hospitals.

Storage cabinets, drawers, and kits shall be easily opened but shall also be easily secured to prevent their coming open in transit. For rapid identification of contents, the use of transparent material for the fronts of some cabinets and drawers may be desirable; otherwise, labeling of the contents on the fronts is recommended. Drawers should be removable.

Patient transfer litters. Each ambulance shall be provided with (1) a wheeled litter, (2) a folding litter, and (3) a collapsible device that enables EMTs to carry a patient over stairways and other narrow spaces where a full-length litter cannot be used (Fig. 46.5). Litters 2 and 3 may be combined as one folding litter. Litters must be easy to move, store, and disinfect. The folding litter should keep the patient above floor level. The wheeled litter, adjustable in height, should be designed so that in the low-riding position the top may be as low as 11 inches but not higher than 15 inches above the floor of the ambulance.

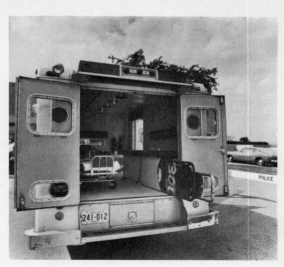

Figure 46.5

An inside view of an approved ambulance shows a litter and spineboard. Note that there is sufficient working space and headroom for EMTs to perform necessary lifesaving functions for a patient while in transit.

Litters shall be equipped with detachable, collapsible, telescoping supports for intravenous-infusion containers.

The head of the litter must be capable of being tilted upward to a sixty-degree, semi-sitting position, and the entire litter must be capable of being tilted into a head-down position of at least ten degrees (for airway care). To permit lying full length in the supine, prone, or lateral position, litters must be at least 69 inches long and 20 inches wide. Most standard litters are 74 to 86 inches long, including handles, and 22 to 23 inches wide. The frame or handles should be designed to permit up to four persons to carry the litter and must provide for fasteners to secure it firmly to the floor or side of the vehicle during transport. Restraining devices must be provided to prevent the patient from falling off the side or sliding off the end during transport. If an X-ray–permeable, removable top from an Emergency Department cart is placed on the litter, the patient can be carried on it and not removed from the top until he is in bed at the completion of initial diagnosis and treatment.

Figures 46.6 and 46.7 illustrate some of the items carried on ambulances as standard and portable equipment.

357

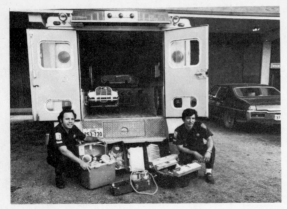

358   Figure 46.6

Some of the standard equipment on an approved ambulance is shown.

Airways. Oropharyngeal airways for adults, children, and infants shall be provided. Airways for mouth-to-mouth ventilation shall also be carried in all sizes. Mouth gags of a commercial type or made from tongue blades taped together and padded shall be provided for use during convulsions to prevent injury to the patient's tongue. For ventilation and oxygenation of patients with tracheostomies, 15-mm tracheostomy tubes and male adapters of various sizes must be available.

Artificial ventilation devices. Portable artificial ventilation devices which operate independently of a supply of oxygen shall be provided. Two units are desirable, one for use in the ambulance and the other for use outside or as a spare. The artificial ventilation device must be a manually operated, self-filling, portable bag-valve-mask unit that delivers air and is capable of oxygen enrichment. When attached to an oxygen supply, with an oxygen reservoir in place, the unit should be capable of delivering almost 100-percent oxygen to the patient. The unit must be easy to clean and decontaminate. It must have one standard universal adapter (15-mm tracheal tube/22 mm-mask). The non-breathing valve must permit inhalation of oxygen during both artificial and spontaneous breathing from the bag.

Masks in several sizes for adults, children, and infants must be available. They shall be transparent, to permit rapid recognition of change of color in the patient and to detect vomiting and abnormalities of breathing (for example, clouding of the mask during exhalation). Oxygen-powered, manually triggered inflation devices are acceptable if properly designed.

Suction equipment. Portable and installed suction equipment must be available. The portable unit must provide vacuum and flow adequate for pharyngeal suction. It shall be fitted with large-bore, non-kinking suction tubing with a rigid pharyngeal suction tip. There must also be sterile suction catheters of various sizes for suctioning via an endotracheal or tracheostomy tube, a nonbreakable collection bottle, and a supply of water for rinsing the tubes.

The installed suction unit must be powerful enough to provide an airflow of thirty liters per minute at the end of the delivery tube and a vacuum of 300 mm Hg when the tube is clamped. The suction force must be controllable for use on children or intubated patients. There shall be an additional set of rigid pharyngeal-suction tips (tonsil suction tips) and sterile tracheal-suction catheters of various sizes.

For tracheal suction a Y-piece or T-piece or a lateral opening shall lie between the suction tube and the suction source for on-off control. The suction yoke, collection bottle, water for rinsing, and suction tube must be readily accessible to the EMT at the head of the litter, and the tube

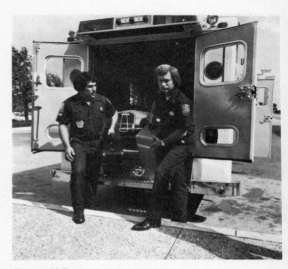

Figure 46.7

EMTs responding to an emergency call take needed equipment with them in "jump bags."

must reach the airway of the patient regardless of his position. Suction apparatus must be easily cleaned and decontaminated.

Oxygen inhalation equipment. There must be two oxygen supplies, one portable, the other installed. The portable unit (300-liter capacity), located near a door for ready use outside, shall be equipped with a yoke, pressure gauge, flowmeter (not gravity-dependent), delivery tube, and oxygen mask. The unit must be capable of delivering an oxygen flow of at least 10 liters per minute. An extra 300-liter-capacity cylinder shall be available.

The installed unit must be supplied by at least 3,000 liters of oxygen contained in two tanks and delivered by a two-stage regulator under pressure of 50 psi (pounds per square inch). There must be yokes, reducing valves, flowmeters (not gravity-dependent), and humidifiers. Delivery tubes must be visible and accessible to the EMT seated at the head of the litter. Delivery tubes must reach to the face of a patient transported in the horizontal position and deliver a continuous flow of at least 10 liters per minute. They shall connect readily to oxygen masks and bag-valve-mask ventilation devices. Oxygen masks (with or without bags) shall be semi-open, valveless, transparent, disposable (or easy to clean and decontaminate), and in sizes for adults, children, and infants.

Equipment for cardiac compression. A spineboard should be readily available. When placed under the patient in bed or on a litter, it provides the necessary resistance for effective external cardiac compression. It should raise the patient's shoulders three to four inches above the level of the litter in order to keep the head in a position of maximum backward tilt and the shoulders and thorax in a straight position without manual support. This position may help maintain an open airway during cardiopulmonary resuscitation given during transportation. A special spineboard may be used, or a long or short spineboard may be supplemented with a tightly rolled sheet under the patient's shoulders and a head stabilizer, like sandbags or a headrest in a doughnut shape. The superiority of mechanical over manual external cardiac compression has not been established. In anticipation of future development of satisfactory equipment, space should be provided for such equipment.

Basic supplies. The following basic supplies must be carried:

1 pillow
2 pillow cases
2 spare sheets
4 towels
6 disposable emesis bags
2 boxes of disposable tissues
1 bedpan
1 thermometer
Disposable drinking cups
2 sandbags
4 blankets
1 blood-pressure apparatus
1 stethoscope

Supplies for splinting of fractures. The following supplies must be carried for the splinting of actual or suspected fractures:

1 hinged, half-ring, lower-extremity splint with a minimum ring size of 9 inches and minimum overall length of 43 inches, with commercial limb-support slings, padded ankle hitch, and traction strap with buckle. A telescoping splint may replace the rigid unit.

Splints for the upper and lower extremities, such as padded boards, of material comparable to four-ply wood in widths of 3 inches and length of 15, 36, and 54 inches. The splints may be cardboard, plastic, or wire ladder, canvas-slotted, lace-on, or inflatable, with number and types to be determined by local option.

Triangular bandages for fractures of the shoulder and upper-arm and for fixation of rigid splints.

Short and long spineboards and accessories (straps and cervical supports) for safe extrication, as well as splinting in case of actual or suspected injuries of the spine.

Supplies for wound dressing. Supplies to be carried for dressing of open wounds and for padding and application of splints include:

Sterile gauze pads of conventional sizes

Universal dressings, approximately 10 × 36 inches, packaged by folding to 9 × 10 inches

Soft roller, self-adhering bandages, 6 inches × 5 yards

Sterile, non-porous dressings for occlusion of sucking wounds of the chest (plastic wrap or aluminum foil is effective)

Adhesive tape, in widths of 3 inches

Safety pins, large

Bandage shears

Supplies for treatment of shock. Equipment for treatment of shock must include:

Sterile intravenous agents, preferably in plastic bags

Sterile, disposable intravenous administration kits (incuding injection kits containing needles, cathether needles, syringes, antiseptic sponges, a venous tourniquet, and tape)

Military Anti-Shock Trousers, commonly referred to as MAST pants (optional)

Supplies for childbirth. In addition to sterile dressings and towels, a sterile kit containing gloves, scissors, and umbilical clamps or tapes shall be carried. For a complete list of the necessary equipment for childbirth, see Chapter 36.

Carrier for transportation of newborn infants. Each ambulance service must be able to obtain immediately from a hospital or other source a portable infant carrier that can either be fastened to the litter or stand alone for transporting newborn infants. The carrier shall permit oxygen enrichment, humidification, control of body temperature, and accessibility to the baby's head for resuscitation. There must be artificial ventilation and sterile tracheal-intubation equipment in appropriate sizes for this purpose. The following additional equipment and supplies should be in the carrier:

Crib
3 hot water bottles
1 quilted pad
1 baby blanket
2 diapers
1 room thermometer
1 rubber suction tube with glass trap (sterilized)

1 umbilical clamp
1 rubber suction bulb
1 rubber funnel with tube
1 portable oxygen cylinder with attachments
1 bottle of 70-percent alcohol

Supplies for treatment of acute poisoning. Activated charcoal and syrup of ipecac in premeasured doses must be provided, as well as drinkable water and equipment for oral administration. There should be equipment for irrigation of the conjunctiva and skin. Snakebite kits shall be carried in areas where the hazard of snakebite exists.

Special equipment for physicians and others specially trained. In anticipation of the occasional presence of a physician at the scene of emergencies and the advanced training of greater numbers of technicians (EMT-Paramedics), in the use of special equipment, space in the ambulance should be provided for the following items in a locked container:

1 tracheal-intubation kit
1 pleural-decompression set
1 drug-injection kit with appropriate drugs
1 large-bore needle with obturator, or a cricothyrotome
1 portable cardioscope with external defibrillator
1 venous cut-down kit
1 "minor" surgical kit
1 sterile urinary catheter

Equipment for safeguarding personnel. A weatherproof compartment accessible from outside the patient compartment shall be provided for equipment to safeguard patients and technicians, control traffic and bystanders, and illuminate work areas. These items are:

12 reflectorized or intermittertly flashing warning devices (replacing the formerly recommended flares, which have caused fires at the accident scene)

2 flashlights, stand-up type, 6V standard lantern, battery-powered

1 fire extinguisher, type BC, dry powder, size 5

2 walkie-talkies (see Chapter 49)

2 pairs of gauntlets, foam-insulated, vinyl-coated, of fluorescent orange

2 self-contained air masks (not oxygen-generating), 1 to be a quick-entry type (30 minutes)

2 portable flood lights, each 300W/120V, with stand, twist-lock–type connectors, and 100-foot cords (if not easily and quickly obtainable from other primary-response vehicles, such as fire company apparatus)

Equipment for release from entrapment or confinement. A weatherproof compartment shall be provided outside the patient compartment for equipment for release from entrapment or confinement. These items are:

1 wrench, 12 inches, adjustable, open-end
1 screw driver, 12 inches, regular blade
1 screw driver, 12 inches, Phillips type
1 hacksaw with 12 wire (carbide) blades
1 vise-grip pliers, 10 inches
1 hammer, 5 pounds, with 15-inch handle
1 fire axe, butt, 24-inch handle
1 wrecking bar, 24 inches
(Hammer, axe, and wrecking bar may be separate or one combination tool)
1 crowbar, 51 inches, pinch-point
1 bolt cutter with jaw opening $1–1\frac{1}{4}$ inches
1 portable power unit with attachments, minimum 4-ton capacity
Shoring blocks
1 shovel, pointed blade (folding type)
1 double-action tin snip, hand-operated, minimum 8 inches
2 ropes, Manila, 50 feet $\times \frac{3}{4}$ inches diameter each
2 pairs gloves (gauntlets, leather)
2 pairs goggles (clear, eye-protective)
2 hard hats
1 "come-a-long" (hand-powered winch), heavy duty (two-ton with rated chain set
1 asbestos blanket
1 air-powered tool with various cutting devices (optional)

Currently, the approved ambulance must carry enough equipment to make it a self-sufficient station for rendering emergency care and providing rescue services.

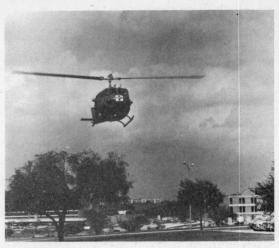

Figure 46.8

A helicopter can often be of great assistance in transporting patients over difficult terrain or congested land traffic or in circumstances requiring more speed than land vehicles can provide.

361

The Helicopter as an Ambulance

General considerations. The capability of helicopters to provide effective transportation for the sick or injured has been proved by both military and civilian groups. Under certain circumstances the helicopter is unsurpassed as transportation to avoid traffic congestion, speed emergency care to a patient in a remote or otherwise inaccessible area, or transport the sick or injured quickly to medical facilities (Fig. 46.8). However, its use is not always feasible because of bad weather, mechanical unreadiness, or lack of appropriate landing space. At this time, reliance must still be placed mainly on surface transportation units.

Despite the demonstrated usefulness of helicopters, financial considerations make it unlikely that any agencies other than governmental ones will operate them on a large scale in the immediate future. In municipal operations they are financially feasible only as multipurpose machines for a variety of missions.

The best way to obtain a helicopter for use as an ambulance in an emergency is through the armed forces.

Capabilities and limitations. The benefits a patient derives from use of a helicopter ambulance instead of a ground ambulance are difficult to assess, and there is no standard against which to measure these benefits. The helicopter should not be used in cases where a surface ambulance is nearby and can transport the patient as quickly as the airborne vehicle. Certainly the use of a helicopter is not indicated unless serious illness or injury is present, but it should be used when such patients are in remote or inaccessible locations, which it can reach much more quickly than a surface vehicle. Generally it should also be used in any circumstances when it can expedite the delivery of trained personnel and medical supplies to the scene.

Despite its speed and ability to fly to its destination in a straight line, a helicopter usually cannot reach the scene of a medical emergency in an urban or suburban area ahead of a ground ambulance dispatched simultaneously from a well-deployed fleet of vehicles. A helicopter often cannot operate in severe weather conditions, and night operations are dangerous in mountainous terrain or near surface obstructions. Furthermore, in highly developed areas, the presence of poles, overhead wires, tall buildings, and heavy street traffic tend to delay or preclude a helicopter landing unless a trained controller is at the scene to point out obstacles, control traffic, and guide the helicopter by means of hand signals or direct voice communication. There is, however, considerable potential for helicopter use in preference to freeways, where surface traffic congestion often can be a serious problem. In an urban or suburban area the helicopter would be the proper response vehicle in only a small percentage of the total number of emergency calls.

Helicopter ambulances would seem to have the greatest potential in rural areas, where the response time of a surface ambulance is relatively long and where the presence of open areas will permit unassisted helicopter landings and takeoffs. But rural areas are also characterized by a relatively small population base. The frequency of occurrence of medical emergencies will therefore be relatively low within the effective operation radius of a helicopter during any given time period.

Because of the infrequent demand for helicopter ambulance service in all potential oper-

ating areas, coupled with the high initial investment cost and relatively high operating costs, the helicopter is an extremely expensive ambulance. A standby helicopter ambulance program, with a helicopter parked at a medical center solely to answer emergency calls, is neither feasible nor recommended. The substantial costs can be justified, however, if the helicopter is operated as a supplement to existing ground ambulance services as well as for law enforcement operations. Its medical emergency service should be combined with other services, such as law enforcement, patrol, firefighting, or search and rescue, always taking care that the medical capabilities and priorities of the system are not sacrificed to less vital uses by other agencies.

Traveling by helicopter imposes a certain degree of vibration and discomfort on the passengers. When comparing this roughness to the vibrations encountered in riding in a surface vehicle, it is necessary to consider the varying quality of roadway smoothness and the twists and turns one may encounter on the ground. Any rough movement, vibration, or sudden jerk of a patient brings further discomfort and often compounds the seriousness of his condition. Compared to a ground ambulance, the helicopter is rated less detrimental to the patient on rural or remote missions but more detrimental on urban missions.

The availability of helicopters for response may be limited for mechanical reasons. The average mechanical "out-of-service" time has been found by the Coast Guard and Army to be approximately 25 percent, producing only 75 percent availability for one helicopter. If two machines are devoted to the mission, availability rises to 94 percent. If three are available, at least one will be able to respond 98 percent of the time. However, as more machines are assigned to the service, costs become astronomical.

Helicopter ambulance design. The type of helicopter selected for ambulance use will have a bearing on the outcome of any helicopter ambulance project. Many different types are available today. Few are suitable for ambulances; none can be considered ideal. Specific design criteria are not available, but studies have recognized certain requirements.

362

In addition to the pilot, the helicopter should be large enough to carry two litter patients, an EMT, and medical equipment and supplies inside the cabin. The equipment and supplies must be easily accessible while in flight and the cabin must have sufficient space to permit access to the patient for care (Fig. 46.9). The patient must

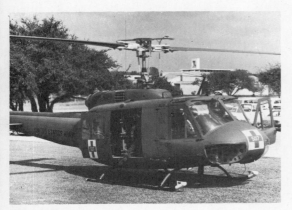

Figure 46.9

The cabin of this standard model helicopter is displayed through the open door. Sufficient space exists to transport two litter patients and render emergency care. The Star of Life emblem is shown on the side of the helicopter.

be isolated from the pilot's compartment to prevent in-flight distractions which could affect flight safety. Low cabin noise and low vibration levels are desirable for maximum patient comfort and for effective monitoring of blood pressure, cardiac function, and other body systems. Turbine power is essential to minimize dispatch time after alert. The operating area will affect performance considerations such as range, speed, and capability for flight at high altitude and by instrument.

Surplus military helicopters. Military surplus planes might appear to be the answer to high helicopter procurement costs. But this "bargain" could have expensive pitfalls, among them the Airworthiness Certificate. Before an Airworthiness Certificate can be obtained for any ex-military aircraft, the buyer—not the Federal Aviation Administration, not the Army, not the people who actually sold the airplane, but the buyer—must obtain on his own an FAA-type certificate; and the buyer must prove that

the plane is in a condition for safe operation (airworthy) before it can be flown. Many military aircraft do not conform to any existing civilian-type certificate, and some can never be made to conform, regardless of modification. The Department of Defense does not represent that surplus aircraft offered for sale are or can be certificated as airworthy. It is difficult, perhaps impossible, to assess the actual airworthiness limitations of a surplus aircraft that has undergone various modifications and replacement of parts, or possibly been subjected to maneuvers that could have overstressed the airframe.

An honest effort must be made to estimate the time and effort that may be required before a surplus helicopter can be certified and pronounced airworthy. The process might take months, even years, and the ultimate cost could exceed that of a comparable used civilian helicopter.

Certification is initiated by application to the nearest FAA-EMDO (Engineering and Manufacturing District Office). These offices are called AEDOs (Aircraft Engineering District Offices) in the FAA Western Region. It would be advisable to consult these experts prior to the purchase of any surplus military aircraft.

Helicopter equipment and personnel. Regardless of whether an ambulance serves on land, sea, or in the air, its essential equipment should be the same and in all ambulances there must be sufficient patient compartment space to allow effective use of the equipment. The air transport of certain types of patients requires special precautions to prevent life-threatening complications. For example, chest injuries with tubes in place must have one-way valves attached to the tubes in order to avoid tension pneumothorax brought on by high altitude in unpressurized aircraft. Nasogastric tubes must be open at all times during flight.

Perhaps the most important factor in aiding the critically ill or injured is timely and proper emergency care at the scene. Not only must there be a trained EMT on board the helicopter, but the pilot must be trained to the same level so he can assist in the care of patients at the emergency site.

Communications. Rapid and reliable com-

363

munication capabilities are an absolute requisite if the potentialities and advantages of helicopter ambulances are to be realized. The greater the number of functions required of the helicopter, the more versatile the radio equipment must be. Two factors are involved: first, the need to alert the operator to dispatch a helicopter and, second, the need for the personnel aboard the helicopter to communicate with the control facility, with personnel at the scene of the accident, and with the hospital during the course of the mission.

The helicopter activity should be alerted by direct landline from the Emergency Medical Services dispatching center or from a designated alternate dispatching center, such as a law enforcement agency. Once alerted and given position information, the regular air-to-ground radio equipment is available for control and relay of additional information to the helicopter. Practical experience has demonstrated that while a direct means of communication from the scene of emergency to the helicopter is desirable, it is not mandatory. Knowledge of hand signals and helicopter landing requirements by the police can often substitute for direct voice communication. Ability to consult with the hospital en route and alert it to the condition of the patient is a valuable capability provided by the air-to-ground radio equipment.

The hospital heliport. When air ambulance service is to be initiated, construction of the hospital heliport or landing area should be planned to be completed by the time the helicopter becomes available. These landing facilities are not costly and require only a clear approach and a small open area with prescribed markings. In some instances the hospital roof can be adapted for use. This heliport might be the most convenient, but the dangers are greater and the construction more costly.

The Federal Aviation Administration has prepared a booklet entitled *Heliport Design Guide*. This excellent reference should be consulted by any community planning a helicopter landing facility.

Use of military helicopters. Military Assistance to Safety and Traffic (MAST) is a program using military helicopters and medical corpsmen

to supplement a civilian Emergency Medical Service. Existing equipment and personnel from active-duty military units are involved. These military personnel work in cooperation with those providing local health care and with law enforcement officials according to a locally developed plan between the civilian and military communities. The program is sponsored by five government agencies forming the MAST Inter-agency Executive Group, with administration assigned to the MAST Inter-agency Coordination Committee. This committee is comprised of representatives from the Departments of Transportation, Defense, and Health, Education and Welfare.

Unfortunately, MAST is available to only a limited number of communities, there being twenty active programs at present. Only existing military units located at existing military bases can participate. No equipment or personnel can be relocated, nor can any new units be established solely to support the MAST program. No additional funding is provided. MAST operations use funds allocated for training, with medical assistance for actual injuries replacing training exercises with simulated injuries. Valuable service is thereby provided to the community, and MAST personnel benefit from realistic experience and motivation. While assistance under the MAST concept is not allowed to interfere with the primary military mission, immediate response from it can be expected except in unusual circumstances.

Many military bases have helicopters and medical personnel but do not have sufficient assets for a firm MAST commitment. The military has traditionally responded to requests for assistance from local communities and it is reasonable to assume that bases not formally committed to MAST will continue to respond on a case-by-case basis. In many cases such assistance can be prearranged by local agreement between civil authorities and the base commander. The scope of military assistance can best be determined on an individual case basis. Military helicopters should be requested only in urgent cases, where existing surface ambulances are unable to accomplish the task quickly or efficiently, where medical help is urgently needed and prevented from reaching the scene, and when suitable public service or commercial helicopters are not available.

The United States Coast Guard has authorized its district commanders to enter into agreements with the states for mutual cooperation and coordination of available facilities providing emergency medical services. Similar agreements might be authorized by state governors for National Guard helicopters to provide assistance in serious emergency medical situations or disasters. Search and rescue services like the Coast Guard maintain helicopters and crews that can be ready to take off in less than five minutes at all times.

Military helicopters suffer reduced readiness outside working hours. Some commands may maintain off-duty standby crews who require up to thirty minutes to return to base and be ready for service. This factor should be remembered when considering whether a military helicopter may be useful in a given situation. It must also be remembered that the military can respond only if its helicopters are not committed to other missions. Civil authorities should therefore always make arrangements for civilian surface vehicles to be dispatched also, regardless of any request for military helicopter assistance.

Maintenance of Safe Emergency Vehicles

The EMT who is an ambulance driver is responsible for the maintenance of the vehicle; it is his job to see that it is safe to use. Daily inspection by the driver should be made of the entire vehicle.

Daily inspection. The following checklist should be observed.

1. A daily inspection of the wheels, tires, brakes, battery, fluid circulation system, lights, warning equipment, and power systems should be made.

2. The best quality puncture-proof tires should be used. They must be checked daily for unusual damage or wear. Emergency tire-inflation units and spare tires must be checked daily. The inflation pressure of the tires must be checked daily.

3. All doors should be checked daily for proper opening, closing, latching, and locking.

4. The air-conditioning, heating, and ventilation systems must be checked daily. Defective water hoses and fan belts must be identified and changed before they rupture or break.

5. The communication equipment in an ambulance is vital in every emergency run. It must be checked daily.

6. The driver should never leave the vehicle with less than a full tank of fuel when he makes his inspection.

7. Inventory should be taken of emergency care supplies, oxygen, and linen. An inventory list should be permanently affixed inside each emergency vehicle.

Run inspection. After each trip, the interior of the vehicle should be cleaned and decontaminated as needed, in accordance with state and local health regulations. Blood, vomitus, and other contaminants must be scrubbed from the floors, walls, and ceiling. The exterior should be washed as needed. Broken windows and torn upholstery should be replaced or repaired without delay.

Thousand mile inspection. Complete servicing every one thousand miles should include oil and filter changes, transmission and differential check, tie rod end inspection, and a check of wheel bearing packing on the front wheels.

CHAPTER 47

Patient Handling and Extrication

GOAL I. Understand the various methods used in the movement of patients.

OBJECTIVES

A. List the methods an EMT working alone can use to move a patient.
B. Describe the standard lifts and carries.
C. Name the specialized methods of handling patients.
D. Describe the handling of sick or injured children.
E. Describe the handling of patients with communicable diseases.

GOAL II. Know how to use the various types of stretchers and litters and know which special type is best for any given injury.

OBJECTIVES

A. Identify the use of each type of stretcher.
B. Describe the use of special and improvised stretchers.

GOAL III. Understand the principles and procedures of rescue operations.

OBJECTIVES

A. Explain the necessity for EMTs to be knowledgeable in rescue operations.
B. List the types of rescue.
C. List the phases of rescue in disaster.
D. Name the areas where specialized rescue is necessary.

GOAL IV. Understand the principles and procedures of extrication.

OBJECTIVES

A. Name the elements to be considered in extrication.
B. Describe the procedures to be used for each type of extrication.

The handling of patients falls into two broad categories. There is the patient who is found in a readily accessible location and who, no matter how serious his injuries, can be moved from the home or building, the sidewalk or street in a routine manner.

Then there is the patient who must be rescued. He may be in a location of difficult access, possibly dangerous to the EMT as well as to the patient. Injuries may or may not be serious, but merely to remove this person from a precarious situation and transport him safely to receive further treatment requires that the EMT exercise special techniques of extrication.

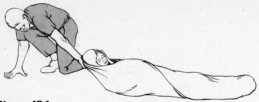

Figure 47.1

The blanket drag is a method by which one person can effectively move a patient. The blanket should be arranged to support the patient's head and neck, as shown.

Both types of patient handling are discussed in this chapter.

368

Basic Patient Handling

After completion of on-the-scene emergency care, the ill or injured patient must be moved from the original position to a stretcher or other carrying device, positioned properly, covered as necessary, and secured by strapping. The loaded stretcher must be moved to and placed aboard an ambulance, and on arrival at the hospital the patient must be transferred to the Emergency Department cart.

Except in the presence of a situation endangering the life of the EMT and the patient as well, movement of the ill and injured should be orderly, planned, and unhurried, so as not to cause further injury or aggravation of the patient's original condition.

For the most part, such movement consists of transfer of the patient from a bed, the floor, or the ground to an ambulance stretcher. It should be carried out by at least two EMTs, with bystanders used as necessary. These recruits must be **instructed in detail** as to their role before actual movement is carried out. The stretcher should be positioned as close as possible to the patient so that movement will be over the shortest distance. Such movement involves lifting, lowering, pulling, and supporting both patient and equipment. If any of these tasks is conducted improperly, discomfort and injury could result to both the patient and the EMTs.

Emergency One-Person Techniques

There are various methods that may be used by a single EMT for patient movement when prompt transfer is necessary because of a hazard to life and when no other assistance is available. For example, it might be necessary for an EMT to act alone in situations such as removing patients from hospital or nursing home fires, or from smoke-filled or contaminated areas, or from buildings in danger of collapse. It must be emphasized that these are emergency movement methods and should not be used if there is time to obtain help. The EMT must be aware that when entrance to a smoke-contaminated area is necessary and a quick-entry mask is not available, then both entrance and exit are best done by crawling, as there is less smoke at the floor level and EMT and patient breathe better air.

The EMT, however, must be familiar with quick-entry masks, and ambulances must carry them if local hazards indicate they might be needed and they are not readily available from other sources. These masks are essential for access to patients in contaminated areas.

Various one-person carries have been well-described and illustrated in many first-aid manuals and emergency care textbooks for years. For the most part, they are of only historic value as they are extremely difficult to carry out and have been replaced by some type of "drag movement" such as the blanket, clothes, or fireman's drag.

The blanket drag. The blanket drag (Fig. 47.1), when properly used, is the most effective one-person carry, as it does afford some support and protection of the patient, with the head being as close to the ground or floor as possible and the extremities in a straight line. If the patient is in bed, he must be moved to the floor before being placed on the blanket. The EMT should cradle the patient's head and shoulders in his own arms while assisting in sliding him to the floor.

The blanket is spread alongside the patient with approximately one-half gathered lengthwise into pleats. The patient's arm opposite the blanket is extended overhead, affording some cushion for the head and allowing the patient to be rolled more easily on one side. The patient is held on his side while the pleated portion of the blanket is pulled close to his back. He is then rolled onto the blanket and on over to the opposite side, with the arm positioned as described above. The pleats are then smoothed out, and the patient is rolled onto his back and wrapped snugly in the blanket with his arms at his sides. The portion of the blanket beneath his head is grasped, and he is dragged to safety. If it is necessary to move the patient down a flight of stairs, the EMT must make certain to support the head and not allow it to bump on the steps.

The clothes drag. A patient may be dragged by his clothing if no blanket is available (Fig. 47.2). The clothes should be grasped behind the patient's neck, being careful not to pull the shirt, blouse, or coat so tight around the neck as to cause an airway obstruction. The patient's head should be supported by the forearm of the EMT and kept as close to the floor or ground as possible. If the patient must be moved down a flight of stairs, the shoulders and head should be cradled in the arms of the EMT, with the head being kept as close as possible to the stairs.

The fireman's drag. The fireman's drag, while somewhat awkward, is another method of moving a patient in an emergency (Fig. 47.3). The patient must be supine with wrists tied together by some suitable piece of material, such as a tie, piece of rope, or a soft belt. The EMT kneels, straddling the patient, places the patient's tied wrists over his own neck, and, by raising the upper part of his body, lifts the patient's shoulders clear of the floor. He then crawls on hands and knees, dragging the patient with him. The disadvantage of this drag is that the patient's head is unsupported and unprotected.

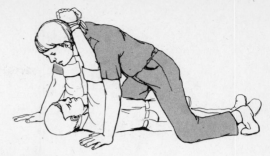

Figure 47.3

The fireman's drag has the disadvantage of providing no support for the patient's head and neck, but if no other method is available, it does enable one person alone to move a patient.

369

Regular Lifts and Carries

Regular lifts and carries are also well-described and illustrated in many first-aid manuals. Movement of a patient, regardless of the number of persons involved in the action, is difficult at best and should not be used over a greater distance than is absolutely essential.

Lifting a patient onto a stretcher should be done by at least two persons (Fig. 47.4). Locking hands under the patient is an excellent way for them to increase their lifting power, maintain effective control of the patient, and be able to maneuver properly. If this method is used, it must first be made certain that the patient does not have an injury of the spine in either the neck or back. A towel or triangular bandage may be used to extend the reach of two attendants beneath the patient's body while still maintaining the same arm strength.

The three-man lift and carry, is a standard technique that has been used for many years. However, even when additional help is available, this carry does not offer adequate neck and back support. Two, three, or four persons have difficulty picking up a patient in their arms and moving simultaneously. In picking up the prone patient, three-point suspension, which is taught in most classes, is an efficient method (Fig. 47.5). There is minimal body movement. The patient is lifted only high enough to put him on the carrying device. Bystanders assisting the EMTs must be **instructed in detail** before the lift is attempted.

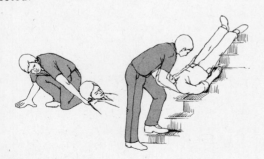

Figure 47.2

The clothing drag enables one person to move a patient when a blanket is not available. Care must be taken to support the patient's head and neck at all times.

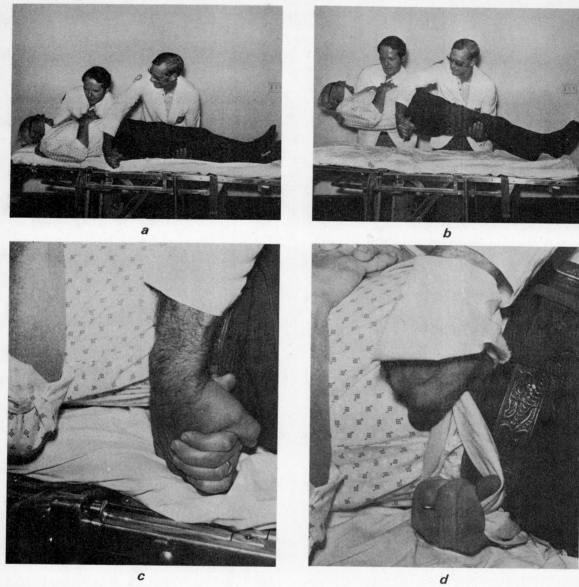

370

a

b

c

d

Figure 47.4 *a–d*

In a two-man pick-up, the EMTs use the locked-hands method (*a–c*) to pick up a routine patient—that is, a patient not seriously ill or injured. If it is necessary to extend their reach, *d*, a towel or triangular bandage may be tied into a loop and used. The technique for the lift is the same and no control or lifting force is lost because of the extension.

Special Transportation Lifts and Carries

All EMTs are on occasion involved in performing special transportation techniques with many variations too numerous to describe here.

In situations in which one cannot use the usual method of sliding a long spineboard beneath the patient along the long axis of the body

(discussed later in this chapter), the straddle load (Fig. 47.6) may be used.

The four-man log-roll, or back-injury roll, is an excellent method of positioning a patient on the long spineboard. Many conditions warrant transporting the patient in the position in which he is found, whether prone or on his side. If it is considered best to position him face-up, the illustrated instructions in Figure 47.7 should be fol-

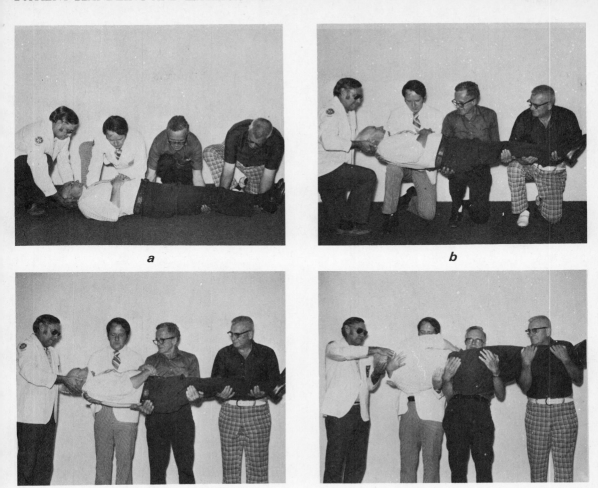

a

b

c

d

Figure 47.5 a–d

In a four-man pick-up, the EMTs are situated at the critical areas of the patient, the head and chest, while the two recruited bystanders are at the buttocks and legs. The bystanders must be instructed in detail as to their actions before the lift is started. *a*, One EMT supports the patient's head. *b*, The patient is then lifted from the floor to the knees of those lifting; *c*, then to their waists, and is carried in that position. *d*, If close quarters or other circumstances demand, the patient may be rolled as a unit against the crew for support.

lowed. As in other lifts and carries, the bystanders assisting the two EMTs must be **instructed in detail** as to their role.

All EMTs will at some time have to utilize a "stair chair." This may be an ordinary household straightback chair or a fold-up litter which is capable of being converted into a chair. The method of loading the stair chair illustrated in Figure 47.8 is used when the patient is too large to be picked up and put into the chair. Note that the patient's legs are elevated and the chairback is placed beneath the buttocks. The patient is then dragged and slid very carefully onto the seat of the chair and the chair is picked up on either side or from the front and back by the two EMTs and raised to a normal seated position. This method of carry can be used with a bed patient. It is very useful in carrying a patient down winding stairs.

Types of Stretchers and Their Uses

Many types of stretchers are available, all with the same basic principles (Fig. 47.9). The familiar standard ambulance cot has wheels and is either of a fixed height or can be raised or

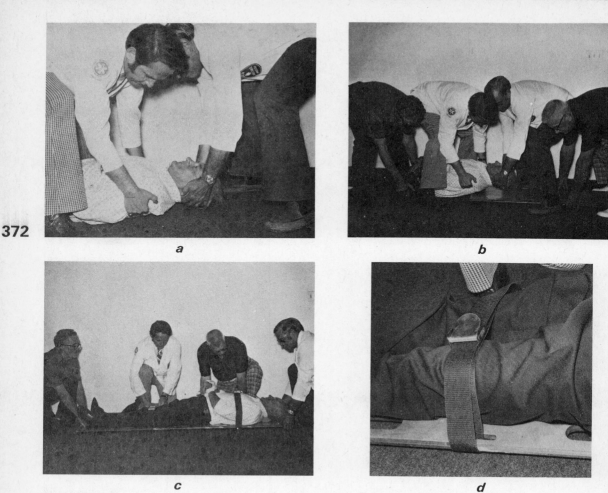

Figure 47.6 a—d

   When it is possible to work on either side of the patient, the straddle slide is useful in maneuvering him onto the long spineboard. In *a*, an EMT with his feet wide apart gently elevates the patient's head while the second EMT straddles the patient and lifts the shoulders. In *b*, one bystander slides the long spineboard between the feet of the EMT and under the patient. The second bystander lifts the patient's hips. In *c*, the patient is secured to the board with straps. In *d*, the strap has been passed through one of the handholds, then across the patient to another handhold, doubled on itself and buckled. This method eliminates the lifting of the board in applying the straps.

lowered. There are handles to assist in rolling, side bars to stabilize the patient, and a comfortable mattress. Spineboards may be carried beneath the mattress to be immediately available for extrication or to provide a firm surface for cardiac compression when placed between the patient and the mattress.

   The split frame or scoop-type stretcher (Robinson, Sarole, or Greene) is efficient, but both sides of the patient must be accessible to make use of it, and it cannot be slid under the patient in the long axis of the body, as can the long spineboard. These scoop stretchers are narrow,

well-constructed, have excellent supportive features, and are compact for storage. In use they are divided longitudinally into halves; the two halves are slid under the patient from each side, the brackets or locking knobs are closed, and the stretcher is loaded with the patient and is ready to be picked up. Pinching of the patient or catching clothing between the stretcher halves is prevented if the patient is gently lifted by the clothes as the stretcher is closed. Once the patient has the stretcher beneath him and has been secured by straps, he may be picked up in the same position in which he was found and even moved

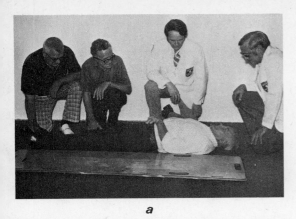

a

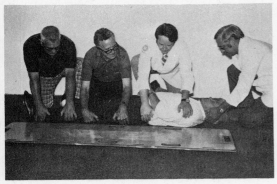

b

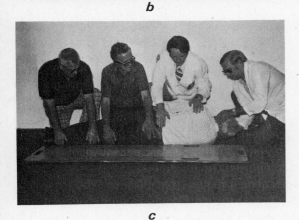

c

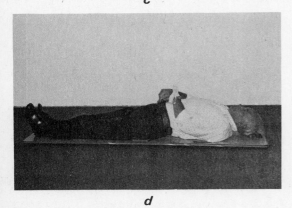

d

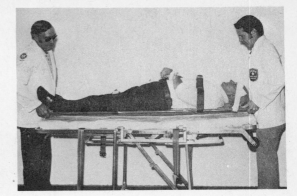

e

Figure 47.7 *a—e*   **373**

The four-man log-roll lift is used for suspected back injuries. In *a*, *b*, and *c*, the patient is rolled onto his side like a log (that is, as a solid unit). The EMTs are at the head and shoulders while the recruited bystanders are at the pelvis and legs. In *d*, the patient has been gently rolled onto the spineboard. In *e*, straps have been used to secure the patient to the board so he can be transported to the stretcher.

down narrow staircases without fear of slipping when the stretcher is tipped as much as ten to fifteen degrees.

There are a number of Emergency Department carts on the market today with a flat, removable top. Some ambulance services equip their ambulances with a spare top from such carts and carry it on the wheeled litter of the ambulance (Fig. 47.10). The patient is placed on this top and at the hospital there is merely an exchange of the tops of the Emergency Department carts. The patient remains on the cart top regardless of where he may be taken in the hospital, even to the X-ray room or operating room, until he is finally placed in a bed.

For difficult terrain or removal from heights or over debris, probably no litter can replace the conventional Stokes basket that has been used for many years by the military services, especially by the Navy and the Coast Guard. Until recently the Stokes basket consisted of a metal frame with chicken wire lining, constructed with a divider which separated the legs. It has now been redesigned as an oblong plastic shell with no leg divider (Fig. 47.11).

One of the difficulties in using the basket stretcher is removing the patient from the basket on delivery to the Emergency Department, as

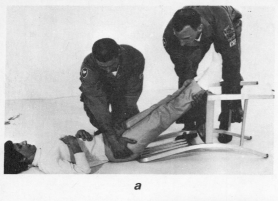

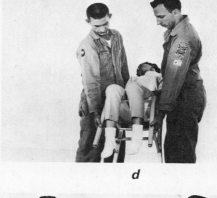

a

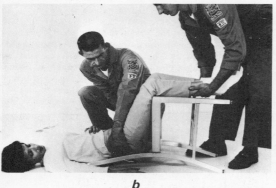

b

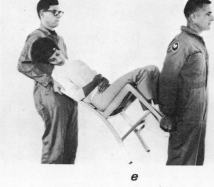

d

e

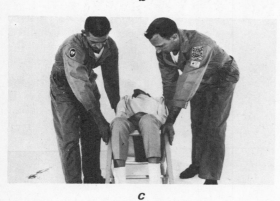

c

Figure 47.8 *a–e*

In the chair lift, the chair is slid under the buttocks of the patient until (*a–b*) he is in a seated position in it although still lying on the floor. Straps may be used to secure the patient to the chair, which is then picked up (*c*) and carried, with the patient seated in it. Two methods of carrying the chair are shown in *d* and *e*.

the patient at times becomes wedged in place. This problem can be overcome by lining the basket with a blanket. The patient is then removed by grasping the rolled-up blanket on either side and lifting.

The folding-type stretcher is commonly carried in ambulances today. It is an aluminum frame with fold-down wheels and legs. This type of stretcher usually rests fairly close to the ground and has a plastic, canvas, or rubber insert between the aluminum rails; it is used as a

second stretcher if more than one litter patient must be transported in the ambulance.

Many years ago the military services determined that their equipment must be standardized, and they produced a folding type stretcher with a D-ring leg that is universally known as the army stretcher. Use of these is prevalent across the country, and they are available by the thousands in civil defense and fire station stockpiles and in major hospitals. This stretcher is excellent in disaster areas as it can be suspended between wooden horses or tables and utilized as an emergency work table. Other advantages are numerous. Many specialized devices have been developed that can be attached to it for holding intravenous sets and traction splints.

Spineboards. Spineboards are a necessary part of ambulance equipment. The short board measures 18 inches wide by 32 inches long. The long board is 18 inches wide by 72 inches long, with two runners on the undersurface which are essential to clear the handholes for easy grasping and to slide the board under the patient. Each board is equipped with two straps, 2 inches by 9 feet, which fasten by friction buckles. While some boards are now being made from fiberglass, exterior plywood in 1/2-inch thickness for the short board and 3/4-inch thickness for the long board is easily worked and makes reasonably priced and efficient units.

The short board is used mostly for extrication of sitting patients, occasionally for a prone patient who is in an awkward position. The long board is an excellent litter for any patient as well as being an efficient extrication device.

Details of construction of both boards are shown in Figure 47.12. In Figure 47.13 the necessary equipment for fixation of the patient's head to the short board is shown. An alternative method of construction and fixation when Velcro fasteners are not used is shown in Figure 47.14.

Improvised stretchers. Various other types of stretchers will be mentioned briefly. A stretcher can be made of two wooden poles and a blanket that will fold around the patient and cradle him. This stretcher is constructed so that each pole may be slid out from under the patient after arrival at the hospital.

It is possible to form a stretcher using only a 40- or 50-foot length of rope. The rope is laid on the ground in a series of tight folds; the patient is then placed on the flat surface formed by the folds. With sufficient help, the looped ends are picked up and the patient is moved (Fig. 47.15). Although a length of rope may not always be available at the scene of an accident, a fire truck is often present, and with every fifty feet of 1½-inch fire hose, a stretcher can be constructed.

On difficult terrain a patient can be handled

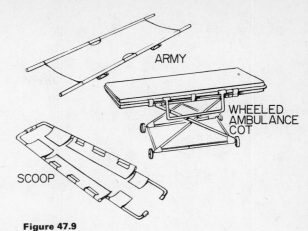

Figure 47.9

Various types of stretchers and cots are shown.

easily with this type of device. Though it is primarily designed for an emergency, it will work satisfactorily in any situation where there are not sufficient stretchers to move patients but where there are ropes or fire hoses.

Handling of Patients with Communicable Diseases

For emphasis, and to dispel fears due to lack of knowledge, some points in handling patients with communicable diseases (Chapter 35) will be repeated here.

When it is known in advance that the patient has a communicable disease, preventive measures can to a great extent protect both the EMT and the ambulance from contamination. Precautions that can be taken include the following:

1. Wear clean coveralls set aside for this purpose.
2. Wear a surgical mask.
3. Remove unnecessary equipment from the ambulance.
4. Use disposable equipment whenever possible (for example, gloves and bed linen).

On termination of the run the coveralls should be turned in for decontamination and the ambulance cleaned and disinfected. The EMT should shower immediately.

When it is not known in advance that the patient has a communicable disease, precautionary

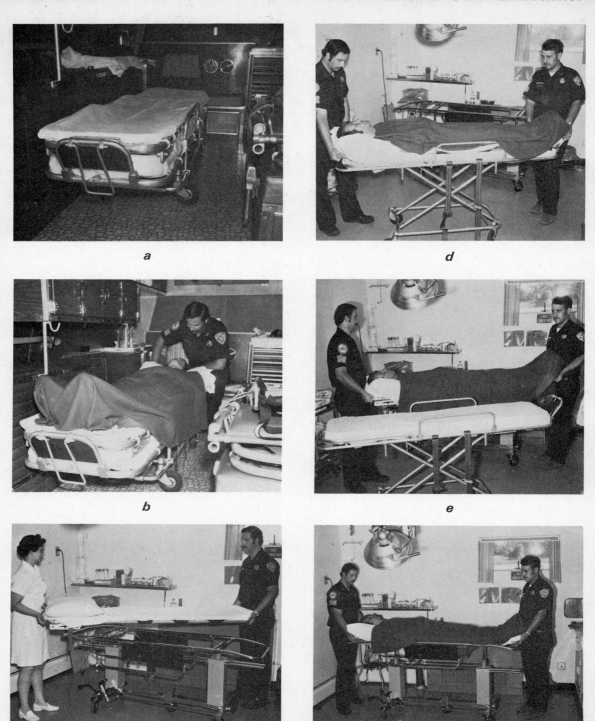

a

b

c

d

e

f

Figure 47.10 *a–f*

    A spare removable top from an Emergency Department cart can be carried on, *a*, the wheeled ambulance stretcher. It does not interfere, *b*, with the positioning of the patient. In the Emergency Department, *c–f*, the tops are interchanged. This method allows movement of the patient through the Emergency Department to any area of the hospital without removing him from the stretcher until he is put into his bed.

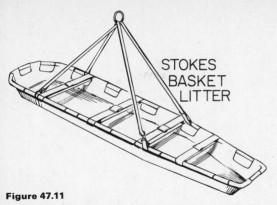

Figure 47.11

A redesigned basket stretcher without the leg divider is shown. It is now made of bright-colored plastic material instead of a metal frame covered with wire mesh.

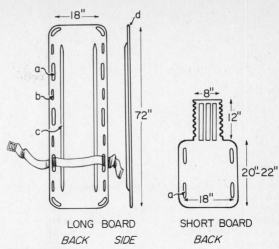

LONG BOARD   SHORT BOARD
BACK   SIDE   BACK

Figure 47.12

These drawings show the details of both long and short spineboards. They are made of exterior plywood, 3/4 inch thick for the long board and 1/2 inch thick for the short board. Finished on both sides, the plywood is sanded, shellacked or varnished, then waxed so the board will slide easily under or behind the patient. In the drawings, *a* marks the handholds, *b* the strap holes, and *c* the runners, which elevate enough that EMTs may slip their fingers under them into the handholds and can pass straps into the strap holes without lifting the board.

The runners are 3/4×3/4 inches with tapered ends and should extend well toward the ends of the board, to prevent tipping should the need for cardiac compression arise. Both ends, *d*, of the long board and the bottom end of the short board are blunt-tapered so the board will slide easily under or behind a patient.

The short board is equipped with a headpiece with notched edges. The notches hold bandages firmly if it is necessary to use this method of stabilizing a patient's head when securing it to the board, as in Figure 47.14. Usually Velcro strips are fastened to the back of the headpiece. Velcro is a fastener material consisting of two strips of nylon tape, one covered with tiny hooks, the other with tiny loops. When the surfaces are pressed together they lock securely, but may be opened easily by peeling apart.

measures against infection can still be taken after exposure.

1. EMTs must be notified and immunized as necessary.
2. The ambulance, equipment, and supplies must be checked, cleaned, and decontaminated.

Handling of Children

In situations in which children are involved, fear of the unknown and inability to communicate are the greatest causes of failure in effective care. Gentle handling, a constant flow of soothing words, and soft speech will often simplify these problems. Equipment being used should be explained simply and promptly. Bleeding areas should be covered quickly as the sight of blood can cause panic in children, as it does in some adults.

Rescue and Extrication

Rescue, by definition, means to free from danger of death or destruction by prompt or vigorous action. One aspect of rescue is extrication, which here means a method by which patients are freed either by means of force or ingenuity from that which binds or holds back.

The problems of rescue may range from simply opening a car door to treat and remove an injured patient to a complex situation with multiple patients in a coal mine disaster or a train wreck. In between, there are many emergency situations requiring rescue and extrication, such as drownings, fires, cave-ins, and mountain skiing or snowmobile accidents. Because of the specialized skills and equipment needed for most complex rescue and extrication work, the EMT cannot be expected to become an expert in every aspect of rescue, nor will the total field be covered in depth in this chapter. The perfect rescue worker would have the skills of a mountain climber, engineer, deep sea diver, and expert skier all in one person.

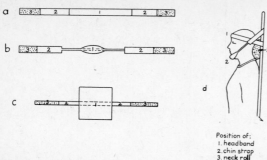

Position of:
1. head band
2. chin strap
3. neck roll

Figure 47.13 *a–d*

Equipment is shown for the headpiece on a short spineboard.

a. The head band is 42 inches long and consists of (1) a center padded section, (2) two sections of thin webbing 2 inches wide, and (3) two end strips of Velcro fastener.

b. The chin strap measures 42 inches long and consists of (1) a regulation football chin strap, (2) two sections of thin webbing 2 inches wide, and (3) two end strips of Velcro fastener.

c. A neck roll measures 32 inches long and consists of (1) a foam rubber roll 8 inches wide and 4 inches in diameter, covered first with plastic and then with stockinette, both of which are disposable and easily replaceable, (2) two strips of thin webbing 1 inch wide, and (3) two end strips of Velcro fastener.

The neck roll is rarely used. It is designed to support the head in the rare fracture-dislocation of the cervical spine, in which the head is fixed in a tilted and flexed position and any attempt to straighten it results in resistance to movement and increased pain.

d. All this equipment is shown in use, securing a head to the spineboard, with the neck supported by a neck roll.

Knowledge of the type and availability of specialized rescue squads in any given area is a function of the dispatch center. Just as the EMT

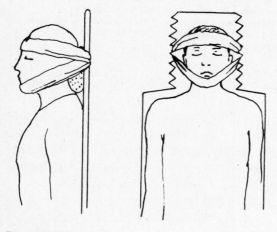

Figure 47.14

If Velcro straps are not available, the head can be stabilized by using a soft roller bandage, which is held in place by the notches on the spineboard.

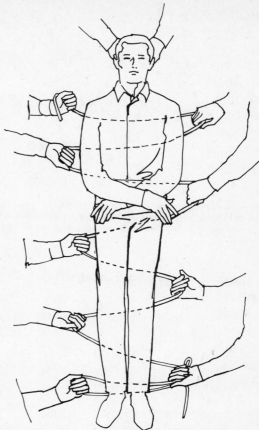

Figure 47.15

An emergency stretcher can be made from 3/4-inch rope or fire hose of 1-1/2 inches diameter. This improvised stretcher can be very useful in lifting heavy patients when there is no other provision for carrying them. Several persons are required to lift and carry it, however, as each loop that is formed must be held.

must have knowledge and skills in certain aspects of rescue and the ambulance must carry certain tools for this purpose, the personnel of specialized rescue squads should have training in emergency care and their vehicles should carry the special equipment necessary to provide such care. Various types of specialized rescue are discussed at the end of this chapter.

Classification of Rescue

Rescue is classified as light (basic), medium, and heavy.

Light rescue is the easiest to carry out and generally can be handled with a minimum of equipment. It involves movement of injured pa-

378

tients from uncomplicated car crashes, from upper floors of buildings by ladder slide and rope lowers, or from lower floors by slide drags and passes.

Medium rescue involves the use of more specialized tools and equipment, such as would normally be found on the rescue truck of a fire department. Medium rescue implies the use of rigging, A-frames, and tripods for casualty handling, as well as the sliding of people from the second and third floors of buildings.

Heavy rescue includes complicated rigging, casualty handling under very difficult conditions, breeching of walls, dis-impaction of vehicles, and all types of rescue normally involved where buildings have been damaged.

Rescue by fire department rescue squads usually falls into the heavy category and the fire department often receives the emergency calls. Though firemen may not have had some of the specialty training needed in many instances, they are skilled at improvising with special techniques that lead to dramatic rescues.

Although the EMT will, with experience, learn much about more complicated extrication techniques, only light rescue will be discussed in this volume.

Light Rescue and Equipment

Light (basic) rescue tools (listed in Chapter 46) must be standard equipment in every ambulance whether it is in rural, suburban, or urban service, and every EMT must be trained in their use. If a rescue vehicle accompanies an ambulance on every call, rescue tools need not be carried in the ambulance. This deviation is the only one permissible to the requirement that every ambulance carry required rescue equipment. The element of time is so critical in life-threatening situations that waiting for tools and equipment cannot be tolerated. Lives that could be saved will be lost if there are such delays.

One of the most frequent situations an EMT will face in extrication will involve entrapped persons following automobile crashes. There are certain considerations in extrication pertinent to all situations. These are:

1. Evaluation of the situation ("size up")
2. Security at the accident scene
3. Access to patients
4. Lifesaving emergency care
5. Disentanglement of patients
6. Preparation of patients for removal
7. Removal of patients

Evaluation of the situation (size-up). Size-up is a term used for years by firefighters. It means simply gathering facts rapidly and analyzing the problem or problems of the incident at hand. It forms a basis for decisions on the extrication process and how it should be carried out. Size-up should start before the scene is reached and should be continuous throughout the extrication process. The dispatcher must obtain all available information about possible problems when he is notified of the incident and should pass this material on to the EMTs at the time of dispatch. He must continue to obtain pertinent information and transmit it during the ambulance run. For example, the problem may be an airplane crash not accessible by road, or someone marooned on a cliff, the descent of which will require special techniques. Or it may be simply an automobile crash.

The time of the incident is important. An accident at school while school is in session may involve more patients, as can one in an apartment building or hotel during the night.

On every ambulance run there must be a leader, usually the senior. This EMT must be able to "keep his cool," to persevere if things do not go exactly as planned, and to have the courage of his convictions as to procedures. But most of all he must have common sense, as extrication is mostly common sense.

On arrival of the ambulance at the scene, this EMT leaves the ambulance with a "jump kit" and continues size-up as he begins work. There can be no specific rules of procedure, as almost every incident is different, but there should be a plan of operation, which should proceed in stages so that nothing is overlooked. A few of the multiple and sometimes conflicting factors the EMT must anticipate and evaluate are listed here.

Is the patient located in a building with stairs

379

which will require a special chair-type stretcher, or is there an elevator?

Is there fire? The presence of fire complicates the extrication process and special units may be required.

The status of vehicles following a crash is important, as the patients' positions and the stability of the vehicles will be involved. Are the vehicles on their wheels, on their sides, or upside down? Unstable vehicles must be secured before any attempt at entry is made. Are patients beneath the vehicles or are they hanging by seatbelts in an upside-down vehicle? Are objects protruding into the vehicle that must be removed? Is equipment necessary for the extrication process available from the ambulance or will special units be required?

Hazards must be looked for and a plan for their control initiated. There may be spilled fuel, electrical wires down, or radiation products present. Radioactive products are being transported more frequently every day. The EMT should recognize and look for the universal radioactive product symbol which these transport vehicles must display (Fig. 42.4).

Downed power lines are a potential danger to both the patient and EMTs alike. The utility company must be notified immediately. Only in extreme circumstances should the EMT attempt to cope with this problem. Unless hot sticks and lineman's gloves and boots, which are sent at regular intervals to utility company laboratories for inspection, are available, and unless the EMTs have been fully instructed in their use, no attempt should be made to cope with power lines before arrival of utility company personnel.

Spilled fuel must be washed away before any power equipment is used and onlookers must be kept away due to the danger of fire from smokers.

The general rule that no patient should be moved before emergency medical care is completed can be disregarded if life and well-being are endangered by circumstances of entrapment. Such patients should be moved out of danger as rapidly as possible without regard for injuries.

Security at the accident scene. The EMT who serves as driver should park the ambulance in a safe place at sufficient distance from the scene to avoid the danger of a second accident. He puts out warning devices if police or other specialized units have not done so. Flares formerly used have been replaced by reflecting or flashing devices because fires have been caused when flares ignited seeping gasoline. The EMT activates the warning lights of the ambulance and enlists the help, if needed, of onlookers for traffic and crowd control. Such persons must be chosen carefully and given explicit instructions about the duties they are to perform. For example, a specific directive could be: "Go down the road a hundred paces and divert traffic."

Gaining access to patients. Gaining access to patients after automobile crashes usually presents no problem. In the great majority of cases the patients have either been ejected at the time of the crash, have removed themselves or been removed by uninjured passengers or by well-motivated but untrained passersby. Such actions can be the source of added injury to the patient and must be curtailed. All EMTs should be active in their own communities in making sure the general public becomes knowledgeable in first aid so that people will know what to do and, more important, what **not** to do to help the sick or injured.

Gaining access to the patient depends on the location and position of the automobile, damage to the vehicle, and the position of the people in it. Access may be as simple as opening the door or as difficult as cutting open an automobile in the dead of night at the bottom of a wooded ravine. Access can involve forcing open doors, cutting off the roof, jacking-up cars, or pulling them apart (Fig. 47.16). Means of access chosen must take into account the patients' injuries.

Lifesaving emergency care. All patients involved must be evaluated. The EMT should make an orderly survey and follow a plan like the one detailed in Figure 4.4. This survey (triage) should not be interrupted except for emergency care of an immediate life-threatening problem, such as:

1. Establish and maintain an airway in the patient
2. Give the patient artificial ventilation

380

3. Control accessible bleeding
4. Give cardiopulmonary resuscitation

In connection with cardiopulmonary resuscitation (CPR), the EMT should remember that the patient must be lying supine on a flat, sturdy surface for cardiopulmonary resuscitation to be effective. The long or short spineboard should be placed beneath or behind such patients and CPR begun as the patient is removed from the vehicle. It is not effective when performed with the patient in a sitting position or on the soft seat of an automobile.

Special problems. Access, disentanglement, and removal from automobiles present special problems which require special instruction. Control of life-threatening problems must be continued and the patient's status re-evaluated continuously.

While major points will be presented here in detail with pictorial examples, EMTs should avail themselves of the special instructional courses in extrication. For example, the Department of Transportation offers an EMT Crash-Victim Extrication Training Course, from which one can utilize either segments or the entire training course.

Methods of gaining access and disentangling automobile parts and debris from around the patient require a great deal of common sense and ingenuity in the use of available methods and tools. While no two automobile crashes are exactly alike, similarities do exist.

Lighting is of utmost importance. It is impossible to work effectively in the dark or with inadequate lighting where injured patients are in serious danger. Besides stand-up flashlights, each ambulance must have floodlights capable of providing light at some distance from the ambulance.

During the gaining of access and disentanglement, great care must be exercised, for at this time the tools are closest to the patient. Heat, noise, and force should be kept to the necessary minimum. Possible injuries the patient may have sustained should be taken into account to avoid making his condition worse. After access is gained and while disentanglement proceeds, additional emergency care should be provided as

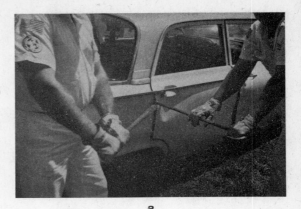

a

381

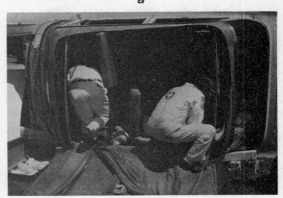

b

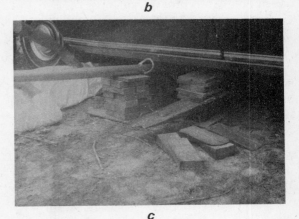

c

Figure 47.16 *a–c*

Access to entrapped patients may involve, *a*, forcing open doors; *b*, cutting off the car roof; *c*, jacking up the car.

other body areas become accessible for treatment.

A knowledge of mechanics and familiarity with the available tools will facilitate access and disentanglement procedures. Prying, either manually or with power equipment, is the method most frequently used on wrecked cars.

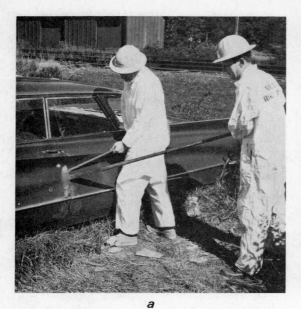

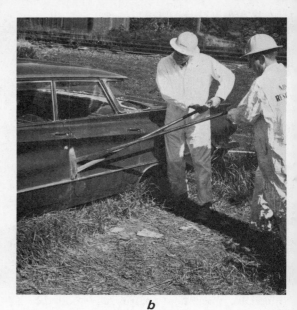

a   *b*

Figure 47.17 *a–b*

   a, A wrecking bar with a thin edge can be used to assist in positioning a larger bar. If a wrecking bar is not available, the larger bar may be driven between the door edge and the jam. *b*, Once an opening is gained, two large bars will give the necessary leverage to spring the door.

Wrecking bars and crowbars will spread metal, open doors, and provide some type of opening into the car (Fig. 47.17).

   Just as it is important to protect the patient from additional injury during the extrication process, the EMTs must protect themselves from injury. The use of safety goggles, hard hats, and work gloves is mandatory.

   When manual force is not sufficient, the hydraulic-powered unit with a spreader attach-ment is used. An opening usually must be made, or one already present enlarged, to accommo-date the jaws of the spreader (Fig. 47.18). After a jammed door has been opened, two EMTs should be able to rotate it completely out of the way by breaking the door check and, at times, the hinges (Fig. 47.19).

   The metal safety lock on the newer cars pre-vents the use of the usual methods in opening doors. An opening is made at the level of the

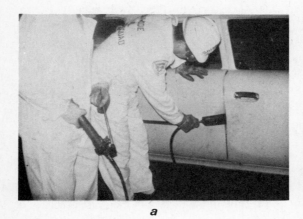

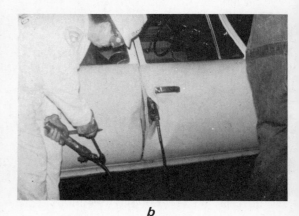

a   *b*

Figure 47.18 *a–b*

   a, The spreader attachment of a hydraulic unit is inserted between door and jamb. *b*, The door lock is snapped or exposed for cutting.

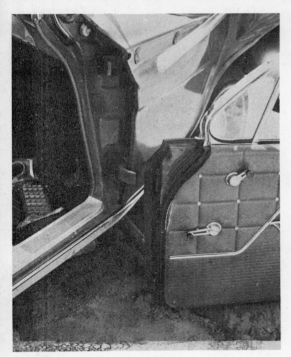

Figure 47.19

As a rule, a car door may be pushed to the full width of its opening. The door in the car pictured above was not broken in the accident; two EMTs broke the lock with bars and snapped the hinges by pushing the door against the jamb to gain access to an injured patient in the front seat. The patient was then easily removed.

tempered bolt by using a spreader to bring the bolt into view and it is then cut off, using the heavy duty air chisel or a large cold chisel and hammer (Fig. 47.20). Another method used by automobile body mechanics is to cut a half-circle around the door handle and turn back the result-

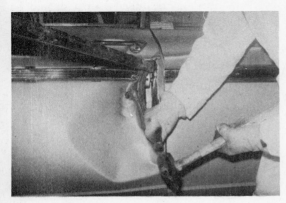

Figure 47.20

The safety lock in newer model cars prevents prying the door open. The bolt is first exposed and then cut off with an air chisel or heavy cold chisel and hammer.

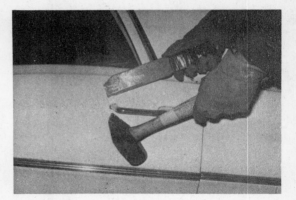

a

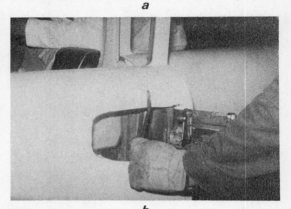

Figure 47.21 *a–b*   *b*

a, A homemade tool made from the spring leaf of an automobile may be used to cut open the door panel at the handle. *b*, This will expose the push rod that will trip the lock, allowing the door to be opened.

ing flap of steel, thus gaining access to the lock. The doorjamb is then struck a heavy blow with a hammer at the lock, which relieves the tension on the bolt and allows the door to be opened (Fig. 47.21).

Release of entrapped patients often involves lifting or pulling the car. At other times, parts of the car **must** be cut away. Needless to say, a knowledge of exactly how to cut away a car is important to avoid injury to an entrapped patient. If such a procedure must be used, the patient should be covered with an asbestos blanket for protection, and the EMT using the cutting tools should be protected with safety goggles and gloves.

If a car is on its side, access through a door or window will allow survey of the patients and necessary lifesaving care, but removing patients through such openings, although possible, is difficult. The top of the automobile may be

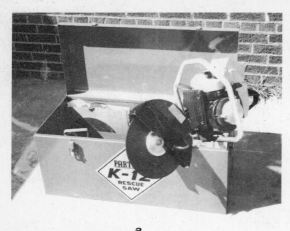

a

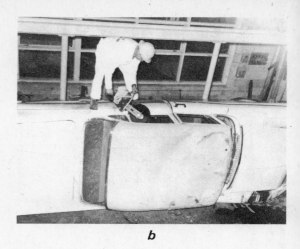

b

384

c

Figure 47.22 *a–c*

a, A gasoline-powered saw with an assortment of blades will cut through metal, concrete, wood, and glass. A disadvantage is the production of sparks, a distinct hazard when gasoline has been spilled. Hosing down the area before operating the saw, or running the blade under a stream of water, will eliminate this hazard. The EMT operating the saw must wear safety goggles. *b*, With the power saw, the top of a car may be turned back in minutes. Cuts are made through the posts instead of the top itself. This is a faster procedure, creates less sparks, and gives more room to attend to the patient inside. *c*, The width of opening possible is shown here. Patients still in the car were treated and covered with an asbestos blanket before the cutting began.

turned down for removal of patients by cutting through the doorposts or the top itself. Doorposts may be cut through by using one of a number of tools: a hacksaw with carbide wire blades (slow), a gas-powered circular saw (dangerous at times if gasoline has been spilled), or a heavy duty, air-powered chisel (Fig. 47.22).

The roof itself may be opened with one horizontal and two vertical cuts. Here again, a number of tools are available to accomplish this end. A simple tool which requires little storage space is a spring-leaf chisel made by grinding one edge of a spring-leaf flat. It is used with a fiber or metal mallet (Fig. 47.23). A pneumatic chisel will do the job more quickly (Fig. 47.24).

Gaining access by pulling part of the car away is accomplished by a heavy duty "come-a-long," which has recently been added to the essential equipment list for ambulances. To free entrapped patients, cars may be pulled from over patients, doors may be pulled open, cars may be pulled apart, and seats may be pulled away (Fig. 47.25).

Disentanglement of the patient. The importance of care in disentanglement of the patient from anything restraining him inside the automobile must be emphasized, even though the primary concern is removal of the patient from the vehicle. Removing or disentangling the vehicle from the patient should be considered if

$\ggg\rightarrow$

Figure 47.24 *a–d*

a, A pneumatic chisel may be powered by a Scott air pack, which furnishes enough air to remove the roof of a car. *b*, One horizontal and two vertical cuts are made and the top is turned down, exposing the crossbars and liner. *c*, The crossbars are cut away. *d*, Removal of the bars and liner gains access to patients inside the car.

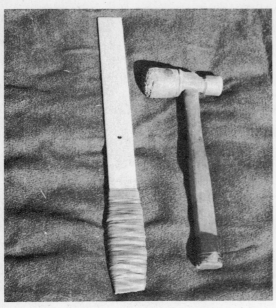

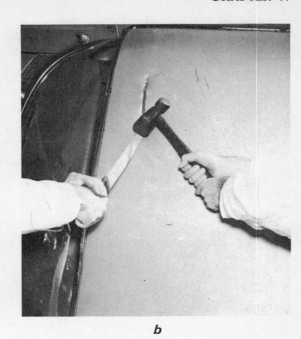

a   b

Figure 47.23 a–b

a, A simple but effective cutting tool is made from a leaf of a car spring. One edge and the end are ground flat to produce a cutting surface and a handle is formed by wrapping the other end with tape. It is used with heavy mallet. *b*, The flat-ground edge peels away a strip of metal and does not bind. This method is not as fast as other methods but it produces no sparks.

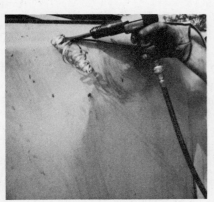

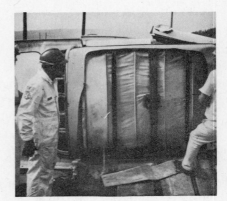

a   b

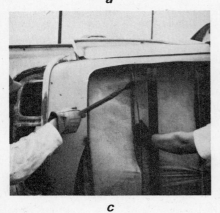

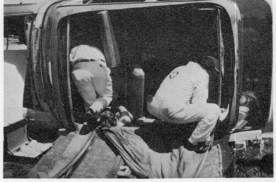

c   d

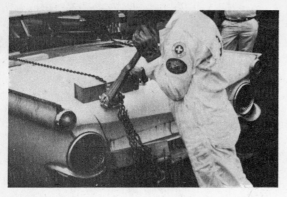

Figure 47.25

A heavy-duty hand-powered winch (a "come-a-long") may be used to pull open doors, pull back seats, or to pull steering wheels away from patients.

doing so is more likely to prevent further injury.

Preparing and "packaging" the patient. Preparation for removal of a patient entails immobilizing all fractures, dressing all wounds, and splinting possible neck injuries, in addition to maintaining continued control of life-threatening problems. Use of standard splints in confined areas is difficult and at times impossible, but simple fixation of upper extremities to the patient's trunk and of lower extremities to each other will suffice until moving the patient enables one to provide adequate splinting of fractures.

Packaging the patient for movement as a unit is best accomplished by means of spineboards (Fig. 47.26). Such packaging converts difficult situations into easy ones. The boards are essential in moving patients with spine injuries and are very helpful in other cases as well.

The short spineboard is used most frequently for stabilization of the sitting patient. The patient's head is supported and the neck immobilized by means of a collar; then the short spineboard is positioned behind the patient (Fig. 47.27). The patient's head is fastened in place using the head band and chin strap with Velcro fasteners or a 6-inch soft roller self-adhering bandage about the forehead if the patient's injuries prevent the use of the conventional straps (Fig. 47.28). If necessary, adhesive strips may be placed across the forehead and upper lip. The patient is secured to the body portion of the board by two 9-foot straps applied across the chest and around the thighs so that the weight of

the body is supported and does not pull down against the fastenings on the head and chin. The patient may then be lifted out with little risk.

If the patient is too large to be handled by two EMTs, he may be removed by means of the long board. It is positioned at right angles to the sitting patient and the patient is turned and slid onto the board (Fig. 47.29). The varnished, hard, polished surface of the board makes the sliding action possible. Once the patient is on the board, the long straps are used for firm fixation so that he can be moved as necessary.

Vertical movement of a patient is no problem when he is secured to the long board (Fig. 47.30). If the patient's injuries demand it, positioning on the side can be easily accomplished with either the long or short board (Fig. 47.31).

So-called scoop stretchers, such as the Sarole, Robinson or Green (Fig. 47.32) function in a similar manner, but all have the disadvantage that they must be applied from both sides of the patient. He cannot be slid onto a scoop stretcher nor may the stretcher be slid beneath the patient from his head or feet, as is possible with the long spineboard.

Traction to drag patients out of entrapment may be accomplished by means of a special rope sling consisting of a 6-foot loop of 1-inch Manila rope with a metal sliding connector, or by using one of the long straps from the spineboard (Fig. 47.33).

Ingenuity, common sense, and mechanical knowledge will solve most extrication problems. Part of the training of the EMT must consist of practice on wrecked cars from junk yards.

The basic principles, skills, and tools used in extrication from automobiles may be used in almost any situation involving entrapment. Simple rescue problems will be encountered, such as removing light debris, freeing a child's foot caught in a tree, or removing patients from minor cave-ins and collapses. A good working knowledge of knot tying, stretcher lashing, basic ladder rescues, and quick-entry masks is essential.

In addition to knot tying, a knowledge of the stretcher lash is useful in situations where the patient must be hoisted or lowered and where specialized equipment, such as a Stokes litter or

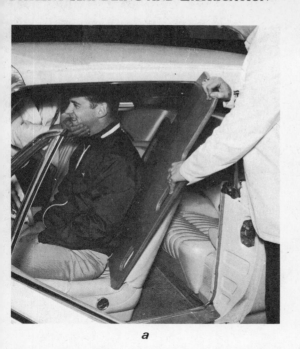

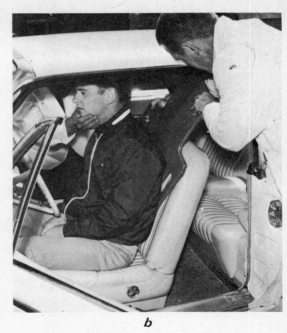

a

b

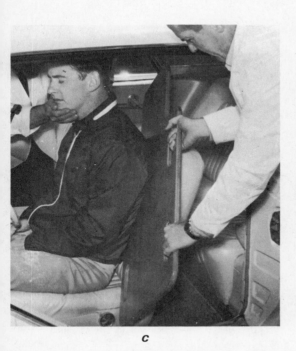

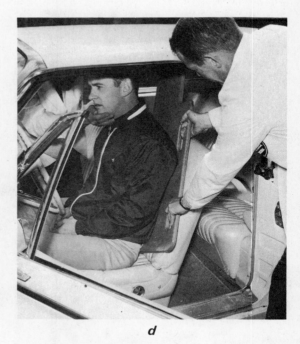

c

d

Figure 47.26 *a–d*

    In positioning the short spineboard behind a patient seated in a car, the EMT must exercise care and ingenuity to avoid disturbing the patient or having to move him before he is properly immobilized. It is possible to maneuver the board through the door and behind the patient. Here, *a*, the board strikes the top of a low doorway, but, *b* and *c*, it may be turned so that either end goes into the car first. It may then be pivoted into an upright position, *d*, and slipped behind the patient, who has remained undisturbed.

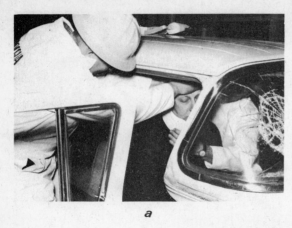

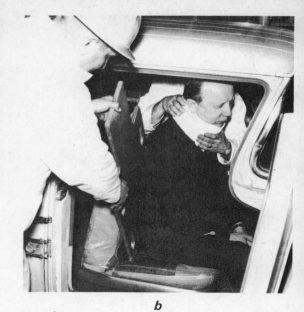

a

388

b

Figure 47.27 *a–b*

   Proper positioning of a spineboard is demonstrated in these pictures, in which the patient has a simulated neck injury. His head is supported by one EMT at all times as a cervical collar is applied and a short spineboard slipped behind the patient.

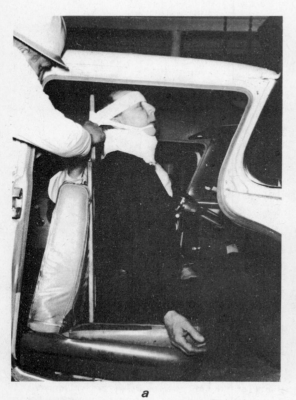

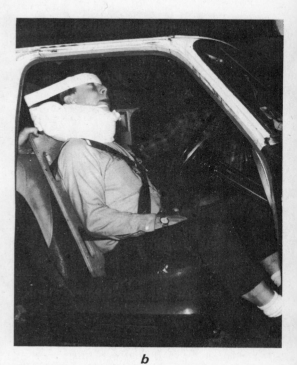

a   *b*

Figure 47.28 *a–b*

   The spineboard in position, the chin strap and head band are secured to it and the patient's head and neck are effectively immobilized.

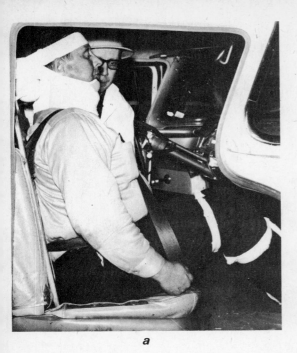

a

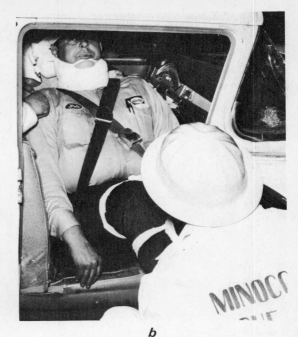

b

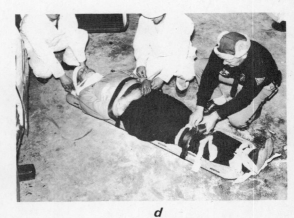

d

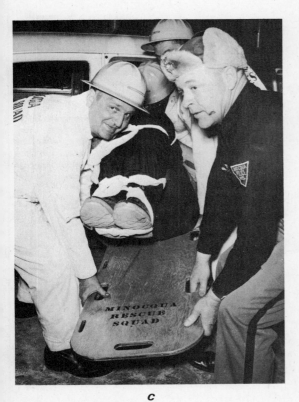

c

Figure 47.29 *a–d*

A patient with a simulated neck injury and fracture of the tibia is too heavy to lift from the car without jostling and possible further injury. *a–b,* His head and neck are immobilized with a cervical collar and secured to the short spineboard. His injured leg is temporarily immobilized by fixation to the opposite leg with triangular bandages. *c,* He may now be laid flat in the seat of the car and a long spineboard slid beneath the short spineboard at his back. He is removed from the car on the long spineboard without difficulty. *d,* The spineboard may be laid on the ground, the leg straps loosened, and the legs straightened. The patient is then again secured to the long spineboard, which has become a litter for him.

390

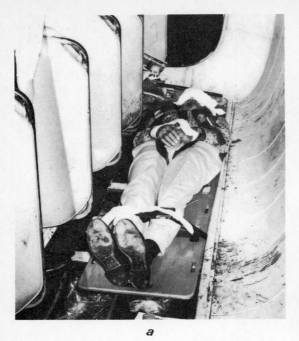

a

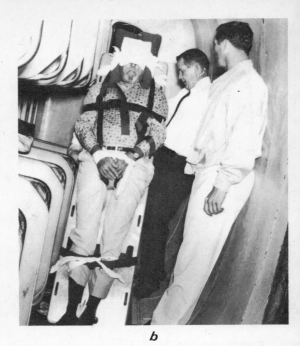

b

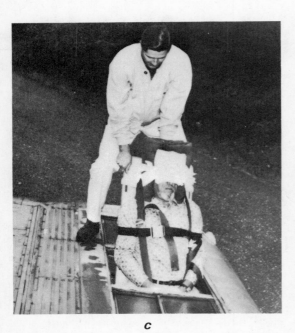

c

Figure 47.30 *a–c*

Use of the long spineboard for vertical movement of the patient is demonstrated. The patient is trapped in an overturned bus. With his weight of 200 pounds, removal from these cramped quarters would be difficult and dangerous without the spineboard. *a,* The long straps go through the handholds on either side at the hips, then, *b,* to the handholds at the end of the board and across the shoulders. The head and neck are secured, as are the wrists. *c,* With the patient thus packaged he may be lifted safely, even in a completely vertical position, through the window of the bus.

a long spineboard, is not available. The stretcher lash with the conventional pole stretcher serves to package the patient in the same way as described in Figure 47.30. The patient is placed on a stretcher, two blankets are wrapped around him, and he is lashed into position (Fig. 47.34).

Ladder Rescue

Basic ladder rescue consists of the one-man forward or backward slide or the twin-ladder slide, where the patient is horizontal (Fig. 47.35), or lowering a stretcher or basket by an aerial

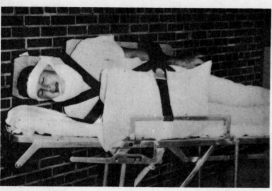

Figure 47.31

When a patient is firmly fixed to a spineboard, he may be transported in almost any position circumstances may make necessary.

ladder. The fireman's basket or rescue knot is used when an injured patient is lowered or when a fireman is lowered to a patient.

Specialized Rescue

In certain situations or disasters, such as snowstorms, floods, or airplane crashes, rescue personnel must often have specialized skills. The first duty of the EMT is to request, if the dispatcher has not already done so, that necessary specialists be brought to the scene. His second duty is to reach the scene himself or stand ready at the first evacuation point to do whatever is necessary. If the specialized rescue personnel have been adequately trained, they will be capable of providing emergency care. In many remote areas they administer drugs such as morphine, apply splints, and treat patients for shock.

Rough terrain and inaccessible areas. Rescue in rough terrain includes hilly or mountainous regions, caves, flooded areas, or situations where road travel is impossible. Conditions may be aggravated by snow, ice, and rain.

The major considerations in rough terrain rescue are:

1. Locate the patient.
2. Provide such immediate care as is necessary.

391

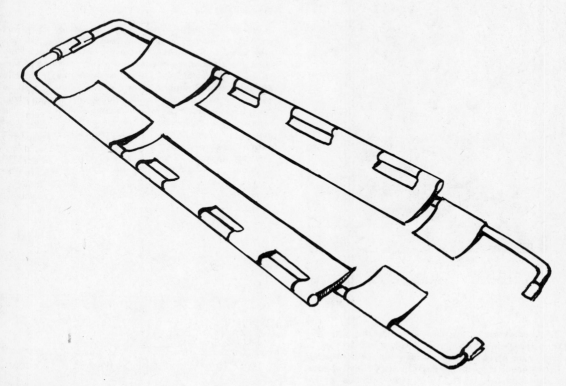

Figure 47.32

Regardless of the manufacturer, all scoop stretchers embody the same principles: they are divided into two halves longitudinally, have locking devices at each end, and must be positioned under the patient from both sides.

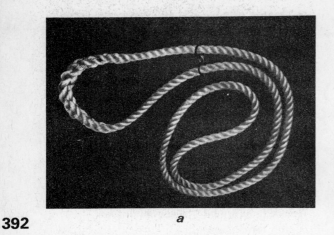

a

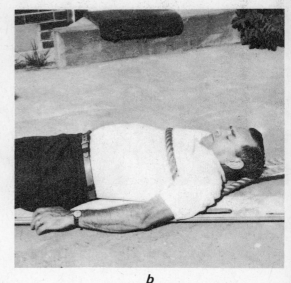

b

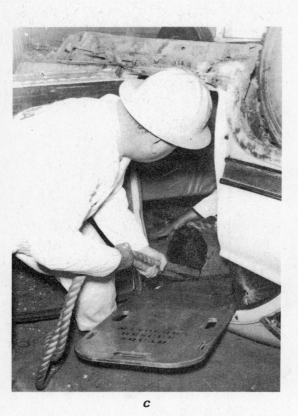

c

Figure 47.33 *a–c*

Where it is difficult to reach the patient and exert sufficient pull to remove him from wreckage, traction may be provided through the use of a sling around his chest. Injuries of the chest will preclude the use of this sling. *a*, A special rope loop (1-inch Manila), 6 feet in diameter, and equipped with a metal slide, should be carried as part of ambulance equipment. A long strap from a spineboard can be put to the same use. *b*, The rope or strap is looped under the patient's arms and across his chest. The loop is kept from slipping over the patient's head by a ring slide, or a triangular bandage if the strap is used. *c*, A patient trapped in a car is fitted with such a sling and gently pulled onto a spineboard.

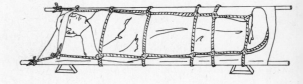

Figure 47.34

If necessary for safety, and when a basket stretcher or long spineboard is not available, the patient may be lashed to the stretcher. He is first wrapped in blankets and then secured to the stretcher with 50 feet of rope. The actual lashing consists of clove hitches on the handles, a series of half-hitches around the patient's body, and a double-locking half-hitch around the feet, followed by a series of half-hitches back up the side of the stretcher.

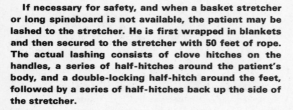

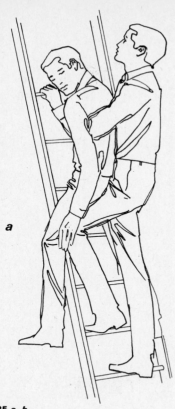

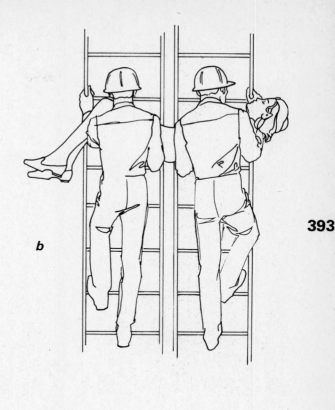

Figure 47.35 a—b

Basic ladder rescues are shown: *a*, **The one-man slide.** *b*, **The two-man, twin-ladder slide.**

3. Exercise all knowledge and use the appropriate equipment to bring the patient out even though no roads are available.

These rescues can involve such techniques as six-man stretcher passes up and down over rough terrain and across streams (Fig. 47.36), and the use of four-wheel-drive vehicles to transport stretchers. Often great ingenuity must be used in suspending a stretcher or padding it so that the patient is provided a reasonably comfortable ride. One technique is to partially inflate innertubes, if they are available, and put them as cushions under the stretcher. This method is far superior to swinging the stretcher on straps, which allows swaying and bouncing to be radiated through the straps with no cushioning effect. A 4- or 5-inch plastic foam padding can also be used to cushion a stretcher.

Helicopters are increasingly used as a quick evacuation means from remote areas or over difficult terrain. They may also be used to trans-

port EMTs to the scene of the emergency. The techniques of boarding and off-loading helicopters and the methods of opening a landing area for a helicopter should be learned and perfected. Standard hand signals for communication with

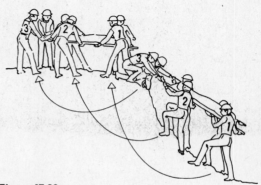

Figure 47.36

The six-man stretcher pass is used when transporting a patient over rough terrain. Recruited bystanders assisting the EMTs must be carefully instructed as to their role.

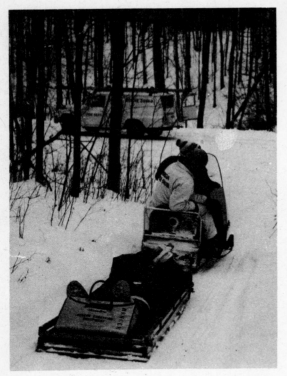

Figure 47.37

In transportation over snow from remote areas, a toboggan sled large enough to accommodate a stretcher, basket litter, or long spineboard can be pulled behind a snowmobile.

394

the helicopter from the ground must be studied and understood. It is never advisable to consider transporting a patient in an open basket beneath the aircraft as there is no possibility of providing emergency care if need should arise during transport.

The increased popularity of the snowmobile has been accompanied by an increased number of accidents involving these vehicles. Often such accidents are in areas accessible only by walking or by using another snowmobile. A special sled 24 inches wide by 7 feet long, with runners fore and aft can be pulled behind a snowmobile, using a rigid hitch. It will accommodate a pole stretcher, a Stokes basket, or a long spineboard for transport of a patient (Fig. 47.37).

Water rescue. Water rescue involves rescue from boats, from the water itself, from marine structures, or from flooding caused by excessive rains or by overflowing dams or reservoirs. EMTs who may be involved with water rescue should have a prearranged plan about what methods of rescue and transportation they will use.

To be efficient in water rescue, the EMT must have a good knowledge of water safety. All personnel involved in water rescue should be trained swimmers or, better, lifesavers. Flotation devices should be worn by rescue workers. These can be lifejackets, water ski belts, or any other mode of flotation.

There are great differences between simply going out in a calm pond to bring in a person who is already hanging onto a flotation device, and attempting to cross a river at flood crest to pick a patient off a bridge, pier, or rock. The ocean front creates additional problems, such as tides and large waves. Personnel working in currents should be attached to shore by a line so that they can be pulled back if necessary. No EMT should go into a boat without wearing a lifesaving device—not carrying it, but actually wearing it. Excessive clothing or heavy boots should be removed if weather conditions permit. These points are made elsewhere in this book in the discussion of water hazards. No harm and perhaps good can come from repeating them here.

Ice rescue. The techniques of movement over thin ice are many and varied. One way uses a skin diver's zippered "wet suit," which can be placed very quickly over the rescuer's clothing. The EMT then runs out over the thin ice with a safety line attached to his body, dives into the water, grabs the patient, and both are pulled to shore.

Another method is to use two sections of a ladder with a line attached to the ladder and also to the EMT, who then walks out on these two sections. The effect is similar to walking on oversized snowshoes.

Phases of Rescue Operations

In disasters where there are multiple patients (as in tornadoes or train wrecks), phases of rescue operations can be established. These phases are distinct and different from emergency care priorities and apply only to extrication operations.

The first phase is to remove lightly pinned casualties, such as those who can be freed by lifting a beam or removing a small amount of debris. In the second phase, remove those who are trapped in more difficult circumstances but who can still be rescued by use of the equipment at hand and in a minimum amount of time.

In the third phase, remove patients where extrication is extremely difficult and where much time can be taken up. The rescue may possibly involve cutting through floors, breaching walls, removing large amounts of debris, or cutting through an expanse of metal. An example would be rescuing a workman from under a heavy piece of machinery in a ditch.

The last phase is removal of dead bodies.

CHAPTER 48

Emergency Driving and Traffic Control at the Accident Scene

397

GOAL I. Understand the importance of safe driving when transporting the sick or injured to the hospital by ambulance.

OBJECTIVES

A. Describe the effects of a speeding ambulance on the patient.
B. Identify the occasions when speed is considered essential in transporting patients.

GOAL II. Understand the factors which contribute to safe driving in responding to emergency calls and transporting the patient to the hospital.

OBJECTIVES

A. Describe the human factors which contribute to unsafe driving.
B. Describe the physical factors which affect control of a vehicle.
C. Name the skills which a driver needs to operate an ambulance safely.

GOAL III. Know and understand the state laws governing ambulance operation.

OBJECTIVES

A. State your state and local laws covering right-of-way privilege.
B. State your state and local laws governing use of lights and siren.

GOAL IV. Understand safe operating procedures at the accident scene.

OBJECTIVES

A. Describe the actions necessary for safe parking of the ambulance at the accident scene.
B. Describe the actions necessary for effective traffic control at the accident scene.

Safe driving is an important phase of transporting the sick or injured. The risk of killing people or causing additional accidents by reckless driving of an ambulance in order to save a few minutes traveling to the hospital cannot be justified. When the EMT takes a turn behind the wheel of the ambulance, he assumes much responsibility. Only one part of this overall responsibility is the prompt transport of the patient to the hospital. Many other factors are equally important. Nor is speed the most important aspect of emergency driving. In general, an emer-

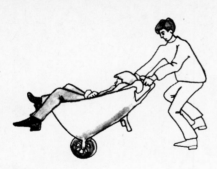

Figure 48.1

A patient who had endured a reckless ride to the hospital in an ambulance was heard to remark he would have preferred to take his chances in a wheelbarrow.

gency mission can be accomplished with far better results if the general rules of defensive driving are narrowed to three words: "Use common sense."

The national data on ambulance accidents are continuously accumulating but are not complete for every state. For the states reporting, an average 10 percent of the ambulances are involved in an accident each year. Another, more revealing, study indicated that only 3 to 5 percent of all ambulance runs were considered true life-or-death emergencies. In a specific series of 2,500 ambulance runs, it was found that haste in transporting the injured person was unnecessary in 98 percent of the cases. Furthermore, no difference in the outcome of the patients' condition would have resulted had 2,455 of these patients been transported to the hospital according to standard driving regulations. Cautious speed combined with the use of lights and sirens did contribute to saving the lives of the other 45 patients. Thus, speed was helpful in less than 2 percent of the cases in this study.

The primary purposes of an EMT on an ambulance are to give emergency care to a person involved in an accident or suffering an illness and to transport him to a hospital. An ambulance driven recklessly at speeds above legal limits has no place in an emergency care program. It is possible that more lives will be lost in accidents caused through reckless driving than will be saved through the proper administration of emergency care and safe transportation to the hospital.

Many accident patients have said that the most frightening part of their experience was not the accident itself but the ride to the hospital in the ambulance (Fig. 48.1). A person in an ambulance traveling at high speed with siren and flashing lights tends to believe his injuries are far more serious than they may actually be.

Panic in onlookers, or in emergency care workers who are not professionals or who are only partly trained, reinforces the belief that speed in transporting the patient to a hospital is all-important. The EMT must remember that he, as a professional, is trained to observe and care for injuries at the scene and to exercise the knowledge gained through training and experience in deciding how a patient should be transported. He makes use of driving judgment similarly gained, and when necessary, calls for police assistance or takes the right-of-way normally given an ambulance to reach his destination as quickly, but safely, as possible.

Factors that Contribute to Inappropriate Driving Speeds

Several factors contribute to the inappropriate use of speed in responding to emergency calls. These can be identified.

Lack of expertise in the dispatcher. Dispatching is a profession which calls for a trained, experienced EMT. Through his working knowledge of emergency calls, the dispatcher is in a position to determine, in the majority of cases, the urgency of the calls received. Dispatchers who are no more than switchboard operators do not make such decisions properly.

Inadequate equipment in the ambulance. If the EMT does not have on hand in the vehicle the emergency equipment and supplies necessary to stabilize the patient, there may be little choice but the most rapid possible transport to the hospital.

Inadequate training of the EMT. If the ambulance attendant is inadequately trained or has no confidence in his ability to care for the patient, again he has little choice but to transport the patient rapidly and to function as a chauffeur rather than as an EMT.

Inadequate driving ability. The EMT driver

who has not been trained in the safe operation of the ambulance will be unaware of the principles governing its proper use. This driver will frequently be inclined to select speed over safety because he does not understand the added risks that speed brings.

In this chapter we shall consider the general principles of safe driving and safe parking, as well as the qualities required in the EMT driver. A comprehensive classroom course of instruction and supervised training on the road are essential to master the techniques and acquire the necessary knowledge for safe ambulance driving.

Factors that Affect Control of a Vehicle

The driver has only two means of controlling the vehicle. He can change its direction or its speed. To accomplish either safely, it is necessary to maintain a continuous rolling contact between the bottom surface of the tires and the surface of the road. The contact points are called the footprint area of the tire. On a typical ambulance the footprint area is approximately 7-1/2 inches wide and 8 inches long for each tire.

Coefficient of friction. The coefficient of friction is a term from physics. It means the frictional force developed when two surfaces pass across one another. Figure 48.2 shows a solid block of rubber weighing 100 pounds being dragged across three different surfaces.

In the first example, 15 pounds of force are required to move the block of rubber; in the second example, 35 pounds of force are required; and in the third example, 100 pounds of force. The coefficients of friction are, thus, 0.15, 0.35, and 1.00. One can readily see that the force required to move the block of rubber varies with the surface across which the rubber is moved. The coefficient of friction is affected by the type and condition of surface on the road and the speed of the vehicle. The practical significance of the coefficient of friction is expressed in the number of feet required to stop a vehicle at a given speed, on a given road, under given conditions.

In terms of distance required to stop, an ambulance traveling on glare ice, where the coeffi-

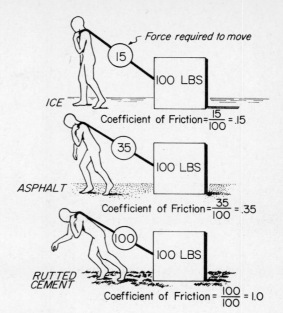

Figure 48.2

The coefficient of friction changes with the surface over which a load is drawn or driven. On a smooth, relatively friction-free surface, only fifteen pounds of force are required to move a 100-pound weight. The coefficient of friction is therefore 15 one-hundredths, or 0.15. On a rough, rutted surface where frictional forces are at a maximum, the coefficient of friction markedly increases. In the third example, one hundred pounds of force are required to move the 100-pound weight; so the coefficient of friction is 100 one hundredths, or 1.00.

cient of friction is of course low, will require many times the distance to stop as that same ambulance will require when traveling at the same speed on a dry concrete surface where the coefficient of friction is higher.

Cold and heat can also affect the coefficient of friction. Soft roads tend to liquefy in very hot weather, reducing the coefficient of friction as compared to that in cold weather. The coefficient of friction may vary widely at different points on the same road, depending on the condition of the surface, its age, and the weather.

A driver must constantly evaluate the road surface with regard to the force the tires can apply to the road at a given speed before skidding will begin. This observation is especially important in turning a corner, where an additional centrifugal force is acting on the vehicle.

If the coefficient of friction on a given road

surface is low—say it is 0.4—and the ambulance weighs 9,200 pounds, the maximum braking force that can be developed by the ambulance tires is $0.4 \times 9,200$ pounds, or 3,680 pounds. If the coefficient of friction for a road surface is higher—say it is 1.00—that same ambulance, weighing 9,200 pounds, can develop a braking force of 9,200 pounds.

Braking. How heavily must brakes be applied to obtain the maximum braking force in order to stop within the shortest distance? If a wheel is stopped suddenly in a panic situation, the braking force drops equally rapidly because of localized heating of the rubber in the tire. The footprint area of the tire in contact with the road surface is actually floating on a layer of molten rubber. Brakes must be applied, but to obtain maximum effect, the tire must rotate sufficiently to keep cool rubber in contact with the road surface. Finally, in a vehicle that has been braked suddenly, the center of gravity of the vehicle continues to move directly forward in a straight line regardless of the steering angle of the front wheel.

Steering. As the steering wheel is turned, a drift angle develops because the center line of the front tires heads away from the direction in which the vehicle is traveling. This angle causes a drag of the tires across the surface of the road, resulting in a cornering force which acts to shove the tire even farther and thereby change the direction of travel of the vehicle, either very slightly or greatly.

Cornering force. To provide cornering force to cause a vehicle to move in a smooth, even turn, front and rear wheels must each supply part of the drag force (traction) on the road. If one should suddenly remove the drag and the cornering force supplied by the tires, the vehicle would continue out of the curve in a straight line, as sometimes happens on icy or wet streets when the tires skid. They lose their traction and thereby their cornering ability. The same situation occurs in panic braking if the brakes lock, causing the tires to lose their rolling contact with the road and thus their traction. Steering ability and control of the vehicle are lost at that same moment.

Drag force. At a high-drift angle with a strong cornering force, there is considerable drag force on the tires because of the scrubbing action of the tire on the road surface. This force has the same effect as applying brakes to the wheels. Drag force alone will act to slow a vehicle as it passes through a corner, and a driver who knows how to take advantage of it can negotiate corners more safely.

A thorough explanation of drag force and its rather sophisticated utilization should be included in driver training courses for the EMT.

Decreasing-radius turns. Expressway entrance and exit ramps are not always constructed with a constant-radius curve (the same degree of curve throughout). Designers of highways are limited by the land available and are sometimes required to plan a decreasing-radius turn (the curve becoming tighter the more one drives into it) to fit into the area they must work with. These curves are usually easily identified by a series of black tire tracks at a point in the curve where it tightens and vehicles try to leave the road. Such hazards should be identified by the EMT and practice runs made over them before undertaking emergency calls.

Hydroplaning. On a wet road a tire tends to displace the water on the surface and make direct contact with the road. But as the vehicle begins to pick up speed above 30 mph, the tire tends to be lifted until there is no direct contact between it and the road surface. The reason is that there is insufficient time for the water on the road surface to be forced out from under the tire. This development is called hydroplaning. At speeds above 55 mph the driver is essentially riding on water and has no control over the vehicle at all.

Tire pressure. It is possible to regulate the cornering forces acting on tires and the footprint area of the tire by raising or lowering the tire pressure. Improved handling of the vehicle can result. Cornering force for a given drift angle of the tire varies with the tire inflation. In general, at lower pressures the footprint area is greater, but excessive wear on the tires may be the result.

Steering characteristics. Vehicles fall into three categories with regard to handling characteristics: understeer, neutral steer, and oversteer. A neutral vehicle has a center of gravity in the middle of the car, making it the easiest of the three to handle. In the understeer vehicle the center of gravity is located forward of the center; in the oversteer vehicle, the center of gravity lies behind the center of the car. In the understeer vehicle, the front tires must develop more cornering force than the rear; in the oversteer vehicle, continuous steering-out of a turn is required because the rear tires must develop more drift angle than the front tires. The oversteer vehicle most closely resembles the modular ambulance.

On an oversteer vehicle the front tires should be somewhat deflated and the rear tires somewhat more inflated in an approximate 40 to 60 ratio front to rear. Test driving is essential for each vehicle to determine the tire inflation which will produce the best handling characteristics.

Factors that Contribute to Safe Driving of Emergency Vehicles

Safe ambulance driving requires training and judgment in the operation of an emergency vehicle. It is important that the driver be familiar with the characteristics of the vehicle with regard to swaying and stopping. Disc booster brakes improve braking efficiency but increase the sway. A driver must know exactly what the vehicle will do and how it will respond to his steering and braking. On an emergency run, his hands should be on the wheel in a comfortable position. He should wear safety belts (both lap and shoulder) and insist that his fellow EMT workers wear them also.

The driver must be constantly alert to changing weather and driving conditions. Warnings of icy or hazardous conditions must be taken seriously. Whether the driver is responding to a call or is inbound to a hospital, he must adjust his speed to the road surface. He should follow specified routes for most routine runs, but have alternate routes developed for various contingencies. During a major disaster it is especially important that all services be coordinated and that vehicles follow assigned routes to hospitals. Should the driver encounter unexpected traffic congestion, he should notify the communication center so other drivers may be advised.

The driver must take account of the flow of traffic. On a 55-mile-an-hour highway where traffic beyond the accident scene has picked up speed, it is logical for the ambulance to proceed at the speed limit. In most instances, on a multi-lane highway the ambulance should stay in the extreme lefthand (fast) lane. Use of this lane offers the least amount of traffic under most conditions and allows other motorists to pull over in a normal righthand manner.

The ambulance driver should always drive defensively. He should not rely on anticipation of what another motorist will do unless a clear visual signal is received. Even then, he must be prepared to use the brakes promptly or to avoid the other car in case of misunderstanding or careless driving.

Care in exercising the right-of-way privilege. Very few emergency cases require extremely rapid transportation. These specific instances have been noted in earlier chapters. State laws vary regarding the right-of-way of an ambulance. Some states allow an emergency vehicle to proceed through a red light after stopping; others, in effect, allow it to go through a red light without stopping at all—a very dangerous practice. The EMT who is the ambulance driver must be familiar with the ambulance right-of-way laws for his state and should exercise the privilege only when necessary.

Care in use of the siren. In some areas, ambulance routes pass through city traffic and city streets. In a well-policed city it is possible that discreet use of the siren will alert a policeman on duty at an intersection so that he may stop other traffic and give the ambulance the right-of-way. However, indiscriminate use of the siren must be avoided. In general it does not help the ambulance driver. A driver in a closed car proceeding at 50 miles an hour with the radio playing and an air conditioner running cannot hear even a penetrating electronic siren until the ambulance is fifty or sixty feet away. If the radio is particularly loud, he may not hear the siren at all.

A radio message to the ambulance dispatcher requesting a police escort, clearance of certain intersections, or police assistance in passing through toll gates or narrow bridges may be more helpful in saving time than use of the siren.

401

Proper planning to save time. If the EMT plans and executes his moves in proper sequence, time will be gained. Speeding up the vehicle another 10 miles an hour will not save as much time as using good judgment in choosing traffic routes or asking for a police escort.

Guidelines for safe driving. The following guidelines should help the EMT in the safe operation of the ambulance.

1. Upon learning of the location of the accident, select the shortest route to the scene.

2. Try to learn the seriousness of the injury or illness in order to decide whether to use warning lights or siren.

3. Avoid routes with heavy traffic congestion. Know alternate routes for each destination during rush hours.

4. When approaching the scene be very careful and alert for pedestrians; curiosity seekers rarely move out of the way.

5. At the accident scene, park in a safe place.

6. When transporting the patient to the hospital, operate the ambulance within the stated speed limits for the area except in the most extreme emergencies.

7. Go with the flow of traffic.

8. Restrain the use of the siren. The patient will be cared for by your fellow EMT until you reach the hospital safely.

9. If it is necessary to use the siren, especially when approaching red lights and stop signs, reduce speed sufficiently to be able to stop the ambulance safely at all times if others do not give way.

10. Never take it for granted that red lights and siren will allow an ambulance to pass through a congested area.

11. Always remember the fellow with his car windows rolled up, the radio playing, and a conversation going on. He is not looking for an ambulance. He cannot hear it. He may have no idea that one is only twenty feet away.

Personal Qualifications of the Ambulance Driver

Not all persons who drive an automobile are qualified to drive an emergency vehicle. Person-nel must be screened carefully. Before an EMT is assigned to a driving position many questions should be satisfactorily answered.

1. Is the driver physically fit? Physicians and emergency workers know from experience that many accidents can be attributed to a physical ailment.

2. Is the driver emotionally fit? Emotions must be given much consideration. The personality of the individual often changes behind a steering wheel. The driver should be calm, able to meet the developments coolly in an emergency situation, and able to adapt his reactions promptly and appropriately to changing circumstances.

3. How will the driver react under emergency conditions? It is necessary not only to know exactly what to do but to be capable of doing it in a tight situation.

The EMT serving as the driver must be aware of important responsibilities and develop the proper attitude for this type of driving. Although an ambulance is usually granted right-of-way privileges, the law is emphatic about the responsibility of the driver. Any idea that an emergency driver can do no wrong must be abandoned. Being able to drive to one's destination without interruption (as granted in right-of-way privileges) and being permitted to pull out of the lane of traffic into the opposite lane are valuable time-saving privileges that must never be abused.

Types of Accidents in Ambulance Driving

An ambulance driver often assumes that motorists and the public will do the right thing when an emergency vehicle is in the vicinity or is following a car. The ambulance driver may take it for granted that motorists will pull to the right-hand curb or travel as close to it as possible. However, this response is often not forthcoming. Instead, the motorist may stop suddenly in front of the ambulance, and if the ambulance is not under control, a serious accident can occur.

Intersection accidents. Intersection accidents are the most frequent and usually the most serious. There are many hazards for which the ambulance driver should be on the alert. If the call is of such urgency that the driver is not waiting for red lights to change, he must still come to a momentary stop at the light and always be watching for the motorist who will drive around traffic that has stopped and enter an intersection without looking, usually at high speed.

Another serious hazard at intersections involves a motorist who has the lights timed so that he arrives when the lights are changing, thereby avoiding a stop. Often he is an experienced driver, perhaps hauling a heavy load which makes it almost impossible for him to stop quickly. He will arrive at the intersection knowing that the light is about to change and expecting to go on through. If the ambulance arrives at the intersection at the same time with the green light in its favor but about to change, and with its driver also expecting to go on through, a collision can scarcely be avoided.

Still another intersection hazard is created if the driver of one emergency vehicle follows another emergency vehicle through an intersection without assessing the situation carefully for himself. A motorist who has waited at the intersection and yielded the right-of-way to the first vehicle will in many instances proceed to drive on into the intersection when the first vehicle has passed. He does not expect a second car close behind. The preventive is for the driver of the second emergency vehicle to expect the unaware motorist and exercise caution himself.

Driving through an intersection when vision is obstructed, without stopping to satisfy oneself that the passage is clear, is dangerous and equivalent to driving blindfolded. There is a possibility of colliding with another vehicle, but even more likely is the possibility of striking a pedestrian who steps from behind some obstruction like a bus or truck.

Safe Parking of Emergency Vehicles

The proper parking of emergency vehicles is necessary to maintain efficient traffic control and flow. Do not park the ambulance beside the accident, for it may block traffic. Pull around in front or behind the accident and park at the side of the road to allow other cars to pass easily.

Park as close to the accident as the immediate need for emergency care indicates. If possible, survey the scene as the ambulance approaches and decide where emergency care can best be given and where to park to unload equipment readily or load patients easily. Where necessary, the ambulance can be temporarily moved into a position to block oncoming traffic so that a patient can be moved safely and quickly. If this maneuver is required, proceed as quickly as possible and do not block traffic longer than is absolutely required. If it is necessary to stop traffic on a multilane highway for any reason, try to stop only one lane at a time.

403

Traffic Control in Emergency Situations

The first responsibility of the EMT at the accident scene is to care for the patients. Only when all the patients have been treated and the emergency situation is under control should the EMT be concerned with the flow of traffic. If the police are delayed in arriving at the scene of an accident, the EMT may then be required to take some action himself.

The purpose of traffic control is to insure an orderly flow. Under ordinary conditions traffic control is a difficult task. Under the conditions that exist at scenes of accidents and disasters, traffic control presents serious additional problems. Passing motorists often try to observe the scene as they drive by, paying little attention to the roadway in front of them. They may even park and return to the scene on foot, creating still another hazard. As soon as possible, appropriate warning arrangements should be made. Reflectors or flashing devices or volunteer flagmen should be placed at sufficient distances to slow oncoming traffic on both sides of the accident. Pedestrians should be moved to a safe distance. Traffic should be directed to unobstructed lanes. Help from wreckers, the power company, and other agencies is needed to clear major obstructions such as fallen trees, broken power lines, and overturned vehicles.

Ordinarily the EMT will direct traffic for only a short time until the police arrive. Remember, the main objective in directing traffic is to forewarn other drivers and to keep the vehicles moving in an orderly manner.

XII

Communications, Records and Reports

CHAPTER 49

Communications

GOAL I. Understand the characteristics of an effective communications system and the need for medical coordination among the dispatcher, the medical facilities, the physician, and the EMT.

OBJECTIVES

A. Describe the role that communication plays in an EMS system.
B. Describe the responsibilities of the EMS dispatcher.
C. Identify the various types of communication equipment used to link the dispatcher, the medical facilities, and the physician with the EMT.

The vital link that ties together the various groups of the Emergency Medical Services system is communication. Its importance cannot be overestimated.

Advances in the development of electronic equipment, medical instrumentation, and the training of EMTs have changed the context of communication relating to Emergency Medical Services. The EMT should understand the structure of the EMS system and its relationship to the community health program and be aware of his responsibilities to each. He must be proficient in the various forms of communication.

Interrelation of Health Care Services

Emergency Medical Services is but one part of the total health care system in a community, and communication and cooperation between all units are essential for any one unit to function to its best capability. An effective EMS communications system depends upon having equipment and trained personnel for direct or indirect exchange of information twenty-four hours a day between the EMS system and the community health care system.

Communication Capability of the EMT

The EMT must be competent in various forms of communication. Efficiency and effectiveness are directly related to ability to communicate with the entire emergency team. He must know the capabilities and limits of the communications system which serves his EMS area and be completely competent in its operation. His effectiveness as a member of the total EMS team is directly related not only to the worth of the system serving that area but to his ability to use it. He must be able to communicate by radio, telephone, lights, siren, flares, hand signals, and written messages and to receive medical information or information relating to command and control of the ambulance. He must be able to transmit concise, accurate reports relating to vehicle status, to conditions at an emergency site, and to the condition and treatment of the patient he is attending.

Communication Capability of the EMS System

An EMS communications system may have

all or part of the capability for the following types of communications:

1. Entry of patient into the system
2. Dispatch of ambulance and supervision in routing it to the emergency scene
3. Intercommunication among emergency units at the emergency scene
4. Communication between the ambulance and hospital, including medical supervision of specialized treatment procedures at the scene and telemetric transmission of the patient's vital signs
5. Communication between the dispatcher and another service unit, such as hospital, police, fire, highway patrol, civil defense, military and other federal agencies, or adjoining EMS systems

408

An effective EMS communication system must provide, on a twenty-four-hours a day basis, the capability to mobilize rapidly and to manage and coordinate all EMS resources. All EMS participants must be able to join in the system, not only for operations in their local areas but to transport patients from one area to another when necessary. EMS communications must satisfy requirements for citizen access, for medical coordination, and for vehicle coordination. Some form of communications center is essential for every EMS system, although the sophistication and characteristics of a system will vary from one area to another. The methods of dispatching and the authority and area of operation will depend on local characteristics and conditions.

Entry into System

One of the most critical points in effective emergency medical care is rapid and proper entry of the patient into the EMS system. The usual method of entry is by telephone, although roadside call boxes, amateur radio operators, and citizens' band radios are being increasingly used. No matter what form of citizen access is used, it must be direct and the system capacity must be sufficient to prevent delays in answering the call. More than one incoming telephone line to the dispatch center should be available and one

other line should be a back-up unlisted number. The crucial first step is the call received by the dispatcher (Fig. 49.1).

Universal emergency number. Implementation of a system using the universal emergency telephone number, 911, can coordinate community resources by using one telephone number for an entire area. The use of a universal emergency number is an excellent concept, which unfortunately has as yet received only limited application. Telephone companies are not willing to install such a service unless all public safety and emergency services in the area agree to cooperate in the system and organize themselves to insure that disposition will be made of every call that is received. Many states have passed legislation requiring installation of 911 systems within a given number of years. Evaluating the multiple services within a community and accomplishing the reorganization required for a central system takes time. However, it seems likely that more and more communities will undertake to comply with the requirements and that a universal number will become an accepted system in this country.

Major Importance of Dispatcher Communications

Communication capability of the dispatcher. The dispatcher establishes the performance level of the EMS communication system. The dispatcher must be trained to extract, interpret, and transmit medical information precisely. He must be thoroughly familiar with the EMS resources in the area, including knowledge of the training levels and capabilities of individual EMTs assigned to ambulances he dispatches. Additionally, he must be completely familiar with the communication system, know the applicable FCC rules, and have a working knowledge of the operational aspects of public safety and public service agencies in the area. He is the focus of all effective EMT activity.

Dispatching may be from an operator at a volunteer operations center, from an ambulance company, or perhaps from someone at a police or fire department dispatch center. In many cases a dispatcher may combine the services required for EMS and fire and police services. The dispatcher who acts solely for EMS frequently also answers the original call for help from the public and thus must be trained to ask for the information needed to initiate a proper response (nature of the illness, degree of injury, or number of patients involved). Additionally, the dispatcher should be a trained EMT or at least knowledgeable about the duties and responsibilities of ambulance personnel and able to communicate in the terminology used in the EMS service. This ability will be especially needed as intercommunication with physicians and hospitals becomes more common.

Dispatching should follow uniform procedures. The first communication between the dispatcher and vehicle should include the nature of the injury or illness, number of persons involved, traffic and road conditions in the area (with special routing if necessary), and any circumstances that might require assistance from police or fire departments or other special services, or that might require precautions to be taken upon arrival at the scene. While special brevity codes are used in many EMS programs and are helpful in day-to-day operations, plain English-language communications are most effective in large-scale disasters or when vehicles from several different systems are involved.

Paging. Paging is a technique utilized to alert and call into action personnel needed to respond to a call for help. It is used extensively in some EMS systems. Specific frequencies are now available for paging both in-hospital and outside the dispatching center. Paging permits EMS personnel to leave the immediate location of the telephone or radio and yet be alerted when needed. Various mechanical devices are used, among them voice public address systems (PA systems), buzzers, flashing lights, and radios. Paging is used most extensively where personnel are not employed exclusively for EMS services, as in a hospital where the EMT has other duties when he is not responding to an emergency call. Paging is also a common method of calling together or alerting personnel in volunteer systems. The dispatcher must be familiar with the paging systems in his area and the details of their operation.

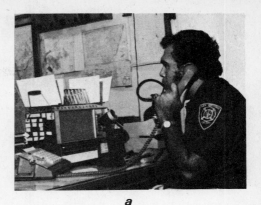

a

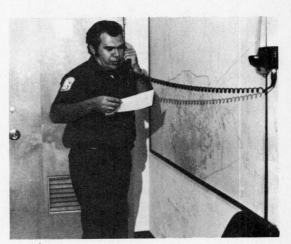

b

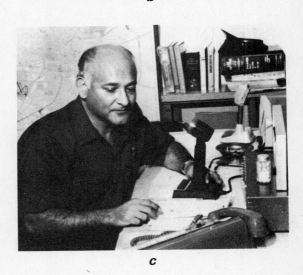

c

Figure 49.1 *a–c*

a, An emergency call is received at the dispatching unit. *b,* A city map is consulted to determine the location of the emergency unit nearest the call. *c,* A summary of the medical problem is relayed to the emergency unit that will answer the call.

409

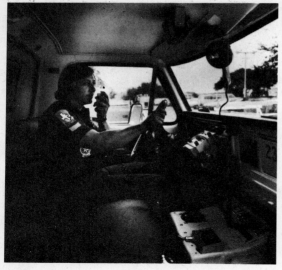

Figure 49.2

An ambulance attendant on duty receives a call from central dispatching.

printed signs. The proper use of these items and of vehicle lights and siren affords effective means of communication in warning or directing traffic, bystanders, and volunteer helpers. In remote or secluded areas the EMT must be able to employ hand, light, and ground signals in rescue operations by plane or helicopter. For communication between EMTs, the ambulance should also be equipped with an intercom system between the driver and the patient compartment and with portable radios (walkie-talkies).

Ambulance personnel's first communication on a call is typically an acknowledgment of the dispatch and a notice that the vehicle is en route to the scene of the incident (Fig. 49.2). Other types of routine communications are reports of the following: departure from the scene of the incident, destination and estimated time of arrival at a hospital, arrival at the hospital, leaving the hospital, return of the vehicle to its service area, and, finally, return of the vehicle to its permanent location (Fig. 49.3). The EMT also communicates with the dispatcher on any special road conditions encountered, as well as the whereabouts of the vehicle, and estimated time of arrival at the scene. Communications from ambulances can also advise on the need for professional assistance or specialized services. The

Paging is also a common method of bringing the physician into the system, since he does not usually devote full time to EMS and may be found at a number of locations in a day's activity. In larger hospitals, specialized teams may be called to report to the Emergency Department or elsewhere in the hospital. Paging may alert a physician so that two-way communication with EMTs in the field can be set up.

The usual type of paging uses coded signals. A particular code will activate a tone selector so that the only person alerted will be the one at the receiver which receives that particular tone. When the individual hears the signal on the receiver, he can press a button and receive the voice communication. Such one-way communication is efficient because a single paging operator can serve many individuals in the field. Two-way communications via the paging device tend to become time-consuming.

Ambulance Communications

In addition to two-way radio facilities, with which every ambulance should be equipped, various supplementary communication devices are essential equipment. Among these are a public address system, lights to signal traffic, and

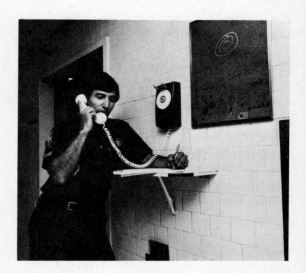

Figure 49.3

After the patient is delivered to the Emergency Department, the EMT reports the termination of the run to the dispatching center.

EMT always should report his arrival at the scene.

Ambulance personnel should have direct radio contact with the Emergency Department of the hospital to describe the nature of the problem, the patient's vital signs, and to request specialized medical advice. When the vehicle does not have a radio on the hospital frequency, communication with the hospital can be provided through the dispatch center by telephone patch or message relay (Fig. 49.4). In some of the newer systems, portable radio units can be carried by the EMT to the side of the patient and direct communication with a physician established and maintained for supervision in diagnostic and treatment procedures.

Walkie-talkie radio units are especially useful for communication between the EMT at a remote scene of injury or illness and the dispatch center, hospital, or supervising physician (Fig. 49.5). The portable unit also allows the EMT to communicate with his vehicle or with other EMTs responding to emergency situations that take them away from the vehicle. Such situations can occur in natural disasters (earthquakes, tornadoes, floods) and large-scale accidents (train wrecks, airplane crashes).

In large cities, it may be necessary for one EMT to leave the vehicle to search for an apartment or the location of an injured person. Walkie-talkie communication should be available to direct the vehicle to the proper location.

Medical Communications

Communication capability requirements of physician. One of the most important criteria for establishing effective communication between a physician and the EMT in the field is that the physician understand the training and capabilities of the EMT and that he be aware of the equipment aboard the vehicle. Physicians who participate in remote supervision of EMTs in the field should themselves serve for a period of time, both day and night, in the field to become acquainted with the special problems of independent duty as distinguished from typical problems and activity in a well-lighted, well-equipped Emergency Department with nurses and ade-

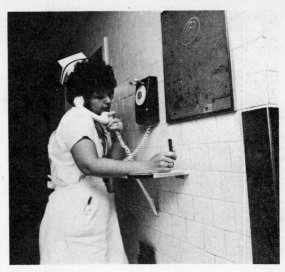

411

Figure 49.4

A nurse at the Emergency Department receives notification from the dispatcher or ambulance attendant of a patient to be expected and a statement of the emergency problem.

quate facilities. In the day-to-day operation of the EMS system, a physician should be available for communication with the EMTs. Established procedures should be defined during the training program to assure standardization and reliability of communication and to minimize errors in following orders and directions of the physician.

Medical coordination ordinarily requires a

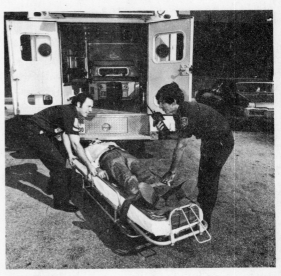

Figure 49.5

In the field the EMT transmits information via walkie-talkie radio to the dispatcher or directly to the hospital.

dedicated channel which is free from interference by other EMS users. The dispatcher, after assigning a channel and establishing the medical communications link, monitors the channel to know when it is clear and available for another assignment. This "real time" method of channel assignment is particularly applicable when several calls occur simultaneously. It provides flexibility in handling multiple incidents and makes maximum use of all frequency channels allocated to EMS.

412

The alternative assignment of channels is by geographic area. This method offers less flexibility but can be justified in areas of low traffic or where an already existing system is in operation.

Telemetry. Telemetry is the transmission of biological data from one site to another through the use of radio. The best-known example of telemetry has been the instant transmission of vital data on the physical condition of astronauts from thousands of miles in space to medical personnel on earth. Telemetry can be used on earth today to send an ECG pattern from a patient in a remote area to a receiving console in a hospital or to transmit other vital information. Since telemetry is ordinarily a part of an advanced EMS program, it will not be further discussed here.

Hospital-to-Hospital Communications

Day-to-day hospital communications are most effectively carried out by telephone (either regular line or hot line) between departments within a hospital or between hospitals. However, radio becomes important in hospital-to-hospital communications in situations where specialized resources are needed, as in a disaster, where there will probably be a failure of telephone lines.

Actually, in times of a disaster, the greatest problem usually is not lack of beds, hospital facilities, or medical resources but the lack of ability to communicate between the scene of the incident and the various medical resources. Unless these links are firmly established in advance, the management of a disaster can become a disaster itself.

Intercommunication with Cooperating Units

The system of communications for a carefully planned EMS system will include the capability for communication among different emergency resources, including police, fire, highway patrol, civil defense, and federal agencies. Of particular importance is the communication needed to effect proper cooperation with special rescue services, such as the Military Assistance to Safety and Traffic (MAST). The new rules and regulations of the Federal Communications Commission now allow federal vehicles and facilities to operate on the radio frequencies common to the newly developed frequencies set aside for EMS system usage.

The necessity to communicate among various EMS systems also is important in disasters involving large areas, where intercommunication with adjoining areas as well as shared frequencies can dispense information among all units concerned with emergency operations.

The dispatcher naturally provides the focus for intercommunication by using direct telephone lines, patching radio to telephone, or utilizing his access to multiple channels.

Federal Communications Commission

The Federal Communications Commission (FCC) is the regulatory agency which governs radio operations within the United States. It also has a controlling function relating to interstate and international telephone and telegraph services which can in some cases be involved in emergency medical services. Its primary function as related to EMS is that it allocates bands of frequencies for different types of radio operations, issues licenses to individual stations and assigns call letters, sets power limitations, and specifies standards of operation for equipment.

Its printed rules and regulations are continuously updated as changes are made; copies of these documents may be purchased from the Government Printing Office, Washington, D.C. These printed rules and regulations are voluminous and, for the most part, quite specific. They are best read and interpreted by persons with communication experience. Their intention is to provide a relatively orderly use of the frequency spectrum by qualified and licensed individuals.

Different localities (geographic areas) and EMS systems have different needs and possible solutions to EMS communication problems. To define the frequencies needed and the communication capability required before the total EMS system is defined is impossible. Therefore, the total EMS system must be defined before the frequencies and the method of communication are established. In rural areas it is not infrequent to find EMS systems operating in conjunction with the local sheriff and other law enforcement agencies. In some portions of the country, volunteer rescue services operate closely in conjunction with volunteer fire departments, even in heavily populated areas.

Definitions

An understanding of the terminology applicable to the FCC rules and regulations and the types of equipment as described by manufacturers is also necessary in order to define the EMS system, since each user must identify his needs and be aware of the special terminology used to describe equipment and system operation. There usually must be close cooperation and communication among technical communication personnel, physicians, and the personnel in the ambulance.

Ambulance repeater—A station in an ambulance for automatic retransmission of radio communications from portable units in the field.

Base station—A land station in the Land Mobile Service which carries on a communications service with land mobile stations. A base station, for example, could be located at a hospital or a dispatching center.

Channel—A frequency or several frequencies used for a specific purpose.

Dedicated line—A line usually used for fixed point-to-point communications. Not usually accessible except from predetermined sites.

Hot line—A direct linkage between predetermined sites as, for example, a dispatching center and a hospital. It is under full control of an individual at each end so that the line is immediately available simply by lifting the receiver. Outside access cannot be obtained except by patching at either end.

Land Mobile Service—A mobile communication service between a base station and land mobile stations, or between land mobile stations.

Mobile repeater station—A mobile station (portable or vehicular) which can retransmit automatically on a mobile service frequency. The communication can originate either from a hand-carried mobile unit or from another mobile station or base station.

Multiplex—The technique whereby two different types of information are transmitted simultaneously on the same frequency.

Patch—A connection between communications systems, for example, a radio communication channel to a regular telephone line.

Scanner—A type of receiving unit in which the frequency being received is automatically and instantaneously changed until a frequency carrying a message is detected, at which time the receiver locks on that frequency and the message can be received. The system allows a single receiver to scan several frequencies and pick out one in which communication is in progress.

Telemetry—The use of telecommunications for automatically indicating a recorded measurement at a distance from the measuring instrument, for example, an ECG sent from an ambulance and received at a hospital.

CHAPTER 50

Records and Reports

GOAL I. Understand the purposes and requirements of EMT reporting and record-keeping.

OBJECTIVES

A. Describe the purposes of EMT reporting and recordkeeping.
B. List the types of information required for medical, legal, community health, and administrative purposes
C. Identify users of information collected through the EMT reporting and recordkeeping system.
D. Identify the importance of EMT reporting and recordkeeping relative to other aspects of EMS.

GOAL II. Know local procedures for reporting and recordkeeping.

OBJECTIVES

A. Name the person or persons who report or record information for your ambulance, and tell what information is recorded and when reported.
B. Summarize local reporting and recordkeeping information requirements and procedures.
C. Demonstrate completion of your local ambulance report form for a hypothetical call.

Adequate reporting and the keeping of accurate records are vital in emergency medical care. They help insure continuity of treatment for the patient and provide data that may be needed for an analysis of his condition as well as for protection of community health, and for administration, research and evaluation, and legal requirements. While these duties are essential for the EMT, they must never come before care of the patient. With experience and alertness, the EMT can learn to obtain most of the information needed from simple observation and questioning while rendering care to the patient at the same time.

General Requirements of the Report Form

Because of the various agencies which derive information from the EMT report form, its requirements are many. Among the types of information sought from it are the following.

Medical purposes. The hospital and the physician will require this information:

Identification and vital statistics of the patient (age, sex, kin)
Description and cause of injuries or nature of the illness

Signs and symptoms of the injury or disease at the scene and in transit

Vital signs of the patient

Emergency care rendered by the EMT at the scene and during transport

Rescue measures or treatment preceding arrival of the EMT

Medicines used by the patient or given by the EMT

Poisons taken (and their containers)

Legal purposes. If the police are not present at the scene of the incident or if they are preoccupied with other duties, the EMT may find it necessary to gather or record information of the following nature:

An account of the circumstances concerning a case of assault, homicide, rape, child abuse, or animal bites

Dying statements, recorded in the exact words uttered, in the presence of a witness if possible

A note of the disposition of the patient's valuables

Suicide notes or other relevant papers

A record of the exact location and position of the patient before moving him

Community health purposes. To protect the patient and others, the following reports are required:

A report to the coroner or medical examiner in the case of sudden or accidental death at the scene or during transport

A report to the community health officer of communicable diseases and of animal bites

A report to appropriate authorities regarding the presence of hazards relating to gas, fire, electricity, chemicals, or radiation

Administrative purposes. An emergency medical service, whether public or private, requires considerable data in administration of its business. Among needed items of information are:

A date/time log of all ambulance runs

Identification of the vehicle and crew making the run

Location of the emergency site and also of

the medical facility to which the patient was transported

Originator of the call for service

Type of service requested

Type of injury or illness reported

Evaluation purposes. To assess and improve the quality of emergency medical services, the reports mentioned in the foregoing paragraphs are often subjected to analysis and statistics are compiled from them. Selected cases may be evaluated by the physician in the Emergency Department and a critique made of the quality of emergency care on any given case or by any given crew.

General Procedures

Procedures for collecting, reporting, and recording emergency care information vary from community to community and depend to some extent on the circumstances existing during the call.

Ideally, recordkeeping and reporting commence with receipt of the request for assistance. The dispatcher completes a dispatch form and transmits the information to an ambulance crew.

Depending upon the circumstances, the crew may report to the dispatcher while en route to the scene. Delays or unusual circumstances should certainly be reported, as the service of other units could be affected by traffic conditions or road blockages. Upon arrival at the scene, the time of arrival, status of the scene, and any need for assistance are also reported to the dispatcher.

Information needed should be obtained and recorded at the scene, time permitting. Because of the pressure of time and the need to render emergency care immediately, the EMT may only jot down brief notes of essential information or details which he feels he might not readily recall when completing the report form later. The status of the patient should be reported to the Emergency Department from the scene if circumstances require it. For example, the need for advice from a physician or information to insure that the Emergency Department will be prepared to receive the patient should be relayed.

En route to the medical facility, the status of the patient and the vehicle may be reported, again depending upon the circumstances. At this time, if possible, the EMT should complete the report form so it will be available to the hospital staff upon arrival.

At the medical facility, the EMT responsible for the patient at the scene and in transit should remain with the patient to provide the attending medical staff a verbal summary of the case and to answer questions. The medical care part of the report should be completed and available at that time.

If all parts of the report (legal, community health, and administrative) have not been completed, they must be finished as soon as possible after transfer of the patient from the responsibility of the EMT. Forms cannot be left to the end of the shift or the day because much information will be lost.

At the end of this chapter (pp. 418–420) an Ambulance Report Form is shown which has been made up from a variety of forms in use in this country (Fig. 50.1). It is a general type which any community or service might adapt to its own requirements. Additional information can be added to it.

The use of effectively designed forms as checklists for the EMT can improve the quality of emergency care in any situation. Certainly the person best able to record information is the person observing moment by moment changes in the patient. This information itself provides the proper background for major medical decisions made at the hospital. While reporting and recordkeeping may not appear to be of much help in an immediate situation, the information has a long-range impact on Emergency Medical Service.

Summary

The principal kinds of information required and the procedures to employ in reporting and recordkeeping may be recalled more easily by the EMT if a rule is attached to each letter of the word RECORD:

Render aid to patient first.

Examine patient, clothing, or purse for medical identification devices.

Collect personal effects of patient, suicide notes, related papers, drug paraphernalia, medicines, and poisons.

Observe and record important facts about the condition of patient and the care provided.

Record statements of patient, relatives, and witnesses.

Determine if possible how the injury occurred and what caused it.

417

Vehicle #_____

Name of Ambulance Service: Crew Identification:

_____   Driver_____

_____   Attendant_____

_____   Attendant_____

- -

Call Date   Month_____Day_____Year_____Call Received_____

Response

Record   Unit Respond_____Lights____Siren____Arrive Scene_____

          Leave Scene _____Lights____Siren____Arrive Hospital_____In Service_____

418

- -

Location of Emergency_____

_____

_____

_____

- -

Name of Patient_____Date of birth_____Sex M   F

Mailing Address_____Religion_____

_____Health insurance_____

- -

Originator	____Central Dispatch	____Fire Dept.	____Hospital	____Other
of	____Police	____Bystander	____Nursing home	
Call	____Relative	____*Physician	____Jail	

*Name_____

- -

Type Accident   ____Auto   ____Diabetic   ____Assault

or Injury   ____Pedestrian   ____Convulsion   ____Attempt suicide

Reported   ____Motorcycle   ____Hemorrhage   ____One down

                 ____Bike   ____OB   ____Unconscious

                 ____Illness   ____MO   ____Unknown

                 ____Chest pains   ____Injury   ____Drowning

                 ____Heart attack   ____Fall

                 ____Overdose   ____Fracture   ____Emergency transport

                 ____Poisoning   ____Burn   ____Routine transport

                 ____Seizure   ____Shooting/Stab

To be filled out by Dispatcher

- -

Figure 50.1

Several characteristics of this sample report form should be noted. The first section is designed to provide the ambulance crew with information concerning the emergency call itself. It may also serve as an evaluation of the report and of the dispatch system. It is completed by the dispatcher.

The remaining parts of the form are completed by the EMT. Section 2 relates to evaluation of the patient and history taking. Section 3 relates to medical care given the patient, and section 4 relates to extrication requirements.

The form shows the orderly sequence of events the EMT should follow from the time he receives the call until he delivers the patient to the medical facility. If used as a checklist by the EMT, it will go far to insure that he consider all aspects of the patient's condition and use all available techniques when rendering emergency medical care.

To be filled out by EMT

EMT Patient Evaluation	Scene	Pulse Rate	Transit		Scene	Respiration	Transit
	_____	Normal	_____		_____	Normal	_____
	_____	Rapid weak	_____		_____	Rapid shallow	_____
	_____	Rapid bounding	_____		_____	Deep gasping labored	_____
	_____	Absent	_____		_____	Frothy blood coughing	_____

	Scene	Blood Pressure	Transit		Scene	Skin Temp. & Color	Transit
	__/__	Time____Time____	__/__		_____	Normal	_____
	__/__	Time____Time____	__/__		_____	Cool, clammy	_____
					_____	Dry, hot	_____
	Scene	Pupils of Eyes	Transit		_____	Red	_____
	_____	Normal	_____		_____	Pale, white, ashen	_____
	_____	Constricted	_____		_____	Blue (cyanotic)	_____
	_____	Dilated	_____				
	R L	Unequal	R L		Scene	State of Consciousness	Transit
	_____	Contact lenses	_____		_____	Alert	_____
	R L	Artificial eye	R L		_____	Confused	_____
	R L	Blind	R L		_____	Unconscious	_____
					R L	Move arms	R L
					R L	Move legs	R L
					R L	Reaction stimuli arm	R L
					R L	Reaction stimuli leg	R L

419

Patient Medical History

_____ Asthma	_____ Epileptic	_____ Pacemaker
R L Blind	_____ Heart condition	_____ Stroke
R L Deaf	_____ Hypertension	_____ Allergic to medications :
_____ Emphysema	_____ Laryngectomee	Identify :_____
		_____
		_____

Emergency Care Rendered by EMT

Scene	Action	Transit		Scene	Action	Transit
_____	Establish airway	_____		_____	Cervical collar	_____
_____	Oropharyngeal	_____		_____	Short backboard	_____
_____	Endotracheal tube	_____		_____	Long backboard	_____
_____	Esophageal obturator	_____		_____	Board splints	_____
_____	Nasal cannula	_____		_____	Inflatable splint	_____
_____	Suction	_____		_____	Traction splint	_____
_____	Oxygen	_____		_____	Scoop type stretcher	_____
_____	CPR	_____		_____	Sealed sucking chest wound	_____
_____	Control bleeding	_____				
_____	OB delivery	_____		_____	Induced vomiting	_____

Rescue &   Scene   Problems
Extrication   ———   Tools needed to gain access to patient
              ———   Tools needed to free patient from entrapment
              ———   Rescue services required other than that available in ambulance
          Identify rescue tools used; _____
                                      _____
                                      _____
                                      _____
                                      _____
                                      _____
                                      _____
                                      _____
                                      _____

420

- -

Anatomical
Sites of
Injuries

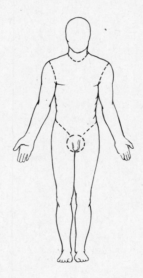

- -

Glossary

It is hoped this glossary will be useful to those with no prior medical knowledge and no experience in emergency medical care work.

Feeling it unnecessary to define every medical term in the book, we have attempted to restrict the list to those words to which the EMT might wish to refer in studying the textbook or perfecting the performance of his duties. Definitions are limited to those particular to the subject matter. To be of immediate assistance to beginners, they have been made as simple as possible. Medical and standard dictionaries should be consulted for amplification of meanings.

Undoubtedly words which should have been included have been overlooked, and definitions which have seemed clear to the writer will be found to be inadequate by the reader. Comments and suggested additions to both words and definitions will be gratefully received and carefully considered for inclusion in future editions.

A

abdomen: The more inferior of the two major body cavities lying between the thorax and the pelvis.

abdominal catastrophe: The most sudden and severe form of an acute abdomen.

abdominal cavity: The space bounded by the abdominal walls, the diaphragm, and the pelvis: It contains the greater part of the organs of digestion, the spleen, the kidneys, and the suprarenal glands.

abduction: Movement of a limb away from the central axis of the body.

abortion: Delivery of the fetus before it is mature enough to survive out of the uterus. Most states define this period as less than twenty weeks of pregnancy. Abortion may be either spontaneous (occurring from natural causes) or induced. A distinction is made between abortion and premature birth. Premature infants are those born after the stage of viability has been reached but before full term.

abrade: To wear away by mechanical action; to scrape away the epidermis.

abrasion: An injury consisting of the loss of a partial thickness of skin from rubbing or scraping on a hard or rough surface. Also called brush burn or friction burn.

absorbent: Having the power to absorb, suck up, or take into itself any gas liquid, light rays, or heat.

access: A way or means of approach; the action of going to or reaching.

acetabulum: The large cup-shaped depression on the external surface of the innominate bone, into which the head of the femur fits.

acetic acid: Vinegar.

acetone: A chemical compound, extremely small amounts of which are found in normal urine. Larger quantities occur in the urine and blood of diabetic persons, sometimes giving a "fruity" odor to the urine and breath of such patients.

acid: Any compound of an electro-negative element with one or more electro-positive hydrogen ions. Acids can cause severe burns. In solution, they have a sour taste.

acidosis: A state characterized by actual or relative decrease of alkali in bodily fluids in proportion to the content of acid. In this state, tissue function is often disturbed, most importantly in the central nervous system.

ketoacidosis: A term given to describe acidosis seen in diabetic patients and associated with an enhanced production of ketone bodies from incomplete metabolism of fats.

acromio-clavicular joint: The union between the clavicle and the scapula and the supporting ligaments.

acromion: The outer end of the spine of the scapula, which projects as a broad, flattened process overhanging the glenoid fossa; it articulates with the clavicle.

activated charcoal: Powdered charcoal which has been treated to increase its powers of absorption.

acute abdomen: A term used to indicate a serious intra-abdominal condition causing irritation or inflammation of the peritoneum and attended by pain, tenderness, and muscular rigidity. The condition occurs in the absence of a traumatic event and usually requires an operation.

Adam's apple: The projection at the front of the neck formed by the largest cartilage of the larynx (thyroid cartilage). Much more prominent in men than in women.

adduction: Movement of a limb toward the central axis of the body or beyond it.

adrenal gland: A flattened body situated in the retroperitoneal tissues at the cranial pole of either kidney; a major endocrine organ whose secretions are essential for life.

afterbirth: The placenta and membranes that are expelled after the birth of a mammal.

air chisel: A chisel attachment for an air hammer powered by air from a Scott pack or a SCUBA tank. Can be used to cut away car roofs, door panels, or door posts.

air embolism: The presence of air bubbles in the heart or blood vessels, usually caused by a wound of one of the large veins of the neck. Air embolism can also result from rapid expansion of air in the lungs, as when a diver ascends in the water too quickly or when one flies too high in an unpressurized plane.

air hunger: Distress in breathing, characterized by rapid or labored respiration.

air passage: Any of several tubes and passages which transmit air from the nose or mouth to the fine bronchioles of the lung. An airway.

air splint: A double-walled plastic tube in which a limb can be immobilized when air is blown into the space between the walls. When the tube is sufficiently inflated, it will form a rigid splint. Inflation should always be by mouth.

airway: Anatomic passage for the transport of air into and out of the lungs.

  lower airway: The passage from the epiglottis to the pulmonary alveoli, including the larynx, trachea, bronchi, and bronchioles.

  upper airway: The passage from the nose, mouth, oropharynx, and nasopharynx to the epiglottis.

airway, artificial: A device to provide and maintain free passage of air through the upper airway.

albumin: A type of simple protein widely distributed throughout the tissues and fluids of plants and animals.

alkali: Any compound of an electro-positive element in combination with an electro-negative hydroxyl ion or similar ion. Alkaline compounds are caustic and can cause severe destruction of tissue.

alkalosis: Alkaline intoxication; an abnormally high alkali reserve (bicarbonate) of the blood and other body fluids, with a tendency for an increase in the pH of the blood. Alkalosis may result from persistent vomiting, hyperventilation, or excessive ingestion of sodium bicarbonate.

allergen: An antigen; any of various sorts of material (microorganisms, toxoids, foreign proteins, and others) that can induce a state of sensitivity when in contact with the tissues of the body.

allergic reaction: A local or general reaction characterized by extreme reactivity of the body to an allergen or antigenic substance. Such reactions include hives, swelling of tissues, and difficulty in breathing.

alpha particle: A positively charged nuclear particle consisting of two neutrons and two protons ejected at high speed in certain radioactive transformations.

aluminum splint: *See* rigid splint.

alveolar ridges: The ridges in either jaw containing cavities or sockets for the teeth.

alveoli: The air sacs of the lungs.

American standard: A safety device for the outlet valves of large gas-filled cylinders to prevent the attachment of a pressure regulator for one gas to the cylinder of another gas.

amino acid: An organic acid in which one of the hydrogen atoms has been replaced by a molecular amine group. Amino acids are the chief components of proteins.

amnesia: Loss or impairment of memory; inability to recall past experiences.

amniotic fluid: A liquid that surrounds the fetus in the uterus and protects it from injury.

amniotic sac: The innermost of the membranes enveloping the fetus in the uterus.

amphetamine: A central nervous system stimulant; a nasal decongestant; closely related in its structure and action to ephedrine or benzedrine.

amputation: The cutting off of a limb, part of a limb, or any other projecting part.

anal canal: The terminal portion of the alimentary canal, extending from the rectum to its distal terminal opening, which is the anus.

analgesics: Agents which can relieve pain.

anaphylactic shock: A condition which develops suddenly, caused by hypersensitivity in the body to drugs or other foreign materials (insect stings, certain foods, inhaled allergens). Violent symptoms include hives, wheezing, tissue edema, broncho spasm, and vascular collapse.

423

anaphylaxis: An unusual or exaggerated allergic reaction of an organism to foreign proteins or other substances.

anesthesia: Loss of sensation in a part of the body or in the body generally induced by a drug.

aneurysm: A permanent, blood-filled dilation of a blood vessel resulting from disease or injury of the blood vessel wall.

angina pectoris: Spasmodic pain characterized by a sense of severe constriction in the chest. It is aggravated or induced by exercise and relieved by rest or medication; associated with an insufficient blood supply to the heart.

angle of Louis: A bony prominence on the breastbone, just inferior to the junction of the clavicle and the sternum and just opposite the second intercostal space.

angulation: The formation of an angle; an abnormal angle or bend in an extremity or organ of the body.

anisocoria: Abnormal, minor inequality of the diameters of the pupils or the eyes.

anoxia: Absence or lack of oxygen; reduction of oxygen in body tissue below required physiologic levels.

antecubital: In front of (anterior to) the elbow.

antecubital fossa: The depression in the skin and soft tissues of the upper extremity anterior to the elbow.

anterior: A term indicating the front part of the body or of any structure.

anticonvulsant: An agent to prevent or arrest convulsions.

antidote: An agent to neutralize a poison or counteract its effects.

antiemetic: A remedy to control nausea and vomiting.

antiseptic: An agent which kills, checks, or retards the growth of disease-producing organisms.

antivenin: An antiserum against an animal or insect venom.

anus: The distal or terminal opening of the alimentary canal.

aorta: The main arterial trunk arising at the heart from which the arterial system proceeds.

aortic valve: The valve at the junction of the aorta and the left ventricle of the heart.

apneic: Characterized by the absence of respiration.

aponeurosis: The end of a muscle where it becomes tendon, serving mainly to connect a muscle with other muscular parts that it moves.

apoplexy: Sudden unconsciousness followed by paralysis, caused by rupture or obstruction of an artery in the brain.

appendicitis: Inflammation of the vermiform appendix.

appendix (vermiform): A wormlike diverticulum from the cecum (right colon).

appreciate: To be fully aware of; to evaluate; to judge with heightened understanding.

apprehend: To perceive, to understand, to anticipate, especially with anxiety or fear.

arachnoid: Resembling a spider's web; a delicate membrane interposed between the dura mater and pia mater and overlying the brain; one of the meninges.

arm: The upper extremity, specifically that segment of the upper extremity between the shoulder and the elbow.

arrhythmia: An abnormal rhythm of the heartbeat.

arterial blood: Oxygenated blood distributed throughout the body in the arteries.

arteriole: A minute arterial branch, especially one just proximal to a capillary.

arteriosclerosis: Hardening of the arteries. A generic term which includes a variety of conditions which cause the arterial walls to become thick and hard and to lose elasticity. *See also* atherosclerosis.

artery: One of the tubular vessels which carries oxygenated blood from the heart to the tissues of the body.

>**brachial artery:** The artery of the arm that is a continuation of the axillary artery, which in turn branches at the elbow into the radial and ulnar arteries.

>**carotid artery:** The principal artery of the neck. It runs upward in the neck and divides into the external and internal carotid arteries to supply the face and head and brain respectively. It can be palpated on either side of the neck.

>**coronary arteries:** The two arteries arising from the aorta, arching down over the top of the heart, and conducting blood to the heart muscle.

>**dorsalis pedis artery:** The artery whose pulse is palpable on the dorsal surface of the foot; it supplies the medial foot and great toe.

>**femoral artery:** The principal artery of the thigh, a continuation of the external iliac artery. It supplies blood to the lower abdominal wall, the external genitalia, and to the lower extremity.

>**maxillary artery:** The artery on either side of the face which supplies blood to the face; it is palpable in front of the angle of the jawbone.

>**popliteal artery:** The continuation of the femoral artery in the popliteal space.

>**posterior tibial artery:** Located posterior to the medial malleolus; it supplies blood to the foot.

>**pulmonary artery:** The major arterial vessel leading from the right ventricle to the lungs.

>**radial artery:** One of the major arteries of the forearm whose pulse is palpable on the lateral wrist at the base of the thumb.

>**temporal artery:** Located on either side of the face just above and in front of the upper portion of the ear. It supplies blood to the scalp.

>**ulnar artery:** A major artery of the foream whose pulse is palpable on the medial wrist at the base of the fifth (little) finger.

articulate: To come together to form joints.

artificial ventilation: Movement of air into and out of the lungs by artificial means.

asphyxia: Suffocation; a condition caused by impaired ventilation and characterized by decreased oxygen and increased carbon dioxide in the blood.

aspirate: To drawn in or out by suction. Thus, one can breathe liquid or other foreign material into the lungs (the child aspirated a button), or such material can be removed from the lungs or elsewhere in the body by mechanical suction (the physician aspirated the button from the child's lungs; blood and pus were aspirated from the wound).

aspirator: An apparatus for removing fluid or other material by suction from a body cavity or opening.

asthma: A condition caused by bronchiolar spasm, characterized by labored breathing, wheezing, a sense of constriction in the chest, and attacks of coughing or gasping.

asystole: Cardiac standstill; absence of any contraction or electrical activity of the heart.

atelectasis: Airlessness of the lungs, caused by failure of the alveoli to expand, or by reabsorption of oxygen from the lungs into the blood.

atherosclerosis: A kind of arteriosclerosis in which the inner layer of the arterial wall is made thick and irregular by deposits of fatty substances and cholesterol. Ultimately it can cause obstruction or destruction of the artery.

atom: The ultimate particle of an element, believed, prior to the 1890s, to be indivisible. The atom is now known to be composed of smaller particles, notably protons, neutrons, and electrons, the first two comprising most of the atomic nucleus.

atomic energy: Energy that can be liberated by changes in the nucleus of an atom, as by fission of a heavy nucleus or fusion of light nuclei into heavier ones.

atrium: Either of the two upper chambers of the heart.

    left atrium: The lesser chamber of the left side of the heart, which receives oxygenated blood from the pulmonary veins, and delivers it to the left ventricle.

    right atrium: The lesser chamber of the right side of the heart which receives unoxygenated blood from the superior and the inferior vena cava, and transmits it to the right ventricle.

audio: Relating to sound waves to which the ear responds. The voice component of a transmitted sound signal.

automatic reaction: An action done without conscious thought, such as breathing.

autonomic nervous system: That portion of the nervous system concerned with the automatic regulation of the activity of cardiac muscle, smooth muscle, and glands.

avulsion: Forcible separation or tearing away of a body part or tissue.

axilla: Armpit.

axillary temperature: The body temperature measured by a thermometer in the axilla with the arm held close to the body for a period of ten minutes.

B

backbone system: A communications system to integrate a number of strategically located base stations into a regional communications system so that a mobile unit anywhere within the service area of the system can communicate with its control center.

bag-valve-mask: A portable artificial ventilation unit consisting of a facemask, a valve, and an inflatable bag.

bag of waters: The amniotic sac and its contained amniotic fluid in which the fetus is enveloped within the uterus.

balanced salt solution: A term describing a solution of water and salts which is so formulated as to resemble normal human blood serum as closely as possible.

ball-and-socket joint: A term describing the type of joint in the hip or shoulder. Such a joint can rotate in a wide range of motions.

band: A term applied to a group of radio wave frequencies.

barbiturate: A sedative or hypnotic agent.

basal cell: The early keratocyte, a cell present in the basal layer of the epidermis.

basal skull fracture: A fracture involving the base of the cranium.

base station: A radio station (transmitter, receiver, and station control) installed at a fixed location and used to communicate with mobile stations.

beeper: A term applied to a selectively activated paging receiver usually carried in one's pocket or on the belt. Upon receiving a page (call) specifically directed to it, the receiver emits a beeping sound.

bends: A disease caused by the pressure of nitrogen gas bubbles in the arteries supplying body tissues. It is characterized by abdominal pain, weakness, joint pains, and occasionally by signs of cerebrovascular occlusion. Also called caisson disease or decompression sickness.

beta particle: An electron, either positively charged (positron) or negatively charged (negatron), which is emitted during beta decay of a radionucleide.

bile: A fluid secreted by the liver and transmitted to the small intestine through the bile ducts. It is required for normal fat digestion and is an end product of the metabolism of red blood cell constituents.

bile ducts: Any of the ducts conveying bile between the liver and the intestine, including hepatic, cystic, and common bile ducts.

biliary system: A ductal system consisting of the gallbladder and the bile ducts connecting the liver to the intestine.

biomedical telemetry: The transmission of biological data from a living subject to a monitoring point by means of radio or wire circuits.

birth canal: The vagina and the lower part of the uterus.

bladder: A musculo-membranous sac serving to collect and store urine.

bladder (gall): *See* gallbladder.

blanch: To become white or pale.

blister: A collection of fluid under the epidermis or within the epidermis.

blood: The "circulating tissue" of the body; the fluid and its suspended, formed elements that are circulated through the heart, arteries, capillaries, and veins. Blood is the means by which (1) oxygen and nutritive materials are transported to the tissues to sustain life, and (2) carbon dioxide and various metabolic products are removed for excretion to cleanse the body.

blood clot: A soft, coherent, jelly-like mass resulting from the conversion of fibrinogen to fibrin, thereby entrapping the red blood cells and other formed elements within the coagulated plasma.

blood pressure: The pressure of the blood on the walls of the arteries, determined by the energy of the heart action, the elasticity of the walls of the arteries, and the volume and viscosity of the blood. *See also* diastolic blood pressure, systolic blood pressure.

blood volume: The total quantity of blood in the body, usually expressed in liters.

blood volume expander: A synthetic solution, administered intravenously to expand blood volume in the treatment of shock.

"bloody show": The mucus and blood that are discharged from the vagina when labor begins, usually one-half to one ounce.

bone: The hard form of connective tissue that constitutes most of the skeleton in most vertebrates.

bony suture: The junction of two bones which have grown together.

Bourdon gauge: A pressure gauge calibrated to record the flowrate of a medical gas from a compressed cylinder.

bowel: *See* intestine.

brachial artery: The artery of the arm that is a continuation of the axillary artery, which in turn branches at the elbow into the radial and ulnar arteries.

bradycardia: Abnormally slow heart rate, generally any rate below sixty beats per minute.

brain: That part of the central nervous system contained within the cranium.

brain contusion: *See* cerebral contusion.

brain stem: The stemlike portion of the brain which connects the brain with the spinal cord.

breech delivery: Delivery of a fetus that presents itself buttocks first or feet first.

bronchial asthma: The common form of asthma.

bronchiole: One of the finer subdivisions of the bronchial tubes, less than one millimeter in diameter, having no cartilage but relatively abundant smooth muscle and elastic fibers in its wall.

bronchitis: Inflammation of the mucous membrane of the bronchial tubes.

bronchus: The two main branches of the trachea that lead into the right and left lungs; any of the larger air passages of the lungs.

burn: A lesion caused by heat or any cauterizing agent.

buttock: The prominence formed by the gluteal muscles on the posterior of either side of the body.

C

caisson disease: *See* bends.

calcaneus: The heel bone.

cannula: A tube that is inserted into a cavity to permit the escape of fluid from the cavity; also a tube inserted into a vessel to permit delivery of fluids or blood.

capillary: Any one of the minute vessels that connect the arterioles and venules, forming a vascular network in all parts of the body.

carbon dioxide: A heavy colorless gas (CO_2) that does not support combustion and dissolves in water to form carbonic acid. It is a normal by-product of body metabolism found in exhaled air.

carbon monoxide: A colorless, odorless, and poisonous gas formed by the incomplete combustion of carbon. Its toxic action when it is inhaled is a result of its strong affinity for hemoglobin and cytochrome, resulting in reduced oxygen transport and blocked oxygen utilization by the body.

cardboard splint. *See* rigid splint.

cardiac: Pertaining to the heart. Sometimes refers to a person who has heart disease, meaning a cardiac patient.

cardiac arrest: A sudden cessation of effective cardiac function, with disappearance of arterial blood pressure.

cardiac arrythmia: *See* arrythmia.

cardiac compression: External heart massage to restore circulation and the pumping action of the heart by artificial means.

cardiac failure: Heart failure; a condition associated with characteristic signs of disturbed cardiac function, such as raised blood pressure, pulmonary edema, and general peripheral edema. Also called congestive heart failure.

cardiac muscle: The muscle of the heart.

cardiac output: The amount of blood pumped out by the heart per minute.

cardiac standstill: Absence of contraction or electrical activity of the heart.

cardiac tamponade: Compression of the heart muscle caused by the accumulation of fluid within the pericardial sac.

cardiogenic: Of cardiac origin.

cardiogenic shock: Shock resulting from decreased cardiac output as a result of primary heart disease; seen in myocardial infarction.

cardiopulmonary resuscitation (CPR): The artificial establishment of circulation of the blood and movement of air into and out of the lungs in a pulseless, non-breathing patient.

cardiovascular: Pertaining to the heart and blood vessels.

carotid artery: The principal artery of the neck arising on the right from the brachiocephalic and on the left from the aortic arch. It runs upward in the neck and divides into the external and internal carotid arteries to supply the face and head and brain respectively. It can be palpated on either side of the neck.

carpal bones: The eight bones of the wrist.

carrier: A person in apparent good health who is infected with some pathogenic organism which in him evokes no manifestations of disease, but which, when accidentally transferred to another, may produce an attack of the disease.

carry: A device or method for carrying patients. *See also* stretcher.

cartilage: A specialized form of connective tissue containing a tough, elastic substance found in joints, at the developing ends of bones, and in specific areas such as the nose and ear.

cartilaginous: Relating to or consisting of cartilage.

catheter: A tube which can be inserted into the body through a passageway to inject or withdraw fluid. Most commonly refers to a tube passed through the urethra into the bladder to drain it of urine in case of retention from any cause.

caustic: Corrosive; exerting an effect resembling a burn.

cecum: A pouch, about 2½ inches in depth, lying below the terminal ileum, into which the ileum opens from one side forming the first part of the large intestine.

cellular hypoxia: A condition resulting from the disturbed function of cells created by enzyme poisoning.

centigrade (Celsius) scale: The temperature scale in which the freezing point of water is zero degrees (0° C) and the boiling point at sea level is one hundred degrees (100° C). *See also* Fahrenheit scale.

centimeter: A unit of measurement equal to about two-fifths of an inch.

central nervous system: That portion of the nervous system consisting of the brain and spinal cord.

central venous pressure: The pressure of the blood in veins which aids in the return of blood to the heart. The pressure is much less than that of the blood in arteries. It is controlled by the blood volume and the capacity of the veins.

centrifugal force: The force that tends to impel a thing or its parts outward from a center of rotation.

cephalic delivery: Delivery of a fetus that presents itself head first. Generally considered to be the normal mode of delivery.

cerebellum: The part of the brain that occupies the posterior cranial fossa behind the brain stem and controls the fine regulation of movement.

cerebral contusion: A bruise of the nervous tissue forming the brain, causing a characteristic symptom response.

cerebral hematoma: A hemorrhage into the substance of the cerebrum.

cerebral vascular accident (CVA): Sometimes called apoplectic stroke, or simply stroke. A condition characterized by impaired blood supply to some part of the brain.

cerebrospinal fluid: The fluid contained within the four ventricles of the brain and the subarachnoid space about the brain and spinal cord.

cerebrum: The main portion of the brain, occupying the upper and anterior part of the cranial cavity. Its two hemispheres, united by the corpus callosum, form the largest part of the central nervous system in man. It is the site of voluntary motor control, the conscious will, and emotions.

cervical spine: The first seven bones of the back, found in the neck.

cervix: The lowermost part of the uterus. The cervix is a tube-like muscular structure forming the lower part of the uterus. It opens into the vagina. The cervix dilates during labor to allow the baby to enter the vagina.

channel: Sometimes used synonymously with "frequency," it is the electronic signal path through which a radio frequency flows.

channel assignment

(by dispatcher): Temporary assignment of a dedicated channel for the time it is needed only.

(by geography): Permanent assignment of a portion of the available channels to a specific area or specific user.

cheek: The side of the face forming the lateral wall of the mouth.

cheekbone: A quadrilateral bone, the zygoma, which forms the prominence of the cheek.

circulatory: Pertaining to the heart, blood vessels, and the circulation of the blood.

circulatory collapse: Failure of the circulation, either cardiac or peripheral.

circulatory hypoxia: A condition resulting from decreased blood flow caused by blood loss, abnormal blood routes, heart failure, arterial obstruction, or venous obstruction.

circulatory system: The body system which consists of the heart and blood vessels.

circumcision: The operation of removing part or all of the foreskin, or prepuce, usually performed a day or two after birth of the male infant.

clammy: Damp and usually cool.

clavicle: The bone articulating with the sternum and scapula; the collarbone.

clinical: A term which refers to the symptoms and course of a disease. The "clinical" course is distinguished from the "findings," which means the anatomical and physiologic effects revealed on laboratory and physical examinations.

clitoris: A small rounded body situated at the most anterior portion of the vulva and projecting between the branched extremities of the labia minora.

closed fracture: A fracture in which there is no communication between the broken bone and the outside environment through the overlying skin.

clot: A coagulation; a thrombus.

cm: Abbreviation for centimeter.

coalesce: To unite into a whole; to mix; to fuse.

coccygeal spine: The lowest segments of the vertebral column, comprising three to five vertebrae which form the coccyx.

429

coccyx: The end of the vertebral column in man, formed by union of four rudimentary caudal vertebrae.

chest: *See* thorax.

chilblain: A chronic injury of the hands or feet characterized by reddish skin, burning, itching, and occasionally chapping and ulceration. It is caused by repeated or prolonged exposure to damp cold.

chill: A feeling of cold with shivering and pallor, accompanied by an elevation of temperature in the interior of the body. Often it is an early symptom of an infectious disease caused by invasion of the blood by bacterial toxins.

chin strap: A strap used to fasten a patient's head to a spineboard.

cholecystitis: Inflammation of the gallbladder.

cholesterol: A fatlike sterol alcohol found in animal fats and oils, milk, and yolk of egg. It can also be found in the body in bile, brain tissue, blood, myelin sheath of nerve fiber, the liver, kidneys, and adrenal glands. In the body it is the major component of gallstones and of the characteristic lesions causing hardening of the arteries.

choroid: The thin, pigmented, vascular coat of the eye extending from the edge of the retina to the optic nerve and carrying the blood vessels for the retina.

chronic obstructive lung disease (chronic obstructive pulmonary disease): A disease caused by the constriction of the major bronchi and bronchioles, resulting in much respiratory distress, especially on respiration.

circuit: The path or course of electricity or other current.

code alert: A means of delivering a specific message or alerting a particular group or team by signaling with voice, bell, light, radio paging, or other means.

coefficient of friction: An expression of the frictional force developed when two surfaces pass across one another; useful in predicting the number of feet required to stop a vehicle at a given speed, on a given surface, under specific circumstances.

coffee grounds vomitus: Vomitus having the appearance and consistency of coffee grounds. It indicates slow bleeding in the stomach and represents the vomiting of partially digested blood.

colic: Of or pertaining to the colon. Also an acute abdominal pain characterized by intermittent cramps, common in infants and young children.

collarbone: The clavicle.

Colles' fracture: A fracture of the distal end of the radius. This fracture can, at times, be accompanied by a fracture of a small fragment of the ulnar styloid process.

colon: That part of the large intestine which extends from the ileo-cecal valve to the rectum.

coma: A state of unconsciousness from which the patient cannot be aroused, even by powerful stimulation.

comatose: In a state of coma.

come-a-long: A hand-operated winch of varying capacity (two-ton capacity is standard for ambulance equipment) used to effect forceful entry, for example, to gain access to a patient trapped in a wrecked car.

comminuted fracture: A fracture in which the bone ends are broken into many fragments.

common bile duct: The duct formed by the union of the common hepatic ducts and the cystic duct; it empties into the duodenum.

communicable disease: A disease which can be transmitted from one person to another.

communicable period: The time during which an infectious agent may be transferred from one host to another.

communication control center: The location from which a communication system is controlled.

communications console: A group of controls, indicators, and monitoring equipment integrated into one functional unit, used to control communication functions.

compartment syndrome: The shocklike state that follows release of a limb after a prolonged period of compression. It is brought about by compression of the arterial blood supply to a muscular compartment.

compound fracture: Open fracture; one in which there is an open wound of the skin and soft parts leading down to the seat of fracture.

concussion: A jarring injury of the brain resulting from a hard blow on the head or from a collision, and causing a variety of transient neurological symptoms.

conduction: The act of transmitting or conveying certain forms of energy, such as heat, sound, or electricity, from one point to another without evident movement in the conducting body.

conductivity: The power of transmitting or conveying certain forms of energy.

conductor: Any substance possessing conductivity.

congestive heart failure: *See* cardiac failure.

conjunctiva: The delicate membrane that lines the eyelids and covers the exposed surface of the optic sclerae.

connective tissue: The body tissue which binds together and is the support of the various structures of the body. It is made of fibroblasts, fibroglia, collagen fibrils, and elastic fibrils.

conscious action: Something occurring as a result of the perceptive attention of the individual, as distinguished from automatic or instinctive response or activity.

consciousness: The state of being conscious. Responsiveness of the mind to the impressions made by the senses.

constriction: Binding or contraction of a part.

contagious disease: An infectious disease transmissible by direct or indirect contact; now synonymous with communicable disease.

contaminated: Soiled with infectious matter.

contaminated with radioactive material: Exposed to and bearing radioactive material on the surface.

continuous duty: A rating applied to receivers and transmitters to indicate their capability for use in a continuous-duty cycle (as opposed to intermittent duty).

continuous telemetry: The transmission of measured data in a continuous, uninterrupted stream, as contrasted to short bursts. Continuous telemetry transmission by radio requires one channel per transmission, whereas burst techniques permit time-sharing of a single communications channel.

contraction: A shortening. In connection with muscles, contraction implies shortening and the development of tension.

contusion: The reaction of body soft tissue to a direct blow. A bruise, characterized by edema and ecchymosis of the tissue.

convection: The conveyance of heat in liquid or gaseous form by the movement of heated particles, as when the warm air of a room ascends to the ceiling. The loss of body heat to the atmosphere when air passes over the body.

convulsion: Abnormal violent and involuntary contractions of the voluntary musculature. A fit or seizure, such as can be precipitated by poison, certain drugs, drug withdrawal, or epilepsy.

core temperature: A body temperature measured centrally, for example from within the esophagus or rectum.

cornea: The transparent tissue layer in front of the pupil and the iris of the eye.

cornering force: The force that results from turning the steering wheel of an automobile and creating a drag of the tires strong enough to shove the tire over, thereby changing the direction of travel of the vehicle.

cornified: Converted into horny tissue; keratinized; describing the most external layer of the epidermis.

coronary arteries: The two arteries arising from the aorta, arching down over the top of the heart, and conducting blood to the heart muscle.

431

coronary artery disease: A disease resulting from an irregular thickening of the inner layer of the walls of the coronary arteries which conduct blood to the myocardium; the lumens of these arteries are narrowed and the blood supply to the heart muscle is reduced.

coronary thrombosis: The obstruction of a coronary artery by a clot.

corrosive: An agent that produces corrosion, as an acid.

corrosion: The wearing away gradually by pressure or by dissolution, as in the case of tissues distended by a tumor or an aneurysm.

cosmic rays: High-velocity particles of enormous energies bombarding earth from outer space. The primary radiation consists of protons and more complex atomic nuclei, which on striking the atmosphere give rise to neutrons, mesons, and other less energetic secondary radiating particles.

costal arch: The fused costal cartilages of ribs 7 to 10; the arch forms the upper limit of the abdomen.

costo-vertebral angle: The angle formed by the spinal column and the twelfth rib; the general anatomic location of the kidneys.

CPR: Abbreviation for cardiopulmonary resuscitation.

cramp: A painful spasm, usually of a muscle; a gripping pain in the abdominal area, colic.

cranial: Relating to the cranium.

cranium: The skeleton of the head, variously construed as including all of the bones of the head except the mandible; those bones forming the vault that lodges the brain.

crepitus: A general term given to describe an abnormal sensation; the grating sensation of the two ends of a broken bone rubbing together; the bubbly sensation of air palpated in tissues; a specific crackling sound heard in the lung with the stethoscope when pneumonia is present.

cricoid cartilage: The lowermost of the laryngeal cartilages.

crico-thyroidotomy: An incision into the lower airway through the crico-thyroid membrane.

cricothyrotome: A surgical instrument used to make an opening into the trachea through the crico-thyroid membrane (fibrous portion of the larynx).

crossbanding: Using VHF equipment to participate in the UHF band of radio frequencies.

crowning (bulging): The bulging-out of the vaginal opening that occurs when the presenting part of the baby presses on it. The presenting part, often the top of the baby's head, may or may not be visible.

crushed chest: *See* flail chest.

current: A stream or flow of fluid, air, or electricity.

cutaneous: Relating to the skin.

CVA: Abbreviation for cerebro-vascular accident.

cyanosis: A bluish or purplish discoloration of the skin due to a lack of oxygen in the blood.

cyanotic: Marked by cyanosis; having a bluish color about the lips or nailbeds.

cyclic: Occurring periodically.

D

D₅W: A solution of 50 grams of dextrose (glucose) in 1,000 ml of sterile water.

D₁₀W: A solution of 100 grams of dextrose (glucose) in 1,000 ml of sterile water.

decerebrate: A condition resulting from a brain injury which renders voluntary muscular control and conscious action impossible. Patients in this state assume characteristic postures and exhibit characteristic signs.

decibel: A unit for expressing the degree of loudness of sound.

decompression sickness: *See* bends.

decontaminate: To rid clothing, bed linen, a room, or vehicle of dangerous substances such as poisonous gases, germs, or the sputum, feces, or urine of a patient; usually used in connection with contagious diseases, also with radioactive contamination.

decreasing-radius turn: A curve that becomes increasingly tighter as one drives into it.

dedicated channel: A radio channel established between the dispatcher and one EMT that is free from interference by other users.

de-energized: Rendered free from electrical current; inert.

defecate: to discharge excrement from the rectum.

defibrillator: Any agent or measure, such as an electric shock, used to stop an incoordinated contraction of the heart muscle and restore a normal heartbeat.

deformity: A deviation from normal shape or size, resulting in disfigurement; may be congenital or acquired.

dehydration: The lack or absence of water or fluid—a serious state in living bodies.

delirium: A condition of extreme excitement, marked by a rapid succession of confused and unconnected ideas, often with delusions and hallucinations.

delirium tremens (DTs): A form of insanity, often temporary, due to alcoholic poisoning, marked by sweating, tremor, restlessness, precordial distress, mental confusion, and hallucinations.

demand-valve unit: An intermittent positive-pressure breathing unit used to assist or control ventilation with a valve connected to the oxygen that opens in response to the patient's inspiratory effort and inflates the lungs until a preset pressure limit is reached. Alternatively, the unit can be manually controlled. Illegal on ambulances unless manual control is provided.

Demerol: Meperidine hydrochloride. A narcotic, analgesic, sedative, and antispasmodic which may produce physiologic and psychic dependence.

demulcent: An agent, such as a mucilage or oil, that soothes and relieves irritation, especially of the mucous surfaces.

depressant: An agent that lowers nervous or functional activity; a sedative.

depressed fracture: A skull fracture with impaction, depression, or sinking in of the fragments.

depression: Dejection, a sinking of spirits; a low area.

dermis: The inner layer of the skin, containing the skin appendages, hair follicles, sweat glands, nerves, and blood vessels.

dextran: A water-soluble polysaccharide used as a synthetic plasma volume-expander in infusions.

dextrose: Glucose.

diabetes: A general term referring to disorders characterized by excessive urine excretion.

diabetes mellitus: A metabolic disease in which carbohydrate utilization is reduced and that of lipid and protein enhanced. It is caused by deficiency of insulin.

diabetic coma: Deep unconsciousness as a result of severe uncontrolled diabetes.

diabetic ketoacidosis: *See under* acidosis.

diabetic patient: A person with excessive amounts of sugar in the blood as a result of inadequate secretion or utilization of insulin by the body.

diagnostic signs: Subjective and objective evidence of a patient's physiologic state and of specific disease processes.

diaphragm: A flat, circular sheet of muscle separating the thoracic and abdominal cavities.

diarrhea: An abnormally frequent discharge of more or less fluid fecal matter from the bowel.

diastole: The dilation, or period of dilation, of the heart, especially of the ventricles; it coincides with the interval between the second and the first heart sounds, sometimes called the resting period.

diastolic blood pressure: Lower blood pressure noted during ventricular relaxation as the heart fills with blood.

digestion: The process or act of converting food into simple chemical substances that can be absorbed by the intestine.

digestive tract: The passage leading from the mouth to the anus through the pharynx, esophagus, stomach, and intestine.

433

dilated pupil: A pupil enlarged from its normal size.

diplopia: Double vision; the condition in which a single object is perceived as two.

direct contact: A means of transmitting a communicable disease directly by touching or being touched by an infected person.

direct-leased land line: A point-to-point telephone line to be used only for a specific purpose or service.

dislocation: The displacement of the ends of two bones at their joint so that the joint surfaces are no longer in proper contact.

disoriented: Having lost the sense of familiarity with one's surroundings.

dispatcher: One who transmits calls to service units, sending vehicles and EMTs on emergency assignments.

distal: Farthest from the center or the median line; in the extremities, farthest from the point of junction with the trunk of the body.

distention: The act or state of being distended or stretched.

dorsalis pedis artery: The artery whose pulse is palpable on the dorsal surface of the foot; it supplies the medial foot and great toe.

dorsiflexion: Turning of the foot or the toes upward.

drag: A general term referring to methods of moving a patient or patients without a stretcher or litter. Usually employed by a single rescuer.

  blanket drag: A method by which one EMT encloses a patient in a blanket and drags him to safety.

  clothes drag: A method by which one EMT can drag a patient to safety by grasping his clothes.

  fireman's drag: A method by which one EMT crawls with a patient, looping the patient's tied wrists over his neck to support the patient's weight.

drag force: The force that causes a scrubbing action or drag of the tire on the road surface when a vehicle is turned, thus slowing the speed of the vehicle.

drape: A sterile covering used about an operative site to decrease the chance of contamination from surroundings; also, the act of placing such a sterile covering about an operative site.

dressing: Sterile gauze or compresses of various sizes applied for protection of a wound and fixed in position; a bandage.

drift angle: The angle that is formed when the steering wheel is turned and the center line of the front tires heads away from the direction in which the vehicle is traveling.

droplet contact: A means of transmitting a communicable disease indirectly by droplets in the spray from an infected person's coughing or sneezing.

drown: To suffocate by submersion, especially in water.

DTs: Abbreviation for delirium tremens.

dumbcane: A tropical American herb (Dieffenbachia seguine) that when chewed causes the tongue to swell. The reaction can be severe enough to cause obstruction of the airway.

duodenum: The first or most proximal portion of the small intestine, extending from the pylorus to the jejunum.

dura mater: The outermost, toughest, and most fibrous of the three membranes covering the brain

dysfunction: Impaired or abnormal function.

dyspnea: Difficult or labored breathing.

E

eardrum (tympanum): A thin, tense membrane forming the greater part of the outer wall of the tympanic cavity and separating it from the external auditory canal; it constitutes the boundary between the outer and the middle ear.

ecchymosis: A discoloration of the skin resulting from subcutaneous and intracutaneous hemorrhage. Bluish in color at first, later it changes to a greenish yellow because of chemical changes in the pooled blood.

eclampsia: The occurrence of one or more convulsions, not attributable to other cerebral conditions such as epilepsy or cerebral hemorrhage, in a patient with pre-eclampsia; a toxic condition of unknown etiology associated with some pregnancies.

edema: A condition in which fluid escapes into the tissues from vascular or lymphatic spaces and causes local or generalized swelling.

egg cell: A female reproductive cell.

ejaculation: A sudden act of expulsion; the expulsion of semen during sexual intercourse.

elastic tissue: A specialized tissue, lying in the lung and the great vessels and large arteries, capable of stretching and recoiling.

electrocardiogram: A graphic tracing of the electric current produced by the excitation of the heart muscle.

electrocution: Death caused by electricity.

electrolyte: A substance that dissociates into ions when in solution and that is capable of conducting electricity. Most common salts are electrolytes.

electron: One of the negatively charged subatomic particles that, distributed about the positively charged nucleus, constitute the atom.

embolism: The blocking of a blood vessel by a clot or other substance carried in the blood stream to that point.

embolus: A blood clot (or other substance such as an air bubble or fat globule) inside a blood vessel which is carried in the blood stream to a smaller vessel where it becomes an obstruction to circulation.

emesis: Vomiting.

emphysema: A disease of the lung characterized by extreme dilation of pulmonary air sacs and poor exchange of oxygen and carbon dioxide in the lung. It causes rapid, shallow breathing and frequently results in a secondary impairment of heart action.

endoscope: An instrument for the examination of the interior of a canal or hollow viscus.

endothelium: A layer of flat cells lining blood and lymphatic vessels; it corresponds to the mesothelium of the serous cavities.

endotracheal: Within the trachea.

endotracheal tube: A tube which can be inserted into the trachea through the nose or mouth as an artificial airway.

energize: To make an electric circuit alive by applying voltage to allow current to flow through it.

enteritis: Inflammation of the intestine, applied chiefly to inflammation of the small intestine, characterized by fluid loss through diarrhea.

envenomation: The act of depositing poisonous toxins.

enzyme: A protein, capable of accelerating or producing by catalytic (helping) action some chemical change in another substance or substrate.

epidermis: The outermost layer of the skin, varying in thickness from 1/200 to 1/20 inch, and containing cornified (keratinized or horny), external protecting cells.

epidural: External to the dura mater.

epidural hematoma: A collection of blood or a clot caused by a laceration or rupture of a meningeal vessel lying external to the dura mater.

epiglottis: The lid-like cartilaginous structure overhanging the superior entrance to the larynx and serving to prevent food from entering the larynx and trachea while swallowing.

epilepsy: A chronic disorder characterized by paroxysmal attacks of brain dysfunction usually associated with some alteration of consciousness. The attacks may remain confined to impaired behavior or may progress to a generalized convulsion.

epileptic patient: A person suffering from a chronic nervous disorder characterized by attacks of unconsciousness or convulsions or both.

epinephrine: A hormone released predominantly in response to hypoglycemia, and causing cardiac stimulation, peripheral vasoconstriction, and bronchodilation.

epiphyseal injury: An injury that results in a break of a bone at the cartilaginous epiphyses, or growth centers at the ends of the long bones. The most common site for these injuries is the distal radial epiphysis.

epiphyseal plate: The disc of cartilage between the shaft and the epiphysis of a long bone during its growth.

epiphysis (epiphyseal plate): A part of a long bone developed from a center of ossification distinct from that of the shaft and separated at first from the latter by a layer of cartilage.

epistaxis: A nosebleed.

epithelium: The purely cellular, avascular layer covering all the free surfaces of the body—cutaneous, mucous, and serous.

erectile tissue: Tissue containing large vascular spaces which fill with blood on stimulation, as in the penis and clitoris.

erythema: Redness of the skin produced by congestion of the capillaries. It may result from a variety of causes, and the cause is usually indicated by a specific term.

erythrocyte: One of the cellular elements found in blood; the red blood cell or corpuscle; the cell in which oxygen is carried in the blood.

eschar: A thick, coagulated crust or slough which develops after a thermal burn or cauterization or laceration of the skin; a scab.

esophagus: The passage leading from the pharynx to the stomach, comprising a muscular tube lined with squamous (skin-like) epithelium.

etiology: The study of causes of disease.

euphoria: A feeling of well-being and "happiness," commonly exaggerated.

evaporation: A change in a compound from liquid to vapor form.

everted: Turned outward.

evisceration: Disembowelling; the protrusion of viscera from any body cavity or through an open wound.

excoriation: A scratch mark or linear break in the skin surface, usually covered with blood or serous crusts.

excretion: The process whereby the residue of food and the waste products of metabolism are eliminated.

expiration: The act of breathing out or expelling air from the lungs.

extension: The act of straightening; the movement by which the two ends of any jointed part are drawn away from each other.

extrication: To free or remove from a difficult situation or position; often used to signify recovery of a patient from a car wreck or other place of entrapment.

eye: The organ of vision.

F

facemask: A device for administration of anesthetic gases or oxygen.

Fahrenheit scale: The temperature scale in which the freezing point of water is thirty-two degrees (32° F) and the boiling point at sea level is 212 degrees (212° F). Zero indicates the lowest Fahrenheit temperature that can be obtained with a mixture of ice and salt. *See also* centigrade scale.

faint: A temporary loss of consciousness, usually of brief duration and not serious.

fallopian tube: A long slender tube that extends from the uterus to the region of the ovary on the same side. It is a passageway for the ovum from ovary to uterus.

436

false motion: Motion of an extremity or a part of the body where ordinarily there should be none, indicative of a fracture. Motion of the two ends of a fractured bone against one another.

fascia: A sheet or band of tough fibrous tissue; fascia lies deep under the skin and forms an outer layer for the muscles and various organs of the body.

fatigue fracture: A fracture in which the bone breaks because of repeated stress that can no longer be tolerated by that particular bone. It can involve bones in the foot or leg.

fatty acid: Any acid derived from fats by hydrolysis.

febrile: Feverish; having a fever.

feces: Excrement or matter discharged from the bowel during defecation, consisting of the undigested residue of the food, intestinal mucosal cells, intestinal mucus, bacteria, and waste material from the food.

femoral artery: The principal artery of the thigh, a continuation of the external iliac artery. It supplies blood to the lower abdominal wall, the external genitalia, and the lower extremity.

femoral condyle: The rounded articular surface at the extremity of the femur, or thigh bone.

femoral nerve: A major peripheral nerve, originating in the lumbosacral plexus.

femoral vein: A continuation of the popliteal vein that becomes the external iliac vein; the major vein draining the leg.

femur: The bone that extends from the pelvis to the knee, the longest and largest bone in the body; the "thigh bone."

fetal death certificate: The certificate required when a baby is born dead (stillbirth). Most states regard stillbirths of less than twenty weeks pregnancy as abortions and may or may not require registration of a birth.

fetus: The developing baby before it is born.

fever: An elevation of body temperature above normal.

fibrillation: uncoordinated contraction of the heart muscle occurring when the individual muscle fibers take up independent, irregular activity; it causes the loss of effective cardiac function.

fibrosis: The formation of fibrous tissue or scar, usually as a reparative or reactive process.

fibula: The outer and smaller of the two bones of the leg, extending from just below the knee to form the lateral wall of the ankle joint.

flail chest: A condition of the chest wall following an injury, characterized by a free segment which moves paradoxically (opposite to normal motion) when the patient breathes; it is caused by fractures of several (at least 3) ribs in two or more places each.

flail segment: That segment of the chest wall in a flail chest injury lying between the rib fractures and moving paradoxically with respiration.

flexible splint: *See* rigid splint.

flexion: The act of bending, or the movement by which the two ends of any jointed part are drawn closer to one another.

flowmeter: A measuring device to measure the rate of flow of any agent introduced into a patient, e.g., oxygen, or intravenous fluid. Specifically, in this text, it is used in connection with the use of oxygen.

flowrate: The rate at which oxygen flows from a cylinder. The flowrate can be adjusted by a flowrate control.

follicle (hair): A deep, narrow pit containing the root of the hair. The duct of the sebaceous gland opens into it.

foot: The distal portion of the vertebrate leg, upon which an individual stands and walks.

foot-drop: Paralysis of the dorsiflexor muscles of the foot and ankle, as a consequence of which the foot falls and the toes drag on the ground in walking.

footprint area: Area of a tire that is in contact with the surface of the road.

forearm: The part of the upper limb of the body between the elbow and the wrist.

foreskin: The free fold of skin that covers the glans penis more or less completely.

four-man log roll (the back-injury roll): A method of placing a patient on a carrying device, usually a long spineboard or a flat litter by rolling him on his side, then back onto a litter.

fracture: Any break in a bone. In a fracture the bones may be separated into several pieces, clearly broken, or only cracked and bent.

basal skull fracture: A fracture involving the base of the cranium.

closed fracture: A fracture in which there is no laceration in the overlying skin and thus no communication between the broken bone and the outside environment.

Colles' fracture: A fracture of the distal end of the radius. This fracture can, at times, be accompanied by a fracture of a small fragment of the ulnar styloid process.

comminuted fracture: A fracture in which the bone ends are broken into many fragments.

compound fracture: Open fracture; one in which there is an open wound of the skin and soft parts leading down to the seat of fracture.

depressed fracture: A skull fracture with impaction, depression, or sinking in of the fragments.

fatigue fracture: A fracture in which the bone breaks because of repeated stress that cannot be tolerated by that particular bone. It can involve bones in the foot or leg.

fracture-dislocation: A fracture of a bone near an articulation with a concomitant dislocation at that joint.

fracture of the hip: A fracture which occurs at the upper end of the femur, close to the hip joint.

greenstick fracture: An incomplete fracture causing partial disruption and bending of a bone; occurs only in a child.

linear fracture: A fracture running parallel to the long axis of the bone.

linear skull fracture: A skull fracture in a straight line.

muscle avulsion fracture: A tearing away of a part of a bone, usually by tendon, ligament, or capsule.

oblique fracture: One which runs obliquely to the axis of the bone.

open fracture (or open dislocation): A fracture or a dislocation having a direct communication with the outside through the skin. There may be a small wound over the fracture or dislocation or the ends of the bone may be protruding through the skin.

pathological fracture: A fracture in which a specific weakness or destruction of bone caused by some process like cancer is the reason for the break.

simple fracture: An uncomplicated fracture. Not compound; the skin not broken over the injury.

spiral fracture: One in which the line of break runs obliquely up one side of the bone.

supracondylar fracture: A fracture of the distal end of the humerus, just above the condyles.

transverse fracture: A fracture whose line forms a right angle with the axis of the bone.

fracture-dislocation: A fracture of a bone near an articulation with a dislocation also at that joint.

frequency: The number of cycles, repetitions, or oscillations of a periodic process completed during a given unit of time.

frontal lobe: The anterior portion of the cerebrum of the brain; the site of emotional control.

frostbite: Local tissue destruction caused by freezing. Deeper destruction than frost nip.

frost nip: Superficial local tissue destruction caused by freezing; it is limited in scope and does not destroy the full thickness of the skin.

fuse: Unite or join together.

fused joint: A joint that forms a solid, immobile, bony structure, as in the skull.

G

galea aponeurotica: The fibrous aponeurosis connecting the occipitalis muscle posteriorly and the frontalis anteriorly and covering the skull; the tissue underlying the scalp.

gallbladder: A pear-shaped, membranous sac on the undersurface of the liver, serving to collect and store bile.

gamma rays: Electromagnetic radiations emitted from radioactive substances; analogous to the X ray.

gangrene: Necrosis due to obstruction of blood supply; it may be localized to a small area or involve an entire extremity.

gas gangrene: A disease originating in a wound infected with clostridium perfringens; it results in rapid local destruction of tissue and death of the patient.

gastric juice: The digestive fluid secreted by the glands of the stomach; it is a thin, colorless liquid of acid reaction, containing mainly hydrochloric acid, pepsin, and mucus.

gastrointestinal tract: The digesting tract of the body including the stomach, small bowel, large bowel, rectum, and anus.

Geiger counter: An instrument consisting of a Geiger-Muller tube and the electronic equipment used in conjunction with it to record the momentary current pulsations in the tube gas produced by the passage of radioactive particles.

genitalia: The reproductive organs.

genital system: The system including all the organs concerned in reproduction.

genitourinary system: System including all the organs concerned in reproduction of the species, and in the formation and voiding of urine.

geographic area use: *See under* channel assignment.

germicidal: Destructive to germs (microbes).

glenohumeral joint: The shoulder joint; the joint between the upper end of the humerus and the scapula.

glenoid fossa: The hollow in the head of the scapula that receives the head of the humerus to make the shoulder joint.

glottis: The vocal apparatus of the larynx, consisting of the true vocal cords and the opening between them.

glucose: One of the simple sugars; free glucose occurs in the blood (normal human concentration, 80 to 120 mg per 100 ml); in diabetes mellitus, it appears in the urine. It is the principal source of energy for man and many other organisms. *See also* dextrose.

gonorrhea: A contagious inflammation of the genital mucous membrane; the most common venereal disease.

grand mal epilepsy: Epilepsy characterized by a generalized convulsive seizure.

granuloma: Any one of a large group of distinctive focal lesions that are granule-like or nodular, are formed as a result of inflammatory reactions, and ordinarily persist in the tissue as slowly smoldering inflammations.

greater trochanter: *See under* trochanter.

greenstick fracture: An incomplete fracture causing partial disruption and bending of a bone; occurs only in a child.

groin: The inguinal region; the topographical area of the abdomen related to the inguinal canal, lateral to the pubic region.

G suit: An inflatable coverall suit which can be used to exert general body compression; originally adapted for astronauts so they could safely endure the force of sufficient acceleration to leave the gravitational pull of the earth.

gullet (esophagus): The passage leading from the pharynx to the stomach, comprising a muscular tube lined with squamous (skin-like) epithelium.

gums: The dense fibrous tissue, covered by mucous membrane, that envelops the alveolar processes of the upper and lower jaws and surrounds the necks of the teeth.

H

Hg: Chemical symbol for mercury.

H_2O: Chemical symbol for water.

half-ring splint: A traction splint with a hinged half-ring at the upper end, which allows the splint to be used on either the right or the left leg.

hallucination: A subjective perception of what does not exist; the individual imagines he sees, hears, or smells that which is actually not present.

hallucinogen: A hallucinatory chemical, drug, or agent, specifically a chemical whose most prominent action is on the central nervous system. An example is mescaline.

hand: The part of the upper limb distal to the forearm; the carpus, metacarpus, and fingers together.

head: The upper extremity of the body, containing the brain and the organs of sight, hearing, taste, and smell.

head band: A band used to fasten a patient's head to a spineboard.

head-tilt maneuver: Procedure for opening the airway to relieve obstruction caused by the tongue. With one hand beneath the patient's neck and one hand on the patient's forehead, the neck is lifted and the head tilted backward as far as possible.

heart: A hollow muscular organ which receives the blood from the veins and propels it into the arteries.

heart attack: *See* myocardial infarction.

heat collapse: *See* heat exhaustion.

heat cramps: Muscle spasms induced by hard work in intense heat accompanied by severe pain; usually caused by depletion of the electrolytes in the body through sweating.

heat exhaustion: A form of reaction to heat, marked by prostration, weakness, and collapse, resulting from unrecognized or unavoidable dehydration.

heat prostration: *See* heat exhaustion.

heat stroke: A condition that results from prolonged exposure to high temperature, characterized by cessation of sweating, extremely high body temperature, and collapse. Extremely serious and often rapidly fatal. Also often called sunstroke.

hematemesis: The vomiting of blood.

hematochezia: The passage of grossly bloody stools or bright red blood from the rectum.

hematoma: A localized mass of extravasated blood that is relatively or completely confined within an organ or tissue, a space, or a potential space; the blood is usually clotted or partly clotted.

hematuria: Any condition in which the urine contains blood or red blood cells.

hemic hypoxia: A condition of insufficient oxygen in the blood related to a diminished capacity of the red blood cells to carry oxygen.

hemithorax: One side of the chest.

hemopneumothorax: Accumulation of air and blood in the pleural cavity.

hemoptysis: Coughing or spitting of blood or of blood-stained sputum.

hemorrhage: The escape of blood from the vessels; bleeding copiously, either internally or externally.

hemorrhagic shock: Shock resulting from hemorrhage sufficient to reduce blood volume markedly.

hemostat: Any agent that arrests, chemically or mechanically, the flow of blood from an open vessel; an instrument for arresting hemorrhage by compression of the bleeding vessel.

hemothorax: Collection of blood in the pleural cavity, outside the lung.

heroin: Diacetylmorphine; an alkaloid prepared from morphine by acetylization. Formerly used for the relief of coughs. Because of the great danger of addiction following use of the drug, its manufacture and importation into the United States is prohibited by federal law.

hinge joint: A joint in which a convexity on one bone fits into a corresponding concavity on the other, allowing motion in one plane only, as in the elbow.

hip: The lateral prominence of the pelvis from the waist to the thigh; more strictly the hip joint.

hip joint: The ball-and-socket joint between the head of the femur and the acetabular fossa.

hives: Red or white raised patches on the skin, often attended by severe itching; a characteristic reaction in an allergic response.

hormone: A chemical substance, produced in the body by a gland or cells of a gland, which has a specific regulatory effect on the activity of another distant organ.

host: The organism which a parasite lives in or on.

hot sticks: Wooden sticks which are rendered non-conductive by special treating; used to manipulate electric wires.

"hot" wire: A wire through which an electric current is passing. A "live" wire.

humeral epicondyle: A projection from the humerus near the articular extremity above or upon the condyle.

humerus: The bone that extends from the shoulder to the elbow.

humidification: The process of adding water to a gas, making it humid or moist.

humidifier: A device used with an oxygen supply to moisten the oxygen and prevent its drying effect on the nose or throat of the patient.

humidity: Moisture or dampness, as of the air.

humor: The extracellular fluids of the body: blood and lymph.

hydraulic-powered unit: A hand-operated hydraulic device, of varying capacity, used with attachments for the forceful raising, pushing apart, or pulling of vehicles or material. Useful in reaching and extricating trapped patients.

hydrochloric acid: The acid of gastric juice. The gas and the concentrated solution are strong irritants.

hydroplaning: Moving over the surface of water; the action of a vehicle skimming over a wet road with the tires not in direct contact with the surface but more or less clear of it because they are riding on a film of water.

hyper-: A prefix meaning excessive, above the normal.

hyperactive: Excessively or pathologically active.

hyperextension: Extension of a limb or part beyond the normal limit.

hyperflexion: Flexion of a limb or part beyond the normal limit.

hypertension: Commonly called high blood pressure; an unstable or persistent elevation of blood pressure above the normal range, which may eventually cause increased heart size and general visceral damage.

hyperthermia: Unusually high fever.

hyperventilation: Increased pulmonary ventilation beyond that needed to maintain the blood gases (arterial levels of oxygen and carbon dioxide) within the normal ranges; the expiration of excessive amounts of carbon dioxide causes a number of symptoms, including dizziness.

hypnotic: Medication causing sleep.

hypo-: A prefix equivalent to sub-, meaning beneath, a lessening or deficiency, the lowest, or least rich, in oxygen (as hypoxia).

hypoglycemia: An abnormally small concentration of glucose in the circulating blood, less than the minimum of the normal range.

hypotension: Commonly called low blood pressure; a blood pressure below the normal range; most commonly it means an acute fall in blood pressure.

hypothalamus: The portion of the brainstem which activates, controls, and integrates peripheral autonomic mechanisms, endocrine activity, water balance, and automatic functions such as sleep.

hypothermia: A body temperature below 98.6° F (37° C).

hypovolemia: Abnormally decreased volume of circulating blood in the body.

hypovolemic shock: Shock caused by a reduction in volume of blood, resulting (1) from hemorrhage or (2) from relaxation of blood vessel walls, causing the vascular system to develop such a large capacity that adequate circulation cannot be maintained.

hypoxia: Low oxygen content in the blood; deficiency of oxygen in inspired air.

hypoxic hypoxia: A condition resulting from decreased oxygen reaching the blood in the lungs.

I

ileocecal valve: The protrusion of the terminal ileum into the large intestine at the ileocolic junction; it protects the terminal ileum from feces forced back from the cecum.

441

ileum: The most distal portion of the small intestine, between the jejunum and the colon.

ileus: An obstruction of the bowel commonly resulting from paralysis of bowel motility caused by peritonitis or other inflammatory processes.

ilium: The expansive superior portion of the hip bone; it is a separate bone in early childhood.

immersion foot: A disorder of the feet following prolonged immersion in water, as after a shipwreck. When first removed from the water, the feet are swollen, cold, waxy white with cyanotic areas, and anesthetic. A short time later the parts become red and hot and the swelling increases.

immobilize: To make incapable of moving.

immune: Resistant to an infectious disease.

immunization: Vaccination; allergization; the process or procedure by which resistance is produced in a person, animal, or plant.

impaled: Pierced with something pointed.

incubation: The development of an infection from the time it gains entry to the body until the appearance of the first signs or symptoms.

incubator: A device, usually a crib, which provides protection and temperature control for a newborn infant.

indirect contact: A means of transmitting a communicable disease indirectly by touching contaminated objects such as soiled dressings or clothing.

infarct: An area of a tissue which is damaged or dies as a result of not receiving a sufficient blood supply; frequently used in the phrase *myocardial infarct* or myocardial infarction (*see under* M).

infect: To enter, invade, or inhabit another organism, causing infection or contamination.

infection: Multiplication of microorganisms in the body proper.

infectious: Capable of being transmitted by infection, with or without actual contact.

inferior: Lower, or toward the lower end.

inferior vena cava: *See under* vena cava.

infrared: Beyond the red end of the spectrum; a section of the electromagnetic spectrum invisible to the eye and characterized by waves of increasing length.

infusion: The administration intravenously by gravity of any of a number of cell-free fluids.

ingestion: The act of taking food, medicine, or other substances, into the body by mouth.

inguinal: Relating to the groin.

inhalation: The drawing of air or other substances into the lungs. Often referred to as inspiration.

injection: The act of forcing a liquid into a part of the body, as into the subcutaneous tissues, the blood vessels, or an organ, through a needle or other tube introduced through the skin.

innocuous: Harmless.

innominate: A term applied to certain structures formed by the fusion of other separate structures.

innominate bone: The bone forming one half of the pelvic girdle and arising from a fusion of the ilium, the ischium, and the pubis.

innominate artery: The brachiocephalic artery in the right giving rise to the right subclavian and right common carotid arteries.

insertion of muscle: The place of attachment of a muscle to the bone which it moves.

inspiration: The act of breathing in or drawing air into the lungs. Often called inhalation.

insulation: A nonconducting substance which offers a barrier to the passage of heat or electricity.

insulin: A protein hormone secreted into the blood, where it regulates carbohydrate metabolism.

insulin shock: Hypoglycemic shock produced by the administration of excessive amounts of insulin; the chief symptoms are sweating, tremor, anxiety, vertigo, and diplopia, followed by delirium, convulsions, and collapse.

integument: A covering or investment; the skin.

442   **internuncial neuron:** Any neuron, in a chain of neurons, which is situated between the primary afferent neuron and the final motor (efferent) neuron.

intertrochanteric area: The area between the two trochanters of the femur.

intervertebral cartilage: *See* intervertebral discs.

intervertebral discs: Layers of fibrocartilage between the bodies of adjacent vertebrae.

intestine: The portion of the alimentary canal extending from the pyloric opening of the stomach to the anus.

   large intestine: The portion of the digestive tube extending from the ileocecal valve to the anus and comprised of the cecum, colon, and rectum. The large bowel.

   small intestine: The portion of the digestive tube between the stomach and the cecum, consisting of three portions: duodenum, jejunum, and ileum. The small bowel.

intoxicate: To excite or stupefy by alcohol or a narcotic, to the point where physical and mental control is markedly diminished.

intracerebral: Within the cerebrum.

intracerebral hematoma: Extravasation of blood within the brain substance.

intracranial: Within the skull.

intramuscular: Within the substance of a muscle.

intravenous: Within a vein.

intravenous agents: Substances, drugs, fluids, or blood products introduced into a patient by way of a vein for the purpose of hydration, to increase the volume of the circulating blood, or to provide faster action of a compound (drug).

intussusception: Telescoping of a segment of the intestine into the next most distal one.

inversion: A turning inward, as of the eyelid, or the foot.

involuntary action: Action performed independent of the will; not voluntary.

involuntary muscle: Muscle not under control of the will. Except in the case of the heart, it is smooth (nonstriated) muscle.

ion: An atom or group of atoms carrying a charge of electricity, either positive or negative. Ions may exist in solid, liquid, or gaseous environments, although those in liquid (electrolytes) are the most common and familiar.

ionization: Dissociation into ions; a process which occurs when a salt or similar substance composed of negatively and positively charged ions is dissolved in water and the two ions separate.

ionization chamber: A chamber for detecting the ionization of an enclosed gas; it is used for determining the intensity of ionizing radiation.

ionize: To separate into ions; to dissociate atoms or molecules into electrically charged atoms or radicals.

ionizing radiation: Radiation which results when a stable, neutral atom is disrupted, releasing individual ions which bear either positive or negative charges.

ipecac: The dried root of *Uragoga* (*Cephaelis*) *ipecacuanha*, a shrub found in Brazil and other parts of South America that can cause vomiting. Available as syrup of ipecac.

iris: The circular pigmented membrane behind the cornea, perforated by the pupil; it is made up of circular muscular fibers and a thin layer of radial muscle fibers; it dilates and constricts the pupil.

ischial tuberosity: A protuberance on the inferior surface of the ischium lateral to the anus and bearing weight when a person is seated.

ischium: The inferior dorsal part of the hip bone; it is a separate bone in early childhood.

islets of Langerhans: Irregular microscopic structures scattered throughout the pancreas and comprising its endocrine portion; insulin is produced in these areas.

IV: Abbreviation for intravenous, or intravenously.

J

jaundice: A condition characterized by the deposition of bile pigment in the skin and mucous membranes, resulting in a yellow appearance of the patient.

jaw thrust maneuver: Procedure for opening the airway. The jaw is lifted and pulled forward to keep the tongue from falling back into the airway. The lower lip is pulled down to force the mouth open.

jejunum: That portion of the small intestine which extends from the duodenum to the ileum.

joint: The articulation, place of union or junction, between two or more bones of the skeleton.

joint capsule: A fibrous sac, with its synovial lining, enclosing a joint.

jugular: Pertaining to the neck.

jugular notch: The bony depression at the superior end of the manubrium sterni.

jugular vein:
   external (bilateral): A major vein draining the scalp and face.
   internal (bilateral): A major vein draining the brain.

jump kit: A closed container fitted with necessary portable equipment and supplies to be used in the emergency care of patients away from the ambulance.

K

keratinize: To become horny or cornified. For example, epidermal skin keratinizes.

ketoacidosis: *See under* acidosis.

keying: Activating a transmitter. When one depresses the "talk" button on the microphone, he keys the transmitter.

kidney: Either of the two retroperitoneal organs in the lumbar region that filter the blood, excreting the end products of metabolism as urine, and regulating salt and water content in the body.

knee: A hinge joint between the femur (thigh bone) and the tibia (leg bone).

kneecap: *See* patella.

Kussmaul respiration: Deep, rapid respiration characteristic of the air hunger seen in diabetic acidosis or coma.

L

labor: The process by which the muscles of the uterus open the birth canal and push the baby down and through so it can be born.

lacerate: To tear or cut roughly.

laceration: A wound resulting from tearing or cutting of body tissue.

lacrimal system: The system pertaining to the tears.
   lacrimal duct: A short canal leading from each lower eyelid to the nose, conducting tears into the nares.
   lacrimal gland: A small gland located in the upper outer angle of the orbit; it secretes tears.
   punctum lacrimale: The small mound at the inner angle of each lower lid containing the upper opening of the lacrimal duct.

ladder splint: A flexible splint consisting of two stout parallel wires and fine crosswires. It resembles a ladder.

landline: A telephone line.

larynx: The musculocartilaginous structure, lined with mucous membrane, situated superior to the trachea and inferior to the root of the tongue, guarding the entrance to the trachea and functioning secondarily as the organ of the voice.

laser: A device that produces a beam of nonspreading, monochromatic, visible light. High energies are concentrated into a narrow beam, and laser-treatment can be completed with so brief a flash that damaging surrounding areas by heat is precluded.

lateral: On the side or to the side; away from the midline.

lateral malleolus: The rounded projection on the lateral side (the outside) of the ankle joint.

leg: The lower limb generally; specifically, that part of the lower limb extending from the knee to the ankle.

444

lens: The transparent body of the eye, through which images are focused on the retina.

lesion: A wound or injury.

lethal: Fatal.

leukocyte: A white blood cell or corpuscle; the cell in which the major defense mechanisms of the blood against bacteria are contained.

levator ani: The muscle that draws the anus upward in defecation and aids in the support of the pelvic floor; the major muscle affording fecal continence.

levator palpebrae: The muscle that raises the upper eyelid.

lid: Either of the two movable conjunctival-cutaneous folds that protect the anterior surface of the eyeball.

ligament: A band of fibrous tissue that connects bone to bone or bone to cartilage, and serves to support and strengthen joints.

linear fracture: A fracture running parallel to the long axis of the bone.

lineman's gloves: Rubber lined leather gloves, especially designed to be nonconductive of electricity.

lipid: Fat.

listless: Characterized by lack of inclination or impetus to exertion.

liter: The basic unit of capacity in the metric system (approximately equal to one quart.)

litter: A stretcher.

live birth certificate: A certificate that a live birth has occurred, regardless of the length of the pregnancy. This registration is required by all states. The certificate may usually be signed by the person attending the birth, not necessarily by a trained medical person.

liver: A large gland situated in the upper part of the abdomen on the right side. All products of absorption in the gastrointestinal tract are initially treated chemically in the liver; bile is produced by the liver; sugar is converted to glycogen and stored in the liver; it possesses a dual blood supply, the hepatic artery, and the portal vein; it is an organ essential for life.

LSD (lysergic acid diethylamide): A serotonin antagonist. It induces schizophrenic-like states in human beings, with hallucinations that are visual rather than auditory. Its use may precipitate psychoses. It is occasionally used in the treatment of chronic alcoholism and psychotic disorders.

lumbar spine: That part of the spine consisting of the most inferior five individual vertebrae located just superior to the sacrum.

lumbosacral plexus: The network of nerves formed by the union of the anterior primary divisions of the lumbar, sacral, and coccygeal nerves.

lumen: The passageway inside a tubular organ; the vascular lumen is the passageway inside a blood vessel.

lung: Either of the pair of organs that aerate the blood. The lungs occupy the lateral cavities of the chest, separated from each other by the heart and mediastinal structures.

lye: A solution of alkaline salts obtained by leaching of wood ashes.

lymph: A clear, transparent, sometimes faintly yellow and slightly opalescent fluid that is collected from the tissues throughout the body. It flows in the lymphatic vessels and through the lymph nodes and is eventually added to the circulation. Lymph consists of a clear liquid portion, varying numbers of white blood cells, and a few red blood cells.

lymph node: One of numerous round, oval, or bean-shaped bodies located along the course of lymphatic vessels. They vary greatly in size (1 to 25 mm in diameter). They function in the defense mechanisms of the body and swell greatly when infected; the characteristic "glands" seen or felt in the neck or in the groin are enlarged lymph nodes.

lymphatic tissues: A three-dimensional network of reticular fibers and cells, the meshes of which are occupied in varying degrees of density by lymphocytes; there are nodular, diffuse, and loose lymphatic tissues.

M

malleolus: The rounded projection on either side of the ankle joint.

mandible: The bone of the lower jaw.

mania: An emotional disorder characterized by great activity, excitement, and unstable behavior.

manubrium sterni: The cranial portion of the sternum, which articulates with the clavicles and the first two pairs of ribs.

mastoid process: The nipple-like projection of the mastoid portion of the temporal bone.

MAST: *See* Military Assistance to Safety and Traffic.

MAST pants: *See* military anti-shock trousers.

maxilla: The irregularly shaped bone that helps to form the upper jaw on either side of the face. It contains the upper teeth and the orbit of the eye, the nasal cavity, and the palate. It is formed by the fusion of several smaller bones.

maxillary artery: The artery on either side of the face which supplies blood to the face; it is palpable in front of the angle of the jawbone.

meatus (urethral, external): (1) In the male, the slit-like opening of the urethra in the glans penis; (2) in the female, the external orifice of the urethra.

medial: In or toward the middle or center.

medial malleolus: The rounded projection on the medial side (the inside) of the ankle joint.

median nerve: A nerve that arises by two roots from the medial and lateral cords of the brachial plexus. Generally, it controls sensation of the central palm, the thumb, and the first three fingers, as well as the ability to oppose the thumb to the fifth (little) finger.

mediastinum: The median or middle area in the thorax, between the lungs, in which lie the heart, great vessels, esophagus, and trachea.

medulla oblongata: The truncated cone of nerve tissue continuous with the pons above and the spinal cord below; it contains ascending and descending tracts and important collections of nerve cells that control vital functions, such as respiration, circulation, and the special senses.

melena: The passage of dark stools stained with blood pigments and digested blood. Characteristically the stools are black and of a sticky tarry consistency.

membrane: A thin sheet or layer of pliable tissue, serving as a covering or envelope of a part or the lining of a cavity.

meninges: The three membranes that envelop the brain and spinal cord: the dura mater, pia mater, and arachnoid.

meningitis: Inflammation of the three layers or membranes that cover the central nervous system. The brain, the spinal cord, or both may be involved.

menopause: Cessation of menstruation in the human female, occurring usually between the ages of forty-eight and fifty.

menses (menstruation): A periodic, physiologic, vaginal hemorrhage, occurring at approximately four-week intervals, and taking its source from the uterine mucous membrane, which is shed. Under normal circumstances, the bleeding is preceded by ovulation.

menstrual flow: The regular monthly vaginal discharge consisting of blood and the shed endometrium (mucous membrane lining of the uterus).

menstrual period: The time of the menstrual flow, usually three to seven days.

mescaline: The most active alkaloid present in the buttons of a small cactus. Mescaline produces effects similar to those produced by LSD: alteration in mood, changes in perception, visual hallucinations, and increases in body temperature and blood pressure.

mesentery: The membranous fold attaching the abdominal organs to the body wall and carrying their blood vessels and nerves.

metabolic functions: Functions relating to metabolism.

metabolic shock: A shock state produced by the excessive loss of fluid and electrolytes; seen in some disease states such as those with excessive vomiting or diarrhea.

metabolism: The sum of all the physical and chemical processes by which living organized substance is produced and maintained by the body and the transformations by which the energy contained in foodstuffs is made available for the uses of the body.

metacarpal bones: The five cylindrical bones of the hand extending from the carpus (wrist) to the phalanges (fingers).

metatarsal bones: The five cylindrical bones of the foot extending from the tarsus (ankle) to the phalanges (toes).

MI: Abbreviation for myocardial infarction.

mid-clavicular line: A line dropped from the mid-point of the clavicle on either side.

middle ear: The tympanic cavity with its ossicles.

military anti-shock trousers (MAST pants): Pressure pants for the control of severe hemorrhage. Used to apply counterpressure over the entire lower half of the body in patients with extensive lacerations or fractures of the lower extremities or fractures of the pelvis or hip joints.

Military Assistance to Safety and Traffic (MAST): A program using military helicopters and medical corpsmen as a supplement to an existing local emergency medical service system for the purpose of providing emergency assistance to civilian patients.

milliliter: A unit of capacity in the metric system; one-thousandth of a liter.

milliroentgen: One thousandth of a roentgen.

mineral acid: A strong acid, such as sulfuric, nitric, or hydrochloric.

miscarriage: Expulsion of the products of conception early in the pregnancy.

ml: Abbreviation for milliliter.

mm: Abbreviation for millimeter.

mobile: A radio designed for installation in and operation from a vehicle, whether in motion or not.

mobile intensive care unit: A vehicle designed to provide specialized emergency care for serious conditions such as cardiac damage or severe trauma, and containing operating room facilities and other special equipment.

molestation: An act of meddling or interfering. Often a result of abnormal sexual motivation or activity.

monitor: A person who receives, and often records, radio messages without transmitting; to listen to radio messages without transmitting.

morphine: A potent drug derived from opium used as a narcotic analgesic.

mortality: Statistically, death rate; the ratio of the number of deaths to a given population in a given situation.

motion sickness: A sensation induced by repetitive motion and characterized by nausea and light-headedness.

motor nerve: An efferent nerve that stimulates a muscle contraction in response to a conscious, willed thought or reflex.

mouth gag: A device for protecting the patient's tongue during a convulsion or for controlling the tongue during the insertion of an artificial airway.

MTF: Medical treatment facility.

mucin: A mucopolysaccharide or glycoprotein, the chief constituent of mucus.

mucous: Pertaining to or resembling mucus; also secreting mucus.

mucous membrane: The lining of body cavities and passages which communicate directly or indirectly with the exterior.

mucus: The opaque, sticky secretion of the mucous membranes, consisting of mucin, epithelial cells, leukocytes, and water, in which various inorganic salts are dissolved.

multiplexing: Transmitting several messages simultaneously on the same radio circuit or channel.

muscle: An organ which by contraction produces a movement of an animal organism. *See also* specific muscles.

447

    cardiac muscle: The muscle of the heart, composed of striated muscle fibers in a syncytium and not under voluntary control.

    involuntary muscle: Muscle that has a characteristic microscopic smooth appearance and that is not under the control of the will.

    voluntary muscle: Muscle that has a characteristic microscopic striped or striated appearance and that normally is under the control of the will.

muscle avulsion fracture: A tearing away of a part of a bone, usually by tendon, ligament, or capsule.

musculoskeletal system: All the bones, joints, muscles, and tendons of the body collectively.

myocardium: The middle and thickest layer of the heart wall; the cardiac muscle.

myocardial contusion: A bruise of the muscular tissue of the heart.

myocardial infarction: The damaging or death of an area of the heart muscle (myocardium) resulting from a reduction in the blood supply reaching that area.

myoglobin: The oxygen-transporting protein of muscle, resembling hemoglobin in function.

myoglobinuria: The excretion of myoglobin in the urine, caused by certain instances of crush syndrome or advanced or protracted ischemia of muscle.

N

nailbed: The area of the corium on which the nail rests.

narcosis: Stupor or general anesthesia produced by a narcotic drug.

narcotic: A drug which, used in moderate doses, produces stupor, insensibility, or sound sleep.

narcotize: To bring under the influence of a narcotic.

nasal bone: Either of the two small oblong bones that together form the bridge of the nose.

nasal cannula: An apparatus for providing supplemental oxygen through a small tubular prong, which fits into the patient's nostril. Usually there are two (called nasal cannulae), one for each nostril.

nasolacrimal duct: The passage leading downward from the lacrimal sac on each side to the inferior meatus of the nose, through which tears are conducted into the nasal cavity.

nasopharyngeal: Relating to the pharynx at the back of the nose.

nasopharynx: The upper portion of the pharynx, above the level of the palate.

National Academy of Sciences: A private society of distinguished scholars in scientific and engineering research, dedicated to the furtherance of science and its use for the general welfare; chartered by the U.S. Congress on March 3, 1863 to serve as an official advisor, upon request and without fee, to the federal government.

National Research Council: Organized by the Academy of Sciences in 1916 in the interest of national preparedness, it served the double purpose of encouraging a broader participation by American scientists and engineers in the service of the academy to the nation.

nausea: Sickness at the stomach; an inclination to vomit.

nebulizer: An apparatus for distributing a liquid in the form of a fine spray or vapor.

neck: The supporting structure of the head, formed by the seven cervical vertebrae and lying between the head and shoulders.

necrosis: The pathologic death of one or more cells, or of a portion of a tissue or an organ, resulting from irreversible cellular damage.

nerve: A cord-like structure comprising a collection of nerve fibers which convey impulses between a part of the central nervous system and some other region of the body or vice versa. *See also* specific nerves.

   cranial nerves: The twelve pairs of nerves connected directly with the brain.

nerve root: One of two bundles of nerve fibers emerging from the spinal cord at each vertebra to join and form a spinal nerve.

net, network: In a communications system, an orderly arrangement of stations interconnected through communications channels which form a coordinated entity.

neural: Relating to any part of the nervous system.

neural observation sheet (neural watch sheet): A chart constructed to provide a convenient record of sequential observations of the neurological status of a patient.

neurogenic shock: A state of shock as a result of generalized vasodilation, produced by action of the nervous system.

neurological: Of or relating to the branch of medical science that has to do with the nervous system and its disorders.

neuron: Nerve cell.

neurotic: A nervous person in whom emotions often predominate over reason.

neurotoxic: Poisonous to nervous tissue.

neutralize: To render neutral; specifically, the chemical combination of hydrogen and hydroxyl ions to form water, thereby rendering each ion harmless.

neutral steer: A term describing the handling characteristics of a vehicle that has a center of gravity in the middle of the car, making it easy to handle.

nitrogen narcosis: A drugged condition which can be created in an individual when the nitrogen in his body is exposed to great pressure, as in a deep dive. Similar to alcoholic intoxication, the condition can even cause a diver to remove his breathing equipment while underwater. Also called "rapture of the deep."

nitroglycerin: A drug (one of the nitrates) which relaxes the muscles in the blood vessels and hence allows dilation of the vessels so that more blood may be carried; it is used to relieve attacks of angina pectoris from spasm of the coronary arteries; one of the vasodilators.

nonconductor: Anything that does not transmit an electrical current or any other source of energy; an insulator.

nuclear energy: The energy contained within the atomic nucleus; atomic energy.

nucleus: Specifically, the central portion of an atom, where most of the mass and all of the positive charge are concentrated.

O

oblique fracture: One which runs obliquely to the axis of the bone.

obstruction: A block or clogging.

occiput: The back of the head.

occlude: To close off, or stop up; obstruct.

occlusive dressing: A dressing or bandage that closes a wound and protects it from the air.

olecranon process: The tip of the elbow.

open fracture (or open dislocation): A fracture or a dislocation having a direct communication with the outside through the skin. There may be a small wound over the fracture or dislocation, or the ends of the bone may be protruding through the skin.

open wound: One in which the affected tissues are exposed by an external opening.

optic nerve: The nerve of sight, which enables visual images to pass to that portion of the brain where they are interpreted.

organic chemical: A substance such as an acid, alkali, salt, or synthetic compound obtained by a chemical process, prepared for use in chemical manufacture, or used for producing a chemical effect. Distinguished from inorganic or mineral.

organic compound: A compound composed of atoms held together by shared electron bonds; an acid made up of molecules containing organic radicals; e.g., acetic acid, citric acid.

organism: Any living thing.

origin of muscle: The place where a muscle is firmly attached to the skeleton, as distinguished from its insertion, which is where it is attached to the bone that it moves.

449

oropharyngeal airway: A device which can be placed in the mouth to make it easier to breathe by lifting the tongue away from the palate.

oropharynx: The central portion of the pharynx, extending from the level of the palate to the vestibule of the larynx.

ossicle: A small bone; specifically, one of the bones of the middle ear.

ovary: One of the two female sexual glands in which the ova are formed.

oversteer: A term describing the handling characteristics of a vehicle that has a center of gravity behind the center of the car, making it necessary to steer continually during a turn since the rear tires must develop more drift angle than the front tires.

ovum: The female reproductive cell which, when fertilized, develops a new member of the same species.

oxygen: A gaseous element existing free in the air. It is absolutely required to support life processes.

oxygen drive: The stimulus to breathe, provided by a low arterial level of oxygen in the blood.

oxygen mask: A device which fits over a patient's nose and mouth to permit the breathing of oxygen. It should be semi-open, valveless, and of transparent plastic.

oxygen toxicity: An unusual condition caused by excessive concentration of oxygen in inspired air, resulting in damage of lung tissue. Ordinarily it is not seen in emergency work.

P

pager: A compact, pocket-carried radio receiver for providing one-way communication, used to locate or direct individuals within a limited area, such as a hospital.

palate: The roof of the mouth; the bony and muscular partition between the oral and nasal cavities.

palpate: To examine by feeling and pressing with the palms of the hands and the fingers.

pancreas: A large, elongated gland situated transversely behind the stomach, between the spleen and the duodenum; it provides a major source of digestive enzymes and is the sole producer of the hormone insulin, regulating the metabolism of sugar.

pancreatitis: Inflammation of the pancreas.

papule: A small, circumscribed, solid elevation on the skin.

paradoxical movement: The motion of the injured segment of a flail chest; opposite to the normal motion of the chest wall.

paralysis: The loss or impairment of motor function in a part.

parasite: An animal or vegetable organism that lives on or in another and draws its nourishment therefrom.

parasympathetic nervous system: The craniosacral portion of the autonomic nervous system generally governing relaxation of sphincters, mobility of smooth muscle, secretions of the gastrointestinal tract, and slowing of the heartbeat.

paraesthesia: An abnormal spontaneous sensation, as of burning, pricking, or numbness.

parietal area: The wall of any cavity.

parietal lobe: The upper central lobe of the cerebrum.

parietal pleura: The portion of the pleura lining the inside of the walls of the thoracic cavity.

party "hot" line: A dedicated telephone line or circuit that serves several parties or locations; though a party line is normally used for emergency or priority traffic, all users have equal priority and may participate in all communications on the circuit.

patella: A triangular sesamoid bone about 5 cm in diameter, situated at the front of the knee; the knee-cap.

pathogenic: Causing disease.

pathological fracture: A fracture in which a specific weakness or destruction of bone caused by some process like cancer is the reason for the break.

pediatric: Relating to the study and treatment of children in health and disease.

pelvic cavity: The lowermost portion of the abdominal cavity, which contains the rectum, urinary bladder, and in the female, the internal sex organs.

pelvis: The bony ring connecting the trunk of the body to the lower extremities.

penis: The male organ of urinary excretion and copulation.

penrose drain: A cigarette drain composed of rubber tubing containing a length of absorbent gauze.

pericardial sac: The fibroserous membrane covering the heart.

pericardial tamponade: Acute compression of the heart from the effusion of fluid into the pericardium or from the collection of blood within the pericardium from rupture of the heart or a penetrating injury.

peripheral nervous system: That portion of the nervous system consisting of the nerves and ganglia outside the brain and spinal cord.

peristalsis: Strong, continuous, wave-like movements which move the intestinal contents from one section of the bowel to the next.

peritoneum: The smooth lining in the abdominal cavity.

peritonitis: Inflammation of the lining of the abdomen.

petit mal epilepsy: Attacks of brief impairment of consciousness.

pH: A symbol used to express acid or alkaline content. On a scale of 14, zero indicates high acidity, 14 indicates high alkalinity, and 7 indicates neutral status.

pharyngeal: Relating to the pharynx.

pharynx: The cavity at the back of nose and mouth; the throat.

phrenic nerve: The motor nerve of the diaphragm.

pia mater: The innermost and most delicate of the three membranes covering the brain and spinal cord.

pin index: A safety attachment on the outlet valve of a gas-filled cylinder.

pit viper: A venomous snake that has a hollow, heat-sensitive pit between eye and nostril. Includes the rattlesnake, copperhead, water moccasin, and fer-de-lance.

placenta (afterbirth): A special organ of pregnancy attached to the wall of the uterus through which the baby receives its nourishment and gets rid of its waste products during pregnancy. After the birth of the baby the placenta is expelled through the birth canal. The placenta is usually one-fifth the size and weight of the baby.

plasma: The liquid portion of whole blood within which the red and white cells lie.

platelet: A disc-shaped element of the blood, smaller than a red blood cell and present to act in initiating clotting.

pleura: The membrane lining the thorax.

pleural space: The potential space existing between the pleural surfaces.

plexus: A network or tangle. In addition to the brachial and lumbosacral plexi, defined below, several other plexi exist in the vascular and nervous systems of the body.

brachial plexus: A network of nerves containing the motor and sensory innervation of the arm.

lumbosacral plexus: A network of nerves containing the motor and sensory innervation of the leg.

pneumothorax: An accumulation of air or gas in the pleural cavity, usually entering after a wound or an injury causing a penetration of the chest wall or a laceration of the lung. *See also* spontaneous pneumothorax.

point tenderness: An area of tenderness limited to two to three centimeters in diameter. It can be identified through pain with gentle pressure. Point tenderness can be located in any area of the body. It is usually associated with acute inflammation, as in peritonitis (abdominal point tenderness), or disruption of tissue (tenderness over a fracture).

polydacron rope: An especially designed rope made from nonconductive plastic (polydacron) material used to manipulate live electric wires.

polydipsia: Frequent, excessive drinking of fluids because of extreme thirst.

451

polyuria: Excessive excretion of urine.

popliteal: Relating to the posterior surface of the knee, a lozenge-shaped space at the back of the knee joint.

popliteal artery: The continuation of the femoral artery in the popliteal space.

posterior tibial artery: Located just posterior to the ankle bone; it supplies blood to the foot.

potassium: An alkaline metallic element, symbol K (kalium), occurring abundantly in nature but always in combination. Its salts are largely used in medicine.

precursor: Anything that precedes another or from which another is derived.

pregnancy: The condition of having a developing fetus within the body.

presenting part: The part of the baby that is born first, usually the head. A head-first delivery is called cephalic delivery. Buttocks or feet first is called a breech delivery.

pressure-compensated flowmeter: An instrument designed to measure the rate of flow of gas from a compressed gas cylinder.

pressure dressing: A dressing through which enough pressure is applied over the wound site to stop bleeding.

pressure point: One of several places on the body where the blood flow of a given artery can be restricted by pressing it against an underlying bone.

pressure splints: Inflatable plastic circumferential splints that may be applied to an extremity and inflated to achieve stability after a fracture.

priapism: Persistent erection of the penis, especially when due to disease, injury, or excessive quantities of androgens and not to sexual desire.

prolapse: To fall out or sink down, said of an organ or other part.

prone: The position of the body when lying face downward.

proton: The unit of positive electricity, forming part (or in hydrogen the whole) of the nucleus of the atom around which the negative electrons revolve.

proximal: Nearest the trunk or the point of origin, said of part of an extremity, or any other structure so situated.

psi: Abbreviation for pounds per square inch.

psilocybin: A hallucinogenic agent obtained from the fruiting bodies of a hallucinogenic fungus and other species of Psilocybe and Stropharia.

psychiatry: The medical specialty dealing with mental disorders.

psychogenic shock: A fainting spell as a result of transient generalized vasodilation in response to a sudden emotional stimulus.

pubic symphysis: The joint formed by union of the bodies of the pubic bones in the median plane characterized by a thick mass of fibrocartilage.

public address system: An apparatus including a microphone and loudspeakers used for broadcasting.

pulmonary alveoli: The air sacs of the lung.

pulmonary artery: The major arterial vessel leading from the right ventricle to the lungs.

pulmonary edema: Abnormal accumulation of fluid in the pulmonary tissues and air spaces.

pulmonary contusion: A bruise of the pulmonary tissue.

pulmonary resuscitation: A technique providing artificial ventilation, either mouth to mouth, mouth to nose, or aided by artificial devices.

pulmonary veins: The four veins that return aerated blood from the lungs to the left atrium of the heart.

pulse: A regular throbbing in the arteries caused by the contraction of the left ventricle of the heart.

punctum lacrimale: The orifice of the lacrimal duct leading to the nose, situated at the inner angle of the lower eyelid.

puncture wound: The penetration of the skin with any sharp or pointed object.

pupil: The opening in the center of the iris of the eye for the transmission of light.

pupillary: Relating to the pupil.

452

R

rad: A measure of the dose absorbed from ionizing radiation. It is equivalent to 100 ergs of energy per gram.

radial artery: One of the major arteries of the forearm; the pulse is palpable at the base of the thumb.

radial head: The circular proximal end of the radius allowing the normal rotatory motion of the forearm with the ulna as axis.

radial nerve: One of the three major nerves of the arm. Descending at the back of the arm closely applied to the humerus and then into the forearm, it is ultimately distributed to the skin at the back of arm, forearm, and hand, the extensor muscles on the back of arm and forearm, the elbow joint and many other joints of the hand.

radiant energy: Any energy which is radiated from any source: electromagnetic waves, radio waves, visible light, X rays, or nuclear radiation.

radiation: The sending forth of light, short radio waves, ultraviolet or X rays, or any other rays for treatment or diagnosis or for other purpose.

radiation sickness: The condition that follows excessive irradiation from any source, whether therapeutic, industrial, or military. In mild forms the reactions are anorexia, nausea, vomiting, malaise, and leukopenia. More severe forms involve reduction or disappearance of leukocytes with risk of infection, and reduction of new red cells leading to anemia. Death can result.

radioactivity: The property of spontaneously emitting rays or subatomic particles of matter with the release of large amounts of energy.

radio patch: An interconnection between radio and telephone communications circuits; radio patch permits direct-voice communication, as opposed to operator relay.

radio-translucent: The ability of any material to allow passage of electric waves or X rays through it.

radius: The bone on the lateral or thumb side of the forearm, so aligned by its head as to describe a circle about the ulna when the hand is rotated.

rale: A sound that can be heard in the chest in cases of disease of the lungs or bronchial tubes.

rape: Sexual intercourse by force.

rapture of the deep: *See* nitrogen narcosis.

rash: A breaking out on the skin, either localized or generalized.

"real time" use: *See* channel assignment (by dispatcher).

recompression: The action of compressing again.

recompression chamber: A pressure chamber so constructed that air under greater-than-atmospheric pressure can be administered to a patient; it is used in the treatment of the bends and in conditions requiring the administration of oxygen under pressure.

rectal temperature: The body temperature measured by a thermometer inserted into the rectum and retained there for one minute. Normally one degree higher than oral temperature.

rectum: The most distal portion of the large intestine, beginning anterior to the third sacral vertebra as a continuation of the sigmoid colon and ending at the anal canal.

reducing valve: A device attached to an oxygen container to control the pressure of the oxygen delivered to a patient; it reduces the pressure from its very high storage level to one suitable for delivery to the patient.

referred pain: Pain perceived as coming from an area remote from its actual origin, such as the arm, elbow, or wrist pain felt in angina pectoris, or the pain above the clavicle, common in diaphragmatic pleurisy.

reflex action: An automatic reaction to a stimulus, such as pulling one's hand away from something hot.

reflex arc: The nervous route utilized in a reflex action, consisting of an afferent (sensory) nerve, internuncial (connecting) nerve, an an efferent (motor) nerve.

renal: Relating to a kidney or the kidneys.

repeater: A radio set used in transmission.

reproductive system: The system that includes all the organs concerned in reproduction.

rescue: The freeing of persons from threatening or dangerous situations by prompt and vigorous action.

  heavy rescue: Rescue activity that involves the use of complicated tools, equipment, and procedures.

  light rescue: Rescue activity by simple means and with minimum of equipment.

  medium rescue: Rescue activity using more specialized tools and equipment than are standard in an ambulance.

rescue tools: Cutting, prying, digging, and pulling tools used to free entrapped persons.

reservoir: The location where infecting organisms live and multiply.

respiration: The exchange of oxygen and carbon dioxide between the atmosphere and the cells of the body.

respiratory shock: Shock induced as a result of an insufficient supply of oxygen in the body or as a result of an inability to breathe.

respiratory system: A system of organs, the function of which is to control the drawing-in and breathing-out of oxygen and carbon dioxide respectively.

resuscitation: The techniques of using assisted breathing to restore adequate ventilation and external cardiac massage to support circulation.

retina: The innermost of the three tunics of the eyeball, supported by the vitreous body against the sclera—the light-sensitive area of the eye where images are projected. Its cells are continous with and form the optic nerve.

retransmission: Employment of a radio communications set for the purpose of rebroadcasting a message on a different frequency simultaneously with the original broadcast by means of an electrically operated linkage device between the receiver and transmitter of the set.

retrograde amnesia: Amnesia in reference to events that occurred before a traumatic event or before the disease that caused the condition.

retroperitoneal: Behind the peritoneum.

rhonchi: Loud rales; especially whistling or snoring sounds produced in the larger bronchi or the trachea.

rib: Any one of the paired arches of bone, twelve on either side, that extend from the thoracic vertebrae toward the median line of the trunk.

rib cage: The thorax.

right atrium: *See under* atrium.

right ventricle: *See under* ventricle.

rigid splint: A splint made of a firm material, either unbending or flexible, to be applied to an injured extremity to prevent motion at the site of a fracture or dislocation. Examples include padded wooden, metal, or plastic splints, and folded-cardboard splints.

"Ringer's lactate": A sterile solution of sodium chloride, potassium chloride, and calcium chloride in water for injection; given as a fluid and electrolyte replenisher by intravenous injection; another balanced salt solution.

Robinson stretcher: A split-frame stretcher.

roentgen: The international unit of X- or gamma-radiation.

roller dressing: A strip of rolled-up material of variable widths.

rotation: The turning or movement of a body round its axis.

rupture: A tear or solution of continuity; a break of any organ or tissue.

S

454

sacral spine: The five fused vertebrae which constitute the sacrum, a part of the pelvic girdle.

sacroiliac joint: The joint or articulation between the sacrum and ilium and the ligaments associated therewith.

sacrum: The triangular bone just below the lumbar vertebrae, formed usually by five fused vertebrae between the two innominate (hip) bones.

"safe residual": The point at which an oxygen cylinder should be replaced to avoid totally depleting its contents. The standard safe residual is 200 psi.

saline solution: A solution of any salt but usually referring to common table salt, sodium chloride.

saliva: The clear, alkaline secretion from the glands of the mouth.

salivary glands: The paired glands of the oral cavity whose combined secretions constitute the saliva; they include the parotid, sublingual, and submandibular glands as well as numerous small glands in the tongue, lips, cheeks, and palate.

salivation: An excess secretion of saliva.

Sarole stretcher: A split-frame stretcher.

scab: A crust formed by the coagulation of blood, pus, serum, or a combination of these on the surface of an ulcer, erosion, or other type of wound.

scapula: The flat, triangular bone at the back of the shoulder; the shoulder blade.

scapular spine: The prominent triangular ridge on the dorsal aspect of the scapula.

sciatic nerve: A major collection of nerve fibers arising from the lumbosacral plexus and subserving most sensation of the lower extremity and motion of the leg and foot.

sclera: The white portion of the eye; the tough outer coat of the eye, which gives protection to the delicate, light-sensitive inner layer.

scrotum: A pouch of thickened skin hanging at the base of the penis in the midline, containing the testes and their accessory ducts and vessels.

SCUBA: Abbreviation for self-contained underwater breathing apparatus.

scuba diving: Remaining under water for long periods by using a self-contained underwater breathing apparatus.

sebaceous gland: A gland of the skin, secreting an oily substance, sebum, and situated in the dermis.

sebum: The secretion of the sebaceous gland; a thick, semifluid substance composed of fat and epithelial debris from the cells of the skin.

secondary infection: An infection occurring in someone already suffering from an infection or from a wound that becomes secondarily infected after the wound was received.

sedative: An agent that quiets nervous excitement; sedatives are designated according to the part or the organ upon which their specific action is exerted, for example, cardiac, cerebral, nervous, respiratory, spinal, and the like.

seizure: An attack; the sudden onset of a disease or of certain symptoms, such as a convulsion.

selective calling equipment: Encoding devices used to alert, or signal, a particular pager unit or group of pager units.

self-contained air masks: Complete units for delivery of air to a rescuer when entering contaminated areas (smoke or poisonous gases); the unit has a tight-fitting mask, controls, and an air supply.

seminal duct: *See* vas deferens.

seminal vesicle: Either of the paired, sacculated pouches attached to the posterior part of the urinary bladder; the duct of each joins the ductus deferens of the same side to form the ejaculatory duct.

sensory nerve: A peripheral nerve that conducts impulses from a sense organ to the central nervous system.

semiconscious: Partly conscious.

septic shock: Shock developing in the presence of, and as a result of, severe infection.

serosa: The outermost layer of most organs, usually continuous with the lining of the body cavities; a thin membrane having the capability to exude plasma in response to injury and to absorb material in solution.

455

sesamoid: A small nodular bone embedded within a tendon or joint capsule.

shadow area: A dead spot in a communicating area where radio contact is difficult or impossible to achieve.

shell temperature: The temperature of the extremities and surface of the body.

shivering: Trembling from cold or fear.

shock: A generalized depression of all body functions caused by progressive failure of the cardiovascular system so that perfusion of tissues and organs is lost.

  anaphylactic shock: A sudden condition caused by hypersensitivity in the body to drugs or other foreign materials (insect stings, certain foods, inhaled allergens). Violent symptoms are produced which include hives, wheezing, tissue edema, pulmonary edema, bronchospasm, vascular collapse, and death.

  cardiogenic shock: Shock resulting from decreased cardiac output as a result of primary heart disease; seen in myocardial infarction.

  hemorrhagic shock: Shock resulting from hemorrhage sufficient to reduce blood volume markedly.

  hypovolemic shock: Shock caused by a reduction in the volume of circulating blood, resulting either from hemorrhage or from relaxation of blood vessel walls so that the peripheral vascular system can contain more blood than normal. Under the latter condition, the volume of blood available for circulation is reduced as effectively as if it were lost from the body.

  insulin shock: Hypoglycemic shock produced by the administration of excessive amounts of insulin; the chief symptoms are sweating, tremor, anxiety, vertigo, and diplopia, followed by delirium, convulsions, and collapse.

  metabolic shock: A shock state produced by the excessive loss of fluid and electrolytes; seen in some disease states such as those with excessive vomiting or diarrhea.

  neurogenic shock: A state or shock as a result of generalized vasodilation, produced by action of the nervous system.

  psychogenic shock: A fainting spell as a result of transient generalized vasodilation in response to a sudden emotional stimulus.

  respiratory shock: Shock induced as a result of an insufficient supply of oxygen in the body or as a result of an inability to breathe.

  septic shock: Shock developing in the presence of, and as a result of, severe infection.

shoulder blade: *See* scapula.

shoulder girdle: The encircling bony structure supporting the upper limbs; comprising the scapula and the clavicle and their central attachments.

shoulder joint: A ball-and-socket joint between the head of the humerus and the glenoid fossa of the scapula.

SIDS (sudden infant death syndrome): Crib death; abrupt and inexplicable death of an apparently healthy infant.

sigmoid colon: The terminal division of the large intestine which makes several turns, roughly resembling the letter S, terminating at the rectum.

simple fracture: An uncomplicated fracture; not compound. The skin is not broken over the injury.

sinus: A general term for spaces, such as the channels for venous blood in the cranium or the air cavities within the cranial bones.

six-man stretcher pass: Method of transporting a patient on a litter over rough terrain; it consists of passing a stretcher by six persons in two parallel rows, the last two persons in the line proceeding ahead each time as the stretcher passes them.

size-up: The rapid gathering of facts and analyzing of the problem or problems of an incident or accident immediately upon arrival at the scene.

skeletal muscle: Striated muscle attached to and moving the bones; generally under voluntary control.

skeleton: The framework of the animal body, especially the bony framework of the body of higher vertebrates.

skin: The outer integument or covering of the body, consisting of the dermis and the epidermis and resting upon the subcutaneous tissue. It forms the largest organ of the body and contains various sensory and regulatory mechanisms.

skull: The bones of the head collectively.

sling and swathe: A bandage in which the arm is placed in a sling and is bound to the chest by a swathe (passing around the chest and over the arm).

slough: To separate from the living tissue, said of a dead or necrosed part.

smooth muscle: Muscle consisting of non-striated cells comprising the walls of the internal organs, blood vessels, hair follicles, and other appendages; generally it is not under voluntary control.

snorkel: A tube housing an air-intake and exhaust pipe which can be used for breathing underwater when one end is projected above the water.

snow blindness: Obscured vision caused by sunlight reflected from snow.

snowmobile: A vehicle for travel over snow and ice; powered by a gasoline motor and propelled by means of an endless tract, it is steered by handlebars controlling two runners in front. It can be used in removing patients from areas of snow and ice which are inaccessible to other land vehicles.

sodium hydroxide: Caustic soda soluble in water; used externally as a caustic.

soft tissue: The non-bony and noncartilaginous tissue of the body.

solar radiation: Radiant energy from the sun.

somatic nerve: One of the nerves of sensation or motion.

source: The object, person, or substance from which an infectious agent passes to a host.

spasm: The sudden, involuntary movement of a muscle accompanied by pain and interfering with function.

sphincter muscle: A muscle that encircles a duct, tube, or opening in such a way that its contraction constricts the opening.

sphygmomanometer: An instrument for measuring blood pressure in the arteries.

spinal canal: A bony channel formed by the vertebral bodies and neural arches that contains and protects the spinal cord.

spinal column: All the vertebrae; the spine; the backbone.

spinal cord: The cord of nervous tissue extending from the brain through the length of the spinal canal; paired motor and sensory spinal nerves branch off from the spinal cord.

spineboard: A wooden or metal device primarily used for extrication and transportation of patients with actual or suspected spinal injuries; also serves as a litter and can be used to raise or lower patients or to provide rigid support during cardiac compression. The long spineboard is six feet; the short board is less than three feet—32 to 34 inches.

spiral fracture: One in which the line of break runs obliquely up one side of the bone.

spleen: A large, glandlike, ductless organ situated in the upper part of the abdominal cavity on the left side.

splint: A device to immobilize an injured part. There are many forms of splints, generally of two types. Traction splints are those that immobilize by applying pull to the injured part; rigid splints are those that immobilize by applying a rigid structure to the injured part.

spontaneous pneumothorax: A pneumothorax occurring from disease of the lung—as for example, an abscess—or from any natural cause; not traumatic.

sprain: The tearing or stretching of the ligaments surrounding a joint as a result of a sudden twisting injury.

sputum: expectorated matter, especially mucus or matter resulting from diseases of the air passages.

squelch: A system for removing objectionable background noise from a p.a. system or radio speaker.

status epilepticus: A condition in which one major attack of epilepsy succeeds another with little or no intermission.

sterile: Aseptic or free from all living microorganisms and their spores; not fertile.

sterilize: To render sterile or free from bacterial contamination; to make an organism unable to reproduce.

sternoclavicular joint: The articulation between the clavicle, the sternum, and the cartilage of the first rib with an articular disc, subdividing the joint into two cavities.

sternum: The longitudinal bone plate forming the middle of the anterior wall of the thorax, articulating above with the clavicles and along the sides with the cartilages of the first seven ribs.

stethoscope: An instrument of various forms, sizes, and materials for detecting sounds generated within any part of the body.

stillbirth: Born dead.

stoma: A small opening; an opening through the throat into the trachea, used for breathing when the larynx has been removed.

stomach: The expansion of the alimentary canal between the esophagus and the duodenum.

stool: Feces, or the matter discharged at a movement of the bowels.

stove-in chest: *See* flail chest.

straddle load: A method for placing a patient on the long spineboard by straddling both board and patient and sliding him onto it.

stress: The application to the body of forces of a damaging nature that tend to disturb its normal state.

stretcher: A device enabling two persons to lift and carry a patient in a lying-down position.

    ambulance stretcher: Carrying device used to transport patients to, from, and in an ambulance, usually wheeled but also portable.

    army stretcher: A folding stretcher made of wooden poles covered with canvas, with short, folding legs.

    basket stretcher: A device originally designed to remove the injured from the holds of ships and called the Stokes basket, it was a long narrow metal basket covered with chicken wire. Now made of plastic without the original leg divider.

    Robinson stretcher: A split-frame stretcher.

    Sarole stretcher: A split-frame stretcher.

    scoop stretcher: A split-frame stretcher.

    split-frame stretcher: A carrying device for patients that is divided longitudinally, slipped beneath the patient from each side, and locked at each end, thus providing both an extrication device and a litter.

    Stokes basket: A basket stretcher shaped like an oblong plastic shell, useful in removing patients from heights, or over difficult terrain or debris.

stretcher lash: A method for using a rope to secure a patient to a stretcher for the purpose of raising or lowering him from heights or depths or transporting over rough terrain.

stroke: A general term referring to a vascular accident within the central nervous system, caused by a clot or hemorrhage in the brain, often resulting in paralysis of one side of the body.

S-tube: An oropharyngeal airway shaped like an S which can be used to prevent the patient's tongue from obstructing his airway while artificial ventilation is being given through the same device.

stupor: A state of suspended or diminished sensibility.

subcutaneous: Beneath the skin; a method of drug administration by hypodermic injection.

subcutaneous emphysema: The presence of air or gas in the subcutaneous tissues of the body.

subdural hematoma: A collection of blood or a clot caused by a laceration or rupture of a meningeal vessel lying between the dura mater and the arachnoid.

substernal: Beneath the sternum.

subtrochanteric area: Area below any trochanter.

458   **sucking chest wound:** A wound of the chest wall through which air passes into and out of the pleural space with each respiration.

suction catheters: Hollow semi-rigid tubes of varying diameters which are used to aspirate material from within the pharynx, trachea, and upper bronchi.

suffocate: To impede respiration; to asphyxiate; to suffer from want of oxygen; to be unable to breathe.

suffocation: The act or condition of suffocating; asphyxiation.

sulfuric acid: A colorless, nearly odorless, heavy, oily, corrosive liquid containing 96 per cent absolute acid. Used occasionally as a caustic.

sunstroke: Heat stroke.

superior: Above, in relation to another structure.

superior vena cava: *See under* vena cava.

supine: Lying on the back with the face upwards.

supracondylar fracture: A fracture of the distal end of the humerus.

swathe bandage: A bandage that passes around the chest, splinting an injured arm to the chest.

swimmer's ear: A non-emergency condition which results from inflammation in the external ear canal created by the growth of infecting organisms, usually picked up during swimming or diving.

sympathetic nerve: One of the nerves of the sympathetic portion of the autonomic nervous system.

sympathetic nervous system: The thoracolumbar portion of the autonomic nervous system; generally acting to stimulate a sphincter contraction, reduce smooth muscle activity, increase heart rate, or activate the organs of the skin.

symphysis pubis: The firm fibro-cartilaginous joint between the two pubic bones.

syncope: A fainting spell.

synovia (synovial fluid): A clear, viscid fluid the function of which is to lubricate the joint.

synovium: The lining membrane of a joint cavity.

syrup of ipecac: A drug which will induce vomiting. *See under* ipecac.

systole: The contraction or period of contraction of the heart, especially of the ventricles; it coincides with the interval between the first and the second heart sounds and is that period in which blood is delivered to the arterial tree.

systolic: Relating to, or occurring during cardiac systole.

systolic blood pressure: The higher blood pressure noted at the moment of ventricular contraction.

T

tachycardia: Abnormally fast heart rate, generally anything over one hundred beats per minute.

talus: The most superior of the tarsal bones and the one which articulates with the tibia and fibula to form the ankle joint.

tamponade: A general term indicating compression. *See also* cardiac tamponade.

tarsal: Relating to a tarsus in any sense.

tarsal bone: One of the seven bones of the ankle.

tarsal plate: The firm framework of connective tissue that gives shape to the upper eyelid.

tarsus: The root of the foot, or instep. The fibrous plates giving solidity and form to the edges of the eyelids; they are often called (erroneously) tarsal cartilages.

telemetry: The measurement of diagnostic signs by electrical instruments and the transmission of them, especially by radio, to a distant place for recording; used for electrocardiograph signals.

telephone "hot" line: A direct, dedicated telephone circuit that connects two or more points for instant communication without dialing.

telephone patch: *See* radio patch.

temperature, body: The temperature of the body. In cold-blooded animals it varies with environmental temperature; in warm-blooded animals it is usually constant within a narrow range. In human beings, 98.6° is considered normal for oral temperature, 99.6° for rectal.

temporomandibular joint: Mandibular joint; the articulation between the head of the mandible and the mandibular fossa and articular tubercle of the temporal bone.

459

temporal artery: Located on either side of the face in front of the ear; supplying blood to the scalp.

tendon: A fibrous cord by which a muscle is attached to bone.

tenesmus: A painful spasm of the anal sphincter with an urgent desire to evacuate the bowel or bladder; involuntary straining with the passage of very little fecal matter or urine.

tension pneumothorax: A condition that develops when air is continually pumped into the chest cage outside the lung and is unable to escape; it is associated with compression of the lung and heart.

testicle (testis): The male genital organ.

testis: A testicle.

thalamus: A constituent of the brain stem; the site of certain involuntary nervous controls in the body.

thermal: Pertaining to or characterized by heat.

thermal conductivity: The power to transmit or convey heat.

thigh: The portion of the lower extremity between the hip and the knee.

Thomas splint: A rigid splint made of either metal or plastic which can provide support for and a steady longitudinal pull on a lower extremity. When traction is applied through the foot and ankle hitch, countertraction is applied against the ischial tuberosity. Rigid bars extend the length of the splint, the upper end is curved, and the leg fits within the framework and is supported by it.

thoracic cage: The chest (refers to the fact that the ribs resemble a cage).

thoracic cavity: The space within the thoracic (chest) walls, bounded below by the diaphragm and above by the neck.

thoracic spine: The vertebrae, usually twelve in number, between the cervical spine and the lumbar spine.

thorax: The upper part of the trunk between the neck and the abdomen; the chest.

thready pulse: A pulse beat that is weak and scarcely perceptible; characteristic of the pulse in shock.

three-man lift (or four-man lift): A method by which a number of persons may lift and move a patient smoothly.

three-point suspension: The distribution of the weight of a patient while he is being moved; trunk, buttocks, and legs are separately supported.

thrombus: A blood clot which forms inside a blood vessel or within the cavity of the heart.

thyroid cartilage: The largest of the cartilages of the larynx.

thyroid gland: A ductless gland lying on the upper part of the trachea; it produces thyroid hormone.

tibia: The shin bone.

tourniquet: A device, such as a bandage, twisted tight around an extremity to arrest bleeding which cannot be controlled by any other means.

toxemia: An abnormal condition associated with the presence of toxic substances in the blood.

toxic: Poisonous.

toxin: A poison; frequently used to refer specifically to a protein produced by some higher plants, certain animals, and pathogenic bacteria which is highly toxic to other living organisms.

trachea: The windpipe; the main trunk for air passing to and from the lungs.

tracheostomy: An opening in the trachea made at an operation; a tube is inserted to maintain an airway. An emergency method of establishing access to the air passage.

tracheostomy tube: A tube used to keep a tracheostomy open.

traction: The act of pulling.

transfusion: The introduction of whole blood or blood cellular components directly into the bloodstream.

transmission: The conveyance of disease from one person to another.

transverse colon: The division of the large intestine that crosses the abdomen, located between the ascending colon and the descending colon.

transverse fracture: A fracture whose line forms a right angle with the axis of the bone.

trauma: An injury inflicted, usually more or less suddenly, by some physical agent.

traumatic asphyxia: Asphyxia occurring as a result of sudden or severe compression of the thorax or upper abdomen or both.

traumatic emphysema: Emphysema occurring as a result of trauma.

tremor: Trembling; shaking.

trench foot: A chronic condition of cold injury affecting the feet of anyone obliged to stand for long periods of time in cold water, snow, or mud; a vascular injury of the feet.

triage: The sorting or selection of patients to determine the priority of care to be rendered to each.

triangular bandage: A piece of cloth cut in the shape of a right-angled triangle, used as a sling for the arm and for other purposes.

trochanter: Either of the two bony prominences developed from independent centers near the upper extremity of the femur, below the femoral neck.

    greater trochanter: The greater of two bony processes below the neck of the femur; a broad, flat, lateral surface serving as a point of attachment for several muscles.

    lesser trochanter: A pyramidal process projecting from the medial and upper part of the shaft of the femur at the line of junction of the shaft and the neck; it receives the insertion of major muscles.

trunk: The body, excluding the head and extremities.

tympanum: The cavity of the middle ear.

U

UHF: Ultrahigh frequency. The radio frequencies between 300 and 3,000 megahertz (MHz).

ulcer: A lesion on the surface of the skin or a mucous surface caused by the superficial loss of tissue, usually with inflammation.

ulna: The inner and larger bone of the forearm, on the side opposite the thumb.

ulnar artery: A major artery of the forearm whose pulse is palpable on the inner wrist at the base of the fifth (little) finger.

umbilical clamp: A device, usually of plastic, used to compress the umbilical cord, allowing it to be cut without endangering the mother or baby from blood loss.

umbilical cord: The rope-like attachment between the placenta and the navel of the fetus, usually about twenty inches in length. Before birth the fetus receives nourishment from the placenta and passes waste back to it through blood vessels in this cord.

umbilicus: The navel; a small depression in the abdominal wall marking the point where the fetus was attached to the umbilical cord.

unconsciousness: Not conscious; "out cold."

understeer: A term describing the handling characteristics of a vehicle that has the center of gravity

460

located forward of the center of the vehicle, making steering more difficult.

universal dressing: A large (9×36 inches) dressing of multilayered material which can be used open or folded or rolled to cover most wounds, to pad splints, or to form a cervical collar.

universal emergency telephone number: 911, a master telephone number which in many areas can be called in case of any kind of emergency.

uremia: The retention of excessive waste products of metabolism in the blood, and the toxic condition produced thereby; usually a result of failure of normal function of the kidney.

ureter: The fibromuscular tube which conveys urine from the kidney to the bladder.

urethra: The membranous canal conveying urine from the bladder to outside the body.

urinary bladder: A musculomembranous bag serving as a storage place for urine until it is discharged from the body.

urinary system: The organs concerned in the formation and voiding of urine. The system consists of the kidneys, ureters, bladder, and urethra.

urine: A fluid waste product of the body, excreted by the kidneys, passed through the ureters, stored in the bladder, and discharged through the urethra.

uterus (womb): The muscular organ that holds and nourishes the fetus. The uterus opens into the vagina through the cervix.

V

vagina: A sheath, or sheathlike structure; the female organ for reception of the penis during sexual intercourse; the lower part of the birth canal during delivery.

vagus nerve: The tenth cranial nerve; it serves the larynx, lungs, heart, esophagus, stomach, and most of the abdominal viscera.

vascular: Relating to or containing blood vessels.

vas deferens: The spermatic duct of a testicle.

vasoconstrictor: An agent that causes narrowing of the blood vessels.

vasodilation: Dilation of the blood vessels.

vein: A tubular vessel which carries blood from the capillaries toward the heart.

femoral vein: A continuation of the popliteal vein that becomes the external iliac vein; the major vein draining the leg.

pulmonary veins: The four veins that return aerated blood from the lungs to the left atrium of the heart.

Velcro: A fastener consisting of two strips nylon tape—one covered with minute hooks, the other with minute loops, which lock securely when pressed together and pull apart easily when one begins separating them at one end.

vena cava: One of the two large veins conducting blood to the right upper chamber of the heart.

inferior vena cava: The venous trunk returning blood from the lower extremities and the pelvic and abdominal viscera.

superior vena cava: The venous trunk returning blood from the upper extremities, head, neck, and chest.

venereal disease: Certain diseases of the sexual system in either male or female, generally acquired through sexual intercourse with an infected partner. The most common venereal diseases are syphilis, gonorrhea, and chancroid.

venipuncture: The puncture of a vein.

venom: A poisonous fluid secreted by snakes, spiders, or scorpions.

venous: Relating to a vein or to the veins.

venous blood: Unoxygenated blood gathered from the body in veins and carried back to the heart.

ventilation: The process of breathing; the constant supplying of oxygen to the body through the lungs and concurrent removal of carbon dioxide.

ventricle: One of the two lower chambers of the heart.

> **left ventricle:** The greater chamber, on the left side of the heart, which propels oxygenated blood out through the aorta into the systemic arterial system.

> **right ventricle:** The lesser chamber, on the right side of the heart, which propels unoxygenated blood through the pulmonary trunk and arteries into the lungs.

ventricular fibrillation: A disorganized twitching of the heart muscle which results in a failure of the heart to pump blood. It is one of the conditions generally associated with cardiac arrest.

Venturi mask: A breathing unit designed to provide a specific concentration of oxygen through a delivery tube connected to a standard facemask.

venule: Any of the small vessels that collect blood from the capillary plexi and join to form veins.

vertebra: Any of the thirty-three bones of the spinal column.

> **cervical:** The upper seven vertebrae, constituting the skeleton of the neck.

> **coccygeal:** The lowest segments of the vertebral column, comprising three to five rudimentary vertebrae which form the coccyx, or tail bone.

> **lumbar:** The five vertebrae between the thoracic spine and the sacrum.

> **sacral:** The five fused vertebrae which constitute the sacrum, a part of the pelvic girdle.

> **thoracic:** The twelve vertebrae between the cervical and the lumbar spine.

vertebral arch: A posterior projection from a vertebra; also called a neural arch.

vertebral body: The round, solid bone forming the front part of each vertebra.

vertebral spine: The posterior projection of each vertebra, also called the spinous process.

vestigial: A small or imperfectly developed bodily part or organ that remains from one more fully developed in an earlier stage of the individual, or in a past generation, or in closely related forms.

VHF: Very high frequency, the radio frequencies between 30 and 300 megahertz (MHz).

virus: The specific agent of a type of infectious disease; specifically, a term for a group of microbes which with few exceptions are capable of passing through fine filters that bacteria cannot pass through.

viscera: The internal organs of the body.

visceral: Relating to the viscera.

visceral pleura: The portion of the pleura covering the lungs.

vital signs: The observable physical signs by which the physical state of an individual can be determined; ordinary vital signs include pulse, blood pressure, respiratory rate, temperature, and level of consciousness.

vitreous humor: A viscous substance contained within the globe of the eye, giving support to its form.

vocal cords: A fold of mucous membrane in the larynx forming the inferior boundary of the ventricle of the larynx; these are activated by air passing over them and their vibrations are the source of the sound which is the voice.

voice box: The larynx.

voluntary: Relating or acting in obedience to the will.

voluntary muscle: A muscle whose action is under the control of the will; all the striated muscles, except the heart, are voluntary muscles.

vomitus: Vomited matter.

vulva: The external genital organ of the female.

W

walkie-talkie unit: A compact, battery-operated radio transmitting and receiving set, which can be carried by a person to provide two-way radio communication.

warning lights: Flashing lights that serve as a signal on an ambulance.

warning signal: An intermittent audible signal of varying tone made by a siren to clear the way for an ambulance. Used when going on a call. Rarely should the siren be used while transporting a patient.

wet suit: A close-fitting full body covering, with zipper fasteners, of rubber, used by underwater divers.

wheal: A swelling on the skin, produced by a sting, an injection, an external force, or an internal reaction (such as hives produced by a food allergy).

wheezing: Breathing with difficulty and noisily.

wind-chill factor: A factor taking into account the relationship of wind velocity to thermometer temperature in determining the effect on a living organism.

windpipe: The trachea.

womb: The uterus.

wrecking bar: A short metal bar chisel-shaped on both ends, one of which is a half circle, used to effect forceful entry to patients trapped in vehicles.

wrist: The region of articulation between the forearm and hand.

X

xiphoid process: The cartilage at the lower end of the sternum.

X ray: Electromagnetic radiation.

Z

zygomatic process of the maxilla: The rough projection from the maxilla that articulates with the zygomatic bone.

zygomatic process of the frontal bone: The massive projection of the frontal bone that joins the zygomatic bone to form the lateral margin of the orbit.

Selected List of Supplementary Reading

One copy (only) of most of the publications listed below may be obtained free from the U.S. Department of Transportation by any qualified organization. Write on your letterhead to:

Robert E. Motley
Rescue and Emergency Services Division
National Highway Traffic Safety Administration
400 Seventh Street, S.W.
Washington, D.C. 20590

Aaron, James E. et al. *First Aid and Emergency Care: Prevention and Protection of Injuries*. New York: McMillan Co., 1972. 411 pp.

American Academy of Orthopaedic Surgeons. *National Workshop on the Training of Emergency Medical Technicians: Recommendations and Conclusions for an Approach to an Urgent Problem*. Pub. no. NA 8–42. Washington, D.C.: U.S. Department of Transportation, National Highway Traffic Safety Administration, 1971.

American Academy of Pediatrics, Committee on Disaster and Emergency Medical Care. *Disaster and Emergenvy Medical Services for Infants and Children*. 2d ed. Evanston, Ill.: American Academy of Pediatrics, 1975. 72 pp.

American College of Surgeons. "Essential Equipment for Ambulances." *Bulletin of the American College of Surgeons* 55 (May 1970): 7–13.

American Heart Association. *Recommendations for Human Blood Pressure Determination by Sphygmomanometers*. New York: American Heart Association, 1967. 23 pp.

———. *Standards for Cardiopulmonary Resuscitation (CPR) and Emergency Cardiac Care (ECC)*. New York: American Heart Assn., 1973. 35 pp.

American Hospital Association. *Emergency Medical Communications System: A Guide for Hospital Participation*. Chicago: American Hospital Association, 1973. 45 pp.

American Medical Association. *Categorization of Hospital Emergency Capabilities: Recommendations of the Conference on the Guidelines*. Pub. no. OP-387. Chicago: American Medical Association. 33 pp.

———. *Developing Emergency Medical Services: Guidelines for Community Councils*. Pub. no. OP-386. Chicago: American Medical Association. 15 pp.

———. *The Wonderful Human Machine*. Chicago: American Medical Association, 1967. 56 pp.

American National Red Cross. *Advanced First Aid and Emergency Care*. Washington, D.C.: American National Red Cross, 1973. 318 pp.

———. *Cardiopulmonary Resuscitation*. Pub. no. 321130. Washington, D.C.: American National Red Cross, 1974. 40 pp.

Baker, G. L. "Design and Operation of a Van for the Transport of Sick Infants." *American Journal of Diseases of Children* 118: 743–47. 1969.

Beckwith, J. Bruce. "The Sudden Infant Death Syndrome." *Current Problems in Pediatrics*, vol. 3 (1973). Reprint by Yearbook Medical Publishers, Chicago. 37 pp.

Crampton, Richard S. *Basic Rescue Cardiology*. Charlottesville, Va.: University of Virginia Medical Center, 1973. 150 pp.

Dreisbach, Robert H. *Handbook of Poisoning: Diagnosis and Treatment*. Los Altos, Calif.: Lange Medical Publications, 1974. 517 pp.

Dubin, Dale. *Rapid Interpretation of EKG's*. 2d ed. Tampa, Fla.: Cover Publishing Co., 1973.

Ellis, Michael D., ed. *Dangerous Plants, Snakes, Arthropods and Marine Life of Texas*. U.S. Department of Health, Education and Welfare, Public Health Service. Washington, D.C.; Government Printing Office, 1974, 277 pp.

Farrington, J. D. The Registry of Ambulance Attendants. *Emergency Medicine Today*. Chicago: American Medical Association, 1972.

Federal Aviation Administration. *Heliport Design Guide*. Pub. no. 150/5390-1A. Washington: Government Printing Office, 1964.

Federal Communications Commission. *Rules and Regulations*. Vols. 2 and 5. Continuously updated. Washington, D.C.: Government Printing Office.

Folsom, Farnham. *Extrication and Casualty Handling*

Techniques. Philadelphia: J. B. Lippincott Co., 1975.

Frazier, Claude A. "The Buzzin' Cousins and How They Sting." *Emergency Medicine* 6 (1974): 27–35.

Gay, George R. "Up, Down, and Out." *Emergency Medicine* 5 (1973), 22–26.

Grant, Harvey, and Murry, Robert. *Emergency Care.* Bowie, Md.: Robert J. Brady Co., 1971. 334 pp.

Gresham, Edwin L. "Stress in the Early Hours." *Emergency Medicine* 6 (1974): 51–67.

Halstead, Bruce W. *Poisonous and Venomous Animals of the World.* Washington, D.C.: Government Printing Office, 1965.

Hanlon, John J. "Emergency Medical Care as a Comprehensive System." *Health Service Report* 88 (1973): 579–87. Reprint by U.S. Department of Health, Education and Welfare, Pub. no. HSA-742026. Washington, D.C.: Government Printing Office.

Henderson, John. *Emergency Medical Guide.* New York: McGraw Hill Book Co. 429 pp.

Huszar, Robert J. *Emergency Cardiac Care.* Bowie, Md.: Robert J. Brady Co., 1974, 267 pp.

International Association of Laryngectomees. *Neck Breathers' First Aid.* New York: American Cancer Society, 1971.

Landau, Barbara R. *Essential Human Anatomy and Physiology.* Glenview, Ill.: Scott, Foresman and Co., 1976.

Miller, Benjamin F. et al. *Encyclopedia and Dictionary of Medicine and Nursing.* Philadelphia: W. B. Saunders Co., 1972. 1089 pp.

Morse, Thomas S. "Step by Step with an Injured Child." *Emergency Medicine* 6 (1974): 121–33.

———. "Transportation of Sick and Injured Children." In *Surgical Pediatrics*, edited by Stephen L. Gans. New York: Grune and Stratton, Inc. 1973.

National Academy of Sciences. *Accidental Death and Disability: The Neglected Disease of Modern Society.* U.S. Department of Health, Education and Welfare, Emergency Health Services, no. A-13. Washington, D.C.: Government Printing Office, 1968. 38 pp.

———. *Medical Requirements for Ambulance Design and Equipment.* U.S. Department of Health, Education and Welfare, Pub. no. (HSA) 74-2035. Washington, D.C.: Government Printing Office, 1974. 24 pp.

———. Committee on Emergency Medical Services and Subcommittee on Ambulance Services. *Advanced Training Program—Emergency Medical Technician: Guidelines and Recommendations.* U.S. Department of Transportation. Washington, D.C.: Government Printing Office, 1973.

National Institute of Health. *Facts about Sudden Infant Death Syndrome.* Pub. no. 72-225. Washington, D.C.: U.S. Department of Health, Education and Welfare.

National Institute of Mental Health. *Emergency Care for Mental Health Crises.* Philadelphia: Charles Press, 1974.

Ohio Department of Education, Ohio State University, Division of Vocational Education, Instructional Materials Laboratory. *Emergency Victim Care.* Columbus, Ohio: Ohio Department of Education, 1971. 352 pp.

Page, James O. *Emergency Medical Services for Fire Departments.* Washington, D.C.: International Firefighters Assn., 1975.

Phibbs, Brendan. *The Cardiac Arrhythmias.* 2d ed. Saint Louis: C. V. Mosby Co., 1973. 206 pp.

Rose, Leonard B., and Rose, Beatrice K. *Fundamentals of Mobile Coronary Care.* New York: Medcom Press, 1974. 123 pp.

Segal, Sydney. "Transfer of a Premature or Other High-risk Newborn Infant to a Referral Hospital." *Pediatric Clinics of North America* 13 (1966): 1195–1205.

———, ed. *Manual for the Transport of High-risk Newborn Infants—Principles, Policies, Equipment, Techniques.* Canadian Paediatric Society, 1972.

Stephenson, Hugh E., Jr., ed. *Immediate Care of the Acutely Ill and Injured.* Saint Louis: C. V. Mosby Co., 1974.

Stringer, Llewellyn W. *Emergency Treatment of Acute Respiratory Diseases.* Rev. ed. Bowie, Md.: Robert J. Brady Co., 1973. 101 pp.

Tarkoff, Mitchell P. "Clues to Pulmonary Function." *Emergency Medicine* 6 (1974): 183–99.

U.S. Department of Health, Education and Welfare. *"911"—The Emergency Phone Number: A Handbook for Community Planning.* Pub. no. 2205-0003. Washington, D.C.: Government Printing Office, 1973. 62 pp.

———. Health Services and Mental Health Administration. *Emergency Medical Services Communications Systems.* Pub. no. (HSM) 73-2003. Washington, D.C.: Government Printing Office, 1972. 38 pp.

U.S. Department of Transportation. *Ambulance Design Criteria.* Pub. no. TD8.2: Aml. Washington, D.C.: Government Printing Office, 1973.

———. *Emergency Medical Services.* Highway Safety Program Manual, vol. 11. Pub. no. 5003-00170. Washington, D.C.: Government Printing Office, 1974.

———. *Emergency Medical Technician—Ambulance: Basic Training Program. Course Guide and Course Coordinator Orientation Program.* Pub. no. TD2.208: EM3/2. Washington, D.C.: Government Printing Office, 1969, 46, pp.

———. *Emergency Medical Technician—Ambulance: Basic Training Program. Instructor's Lesson Plans.* Pub. no. TD2.208: EM3/3. Washington, D.C.: Government Printing Office, 1970. 344 pp.

———. *Emergency Medical Technician—Ambulance:*

Job Description. Washington, D.C.: Government Printing Office, 1972.

———. *Emergency Medical Technician—Ambulance: Patient Handling Manual.* Pub. no. TD8.8:EM3/3. Washington, D.C.: Government Printing Office.

———. *Emergency Medical Technician—Ambulance: Refresher Training Program Course Guide.* Pub. no. TD8.8:EM3. Washington, D.C.: Government Printing Office.

———. *Emergency Medical Technician—Dispatcher: Training Course.* Pub. no. TD8.8:D63. Washington, D.C.: Government Printing Office.

———. *Emergency Medical Technician: Crash-victim Extrication Training Course. Course Guide.* Pub. no. 5003–00164. Washington, D.C.: Government Printing Office.

———. *Emergency Medical Technician: Crash-victim Extrication Training Course. Course Coordinator's Guide.* Pub. no. 5003–00165. Washington, D.C.: Government Printing Office.

———. Federal Specifications—Ambulance—Emergency Care Vehicles. Pub. no. KKK-A-1822. January 2, 1974, 40 pp. Amendment no. 1, June 25, 1975. 7 pp. Washington, D.C.: U.S. Department of Transportation, National Highway Traffic Safety Administration.

———. *A Helicopter Ambulance Service. Do You Need It? Can You Justify It? Can You Afford It?* Washington, D.C.: Government Printing Office, 1973.

———. *Helicopters in Emergency Medical Services: Experiences to Date.* Pub. no. TD8.2:H36. Washington, D.C.: Government Printing Office, 1972.

Vogt, F. B. "Communication Systems for Emergency Medical Services." *Emergency Medical Services* 1 (1972): 18–24.

———. "Why Can't People Plan Communications Systems?" *Emergency Medical Services* 3 (1974) 9–16.

Warren, James V. "Ten Tips to Help You Make Better Use of Your Stethoscope." *Medical Opinion* 3 (1974): 31–37.

Index

468

470

472

474

478

480

Important Telephone Numbers

Fill in telephone numbers for places you may need to call in an emergency.

Keep this book in a convenient location. A second list by the telephone would be advisable. Remember that one minute saved in calling for help or getting advice may mean saving a life.

Ambulance services _____

_____

_____

Antivenin Index
(Oklahoma City Zoo)
Weekdays   (405) 424-3344
Nights and weekends (405) 271-5424

Blood Bank _____

Civil Defense Department
(local)   _____

Decompression advice
Brooks Air Force Base (512) 536-3278
Navy Experimental
Diving Unit   (904) 234-4355

Decompression unit
(where to get one) _____

Electric Department _____

Emergency Departments of
local hospitals   _____

_____

Fire Department _____

Gas Department _____

Geiger counter
(where to get one) _____

Health Departments
Local   _____

State   _____

Helicopter (where to get one) _____

Legal Aid Society _____

Medical Society (local) _____

Mental hospitals
Local   _____

State   _____

Military training center
(nearest one)   _____

Nuclear Regulatory Commission (NCR)
Local   _____

National   _____

Poison Control Centers
Local   _____

National   _____

Police
Emergency   _____

Traffic   _____

Premature infant carrier
(where to get one) _____

Red Cross (local) _____

Rescue squads (local) _____
(Other than ambulance
services or fire and
police departments) _____

Visiting Nurses Association _____

Water Department _____

Other useful numbers _____

_____

_____

NOTES

NOTES

NOTES

NOTES

NOTES

NOTES